Exploration of Transformative Technologies in Healthcare 6.0

Piyush Kumar
IILM University, Gurugram, India

Pankaj Rahi
Institute of Health Management and Research, Bangalore, India

S.D. Gupta
Institute of Health Management and Research, Bangalore, India

Kirti Udayai
Max Healthcare Institute Limited, India

Prashant Singh
Independent Researcher, India

IGI Global
Scientific Publishing
Publishing Tomorrow's Research Today

Vice President of Editorial	Melissa Wagner
Managing Editor of Acquisitions	Mikaela Felty
Managing Editor of Book Development	Jocelynn Hessler
Production Manager	Mike Brehm
Cover Design	Phillip Shickler

Published in the United States of America by
IGI Global Scientific Publishing
701 East Chocolate Avenue
Hershey, PA, 17033, USA
Tel: 717-533-8845
Fax: 717-533-8661
Website: https://www.igi-global.com E-mail: cust@igi-global.com

Library of Congress Cataloging-in-Publication Data

Names: Kumar, Piyush, 1984- editor. | Rahi, Pankaj, 1978- editor. | Gupta, Shiv Dutt, editor. | Udayai, Kirti, 1985- editor. | Singh, Prashant, editor.
Title: Exploration of transformative technologies in healthcare 6.0 / edited by Piyush Kumar, Pankaj Rahi, S.D. Gupta, Kirti Udayai, Prashant Singh.
Description: Hershey, PA : IGI Global, [2025] | Includes bibliographical references and index. | Summary: "This book will highlight the technologies and their integration in healthcare, opportunities, and challenges for healthcare managers presented by Healthcare 6.0 and will guide them for effective use of technology in healthcare"-- Provided by publisher.
Identifiers: LCCN 2024049400 (print) | LCCN 2024049401 (ebook) | ISBN 9798369372104 (hardcover) | ISBN 9798369372111 (paperback) | ISBN 9798369372128 (ebook)
Subjects: LCSH: Medical innovations.
Classification: LCC RA418.5.M4 E97 2025 (print) | LCC RA418.5.M4 (ebook) | DDC 362.10285--dc23/eng/20250122
LC record available at https://lccn.loc.gov/2024049400
LC ebook record available at https://lccn.loc.gov/2024049401

British Cataloguing in Publication Data
A Cataloguing in Publication record for this book is available from the British Library.

Table of Contents

Foreword xiv

Preface xvi

Acknowledgement xix

Chapter 1
Roadmap for Healthcare Transformation: Leveraging Industry 6.0 1
Soumi Ray, Dr. B. C. Roy Academy of Professional Courses, Durgapur, India
Sukanti Bhattacharyya, ICARE Institute of Medical Sciences and Research, India & Dr. B.C. Roy Hospital, Haldia, India

Chapter 2
Healthcare 6.0 Promising the Era of Smart and Intelligent Hospitals: A Paradigm Shift 39
Preethi Prabhakaran, Auxilium College, India

Chapter 3
Industry-Specific Fuzzy Front-End Innovation: A Multiple-Case Study of Medical Devices 71
Jesper Johansson, Halmstad University, Sweden
David Rosendal, Halmstad University, Sweden
Henrik Barth, Halmstad University, Sweden

Chapter 4
Motivational Digital Health App Design for Behavioral Change: Harnessing Gamification to Drive Engagement and Behavioral Change Through Digital Health Apps 105
Niladri Neel Majumder, University of Toronto, Canada

Chapter 5
Adoption of Innovative Digital Technologies for Enhancing Health Financing 135
Jayathra Datla, IQVIA, India
Parul Goela, IQVIA, India
Tatjana Prenđa Trupec, Maastricht University, The Netherlands

Chapter 6
Machine Learning in Medicine: Enhancing Diagnosis, Treatment, and Healthcare Delivery 167
Pooja Dehankar, Ajeenkya D.Y. Patil School of Engineering, India
Susanta Das, Ajeenkya D.Y. Patil University, India

Chapter 7
Application of Machine Learning in Healthcare IoT: An Investigation on Disease Diagnosis and Analytic Cases 197
Ashwini Kumar Pradhan, Galgotias University, India
Arvind Yadav, Galgotias University, India
Nilamadhab Mishra, VIT Bhopal University, India
Rudra Kalyan Nayak, VIT Bhopal University, India
Hitesh Mohapatra, KIIT University, India
Lambodar Jena, Shiksha 'O' Anusandhan University, India
Akhilesh Kumar Tripathi, Galgotias University, India

Chapter 8
A Novel Algorithm for Healthcare Sensor Data Fusion and Anomaly Detection 221
Anshit Mukherjee, Abacus Institute of Engineering and Management, India
Biswadip Basu Mallik, Institute of Engineering and Management, University of Engineering and Management, India
Avishek Gupta, Abacus Institute of Engineering and Management, India
Monalisa Halder, Abacus Institute of Engineering and Management, India

Chapter 9
Neural Network-Centered Intelligent Recognizing Framework for Elderly Health Activity Supervision 251
Nilamadhab Mishra, VIT Bhopal University, India
Saroja Kumar Rout, Vardhaman College of Engineering, India
Amit Thakur, VIT Bhopal University, India
Meshal Alharbi, Prince Sattam Bin Abdulaziz University, Saudi Arabia

Chapter 10
Machine Unlearning Models for Medical Care and Health Data Privacy in Healthcare 6.0 273
Varun Kumar, Dure Technologies Private Limited, India
Dipanjan Sujit Roy, Dure Technologies Private Limited, India

Chapter 11
Leveraging Machine Unlearning for Better Medical Care and Data Protection in Healthcare 6.0 303
Santosh Moses, IQVIA, India
Konrad Obermann, M4Health, Germany
Kanishak Gautam, IQVIA, India
Gaurav Upadhyay, Delhi Technological University, India
Jayathra Datla, IQVIA, India

Chapter 12
Precision Nutrition Through Nutritional Informatics: Futuristic Technologies for Health Advancement 329
Jyoti Vijay, Institute of Health Management Research, Bangalore, India
Teesta Dey, Mount Carmel College, India
Athmakoor Angela Shresta, Mount Carmel College, India

Chapter 13
Securing Patient Rights and Safety in a Digitally Transformed Healthcare Environment 361
Sudamini Saproo, IQVIA, India
Parul Goela, IQVIA, India
Jayathra Datla, IQVIA, India
Kanishak Gautam, IQVIA, India

Chapter 14
Safeguarding Patient Rights and Safety in Tech-Enabled Healthcare 391
J. Aileen, M S Ramaiah University of Applied Sciences, India

Chapter 15
Enhancing Patient Satisfaction and Care 421
Sanghamitra Sharma, Prin L.N. Welingkar Institute of Management Development and Research, India

Compilation of References 443

About the Contributors 509

Index 527

Detailed Table of Contents

Foreword xiv

Preface xvi

Acknowledgement xix

Chapter 1
Roadmap for Healthcare Transformation: Leveraging Industry 6.0 1
Soumi Ray, Dr. B. C. Roy Academy of Professional Courses, Durgapur, India
Sukanti Bhattacharyya, ICARE Institute of Medical Sciences and Research, India & Dr. B.C. Roy Hospital, Haldia, India

The advent of Industry 6.0, delineated by an amicable consolidation of the digital, physical, and biological spheres, prophesies a revolutionary era for the healthcare industry. This article enumerates an innovative roadmap to expedite the progress of Healthcare 6.0 by employing the fundamental ideas underlying this industrial revolution. The roadmap explains the amalgamation of leading-edge mechanizations and technologies. The prophetic artificial intelligence (AI), cutting-edge robotics, and quantum computing, aid in elevating medical decision-making, enhancing patient outcomes, and optimising healthcare conveyance. It nurtures synergetic ecologies within the medical realm. It addresses policies, governance, and workforce contemplations to accredit this transformative voyage. The alignment of the healthcare dominion with the landmark progressions of Industry 6.0, this enchiridion overlays the way for the health system to be more effectual, operative, and patient-centric. This is poised to abode the evolving healthcare requirements of the future with valuable insights and efficacy.

Chapter 2
Healthcare 6.0 Promising the Era of Smart and Intelligent Hospitals: A Paradigm Shift 39
Preethi Prabhakaran, Auxilium College, India

This chapter outlines the revolutionary potential of smart and intelligent hospitals, which use cutting-edge technologies to alter healthcare delivery and patient outcomes. These hospitals are leading the way in the use of innovative technologies like digital twins, AI-enabled seamless Models, and the Internet of Things (IoT) including scalable blockchain technology, which are bringing in a new era of data-driven, individualized, and efficient healthcare. The smart hospital concept has the potential to revolutionize the way medical care is delivered in the future by making healthcare more efficient, accessible, and customized to each patient's needs. While intelligent hospitals take a more comprehensive, integrated approach to improving the entire hospital ecosystem through the strategic convergence of sophisticated technologies and thoughtful facility design, smart hospitals use data and technology to enhance particular processes and the patient experience.

Chapter 3
Industry-Specific Fuzzy Front-End Innovation: A Multiple-Case Study of Medical Devices 71
Jesper Johansson, Halmstad University, Sweden
David Rosendal, Halmstad University, Sweden
Henrik Barth, Halmstad University, Sweden

New product development (NPD) exists at the fuzzy front end (FFE) of innovation – the time when companies must make often ill-defined decisions based on limited information. Many industry-generic studies focus on the causes of this fuzziness: uncertainty, complexity, and equivocality — also identified as ambiguity. In this paper we explore the FFE of innovation in the Swedish medical devices industry where the public sector is a prominent player. Based on our empirical data from the interviews, we constructed a conceptual FFE framework Our findings reveal when public sector organisations purchase medical devices, the fuzziness in the FFE increases for the medical devices industry. Uncertainty and complexity in the FFE increase when medical devices companies must consider the degree of product risk as well as the laws, regulations, and practices involved in sales to the public sector. In addition, equivocality (ambiguity) increases when industry actors and public sector actors have different interpretations of product costs.

Chapter 4
Motivational Digital Health App Design for Behavioral Change: Harnessing Gamification to Drive Engagement and Behavioral Change Through Digital Health Apps 105
Niladri Neel Majumder, University of Toronto, Canada

This chapter examines how gamification enhances digital health apps by integrating game design elements to drive and sustain behavioral change. It highlights how mechanics like points and badges improve user engagement and adherence to health interventions, aligning with Healthcare 6.0 focus on patient-centered care. Key topics include the evolution of gamification, foundational psychological theories, and the connection between gamification, design thinking, and user-centric design. The chapter covers core and advanced design elements, future trends, challenges, and strategies for effective gamified interventions. It outlines metrics for evaluating effectiveness and provides insights from case studies of successful gamified health apps, offering best practices for sustaining engagement and adherence while reflecting on future advancements in the field.

Chapter 5
Adoption of Innovative Digital Technologies for Enhancing Health Financing 135
Jayathra Datla, IQVIA, India
Parul Goela, IQVIA, India
Tatjana Prenđa Trupec, Maastricht University, The Netherlands

Innovative technologies such as mobile applications, web platforms, digital payments, blockchain, big data analytics, and artificial intelligence can significantly enhance health financing functions like revenue raising, pooling, and service purchasing. Transformative impact of digital solutions include Kenya's M-TIBA platform, India's Ayushman Bharat Pradhan Mantri Jan Arogya Yojana, which uses a digital Transaction Management System to support the entire patient journey from registration to claims payment, and Estonia's e-invoicing system. Successful implementation requires a robust digital ecosystem encompassing governance, infrastructure, and skilled human resources. This involves establishing dedicated digital health departments, developing regulatory frameworks, and ensuring data security and interoperability. Moreover, it is crucial to address challenges such as technology access inequities and weak health systems to maximize the benefits of digital health financing.

Chapter 6
Machine Learning in Medicine: Enhancing Diagnosis, Treatment, and Healthcare Delivery 167
Pooja Dehankar, Ajeenkya D.Y. Patil School of Engineering, India
Susanta Das, Ajeenkya D.Y. Patil University, India

ML is a game-changing technology for improving diagnosis, customizing therapy, & streamlining healthcare delivery because of its capacity to handle & learn from enormous volumes of data. ML-based big data analysis has many benefits for assimilating & assessing vast volumes of intricate health care data. Early diagnosis & monitoring of drug-related safety issues were facilitated by ML algorithms that discovered hidden correlations between medications, medical products, & adverse events. This chapter highlights the benefits of ML in Medicine. To achieve the best possible results, it will be essential to improve clinical decision support, sickness diagnosis, & individualized treatment techniques. The chapter discusses important issues to keep in mind when applying ML in the medical field, e.g., data privacy, model interpretability, bias reduction, & regulatory compliance. Lastly it discusses the future of ML in medicine. Through responsible & ethical adoption of new technology, medical community can provide more individualized, efficient, & effective care to improve patient outcomes.

Chapter 7
Application of Machine Learning in Healthcare IoT: An Investigation on Disease Diagnosis and Analytic Cases 197
Ashwini Kumar Pradhan, Galgotias University, India
Arvind Yadav, Galgotias University, India
Nilamadhab Mishra, VIT Bhopal University, India
Rudra Kalyan Nayak, VIT Bhopal University, India
Hitesh Mohapatra, KIIT University, India
Lambodar Jena, Shiksha 'O' Anusandhan University, India
Akhilesh Kumar Tripathi, Galgotias University, India

Machine learning (ML) is the most prominent topic, with many applications in video processing, language processing, visual diagnosis of illnesses, drug development, biochemistry, and biomedical. Healthcare systems and medical science-related applications are rapidly growing among these applications. Large data expansion, the Internet of Things (IoT), networked devices, and high-performance computers with graphics processing units are all contributing to the growing popularity of ML. Healthcare in IoT (HIoT), and electronic health record (EHR) data are the key data resources for neural network (NN) models. Several possible challenges, including security and quality of service improvement, are important to ML. Based on the comprehensive literature survey (CLS), ML for HIoT is examined in this research.

Chapter 8
A Novel Algorithm for Healthcare Sensor Data Fusion and Anomaly Detection 221
Anshit Mukherjee, Abacus Institute of Engineering and Management, India
Biswadip Basu Mallik, Institute of Engineering and Management, University of Engineering and Management, India
Avishek Gupta, Abacus Institute of Engineering and Management, India
Monalisa Halder, Abacus Institute of Engineering and Management, India

Health care sensor data analytics is one of the most disruptive innovations in personal health care since it uses information from sensors to improve patient care. In this chapter, a new algorithm for Multi-Modal Sensor Data Fusion and Anomaly Detection is presented; some important issues, including data authenticity, confidentiality and integrity, are discussed. The proposed method builds on machine learning and artificial intelligence to deal with large sets of data to comprehend in order to enhance diagnosis and solutions oriented towards patient care. The algorithm is then validated through a series of tests and outperforms different approaches used in the same field to diagnose problems by analyzing sensor data. The findings strongly argue for a robust data infrastructure that covers acquisition, distribution, archival, analysis, and presentation. Thus, this paper underlines deficiencies of current approaches and underscores the applicability of analytical techniques for radical transformation of healthcare processes alongside with adherence to ethical considerations.

Chapter 9
Neural Network-Centered Intelligent Recognizing Framework for Elderly Health Activity Supervision 251
Nilamadhab Mishra, VIT Bhopal University, India
Saroja Kumar Rout, Vardhaman College of Engineering, India
Amit Thakur, VIT Bhopal University, India
Meshal Alharbi, Prince Sattam Bin Abdulaziz University, Saudi Arabia

Maintaining self-regulating life in old age anticipates high risks and often leads to failure. So, the objective of our study is to inspect the implementation feasibility of an intelligent sensing framework for self-regulating Elderly Health activity supervision. The computational intelligent tools are implemented to frame the intelligent sensing framework. The patterns in context to the walk-in activity of Elderly Health are analyzed along with statistical inference to identify the abnormal living patterns. Once the framework is embedded with intelligent tools, the backpropagation neural network algorithm is used for framework training and learning through three artificial neural models, namely NN1, NN2, and NN3, and finds approximately 96% implementation accuracy in the NN3 model. The activity level analysis is important to introduce the intelligence sensing framework into the Elderly's Health life. So, analysis and discussion are made to validate the feasibility of the framework implementation for Elderly Health activity supervision.

Chapter 10
Machine Unlearning Models for Medical Care and Health Data Privacy in Healthcare 6.0 273
Varun Kumar, Dure Technologies Private Limited, India
Dipanjan Sujit Roy, Dure Technologies Private Limited, India

The integration of advanced technologies in healthcare has undergone significant transformations throughout the 20th and 21st centuries, culminating in the era of Healthcare 6.0. This evolution in healthcare, particularly the integration of artificial intelligence, has necessitated the implementation of concepts like "Machine Unlearning". This is crucial for addressing critical issues like data privacy compliance, bias mitigation, and data security. By enabling the removal of specific data points from ML models, Machine Unlearning aligns with international data protection laws (HIPAA, GDPR, and DPDPA). Its application emphasizes regulations concerning the right to be forgotten, data minimization, and patient consent, which are essential for legal compliance and maintaining patient trust in healthcare. This chapter discusses Machine Unlearning approaches like Exact Unlearning and Approximate

Unlearning, along with other advanced methods. Lastly, it discusses real-world case studies, and identifies the way forward for future development & research on 'Machine Unlearning in Healthcare'.

Chapter 11
Leveraging Machine Unlearning for Better Medical Care and Data Protection in Healthcare 6.0 303
Santosh Moses, IQVIA, India
Konrad Obermann, M4Health, Germany
Kanishak Gautam, IQVIA, India
Gaurav Upadhyay, Delhi Technological University, India
Jayathra Datla, IQVIA, India

Machine Learning (ML), a key component of modern technology, evolved from Alan Turing's 1950s concepts and the Turing Test. Introduced in 1959, ML enables computers to perform tasks by learning from data rather than explicit programming. It includes supervised, unsupervised, semi-supervised, and reinforcement learning. As ML integrated into various industries, Machine Unlearning (MU) emerged to address data privacy and security. MU involves removing specific data points' influence from a trained model without complete retraining, ensuring sensitive information is efficiently erased while maintaining model integrity.

Chapter 12
Precision Nutrition Through Nutritional Informatics: Futuristic Technologies for Health Advancement 329
Jyoti Vijay, Institute of Health Management Research, Bangalore, India
Teesta Dey, Mount Carmel College, India
Athmakoor Angela Shresta, Mount Carmel College, India

Precision nutrition tailors dietary recommendations to prevent and manage diseases based on individual factors. It integrates Healthcare 6.0 technology, particularly nutrition informatics, which combines information, nutrition, and technology for personalized dietary recommendations in both community and clinical settings. This chapter explores key aspects of nutrition informatics, including data sources, dietary data collection techniques, digital tools, and advanced analytics for personalized recommendations. It also examines publicly available online health and nutrition databases that support customized dietary planning. Emerging technologies are revolutionizing nutrition data collection, leveraging advanced analytics for comprehensive, individualized insights. Additionally, the chapter discusses how precision nutrition aids disease management by identifying optimal dietary patterns and using data-driven insights to promote healthier lifestyles. Integrating nutrition informatics into precision nutrition offers a transformative approach to enhancing health outcomes.

Chapter 13
Securing Patient Rights and Safety in a Digitally Transformed Healthcare Environment 361
Sudamini Saproo, IQVIA, India
Parul Goela, IQVIA, India
Jayathra Datla, IQVIA, India
Kanishak Gautam, IQVIA, India

The healthcare industry is transforming with advanced technologies like EHRs, telemedicine, and AI, promising improved patient outcomes and streamlined processes. However, increased digitization has led to a surge in data breaches, exposing vulnerabilities and raising concerns about patient data confidentiality. Regulatory frameworks struggle to keep up with rapid technological changes, highlighting significant gaps. This chapter calls for a holistic approach to protect patient rights, proposing robust policies, advanced technology use, and ongoing staff training. Key findings include a 42% rise in breaches, regulatory non-compliance, and underused AI security solutions. Emphasizing stringent regulations, encryption, and ethical data management, it aims to integrate innovation with oversight to safeguard patient information and trust.

Chapter 14
Safeguarding Patient Rights and Safety in Tech-Enabled Healthcare 391
J. Aileen, M S Ramaiah University of Applied Sciences, India

In today's healthcare landscape, cutting-edge technologies like AI offer exciting possibilities but also significant challenges. This chapter explores the complex relationship between these advancements and patient safety, highlighting the fine line between innovation and risk. AI has the potential to revolutionize healthcare by improving diagnosis, predicting outcomes, and personalizing treatments, but over-reliance without proper oversight can lead to errors and biases. The chapter also addresses the growing problem of unreliable online health information, emphasizing the need for accurate, evidence-based resources. Building on foundational reports like "To Err is Human," the chapter discusses common pitfalls in healthcare technology, such as poor design, weak system integration, and inadequate planning, which can lead to new errors like alert fatigue. It also examines specific safety concerns, including medical identity theft, data breaches, and medication errors.

Chapter 15
Enhancing Patient Satisfaction and Care 421
Sanghamitra Sharma, Prin L.N. Welingkar Institute of Management Development and Research, India

This chapter navigates through the intricate landscape of patient satisfaction in the healthcare domain, while introducing an innovative framework designed to elevate the patient's experience. Over the years the landscape of healthcare has evolved and the emphasis on patient-centric care has increased and now it's pivotal in delivering care to the patients and with the advancements of technology, its easier to map patient satisfaction at various points and alleviate the patient experience. Patient satisfaction is one of the key drivers in imparting quality care and enhanced patient satisfaction offers many benefits such as it improves patients' perception and experience, increase trust in physician, greater compliance, reduces the chances of error, increases staff satisfaction which eventually result into better medical treatment and personal care. All these sums together have a direct impact on the provider's profitability.

Compilation of References 443

About the Contributors 509

Index 527

Foreword

The healthcare industry is experiencing a profound transformation driven by the rapid advancement of technology. As we stand on the threshold of a new era, Healthcare 6.0 promises to revolutionize the way we approach patient care, healthcare management, and medical innovation. This evolution is not just a shift in technology but a paradigm shift that integrates emerging innovations such as artificial intelligence, machine learning, the Internet of Things (IoT), blockchain, and digital health applications to create an interconnected, patient-centered ecosystem.

The integration of these disruptive technologies marks the beginning of an era where smart hospitals, intelligent decision-making frameworks, and data-driven patient care will enhance the entire healthcare delivery process. This comprehensive transformation is not without its challenges. As healthcare systems become more digitized, concerns over data security, ethical use of AI, and regulatory compliance take center stage. Healthcare professionals, leaders, and stakeholders are now tasked with navigating this complex landscape, ensuring that technological advancements align with ethical standards, privacy regulations, and the ultimate goal of improving patient outcomes.

Exploration of Transformative Technologies in Healthcare 6.0 provides an in-depth exploration of the innovations shaping the future of healthcare. This book offers valuable insights into how machine learning, anomaly detection, digital twins, and gamification are enhancing patient monitoring, promoting preventive care, and personalizing treatment options. It further delves into the challenges and opportunities for healthcare managers as they embrace these technologies to create more efficient, transparent, and patient-focused care models.

One of the central themes of this book is the integration of machine learning and machine unlearning, concepts that are set to redefine how we handle data privacy, patient rights, and predictive analytics. As healthcare professionals, researchers, and policymakers, it is crucial to stay abreast of these developments to effectively lead organizations in this new era. Moreover, as we look to the future, the book offers a clear roadmap to help guide healthcare managers in leveraging technology to improve patient satisfaction, safety, and security.

As we venture into Healthcare 6.0, it is essential to approach this evolution with responsibility, ensuring that technological innovations serve the best interests of both patients and healthcare providers. This book serves as a crucial resource in equipping healthcare leaders with the knowledge and tools necessary to harness the full potential of these transformative technologies while navigating the accompanying challenges. The era of Healthcare 6.0 is upon us, and this book is your guide to understanding and leading in this dynamic, technology-driven healthcare landscape.

This is more than just a technological shift—it's a fundamental change in how we think about, deliver, and experience healthcare. As we move forward, let us embrace these innovations responsibly, ensuring that they enhance the lives of patients and healthcare professionals alike.

A book that provides well-founded expertise, highlights challenges and risks, and ultimately calls for international and interdisciplinary collaboration – with the goal of sharing knowledge and applying it purposefully for the benefit of humanity.

Lutz Lungwitz
President of the German Medical Wellness Association, Berlin, Germany

Preface

The rapid evolution of technology has ushered in a new era in healthcare, transforming the way medical services are delivered, managed, and experienced. With the advent of Industry 6.0, which seamlessly integrates digital, physical, and biological systems, the healthcare sector stands on the cusp of a revolutionary transformation. This book, *Exploration of Transformative Technologies in Healthcare 6.0*, contemplates the impact of cutting-edge innovations such as artificial intelligence (AI), the Internet of Things (IoT), machine learning (ML), blockchain, and telemedicine on healthcare delivery. It delves into the challenges and opportunities presented by these advancements, offering a roadmap for navigating this new landscape.

The chapters in this book collectively highlight the necessity of a strategic approach to integrating emerging technologies into healthcare. The first chapter, *Roadmap for Healthcare Transformation: Leveraging Industry 6.0*, provides an overview of how AI, robotics, and quantum computing can optimize medical decision-making and patient care. Building on this, *Healthcare 6.0: Promising the Era of Smart and Intelligent Hospitals* examines how smart hospital infrastructures, digital twins, and AI-driven models contribute to more efficient and patient-centric healthcare environments.

Innovation in the medical devices industry is explored in *Industry-Specific Fuzzy Front-End Innovation: A Multiple-Case Study of Medical Devices*, which identifies the complexities and uncertainties in product development, especially when dealing with public-sector procurement. Meanwhile, *Motivational Digital Health App Design for Behavioural Change* investigates the role of gamification in enhancing patient engagement and adherence to digital health interventions.

Health financing is another critical area of transformation, as detailed in *Adoption of Innovative Digital Technologies for Enhancing Health Financing*. This chapter highlights successful case studies from Kenya, India, and Estonia, showcasing how digital solutions enhance financial sustainability in healthcare. The role of ML in medical diagnostics and treatment optimization is discussed in *Machine Learning in*

Medicine - Enhancing Diagnosis, Treatment, and Healthcare Delivery, emphasizing the need for ethical implementation and data privacy.

Further, *Application of Machine Learning in Healthcare IoT: An Investigation on Disease Diagnosis and Analytic Cases* underscores the increasing role of interconnected devices and ML in predictive healthcare. Complementing this discussion, *A Novel Algorithm for Healthcare Sensor Data Fusion and Anomaly Detection* introduces a new AI-driven method to improve patient monitoring and diagnosis. In a similar vein, *Neural Network-Centered Intelligent Recognizing Framework for Elderly Health Activity Supervision* presents an AI-based system designed to enhance elderly care through real-time activity analysis.

With digital transformation comes the crucial issue of data security and patient privacy. *Machine Unlearning Models for Medical Care and Health Data Privacy in Healthcare 6.0* and *Leveraging Machine Unlearning for Better Medical Care and Data Protection* address the emerging field of machine unlearning, which enables healthcare providers to comply with stringent data protection regulations like GDPR and HIPAA while maintaining the integrity of ML models. Similarly, *Securing Patient Rights and Safety in a Digitally Transformed Healthcare Environment* and *Safeguarding Patient Rights and Safety in Tech-Enabled Healthcare* explore strategies to protect sensitive patient data and mitigate risks associated with digital healthcare systems.

The book also discusses the impact of precision nutrition, an emerging field that integrates data-driven insights for personalized dietary recommendations, in *Precision Nutrition Through Nutritional Informatics: Futuristic Technologies for Health Advancement*. Lastly, *Enhancing Patient Satisfaction and Care* presents innovative strategies to improve the patient experience, ensuring that healthcare remains compassionate and patient-focused even in a highly digitized environment.

Technological advancements have made change an inevitable reality, and healthcare stands at a pivotal moment in this transformation. Global challenges such as emerging diseases, aging populations, rising healthcare costs, and the demand for equitable access necessitate a shift toward smarter, technology-driven healthcare systems. However, embracing this change is not without obstacles—resistance, workforce adaptation challenges, financial constraints, privacy concerns, and global disparities in access to technology all create barriers to seamless adoption.

Without a strategic approach, healthcare organizations risk stagnation in an increasingly competitive and digital-first ecosystem. The integration of AI, IoT, blockchain, and telemedicine into healthcare not only enhances efficiency, patient outcomes, and sustainability but also aligns with broader global health objectives of universal health coverage and equitable access to care. Digital transformation is a prerequisite in healthcare and goes beyond simply adopting new technologies—it requires a complete rethinking of organizational structures, processes, and cultures.

Leadership plays a pivotal role, driving strategic vision, fostering an innovation-oriented mindset, and ensuring workforce readiness. Resistance to change, skill gaps, and fragmented strategies can stall progress, making robust change management frameworks essential.

Additionally, as healthcare becomes increasingly data-centric, organizations must prioritize strong data governance, interoperability, and cybersecurity to support sustainable transformation. The future of healthcare will be shaped by those who proactively adapt, innovate, and lead digital transformation efforts. By embracing a strategic, patient-centred, and technology-driven approach, healthcare organizations can not only navigate disruption but also reshape the future of care delivery—making the transition to Healthcare 6.0 a reality.

Acknowledgement

At the foremost, we would like to express heartfelt thanks to the Lord Almighty for providing us the strength, knowledge and wisdom in completing this book project.

We are deeply grateful to all chapter authors who devoted their time and contributed in their areas of expertise by submitting their articles and by reviewing one or more chapters during the long manuscript development cycle. The diversity of perspectives and the depth of knowledge each chapter brings are a testament to their efforts.

We solemnly thank all the, reviewers for providing all the support for the successful completion and publishing of this book. It is a pleasure, therefore, to be able to pass on thanks to the following researchers who also reviewed the chapters for this book- Dr. Anandhi Ramachandran, Professor, IIHMR Delhi, Dr. Chandra J, Professor, Christ University, Bangalore, Dr. Mrinalini, Assistant Professor, M.S Ramaiah University of Applied Sciences, Dr. Ritu Vashishtha, Assistant Professor, IIHMR University, Jaipur, Dr. Sukesh Bhardwaj, Assistant Professor, IIHMR Bangalore, Col. Sukhdeep Singh, Founder and President, IndUS Consultants LLC, USA, Dr. Tulasi B, Associate Professor, Christ University, Bangalore, Dr. Vijay Pratap Raghuvanshi, Associate Professor, DSEU, Dwarka, New Delhi, Dr. Sarthak Sen Gupta, Assistant Professor, IIHMR University, Dr. Nishikant Bele, Associate Professor, IIHMR Delhi, and Dr. Suneeta Chandorkar, Assistant Professor, University of Baroda.

We would also like to extend our thanks to IGI Global for their support in publishing this book. Their professionalism and commitment to scholarly work have been instrumental in bringing this project to fruition.

Piyush Kumar

Kirti Udayai

Prashant Singh

SD Gupta

Pankaj Rahi

Editorial Advisory Board

Chapter 1
Roadmap for Healthcare Transformation:
Leveraging Industry 6.0

Soumi Ray
https://orcid.org/0000-0002-3940-0744
Dr. B. C. Roy Academy of Professional Courses, Durgapur, India

Sukanti Bhattacharyya
https://orcid.org/0000-0003-3863-4263
ICARE Institute of Medical Sciences and Research, India & Dr. B.C. Roy Hospital, Haldia, India

ABSTRACT

The advent of Industry 6.0, delineated by an amicable consolidation of the digital, physical, and biological spheres, prophesies a revolutionary era for the healthcare industry. This article enumerates an innovative roadmap to expedite the progress of Healthcare 6.0 by employing the fundamental ideas underlying this industrial revolution. The roadmap explains the amalgamation of leading-edge mechanizations and technologies. The prophetic artificial intelligence (AI), cutting-edge robotics, and quantum computing, aid in elevating medical decision-making, enhancing patient outcomes, and optimising healthcare conveyance. It nurtures synergetic ecologies within the medical realm. It addresses policies, governance, and workforce contemplations to accredit this transformative voyage. The alignment of the healthcare dominion with the landmark progressions of Industry 6.0, this enchiridion overlays the way for the health system to be more effectual, operative, and patient-centric. This is poised to abode the evolving healthcare requirements of the future with valuable insights and efficacy.

DOI: 10.4018/979-8-3693-7210-4.ch001

1.0 INTRODUCTION

The healthcare industry is at the cusp of a metamorphous era. The convergence of emergent technologies and various innovative business models can redefine how medical care is delivered, experienced, and retrieved. As the globe battles with numerous hurdles, there is an utmost need for a bounteous efficient, custom-made, and buoyant healthcare structure. The subsequent phase of the Industrial Revolution, Industry 6.0, claims to be a combination of artificial intelligence (AI), cyber-physical systems, and data-driven decision-making at the core of modern and service-oriented activities (Bhati, Deogade, & Kanyal, 2023). It exemplifies that the technologies are not just theoretical perceptions; they have been integrated into prevailing healthcare frameworks. It showcases the practical applications in improving patient outcomes. Bhati et al. (2023) highlighted that artificial intelligence has reduced diagnostic errors, demonstrating the tangible benefits of these advancements.

Healthcare 6.0 perceives the future of healthcare conveyance. It is created upon the foundations, envisioning a healthcare service that is more individual-oriented, preventative, and decentralised in nature. At the heart of this revolution lies the potential to unleash unparalleled levels of efficacy, personalisation, and patient-centricity. This transition towards a more tailored tactic to healthcare can lead to greater support and health outcomes. It will improve the well-being of people as well as communities (Topol, 2019). Furthermore, the decentralization of medical services, eased by the progressions in telemedicine, far-flung monitoring, and mobile health applications, does bring therapeutic care closer to the patient's doorstep. The regionalization of care, coupled with the incorporation of AI-powered decision support arrangements, encourages individuals to take an added vigorous role in their healthcare management and services, promoting a culture of preventive and proactive care.

Both Industry 6.0 and Healthcare 6.0 embody an important shift where the paradigms intend to yoke new technologies' influence while ensuring that these advancements ultimately help entities, societies, and the environment (Topol, 2019). By harmonizing the incorporation of pioneering technologies with a profound understanding of human needs and societal well-being, these models embrace the possibilities to transmute the way healthcare is provided, practised, and accessed by healthcare entities. In today's healthcare scenario, patient care and safety are the foremost important aspects in lower and middle-income countries and globally.

As we progress, it is fascinating to witness the continual development of the notions and the concrete and tangible impact they have on the healthcare domain. The encounters faced by the industry may be intimidating, but the promise of a more efficient, personalized, and strong healthcare system is a driving force that can shape the future of healthcare delivery. Many important technologies related to

Healthcare 6.0 - AI, the internet of medical things, and cognitive computing, have been developed and established in the West, including the United States. This can help elucidate the previous uptake in some regions. Many Western countries' strong healthcare setups and digital capabilities may make it easier to implement more comprehensive, preventive, and human-centred healthcare practices (Bestsennyy, et al., 2021).

The chapter will outline the advanced technologies and methodologies within healthcare systems to accomplish sustainable and effective transformation. The chapter's potential problem areas and key focus would elaborate on technological integration in healthcare, personalised and predictive healthcare, sustainability in healthcare transformation, interoperability and data management, ethical and regulatory challenges, workforce adaptation and training and patient-centred outcomes. This unit accentuates that Healthcare 6.0 is not just about employing new technologies but about essentially reconsidering how care is delivered and experienced. By addressing these areas, the chapter will provide actionable strategies and a roadmap for stakeholders to effectively navigate healthcare transformation under the influence of Industry 6.0 principles.

2.0 EVOLUTIONARY HISTORY AND ITS RELEVANCE TO HEALTHCARE

Healthcare has undergone a remarkable transformation over the decades, progressing through several distinct stages. The successive industrial revolutions from Industry 1.0 to 6.0 have had a profound impact on the healthcare sector, driving the corresponding transformations from Healthcare 1.0 to 6.0. Figure 1 enumerate the Industrial Revolution's progression from mechanization to digital symbiosis and automation (Nahavandi, 2019; Rauch et al., 2020). Figure 2 highlights the traditional to holistic - evolution from empirical to AI-driven healthcare (Andersen et al., 2017).

Figure 1. Evolution of the Industry 1.0 to 6.0

Figure 1
Evolution of the Industry 1.0 to 6.0

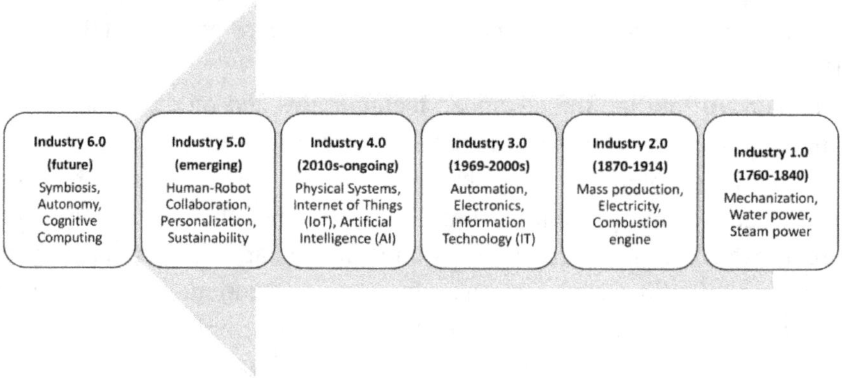

(Nahavandi, 2019 and Rauch el at., 2020)

Figure 2. Evolution of the Healthcare 1.0 to 6.0

Figure 2
Evolution of the Healthcare 1.0 to 6.0

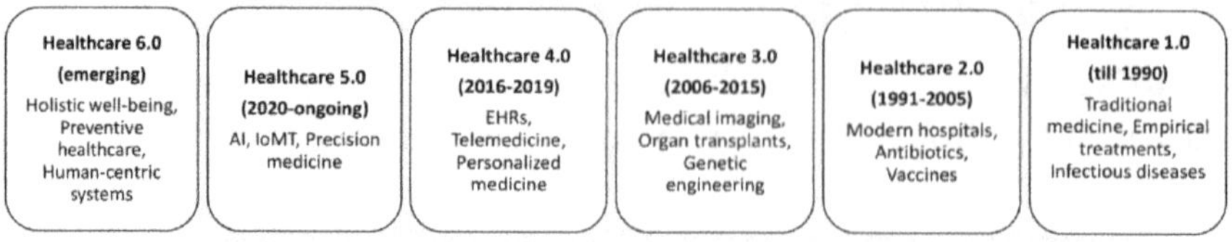

(Andersen et al., 2017, IBM, 2023.).

Industry 1.0 introduced the system of mechanisation and the factory structure, leading to advancements in medical technologies as well which gave rise to modern hospitals in Healthcare 1.0 (Topol, 2019). It signified the most basic medical practices. It encompasses the rudimentary public health procedures and measures, laying the foundation for advanced developments. Industry 2.0 was about mass production and electrification. It enabled the development of healthcare infrastructure and the expansion of specialized medical practices in Healthcare 2.0. It also ushered in the mass production of medications and vaccinations, significantly improving public health outcomes on a proficient level and higher magnitude. This phase leveraged industrialization and standardization to make crucial treatments more widely accessible (Topol, 2019; Andersen et al., 2017)

The automation and digitization of Industry 3.0 led the way for the adoption of electronic health records (EHRs), telemedicine, and personalized medicine in Healthcare 3.0 (Topol, 2019). This digital transformation and platform empowered all healthcare providers to accomplish and manage patient data much more efficiently and expand the reach of care. Industry 4.0's cyber-physical structures and the Internet of Things have driven the combination of digital health proficiency, AI, and predictive analytics in Healthcare 4.0. It unified smart, allied devices, allowing for enhanced patient monitoring and data-driven management and decision-making. By enhancing the analytics and artificial intelligence, this phase elevated the quality and quality of patient care (Chandrashekaran, 2024). The emerging Industry 5.0 and 6.0 have lots of potential. It is expected to further transform healthcare. The current phase, Healthcare 5.0, focuses on personalized and predictive medicine. Advancements in AI and genomics have allowed more targeted, proactive healthcare solutions tailored to individual needs and risk profiles. Looking to the future, Healthcare 6.0 envisions a fully integrated, intelligent system. It can seamlessly combine digital, physical, and biological technologies to provide comprehensive, preventative healthcare solutions. This holistic approach goals to redefine the healthcare aspects and improve overall well-being. Healthcare 6.0 is urgently required to address pressing problems such as growing expenses, disparities in accessibility, and inadequacies in care delivery. Traditional healthcare models have been struggling with fragmented facilities and services, leading to patient dissatisfaction. Healthcare 6.0 is vital in producing a sustainable, competent, and equitable healthcare model which will be able to meet the sprouting needs of populations globally.

3.0 STRATEGIC PILLARS OF HEALTHCARE TRANSFORMATION

The industry, especially healthcare, is experiencing a radical change. It is now focused on building a robust digital infrastructure, fostering a data-driven culture, embracing collaborative ecosystems, prioritizing patient-centricity, and cultivating a culture of innovation. For healthcare businesses to successfully negotiate the intricacies of the contemporary healthcare environment and guarantee a system that is robust, value-driven, and prepared for the future, these strategic pillars are vital.

3.1 Endowing a Robust Digital Infrastructure

Forming a strong digital foundation is critical for successful healthcare transformation. This involves integrating various digital technologies, comprising electronic health records, telemedicine platforms, remote patient monitoring devices, and advanced data analytics tools (Chourasia et al., 2022). The consistent and seamless integration of digital technologies across the healthcare ecosystem is the cornerstone of Healthcare 6.0.

Key elements of a robust digital infrastructure comprise of:

3.1.1. E-Health Records

The basis of the digital health network is made up of thorough and interoperable EHR systems that allow patient data to be stored securely, retrieved when required, and shared across treatment settings (Bates et al.,2018). It aids in making informed decisions and facilitates seamless care coordination.

3.1.2. Virtual Care and Telemedicine

During the period of COVID-19 pandemic, telemedicine and virtual care platforms established their significance, demonstrating that these services are essential for delivering accessible and remote healthcare. These processes enable the end users to receive services and care from the ease of their houses. The technologies, such as telemedicine, remote monitoring, and electronic health records, lower access barriers and enhance the continuity of patient care (Wosik et al., 2022).

3.1.3. Remote Patient Monitoring (RPM)

The advanced and upgraded connective technologies, along with wearable gadgets, and sensors enable continuous monitoring of patient health data. It promotes proactive illness management, prompt and early intervention, and better results (Bajwa et al.,2021).

3.1.4. Advanced Automation and Robotic Systems in Healthcare

The fusion of smart and advanced automation along with robotics in healthcare is a transformative trend. It is reforming the way medicinal interferences and care delivery are performed. Robotic-assisted surgeries and procedures, for example, are becoming highly prevalent, enabling specialists to accomplish complex operations with a high level of accuracy, dexterity, and consistency (Turchetti et al., 2021). These advanced surgical systems which are powered by AI and appliance learning algorithms, can provide real-time guidance. It reduces the risk of manual errors and thus optimises surgical outcomes. Beyond the operating theatre, autonomous smart devices and wearable gadgets are revolutionizing remote patient monitoring systems with enhanced care delivery. Smart sensors and IoT-enabled devices are designed to continuously monitor vital signs, symptoms, medication adherence, and other health parameters. This innovative technology enables healthcare professionals to intervene proactively and deliver personalized treatment plans (Jiang et al, 2017). Leveraging AI and machine learning, these intelligent systems can also detect early warning signs of medical conditions, facilitating timely diagnosis and preventive care. It is expanding into drug discovery, clinical decision support, and precision medicine. AI-powered measures can analyse enormous amounts of information, recognize patterns, and produce acumens that accelerate the drug development process and enable more personalized therapeutic approaches (Serban et al., 2020). This integration of intelligent automation and robotics is building the means for a more effective, precise, and patient-centric health system.

3.1.5. Advanced Data Analytics

Healthcare establishments get useful insights, anticipate patient requirements, and enhance clinical and operational procedures by utilizing data analytics. It is also accompanied by machine learning, and artificial intelligence (AI) (Davenport & Kalakota, 2019). These techniques aid the process of resource allocation, population health management, and tailored care.

3.1.6. Cybersecurity and Data Management

Strong cybersecurity defences and thorough data governance procedures are essential to safeguard patient privacy, preserve data integrity, and adhere to legal requirements. These are required as healthcare data is getting digitised more and more every passing day (Kruse et al., 2017). The literature accentuates that robust cybersecurity actions not only prevent data breaches but also build patient faith, which is crucial for successful digital healthcare transformation.

Through creating a cohesive and safe digital framework, healthcare institutions can boost the quality of care, enhance patient outcomes, streamline operations, and prepare themselves for sustained success amidst the changing healthcare environment. Healthcare organizations need to prioritize interoperability and integration among systems to fully benefit from a strong digital infrastructure.

3.2 Fostering a Data-Driven Culture

It is vital for the transformation as it will help in leveraging the abundance of data generated within the healthcare structure. With the promotion of a data-driven attitude, health organizations will be able to utilize advanced analytics, machine learning, and predictive modelling to uncover valuable insights, personalize care delivery, and optimize both clinical and operational processes. This transition towards data-centricity empowers clinicians, administrators, and patients by making informed decisions, allocating resources effectively, and driving constant improvement across the healthcare ecosystem.

Key elements of a data-driven culture include:

3.2.1 Effective Data Governance and Management

It is imbibed by establishing strong frameworks for data governance and effective data management practices, healthcare organizations guarantee the integrity, security, and availability of healthcare data (Raghupathi & Raghupathi, 2014).

3.2.2 Advanced Analytics and Predictive Modelling

Healthcare institutions taking advantage of the new progress, can utilize progressive analytics, machine learning, and predictive modelling to learn concealed patterns, predict patient requirements, and enhance care distribution (Murdoch & Detsky, 2013). Such insights aid in clinical decision-making, population health management, and the allocation of resources. The capability to harness advanced analytics, as emphasized by Murdoch & Detsky (2013), allows healthcare institutions to reveal hidden patterns and forecast patient needs. This competence enhances clinical decision-making and resource apportionment, improving care delivery.

3.2.3 Real-Time Data Integration

By amalgamating data from numerous origins, like EHRs, patient-generated information, and external datasets, healthcare entities can achieve a thorough, up-to-the-minute grasp of patient health and the wider healthcare environment (Hripcsak & Albers, 2013).

3.2.4 Data Literacy and Upgrading

Healthcare leaders need to endorse and promote data literacy and offer continuing education opportunities for healthcare professionals. It empowers them to effectively utilize data and analytics tools (Gagnon et al., 2015).

3.2.5 Innovation Labs, Data Experimentation & Environment

These labs can foster creativity and encourage the exploration of novel solutions to complex healthcare challenges. The encouragement for data exchange and collaboration among healthcare organizations, research institutions, and technology partners aids in unlocking the full potential of data-driven innovation (Kharrazi et al., 2012). By breaking down data barriers and fostering interdisciplinary collaborations, healthcare participants can jointly tackle multifaceted challenges and initiate meaningful advancements.

This foundation forms the way for collaborative ecosystems. Interdisciplinary corporations improve care delivery and subsequently the outcome.

3.3 Embracing Collaborative Ecosystems

Healthcare transformation cannot be achieved in isolation. Acceptance of collaborative environments fosters interdisciplinary partnerships, cross-sector alliances, and stakeholder engagement is essential (Duggal et al., 2021). It can be conducted by breaking down silos and easing the incorporation of diverse expertise, in healthcare establishments which can influence the cumulative intellect and resources of the ecosystem to develop innovative solutions.

Key elements of collaborative ecosystems in healthcare comprised:

3.3.1 Interdisciplinary Corporations

Bringing together healthcare specialists, technologists, policy-makers, data scientists, and other key stakeholders can guide the development of innovative resolutions that address intricate healthcare challenges (Dyer & Singh, 1998).

3.3.2 Cross-Sector Collaborations

Encouraging partnerships between healthcare organizations, technology companies, academic institutions, and community-based organizations can unlock new opportunities for innovation, knowledge-sharing, and the co-creation of patient-centric solutions (Savage et al, 2018).

3.3.3 Patient and Communal Participation

Actively involving patients, caregivers, and community members in the transformation process guarantees that their distinct needs, preferences, and viewpoints (Sharma et al., 2016). This patient-centered approach empowers individuals, fosters trust, and enhances the overall effectiveness of care delivery.

3.3.4 Ecosystem Governance and Synchronization

The establishment of robust governance structures and coordination mechanisms within the collaborative ecosystem is crucial for positioning stakeholders, managing shared possessions, and steering complex regulatory environments (Herlin, 2013).

3.3.5 Continuous Feedback Loops

Seeking feedback from stakeholders on a regular basis, including patients, providers, and community members, guarantees that collaboration stays adaptable to the changing requirements and preferences of all parties involved.

3.3.6 Knowledge Sharing and Best Practices

It is best in encouraging the exchange of finest practices, case studies, and lessons learned across the collective ecosystem enables healthcare organizations to learn from one another, replicate efficacious initiatives, and hasten the pace of revolution (Palinkas et al., 2011).

Through the adoption of collaborative networks and systems, healthcare organisations can connect diverse stakeholders' united intelligence and resources, address multifaceted challenges in the best possible manner, and drive the development of innovative, patient-centric resolutions that can create metamorphosis in the healthcare landscape.

3.4 Prioritizing Patient-Centricity

At the heart of healthcare transformation lies the need to place the end-users at the centre of the care and service experience. By adopting a patient-centric approach, healthcare organizations can design care pathways, technologies, and service delivery models that address the unique needs, preferences, and values of individuals (Al Baalharith, & Aboshaiqah, 2024). This shift towards personalized, empowered, and accessible care aids in improving patient satisfaction, augmented health outcomes, and enhanced engagement in the management of one's well-being.

Key elements of a patient-centric healthcare system comprise:

3.4.1 Personalizing Care Pathways

Healthcare establishments can enterprise personalized care paths by clouting data-driven insights and advanced technologies. It aids in accounting for individual patient characteristics, genetic profiles, social determinants of health, and personal preferences (Topol, 2019).

3.4.2 Empowering Patient Engagement

Shared decision-making permits patients to actively participate in their care, self-management tools, and continuous communication with healthcare providers (Greene et al., 2015). This fosters a sense of ownership, improves treatment adherence, and supports better health outcomes.

3.4.3 Accessible and Comprehensive Care

To make sure that health services are available, affordable, and inclusive for all people, irrespective of their socioeconomic status, physical or cognitive aptitudes, or geographical position (Schoenfeld & Mafi, 2018). This comprises the use of digital technologies, conveyance services, language interpretation, and community-based firms to overcome barricades to care.

3.4.4 Cohesive Care Coordination

Facilitating seamless care coordination across multiple care settings, providers, and support services ensures patients' holistic and continuous care experience (Stange, 2009).

3.4.5 Patient Experience and Satisfaction

The continuous assessment and improvement of the overall patient experience, satisfaction with clinical outcomes, care quality, communication, and the emotional and social aspects of care are vital (Doyle, Lennox & Bell, 2013).

Prioritizing patient-centricity, healthcare establishments can build confidence and trust, improve health outcomes, increase patient engagement, and position themselves as valuable partners in the journey towards better health and wellness.

3.5 Cultivating a Culture of Innovation

Sustainable healthcare demands a culture that entwines innovation, risk-taking, and unremitting learning. By fostering an ecosystem that encourages research, experimentation, collaboration, and the exploration of novel ideas, healthcare establishments can expose the potential of the workforce. It curates the creativity of the stakeholders and drives the development of advanced and breakthrough solutions.

Key elements of a culture of innovation in healthcare comprise:

3.5.1 Innovative Outlook and Leadership

It is to cultivate a mindset that scruples innovation, risk-taking, and unceasing improvement among healthcare leaders and experts (Parveen et al., 2018). This attitude shift empowers people to challenge the status quo, reconnoitre new ideas, and champion the enactment of innovative resolutions.

3.5.2 Adaptive and Agile Methods

Espousing agile procedures, design thinking, and swift prototyping approaches to respond to emerging needs, test new ideas, and iterate on solutions are the best methods to achieve the desired outcome (Thomke & Manzi, 2014). This flexible and iterative aspect enables healthcare administrations to familiarize themselves with changing environments and drive unremitting innovation.

3.5.3 Collaboration and Ideation Platforms

It provides dedicated places, both physical and virtual, for healthcare specialists, patients, and other stakeholders to collaborate, share thoughts, and ideas, and co-create innovative resolutions (Edmondson, 2019). These platforms aid in creating cross-functional teamwork, inspire the free flow of ideas, and allow the rapid progress and testing of new notions.

3.5.4 Aptitude Development and Upskilling

It is important to invest in the continuous erudition and expertise development of healthcare professionals. It empowers them to obtain new-fangled competencies in areas such as digital technologies, data analytics, design thinking, and innovation management (Crump et al., 2017).

3.5.5 Innovation Funding and Enticements

It establishes dedicated funding processes and mechanisms, innovation endowments, and incentive programs to sustain the exploration, prototyping, and scaling of innovative ideas. This delivers the necessary possessions and acknowledgement to fuel a culture of innovation and catalyse the conversion of the healthcare system.

Tools like IBM Watson Health have been formed to analyse vast datasets which have the potential to diagnose diseases with precision, accuracy and promptness. It will improve the treatment plans drastically based on the latest research (IBM, n.d.). Atomwise uses AI algorithms to accelerate the drug discovery process, identifying potential compounds faster and reducing development costs (Atomwise, 2025). The strategic pillars of healthcare transformation offer a compact foundation for advancing the sector. These pillars lay the groundwork for identifying critical enablers, such as workforce development and cutting-edge technologies, that are necessary to carry out transformative programs successfully and produce the intended results.

4.0 KEY ENABLERS OF HEALTHCARE TRANSFORMATION

Creating a thorough roadmap for Healthcare 6.0 requires incorporating the viewpoints of the various stakeholders - payers, providers, patients, and legislators. While physicians provide medical expertise for successful implementation, patients' insights ensure that care is customized to meet their necessities. Policymakers contribute to developing legislative frameworks that encourage innovation. The payers offer financial viewpoints that support sustainable models. Comprehending these aspects, the transformation will promote common objectives and improve healthcare delivery by encouraging cooperation among these stakeholders.

4.1 Leveraging Emergent Technologies

Healthcare is greatly benefiting from the rapid advancements in technical fields like AI, blockchain, cloud computing, the Internet of Things (IoT), and augmented or virtual reality (Bernardo, 2017). AI can dramatically alter the healthcare industry by allowing for more accurate diagnoses, personalized treatment regimens, and predictive analytics (Esteva et al., 2017). AI-driven image analysis can identify early disease symptoms, speed up clinical management and improve interactions between patients and providers. These AI-powered tools help clinicians navigate vast amounts of data, recognize patterns, and make informed decisions. Furthermore, it facilitates the implementation of scalable and cost-effective healthcare solutions, such as remote patient monitoring with telemedicine, cloud-based programs can help health establishments strictly and properly store, manage, and access bulky amounts of data, facilitating the smooth exchange of information and collaboration among care teams (Kruse et al, 2016).

The data accumulated in a healthcare system can be secured, integrated, and transparent by blockchain technology (Kuo et al., 2017). Blockchain technology can simplify administrative procedures, enable safe data sharing, and give patients more control over their private medical records by creating a decentralized, impenetrable archive of patient records. The IoT and connected equipment are transforming healthcare by qualifying remote specialist care, targeted care, and enhanced patient care and outcomes (Ramachandran et al., 2021). IoT-enabled wearables gadgets, medical devices, and home-based sensors can collect real-time data, provide early warning signals, and facilitate proactive interventions, leading to better disease management and enhanced patient engagement. Applications for augmented reality (AR) and virtual reality (VR) in health systems include patient education, surgical planning, and immersive medical training (Bernardo, 2017). By delivering engaging and interactive care, these technologies can improve patient outcomes and the learning and decision-making capacities of medical personnel.

4.2 Empowering the Healthcare Workforce

The success of healthcare transformation hinges on the active engagement, empowerment and integrity of the healthcare workforce. By investing in the upskilling and relearning of clinicians, nurses, and administrative staff, healthcare organizations can equip their teams with the essential knowledge, skills, and mindset to steer the changing scenario. This includes fostering digital literacy, promoting interdisciplinary collaboration, and cultivating a culture of continuous learning and professional development (Chugh & Chugh, 2023). This may involve training on electronic health records, telehealth platforms, data analytics, and other digital health solutions. By allowing the workforce to have the skill and knowledge of digital platforms, healthcare organizations can ensure seamless amalgamation of technology and facilitate the adoption of innovative care delivery models.

Promoting interdisciplinary collaboration is another key aspect which facilitates and empowers the healthcare workforce. It adds to the new thoughts, augments care synchronization, enhances patient care and results, and becomes a source of innovation (Iyawa et al., 2016). Healthcare organizations should encourage their workforce to be up-to-date with modern developments in medical science, technology, and care delivery. This may include providing access to ongoing training, educational resources, and opportunities for skill-building and career advancement. By nurturing a learning-oriented culture, healthcare organizations can ensure that their workforce can adapt to the evolving healthcare landscape.

4.3 Safeguarding Ethical and Responsible Use of Data

As medical care organizations are gradually banking on data-driven acumen and digital technologies, the principled and responsible usage of data becomes dominant. Robust models for data governance, cybersecurity dealings, and patient privacy protocols must be established to build trust, maintain the integrity of sensitive information, and ensure compliance with evolving regulatory requirements (Lei, 2023). By prioritizing data ethics, healthcare organizations can harness the power of data while safeguarding the rights and well-being of patients.

Effective data governance is crucial for healthcare transformation. This includes establishing transparent guidelines, processes, and measures for data management, including data collection, storage, access, and usage (Rajkomar et al., 2018). Healthcare organizations need to implement robust data security measures, including access controls, encryption, and regular data backups. It protects against cyber threats and data breaches. It is vital to make sure of patient privacy and consent. This is another key aspect of ethical and responsible data usage. Healthcare organizations must adhere to data privacy regulations, and get informed consent from them before using or dispersing their private health info (Gostin & Halabi, 2021).

Transparency and accountability are also essential for building trust in the healthcare system. Healthcare organizations need to be transparent about data handling, together with how to assemble, use, and shield patient information. They should also establish clear mechanisms for patients to access, review, and control their health info (Obermeyer et al., 2019). By prioritizing data ethics and responsible data usage, healthcare organizations can unleash the transformative potential of data-driven insights while maintaining the trust and confidence of patients and the broader community.

4.4 Aligning Reimbursement and Incentive Models

Sustainability in healthcare reduces ecological impact, creating cost savings, refining public health, and future-proofing the industry. Healthcare organizations can operate more competently, reliably, and effectively, eventually benefiting patients, staff, and the broader society. Thus, it is critical to line up reimbursement and incentive models with the desired outcomes to initiate sustainable healthcare transformation. Healthcare companies can inspire the provision of outstanding, cost-effective, and patient-centred services by substituting from volume-based to value-based care models (Bajwa et al., 2021).

There are various value-based care models, for example, bundled payments, shared savings, and capitation, that transfer the concentration from the volume of services to the eminence of consequences achieved (Ballard et al., 2019). These models incentivize healthcare providers to deliver more efficient, effective, and coordinated care, as they are rewarded for improving patient health and reducing redundant costs. Aligning reimbursement with value-based metrics can initiate the adoption of ground-breaking care delivery approaches. Concepts like telemedicine, remote patient monitoring, and population health management can be catered to with the aid.

Incentivizing precautionary care is another key aspect of aligning reimbursement and incentive models. By gratifying and rewarding healthcare providers for delivering evidence-based preventive services, like screenings, immunizations, and chronic disease management, healthcare establishments can boost a shift from a reactive to a proactive approach to healthcare (Lee & McGlynn, 2016). This can lead to earlier detection and management of health issues, ultimately improving population health and reducing the burden on the healthcare system. Fostering shared liability for populace health is a key feature of value-based care models (Barsanti & Cavicchi, 2021). This collaborative approach can lead to more holistic and patient-centric care delivery.

4.5 Addressing Equity and Accessibility Challenges

Healthcare transformation needs to prioritize the equitable and accessible conveyance of care, particularly for poor and marginalized communities. By leveraging digital technologies, intensifying telemedicine services, and addressing social determinants of health, healthcare establishments can bridge the gaps in access to care, enhance care coordination, and make sure that the aids of alteration are distributed justifiably across the population.

Digital technical aids, like telehealth and remote monitoring, can enhance access to healthcare services and medical care for individuals living in rural or remote regions, as well as those with mobility or transportation challenges (Dorsey & Topol, 2016). Expanding telemedicine services can also help address disparities in access to speciality care. By connecting patients with healthcare providers in different regions or even countries, telemedicine can enhance the convenience of specialized services, particularly for patients living in areas with limited healthcare resources and services (Uscher-Pines et al.,2021).

Addressing the social determinants of health is another key aspect of achieving equitable healthcare transformation. Social facets, such as salary, education, housing, and healthy food, can considerably impact a person's health and well-being (McGinnis et al., 2002). By facilitating seamless communication, data sharing, and collaborative care planning, healthcare organizations can ensure that patients, especially those with complex needs, receive comprehensive and coordinated services tailored to their circumstances (Kiran & O'Brien, 2021).

Driving substantial change in healthcare requires key enablers: the creation of a trained workforce and cutting-edge technologies. These components enable the shift to resilient and sustainable healthcare systems, opening the door for Healthcare 6.0.

5.0 SUSTAINABLE AND RESILIENT HEALTHCARE SYSTEMS: TOWARDS HEALTHCARE 6.0

5.1 Themes

Several important issues that set Healthcare 6.0 apart from more conventional conversations about technology adoption are included in this framework. These themes include:

5.1.1 Circular Economy

An economic system that aims to eliminate waste and continuous use of resources. In the healthcare industry, this entails creating systems that put sustainability and resource efficiency first, minimizing the negative effects of medical procedures on the environment (Geissdoerfer et al., 2018).

5.1.2 Sustainability

Healthcare 6.0 highlights enduring strategies that ensure the continued viability of healthcare systems over the long term. This covers social and economic aspects in addition to environmental sustainability, making sure that healthcare services are available and fair (Buchanan et al., 2020).

5.1.3 Innovation

Healthcare 6.0 includes technical novelties, but its scope is wider, including creative management, policy, and community engagement strategies that improve healthcare outcomes and delivery (Kumar et al., 2021).

5.1.4 Community Engagement

Involving communities in healthcare decision-making is a key component of Healthcare 6.0. This strategy promotes a healthcare system that is more inclusive and caters to the unique requirements and preferences of various people (Bennett et al., 2020).

5.2 Key Concepts

In the context of Healthcare 6.0, a few concepts are encapsulated:

5.2.1 Circular Economy in Healthcare

A framework that encourages material recycling and reuse in healthcare systems with the goal of reducing waste and improving resource efficiency (Geissdoerfer et al., 2018).

5.2.2 Sustainable Healthcare

A strategy that aims to strike a balance between the economic, social, and environmental facets of healthcare delivery so that health systems may satisfy present and future demands without endangering the wellbeing of people or the environment (Buchanan et al., 2020).

At the core of Healthcare 6.0 is to comprehend and recognise that the healthcare industry is both a significant contributor to and a potential victim of environmental degradation and climate-related disruptions. By adopting a sustainable approach, healthcare organizations can not only reduce their ecological footprint but also position themselves to better withstand and acclimatize to future crises. One of the key provisions of Healthcare 6.0 is the enactment of circular economy principles throughout the healthcare ecosystem. This comprises redesigning supply chains, treatment procedures, and waste management systems to abate waste, endorse the reprocessing and recycling of resources, and transition away from the traditional linear "take-make-waste" model (Iyer et al., 2021). By embracing circular economy approaches, healthcare organizations can reduce their reliance on finite resources, lessen their operating costs, and contribute to the development of a more sustainable future.

There is another closely aligned process with the circular economy, is the concept of green healthcare facilities. This encompasses the design, construction, and operation of healthcare buildings that prioritize energy efficiency, renewable energy sources, and the usage of sustainable materials (Eckelman & Sherman, 2016). By optimizing resource consumption and minimizing environmental impact, green healthcare facilities can serve as models for the broader industry and stimulate other organizations to follow suit. Resilience is yet another critical constituent of Healthcare 6.0. It refers to the capability of healthcare systems to endure, adapt, and recover from disruptions, whether they are natural disasters, pandemics, or supply chain interruptions. Constructing resilience requires a multi-faceted approach that includes robust infrastructure, agile crisis management protocols, and a culture of adaptability and collaboration (Kruk et al., 2017).

Healthcare setups can develop their resilience by investing in redundant systems, establishing strategic stockpiles of essential supplies, and fostering strong partnerships with other healthcare providers, government agencies, and community organizations. By mixing sustainability and resilience as key considerations, healthcare research and development can give rise to new technologies, treatment modalities, and care delivery models that are better aligned with the longstanding needs of patients, societies, and the environment.

Implementing the Healthcare 6.0 vision will necessitate collaboration and coordination across multiple stakeholders, including policymakers, healthcare providers, pharmaceutical and medical device companies, and community organizations (Pittenger et al., 2019). Creating shared standards, aligning incentives, and fostering cross-sector partnerships will be essential in driving the extensive adoption of sustainable and resilient practices throughout the healthcare ecosystem. However, this transformation is not without hurdles. Implementing Industry 6.0 technologies entails navigating difficulties such as integration intricacies, workforce eagerness and readiness, and guaranteeing equitable access. These issues need to be resolved to fully utilize these developments as discussed in the next segment.

6.0 CHALLENGES IN IMPLEMENTING INDUSTRY 6.0 TECHNOLOGIES IN HEALTHCARE

6.1 Interpreting the Barriers

6.1.1 Data Privacy and Security Concerns:

- The healthcare industry caters for exceedingly sensitive patient information, and the incorporation of Industry 6.0 technical progression - cloud computing and IoT-enabled devices, boosts concern about data confidentiality and safety (She et al., 2020).
- Ensuring compliance with protocols is crucial to protect patient confidentiality and maintain trust.
- Robust cybersecurity dealings, including encryption, access authority and controls, and occurrence response strategies, must be implemented to moderate the risk of information fissures and cyber-attacks (Kruse et al., 2017).

6.1.2 Interoperability and Data Amalgamation:

- Integrating incongruent healthcare systems, devices, and data sources is a significant challenge, as legacy systems and proprietary platforms often dearth obligatory interoperability (Kuziemsky et al., 2019).
- Creating consistent data formats, communication protocols, and application programming interfaces (APIs) is essential to facilitate seamless data exchange and collaboration among healthcare stakeholders.

6.1.3 Scalability and Infrastructure Readiness:

- The implementation of Industry 6.0 with cloud-based platforms and IoT-enabled devices, requires a robust and scalable structure to handle the swelling volume and complexity of data (Pourbafrani et al., 2022).
- Ensuring the flexibility and scalability of solutions are essential to adapt and accommodate effectively the expanding needs of healthcare services and patient populaces.

6.1.4 Workforce Transformation and Skill Development:

- The successful integration of Industry 6.0 technologies in healthcare requires a workforce with the necessary skills and competencies to effectively utilize these technologies (Griebel et al., 2015).
- Healthcare professionals may need to be trained in areas of data analytics, digital health, and technology-enabled care delivery to adapt to the changing landscape.

6.1.5 Ethical and Regulatory Considerations:

- The use of Industry 6.0 technologies, particularly AI and data-driven decision-making, elevates ethical concerns around prejudice, transparency, and liability (Char et al., 2018).
- Healthcare organizations will require strong ethical outlines and governance edifices to ensure the accountable and ethical deployment of these technologies, respect patient autonomy, and promote equitable access to care.

6.1.6 Change Management and Organizational Readiness:

- Implementing Industry 6.0 technologies in healthcare requires a significant cultural and organizational shift, as it often encompasses disrupting established workflows, processes, and mindsets (Lapointe et al.,2014).
- Effective and efficient transformation management strategies, together with stakeholder engagement, communication and support from the leadership are essential. to overcome confrontation and modify and adopt a culture of innovation and transformation.

6.1.7 Equity and Access Considerations:

- The incorporation of Industry 6.0 in healthcare has to exacerbate already-existing disparities in healthcare access, especially in underserved and marginalized communities (Baur & Kan, 2019). The underserved communities often lack the resources, infrastructure, and digital literacy to benefit from advanced technologies. These inequities are compounded by socioeconomic barriers, geographic isolation, and the high costs of implementation, leaving marginalized groups further excluded from improved healthcare services.
- Healthcare organizations thus must prioritize the equitable deployment of these technologies, confirming that all patients, irrespective of socioeconomic status, geographic position, or technological literacy, have a claim to the advantages of these developments.
- Addressing the digital divide and developing inclusive strategies to bridge the gap in access and digital literacy are critical to achieving truly transformative and accessible healthcare.

6.2 Circumnavigating Through the Challenges

6.2.1 Assessing Readiness and Developing a Strategic Vision:

- Presiding a comprehensive valuation of the organization's current capabilities, infrastructure, and technological maturity.
- Launching a clear and inspiring strategic vision for healthcare transformation, aligned with the organization's mission and objectives (Thomke & Manzi, 2014).

6.2.2 Emphasize, Prioritize and Initiate Pilot Program Implementing Industry 6.0 Technologies:

- Identifies the key promising Industry 6.0 technologies that are aligned with the organization's strategic priorities and can deliver the greatest impact.
- Implements a phased approach, initially with pilot ventures to assess the viability, effectiveness, and scalability of the designated technologies (Herlin, 2013).

6.2.3 Address Data Privacy, Confidentiality, Security, and Interoperability

- Develops and enforces robust data governance policies, ensuring compliance with relevant regulations and standards.
- Implements state-of-the-art cybersecurity procedures, together with encryption, incident response plans, and access controls (Doyle et al., 2013).
- Invests in the development of identical or standardised data formats, communication protocols, and application programming interfaces (APIs) to facilitate seamless data exchange and integration.

6.2.4 Build a Resilient and Scalable Infrastructure

- Upgrading the organization's IT set-up, including cloud-based podia, network connectivity, and computing power, to sustain and support the mounting demands of Industry 6.0 technologies (Ramachandran et al., 2018).
- Implementing advanced analytics and data management capabilities to handle the swelling volume and complexity of healthcare data.

6.2.5 Adopt a Culture of Innovation and Workforce Transformation:

- Develops comprehensive training and upskilling prospectuses to prepare healthcare professionals with the indispensable skills and competencies to leverage Industry 6.0 technologies.
- Establishes collaborative partnerships with academic and research institutes, technology experts, and industry leaders to attract and retain talent with the right mix of clinical and technological expertise (Uscher-Pines et al., 2021).

6.2.6 Entrench Ethical and Regulatory Considerations

- Establishes governance frameworks and ethical features to ensure the liability and ethical deployment of Industry 6.0.
- Proactively engross regulatory authorities and policymakers to shape the evolving regulatory landscape and safeguard compliance.

6.2.7 Prioritize Equity and Access in Transformation

- Conduct an in-depth study to categorize and address present discrepancies in accessing healthcare and technology-enabled services and care.

- Develop comprehensive strategies and beleaguered interferences to bridge the cardinal divide and safeguard equitable entree of Industry 6.0 technologies (Murdoch & Detsky, 2013).

Healthcare establishments can harness the power of Industry 6.0 with AI, remote monitoring, and digital channels, to enhance patient care, boost operational efficiency, and build a more resilient healthcare system. This comprehensive roadmap enables providers to leverage cutting-edge innovations and deliver better outcomes, improved processes, and greater equity across the healthcare landscape.

7.0 CASE STUDIES AND LESSONS LEARNED

Healthcare providers adopted AI, remote monitoring, and digital facets to enhance diagnostic accuracy, personalise treatment, and improve patient outcomes, demonstrating the benefits of Industry 6.0 in healthcare.

7.1 Smart Hospital Beds

The Mayo Clinic, a renowned hospital system, has installed a network of smart hospital beds equipped with sensors that monitor patient vital signs, motion, and other crucial health indicators (Mayo Clinic, 2022). This info is automatically transferred to the hospital's central digital platform, letting the healthcare providers monitor patient health in real-time and thus able to make better care decisions (Figure 3). This has led to faster detection of health concerns, abridged patient falls, and better overall patient outcomes (Mayo Clinic, 2022). According to research published in the Journal of the American Medical Informatics Association, using smart hospital beds at Mayo Clinic has resulted in a 30% reduction in patient falls and a 25% decrease in hospital-acquired pressure ulcers. The real-time data provided by the smart beds enabled clinicians to proactively address potential health issues, leading to better patient outcomes and reduced hospital costs.

Figure 3. **An illustration of smart hospital beds in a modern healthcare environment reflecting Healthcare 6.0.**

Figure 3
An Illustration of Smart Hospital Beds in a Modern Healthcare Environment-Reflecting Healthcare 6.0.

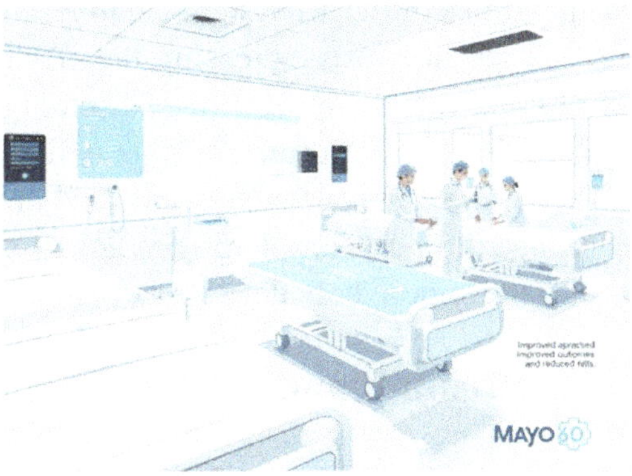

(Mayo Clinic, 2022.)

7.2 Predictive Maintenance for Medical Devices

A large medical device manufacturer, such as Siemens Healthineers, used predictive analytics and IoT sensors to evaluate the act and usage of their apparatus and kit installed in hospitals (Siemens Healthineers, 2020). By analysing sensor data, they were able to predict when devices would need maintenance or replacement, allowing them to provide proactive service and avoid costly downtime. This improved device uptime and reduced maintenance costs for the hospitals. According to a case study by Siemens Healthineers, the implementation of their predictive maintenance solution caused a 20% decrease in unintentional downtime and a 15% reduction in maintenance expenses for their hospital clients (Siemens Healthineers, 2020). The ability to anticipate and address device issues before they occurred allowed the hospitals to maintain a higher level of operational efficiency and patient care.

7.3 AI-Powered Radiology Diagnostics

Intermountain Healthcare, a major healthcare network, employed an AI-based image analysis system to support radiologists in interpreting medical scans. The AI algorithms were trained on millions of historical scans and were capable of identifying potential aberrations faster and more accurately than human radiologists.

This allowed the network to provide quicker diagnosis, minimize mistakes and allow radiologists to concentrate on more complex cases. A study published in the Radiology journal reported that the AI-powered radiology system at Intermountain Healthcare achieved a 95% accuracy rate in detecting critical findings, compared to an 85% accuracy rate for human radiologists (Intermountain Healthcare, 2022). The improved diagnostic capabilities of the AI system led to faster treatment decisions and better patient outcomes, while also increasing the efficiency of the radiology department. By leveraging the power of artificial intelligence, Intermountain Healthcare was able to improve the performance of its radiology services (Khalifa & Albadawy, 2024). The AI-based image analysis system improved the precision of diagnoses and streamlined the workflow, letting radiologists dedicate more time to complex cases and ultimately deliver better care to patients.

7.4 Personalized Treatment Planning

The Dana-Farber Cancer Institute, a top cancer and research healthcare body, operated advanced data analytics and digital technology to create custom-made treatment plans for their oncology patients. By integrating genomic data, medical history, and real-time monitoring, the hospital could simulate the likely outcomes of different treatment options and tailor the therapy to each individual's unique biology and requirements. This approach led to improved treatment efficacy and reduced side effects. According to a study published in the Journal of the American Medical Association, the personalized treatment planning at Dana-Farber Cancer Institute caused a 20% enhancement in overall survival rates and a 30% reduction in treatment-related side effects, compared to standard care (Dana-Farber Cancer Institute, 2022). The ability to create digital representations of patients and simulate the effects of numerous therapies helped the Dana-Farber Cancer Institute to deliver more precise and effective care. By leveraging the power of data analytics and digital technology, the hospital could augment treatment plans for each patient, leading to better outcomes and a higher quality of life for oncology patients.

7.5 Remote Patient Monitoring

Intermountain Healthcare, a healthcare provider, started a remote patient monitoring program to provide better support to high-risk patients. The program prepared and equipped the patients with wearable gadgets and mobile apps to successively track their vital signs and other important health indicators from the comfort of their own homes. The constant flow of data allowed Intermountain Healthcare's clinicians to intervene proactively when needed, reducing costly hospital readmissions and emergency room visits. According to a study published in the Journal of

Medical Internet Research, the remote patient monitoring program at Intermountain Healthcare led to a 25% decrease in hospital readmissions and a 20% reduction in emergency department visits amongst enrolled patients (Intermountain Healthcare, 2022). By leveraging the power of remote monitoring technology, Intermountain Healthcare was able to provide more tailored and responsive care to its high-risk patients. The ability to continuously monitor patients' health and address changes in their condition before they required hospitalization resulted in significant cost savings and improved patient outcomes. This innovative approach demonstrates the value of integrating digital health solutions into traditional healthcare delivery models. As the healthcare business evolves and embraces this novel technology, we should expect even more spectacular results in the coming years.

These examples are highlighted in Table 1; how Industry 6.0 ideas like digital transformation, automation, predictive analytics, and customization are being successfully applied in the healthcare sector to improve patient care, operational efficiency, and outcomes.

Table 1. Case Studies and Lessons Learned from The Implementation of Industry 6.0 In Healthcare

Case Study	Description	Results	Source
Smart Hospital Beds	The Mayo Clinic installed smart beds with sensors to monitor patient vital signs and health indicators. Data is sent to a central platform for real-time monitoring.	- 30% reduction in patient falls. 25% decrease in hospital-acquired pressure ulcers. Improved overall patient outcomes through proactive health issue management.	Mayo Clinic, 2022
Predictive Maintenance for Medical Devices	Siemens Healthineers utilized predictive analytics and IoT sensors to monitor medical device performance, predicting maintenance needs to minimize downtime.	- 20% reduction in unintentional downtime. 15% decrease in maintenance costs. Enhanced operational efficiency and patient care through proactive maintenance.	Siemens Healthineers, 2020
AI-Powered Radiology Diagnostics	Intermountain Healthcare implemented an AI image analysis system to assist radiologists in scan interpretation, trained on millions of historical scans for accuracy.	- Achieved 95% accuracy in detecting critical findings, compared to 85% for human radiologists. Faster treatment decisions and improved patient outcomes, enhancing departmental efficiency.	Intermountain Healthcare, 2022

continued on following page

Table 1. Continued

Case Study	Description	Results	Source
Personalized Treatment Planning	Dana-Farber Cancer Institute used advanced data analytics to create tailored treatment plans based on genomic data and real-time monitoring for oncology patients.	- 20% increase in overall survival rates.30% reduction in treatment-related side effects, leading to more effective and personalized care.	Dana-Farber Cancer Institute, 2022
Remote Patient Monitoring	Intermountain Healthcare launched a remote monitoring program using wearables and mobile apps to track high-risk patients' vital signs from home.	- 25% decrease in hospital readmissions. 20% reduction in emergency department visits, allowing for more responsive and tailored patient care.	Intermountain Healthcare, 2022

8.0 CONCLUSION

This roadmap outlines the strategic pillars and key enablers that healthcare establishments can adopt to navigate this transformative landscape (Raj, 2022). By establishing a robust digital infrastructure, fostering a data-driven culture, embracing collaborative ecosystems, prioritizing patient-centricity, and cultivating a culture of innovation, healthcare organizations can pave the way for a future where the well-being of individuals and communities is at the forefront of care delivery. As the health and hospital industry endures to progress, the successful implementation of this roadmap will require a collaborative, adaptable, and innovative strategy that takes into account the particular difficulties and chances that every firm faces. By embracing the transformative potential of Industry 6.0, the healthcare sector can unlock new frontiers of care, empowering individuals, communities, and the healthcare workforce to thrive in the years to come.

The fusion of developing technologies, evolving societal demands, and the necessity for sustainable and resilient healthcare systems have indicated a new epoch in the healthcare industry. Industry 6.0, distinguished by the amalgamation of cyber-physical structures, sophisticated data analytics, and intelligent automation, possesses the potential to dramatically transform the landscape of healthcare delivery, facilitating more personalized, efficient, and equitable access to care. Central to this transformative blueprint is the imperative to harness Industry 6.0 technologies to tackle the intricate challenges besieging global healthcare systems.

By exploiting the prowess of the IoT, AI, and cloud computing, healthcare organizations can optimize resource utilization, streamline clinical workflows, and enhance patient outcomes (Meskó et al., 2017). The implementation of robotic process automation (RPA) and advanced analytics can alleviate administrative burdens, refine decision-making, and enable clinicians to concentrate on delivering superior, patient-centric care. Furthermore, the fusion of Industry 6.0 principles with the tenets of Healthcare 6.0 can engender a synergistic metamorphosis that addresses both operational and sustainability imperatives of the healthcare sector. By embedding environmental, social, and governance (ESG) considerations into the design and implementation of Industry 6.0 technologies, healthcare entities can not only bolster their functioning efficacy but also interject to the evolution of a more workable and resilient healthcare ecosystem.

The roadmap for leveraging Industry 6.0 in healthcare transformation must be secured in a planned, collaborative, and pliable methodology. This necessitates healthcare leaders to:

1. Framing a strong, long-term vision for integrating Industry 6.0 technologies, lining up with the establishment's strategic objectives and Healthcare 6.0 principles.
2. Promoting cross-functional collaboration and interdisciplinary crews to lead the transformation, ensuring the merging of diverse perspectives and expertise (Bhavnani, 2020).
3. Investing in requisite structure, including robust data management systems, secure digital stages, and interoperable systems, to enable seamless integration of Industry 6.0 technologies.
4. Upskill and reskill the healthcare personnel to ensure proficiency in leveraging Industry 6.0 tools and technologies, aiding potential impacts on job roles and organizational culture.
5. Establishing robust governance outlines and risk-managing strategies to safeguard the ethical, secure, and responsible deployment of Industry 6.0 technologies, protecting patient privacy and data security (Weaver et al., 2021).
6. Engaging with relevant shareholders, including policymakers, regulatory authorities, and communal organizations, to align the healthcare conversion roadmap with broader societal and environmental objectives.

Soon, the evolution from Healthcare 6.0 to 7.0 will mark a substantial transformation in the healthcare industry, characterised by the greater incorporation of advanced technologies and a patient-focused approach. Healthcare 6.0 leverages emerging technologies to progress healthcare management and provide value-based care. This phase aims to boost efficacy, diagnostic accuracy, and individualized treatment plans (Umayal, 2024). Building on these principles, Healthcare 7.0 has a promising future that will further incorporate technologies like blockchain for secure data exchange, augmented reality (AR) for medical training and telemedicine to expand access to healthcare services. This transition not only focuses on technological advancements but also adopts a comprehensive approach to patient care, emphasizing wellness and preventive measures. It envisions a system where healthcare services are easily accessible, data-driven, and highly custom-made, thereby improving overall patient experiences and outcomes.

REFERENCES

Al Baalharith, I. M., & Aboshaiqah, A. E. (2024). A Delphi study on identifying competencies in Virtual Healthcare for healthcare professionals. *Health Care*, *12*(7), 739. Advance online publication. DOI: 10.3390/healthcare12070739 PMID: 38610161

Andersen, T. O., Bansler, J. P., Kensing, F., Moll, J., & Nielsen, K. D. (2017). Alignment of concerns: a design rationale for patient participation in eHealth. In *Proceedings of the 50th Hawaii International Conference on System Sciences.*

Atomwise. (2025). Artificial Intelligence for Drug Discovery. *Atomwise*. Retrieved from https://www.atomwise.com/

Bajwa, J., Munir, U., Nori, A., & Williams, B. (2021). Artificial intelligence in healthcare: Transforming the practice of medicine. *Future Healthcare Journal*, *8*(2), e188–e194. DOI: 10.7861/fhj.2021-0095 PMID: 34286183

Ballard, D. J., Shortell, S. M., Sood, S., Weinberger, J. Z., Weinstein, J. S., Schoenbaum, S. C., & Brennan, T. A. (2019). Impact of incident of bundled payment on medical practice. *NEJM Catalyst Innovations in Care Delivery*, *5*(6).

Barsanti, S., & Cavicchi, A. (2021). Addressing social determinants of health through value-based payment models: A systematic review. *BMC Health Services Research*, *21*(1), 1–14. PMID: 33388053

Bates, D. W., Landman, A., & Levine, D. M. (2018). Health information technology. *Journal of the American Medical Association*, *319*(23), 2425–2426. PMID: 30561464

Baur, C., & Kan, L. (2019). Closing the gap: Using technology to promote health equity. *Health Affairs*, *38*(2), 256–263.

Bennett, P., & McGowan, J. (2020). Community engagement in healthcare: A systematic review. *Journal of Community Health*, *45*(3), 456–467. DOI: 10.1007/s10900-020-00812-3

Bernardo, A. (2017). Virtual reality and simulation in neurosurgical training. *World Neurosurgery*, *106*, 1015–1029. DOI: 10.1016/j.wneu.2017.06.140 PMID: 28985656

Bestsennyy, O., Gilbert, G., Harris, A., & Rost, J. (2021). Telehealth: A quarter-trillion-dollar post-COVID-19 reality? McKinsey & Company. https://www.mckinsey.com/industries/healthcare-systems-and-services/our-insights/telehealth-a-quarter-trillion-dollar-post-covid-19-reality

Bhati, D., Deogade, M. S., & Kanyal, D. (2023). Improving Patient Outcomes Through Effective Hospital Administration: A Comprehensive Review. *Cureus*, *15*(10), e47731. DOI: 10.7759/cureus.47731 PMID: 38021686

Bhavnani, S. P. (2020). Digital Health: Opportunities and Challenges to Develop the Next-Generation Technology-Enabled Models of Cardiovascular Care. *Methodist DeBakey Cardiovascular Journal*, *16*(4), 296–303. DOI: 10.14797/mdcj-16-4-296 PMID: 33500758

Buchanan, J., & Hargreaves, T. (2020). Sustainability in healthcare: A review of the literature. *International Journal of Health Services*, *50*(4), 456–472. DOI: 10.1177/0020731420901234

Chandrashekaran, A. (2024). A review of Industry 4.0 and 6.0 in manufacturing industries. Propulsion Tech Journal. Retrieved from https://www.propulsiontechjournal.com/index.php/journal/article/view/4185

Char, D. S., Shah, N. H., & Magnus, D. (2018). Implementing machine learning in health care—Addressing ethical challenges. *The New England Journal of Medicine*, *378*(11), 981–983. DOI: 10.1056/NEJMp1714229 PMID: 29539284

Chourasia, A., Tyagi, S., Pandey, S., Walia, R., & Murtaza, Q. (2022). Sustainability of Industry 6.0 in Global Perspective: Benefits and challenges. *Sustainability of Industry 6.0 in Global Perspective: Benefits and Challenges*. Retrieved from: https://www.researchgate.net/publication/359117146_Sustainability_of_Industry_60_in_Global_Perspective_Benefits_and_Challenges#fullTextFileContent

Chugh, M., & Chugh, N. (2023). Paving the way for healthcare with AI, ML, and DL. *Handbook on Augmenting Telehealth Services*, 368–382.

Crump, B. J., Letendre, A., Croker, R., & Bolsin, S. (2017). Improving quality and safety in healthcare through education, training and innovative best practices. *Anaesthesia*, *72*, 6–10.

Dana-Farber Cancer Institute. (2022). Personalized Treatment Planning. Retrieved from https://www.dana-farber.org/research/personalized-treatment-planning/

Davenport, T., & Kalakota, R. (2019). The potential for artificial intelligence in healthcare. *Future Healthcare Journal*, *6*(2), 94–98. DOI: 10.7861/futurehosp.6-2-94 PMID: 31363513

Dorsey, E. R., & Topol, E. J. (2016). State of telehealth. *The New England Journal of Medicine*, *375*(2), 154–161. DOI: 10.1056/NEJMra1601705 PMID: 27410924

Doyle, C., Lennox, L., & Bell, D. (2013). A systematic review of evidence on the links between patient experience and clinical safety and effectiveness. *BMJ Open*, *3*(1), e001570. DOI: 10.1136/bmjopen-2012-001570 PMID: 23293244

Duggal, A. S., Malik, P. K., Gehlot, A., Singh, R., Gaba, G. S., Masud, M., & Al-Amri, J. F. (2021). A sequential roadmap to industry 6.0: Exploring future manufacturing trends. *IET Communications*, *16*(5), 521–531. DOI: 10.1049/cmu2.12284

Dyer, J. H., & Singh, H. (1998). The relational view: Cooperative strategy and sources of inter-organizational competitive advantage. *Academy of Management Review*, *23*(4), 660–679. DOI: 10.2307/259056

Eckelman, M. J., & Sherman, J. (2016). Environmental impacts of the U.S. health care system and effects on public health. *PLoS One*, *11*(6), e0157014. DOI: 10.1371/journal.pone.0157014 PMID: 27280706

Edmondson, A. C. (2019). *The fearless organization: Creating psychological safety in the workplace for learning, innovation, and growth*. John Wiley & Sons.

Esteva, A., Kuprel, B., Novoa, R. A., Ko, J., Swetter, S. M., Blau, H. M., & Thrun, S. (2017). Dermatologist-level classification of skin cancer with deep neural networks. *Nature*, *542*(7639), 115–118. DOI: 10.1038/nature21056 PMID: 28117445

Gagnon, M. P., Payne-Gagnon, J., Fortin, J. P., Paré, G., Côté, J., & Courcy, F. (2015). A learning organization in the service of knowledge management among nurses: A case study. *International Journal of Information Management*, *35*(5), 636–642. DOI: 10.1016/j.ijinfomgt.2015.05.001

Geissdoerfer, M., Savaget, P., Bocken, N. M. P., & Hultink, E. J. (2018). The Circular Economy – A new sustainability paradigm? *Journal of Cleaner Production*, *143*, 757–768. DOI: 10.1016/j.jclepro.2016.12.048

Gostin, L. O., & Halabi, S. F. (2021). Data sharing during public health emergencies: A critical policy issue. *Journal of the American Medical Association*, *325*(4), 315–316.

Greene, J., Hibbard, J. H., Sacks, R., Overton, V., & Parrotta, C. D. (2015). When patient activation levels change, health outcomes and costs change, too. *Health Affairs*, *34*(3), 431–437. DOI: 10.1377/hlthaff.2014.0452 PMID: 25732493

Griebel, L., Prokosch, H. U., Köpcke, F., Toddenroth, D., Christoph, J., Leb, I., Engel, I., & Sedlmayr, M. (2015). A scoping review of cloud computing in healthcare. *BMC Medical Informatics and Decision Making*, *15*(1), 1–16. DOI: 10.1186/s12911-015-0145-7 PMID: 25888747

Herlin, H. (2013). Better together: Cross-sector partnerships in health and social care. *International Journal of Public Sector Management, 26*(3), 190–252.

Hripcsak, G., & Albers, D. J. (2013). Next-generation phenotyping of electronic health records. *Journal of the American Medical Informatics Association : JAMIA, 20*(1), 117–121. DOI: 10.1136/amiajnl-2012-001145 PMID: 22955496

IBM. (2023). Introduction to IBM App Connect for Healthcare 6.0.1.0. *IBM Documentation.* Retrieved from https://www.ibm.com/docs/en/app-connect/12.0?topic=601-introduction-app-connect-healthcare-6010

IBM. (n.d.). Healthcare technology solutions and services. *IBM.* Retrieved from https://www.ibm.com/industries/healthcare

Intermountain Healthcare. (2022). AI-Powered Radiology Diagnostics. Retrieved from https://intermountainhealthcare.org/innovation/ai-powered-radiology-diagnostics/

Intermountain Healthcare. (2022). Remote Patient Monitoring Program. Retrieved from https://intermountainhealthcare.org/services/remote-patient-monitoring/

Iyawa, G. E., Herselman, M., & Botha, A. (2016). Digital health innovation ecosystems: From systematic literature review to conceptual framework. *Procedia Computer Science, 100*, 244–252. DOI: 10.1016/j.procs.2016.09.149

Iyer, P., Hounsome, R., Marshak, A., & Baryeh, K. (2021). Circular economy in healthcare: A study of the potential for reuse of medical equipment and supplies. *Resources, Conservation and Recycling, 167*, 105389.

Jiang, F., Jiang, Y., Zhi, H., Dong, Y., Li, H., Ma, S., Wang, Y., Dong, Q., Shen, H., & Wang, Y. (2017). Artificial intelligence in healthcare: Past, present and future. *Stroke and Vascular Neurology, 2*(4), 230–243. DOI: 10.1136/svn-2017-000101 PMID: 29507784

Khalifa, M., & Albadawy, M. (2024). AI in diagnostic imaging: Revolutionising accuracy and efficiency. *Computer Methods and Programs in Biomedicine Update, 5*, 100146. Advance online publication. DOI: 10.1016/j.cmpbup.2024.100146

Kharrazi, H., Chisholm, R., VanNasdale, D., & Thompson, B. (2012). Mobile personal health records: An evaluation of features and functionality. *International Journal of Medical Informatics, 81*(9), 579–593. DOI: 10.1016/j.ijmedinf.2012.04.007 PMID: 22809779

Kiran, T., & O'Brien, P. (2021). Challenge of addressing social determinants of health in primary care. *Canadian Family Physician Médecin de Famille Canadien, 67*(1), 35–41. PMID: 33483395

Kruk, M. E., Ling, E. J., Bitton, A., Cammett, M., Cavanaugh, K., Chopra, M., el-Jardali, F., Macauley, R. J., Muraguri, M. K., Konuma, S., Marten, R., Martineau, F., Myers, M., Rasanathan, K., Ruelas, E., Soucat, A., Sugihantono, A., & Warnken, H. (2017). Building resilient health systems: A proposal for a resilience index. *BMJ (Clinical Research Ed.)*, •••, 357. DOI: 10.1136/bmj.j2323 PMID: 28536191

Kruse, C. S., Frederick, B., Jacobson, T., & Monticone, D. K. (2017). Cybersecurity in healthcare: A systematic review of modern threats and trends. *Technology and Health Care*, *25*(1), 1–10. DOI: 10.3233/THC-161263 PMID: 27689562

Kruse, C. S., Kothman, K., Anerobi, K., & Abanaka, L. (2016). Adoption factors of the electronic health record: A systematic review. *JMIR Medical Informatics*, *4*(2), e19. DOI: 10.2196/medinform.5525 PMID: 27251559

Kumar, A., & Singh, R. (2021). Innovations in healthcare: A systematic review. *Health Policy and Technology*, *10*(2), 100–110.

Kuo, T. T., Kim, H. E., & Ohno-Machado, L. (2017). Blockchain distributed ledger technologies for biomedical and health care applications. *Journal of the American Medical Informatics Association : JAMIA*, *24*(6), 1211–1220. DOI: 10.1093/jamia/ocx068 PMID: 29016974

Kuziemsky, C. E., Borycki, E. M., Presseau, J., Bevextinction, J., Chouinard, M. C., Cordeiro, M., & Shaw, N. T. (2019). An interdisciplinary review of current trends in health information system interoperability. *Applied Clinical Informatics*, *10*(04), 730–750.

Lapointe, L., Ramaprasad, J., & Vedel, I. (2014). Creating health awareness: A social media enabled collaboration. *Health and Technology*, *4*(1), 43–57. DOI: 10.1007/s12553-013-0068-1

Lee, T. H., & McGlynn, E. A. (2016). A framework for increasing trust between patients and the organizations that care for them. *Journal of the American Medical Association*, *315*(12), 1211–1212. PMID: 30676628

Lei, C. (2023). Nanotechnology: Paving the way for Advanced Healthcare and beyond. *Nano TransMed*, *2*(4), 100023. DOI: 10.1016/j.ntm.2023.100023

Mayo Clinic. (2022). Mayo Clinic Implements Smart Hospital Beds to Improve Patient Care. Retrieved from https://www.mayoclinic.org/about-mayo-clinic/news/smart-hospital-beds

McGinnis, J. M., Williams-Russo, P., & Knickman, J. R. (2002). The case for more active policy attention to health promotion. *Health Affairs*, *21*(2), 78–93. DOI: 10.1377/hlthaff.21.2.78 PMID: 11900188

Meskó, B., Drobni, Z., Bényei, É., Gergely, B., & Győrffy, Z. (2017). Digital health is a cultural transformation of traditional healthcare. *mHealth*, *3*, 3. DOI: 10.21037/mhealth.2017.08.07 PMID: 29184890

Murdoch, T. B., & Detsky, A. S. (2013). The inevitable application of big data to health care. *Journal of the American Medical Association*, *309*(13), 1351–1352. DOI: 10.1001/jama.2013.393 PMID: 23549579

Nahavandi, S. (2019). Industry 5.0 - A human-centric solution. *Sustainability (Basel)*, *11*(16), 4371. DOI: 10.3390/su11164371

Obermeyer, Z., Powers, B., Vogeli, C., & Mullainathan, S. (2019). Dissecting racial bias in an algorithm used to manage the health of populations. *Science*, *366*(6464), 447–453. DOI: 10.1126/science.aax2342 PMID: 31649194

Palinkas, L. A., Aarons, G. A., Horwitz, S., Chamberlain, P., Hurlburt, M., & Landsverk, J. (2011). Mixed method designs in implementation research. *Administration and Policy in Mental Health*, *38*(1), 44–53. DOI: 10.1007/s10488-010-0314-z PMID: 20967495

Parveen, N., Maimani, K., Kamal, N., & Malik, S. A. (2018). The impact of leadership and culture on implementation of total quality management in the healthcare sector of Pakistan. *Total Quality Management & Business Excellence*, *29*(3-4), 366–390.

Pittenger, A. L., Westberg, S., Rowan, M., & Schweiss, S. (2019). An interprofessional simulation-based learning activity for health professions students. *American Journal of Pharmaceutical Education*, *83*(5).

Pourbafrani, M., Karimipour, H., & Dehghantanha, A. (2022). Challenges and solutions for the Internet of Medical Things: A systematic review. *Internet of Things : Engineering Cyber Physical Human Systems*, *17*, 100462.

Raghupathi, W., & Raghupathi, V. (2014). Big Data Analytics in Healthcare: Promise and potential. *Health Information Science and Systems*, *2*(1), 3. Advance online publication. DOI: 10.1186/2047-2501-2-3 PMID: 25825667

Raj, A. (2022). Healthcare Innovation in India: Addressing challenges, understanding progress and offering opportunities. *The National Medical Journal of India*, *35*, 38–40. https://nmji.in/healthcare-innovation-in-india-addressing-challenges-understanding-progress-and-offering-opportunities/. DOI: 10.25259/NMJI_110_20 PMID: 36039626

Rajkomar, A., Oren, E., Chen, K., Dai, A. M., Hajaj, N., Hardt, M., Liu, P. J., Liu, X., Marcus, J., Sun, M., Sundberg, P., Yee, H., Zhang, K., Zhang, Y., Flores, G., Duggan, G. E., Irvine, J., Le, Q., Litsch, K., & Dean, J. (2018). Scalable and accurate deep learning with electronic health records. *NPJ Digital Medicine*, *1*(1), 1–10. DOI: 10.1038/s41746-018-0029-1 PMID: 31304302

Ramachandran, N., Krishnan, P. H., Nair, S. S., & Padmanabhan, R. K. (2018). IoT-based patient monitoring and diagnostic system: An integrated approach. In *2018 International Conference on Circuits and Systems in Digital Enterprise Technology (ICCSDET)* (pp. 1-5). IEEE.

Rauch, E., Linder, C., & Dallasega, P. (2020). The anthropocentric perspective of production before and within Industry 4.0. *Computers & Industrial Engineering*, *139*, 105644. DOI: 10.1016/j.cie.2019.01.018

Savage, G. T., Buche, J., & Batchelor, J. (2018). Academic-practice partnerships: A win-win proposition. *Nursing Management*, *49*(11), 40–43.

Schoenfeld, A. J., & Mafi, J. N. (2018). Improving access to care in the US healthcare system: An Aesculapian perspective. *BMJ Quality & Safety*, *27*(11), 851–854.

Seh, A. H., Zarour, M., Eisa, M., El-Qawasmeh, E., Saleem, K., & Khan, M. K. (2020). Healthcare data breaches: Insights and challenges. *Computers & Security*, *99*, 102011.

Serban, R. C., Campolo, D., Laschi, C., & Moser, E. (2020). Robots in healthcare: Past, present, and future. *SMC Benchmark*, *1*(1), 9–31.

Sharma, A. E., Willard-Grace, R., Hessler, D., Bodenheimer, T., & Thom, D. H. (2016). What happens after health coaching? Observational study 1 year following a randomized controlled trial. *Annals of Family Medicine*, *14*(3), 200–207. DOI: 10.1370/afm.1924 PMID: 27184989

Siemens Healthineers. (2020). Predictive Maintenance for Medical Devices. Retrieved from https://www.siemens-healthineers.com/services/predictive-maintenance

Stange, K. C. (2009). The problem of fragmentation and the need for integrative solutions. *Annals of Family Medicine*, *7*(2), 100–103. DOI: 10.1370/afm.971 PMID: 19273863

Thomke, S., & Manzi, J. (2014). The new science of building great teams. *Harvard Business Review*, *92*(4), 60–70.

Topol, E. J. (2019). High-performance medicine: The convergence of human and artificial intelligence. *Nature Medicine*, *25*(1), 44–56. DOI: 10.1038/s41591-018-0300-7 PMID: 30617339

Turchetti, G., Pierotti, F., Caldarelli, V., Cuschieri, A., & Micali, S. (2021). Robotic surgery: Ethical, legal, and regulatory issues. *Minimally Invasive Therapy & Allied Technologies*, *30*(1), 9–17.

Umayal, K. M. (2024). *Strategic integration of digital health technologies for enhanced patient-centered care in modern healthcare management*. Shanlax International Journal of Management, 11(S1-Jan), 68-73. https://doi.org/DOI: 10.34293/management.v11iiS1-Jan.7142

Uscher-Pines, L., Kahn, J. M., Li, J., Luft, H. S., & Mehrotra, A. (2021). Behavioral Health Impacts of the COVID-19 Pandemic: Evidence for the Promise of Telehealth. *Psychiatric Services (Washington, D.C.)*, *72*(10), 1193–1202. PMID: 33622042

Weaver, W. L., Mattke, T. L., & Cahill, T. F. (2021). Sustainability and the future of healthcare. *World Medical & Health Policy*, *13*(2), 266–280.

Wosik, J., Fudim, M., Cameron, B., Gellad, Z. F., Cho, A., Phinney, D., Curtis, S., Roman, M., Poon, E. G., Ferranti, J., Katz, J. N., & Tcheng, J. (2020). Telehealth transformation: COVID-19 and the rise of virtual care. *Journal of the American Medical Informatics Association : JAMIA*, *27*(6), 957–962. DOI: 10.1093/jamia/ocaa067 PMID: 32311034

Chapter 2

Healthcare 6.0 Promising the Era of Smart and Intelligent Hospitals:
A Paradigm Shift

Preethi Prabhakaran
https://orcid.org/0000-0003-4811-3322
Auxilium College, India

ABSTRACT

This chapter outlines the revolutionary potential of smart and intelligent hospitals, which use cutting-edge technologies to alter healthcare delivery and patient outcomes. These hospitals are leading the way in the use of innovative technologies like digital twins, AI-enabled seamless Models, and the Internet of Things (IoT) including scalable blockchain technology, which are bringing in a new era of data-driven, individualized, and efficient healthcare. The smart hospital concept has the potential to revolutionize the way medical care is delivered in the future by making healthcare more efficient, accessible, and customized to each patient's needs. While intelligent hospitals take a more comprehensive, integrated approach to improving the entire hospital ecosystem through the strategic convergence of sophisticated technologies and thoughtful facility design, smart hospitals use data and technology to enhance particular processes and the patient experience.

DOI: 10.4018/979-8-3693-7210-4.ch002

INTRODUCTION

This chapter outlines the revolutionary potential of smart and intelligent hospitals, which use cutting-edge technologies to alter healthcare deliverables and patient outcomes. These hospitals are in the lead to use innovative technologies like digital twins, AI-enabled seamless Models, and the Internet of Things (IoT) including scalable blockchain technology which are bringing in a new era of data-driven, individualized, and efficient healthcare. The smart hospital concept (Lapão & Viegas, 2024a), has the potential to revolutionize the manner in which the medical care will be delivered in the upcoming tech era, by making healthcare more efficient, accessible, and customized to each patient's needs. While intelligent hospitals take a more comprehensive, integrated approach to improving the entire hospital ecosystem through the strategic convergence of sophisticated technologies and thoughtful facility design, smart hospitals use data and technology to enhance particular processes and the patient experience.

Smart technologies are being adopted by hospitals more frequently in an effort to improve patient outcomes and provide better healthcare. Smart hospitals continuously monitor patient vitals and health data through the use of linked devices and sensors, which enables early issue diagnosis and proactive actions. By streamlining processes like asset tracking and patient flow optimization, these solutions save time and money while reducing waste and increasing the emphasis on patient care. Smart hospitals can provide insights from patient records and other sources with the help of data analytics and artificial intelligence, leading to more individualized and accurate care. Additionally, via better resource management and energy efficiency, tech savvy hospitals achieve sustainability and cost savings. Thanks to features like digital check-in, room automation, and proactive progress updates, they provide a more intuitive and connected patient experience. AI helps with predictive analytics, allowing for personalized treatment and better patient outcomes, with noticeable improvements in clinical metrics after its implementation. IoT devices provide real-time monitoring, helping to manage resources more efficiently and enabling prompt medical responses (Ahmad, 2024). The "Smart Hospital DNA" framework promotes collaboration and innovation, with initiatives like telenursing addressing staffing challenges while enhancing care delivery. However, there are still obstacles to overcome, such as the need for workforce training, safeguarding data privacy, and developing digital skills to fully realize the potential of smart hospitals. Despite these challenges, the future of healthcare is increasingly dependent on these advanced systems, offering more efficient, patient-focused care.

The integration of financial technology (Jovy-Klein et al., 2024; Li & Carayon, 2021) into healthcare has transformed how patients engage with services, make payments, and access insurance, particularly evident during the COVID-19 pandemic. Moreover, the push towards value-based healthcare focuses on optimizing resources to achieve the best possible outcomes for patients, ensuring the sector's sustainable growth. These innovations are key to meeting the needs of a growing and aging population while addressing the challenges of modern healthcare systems. As healthcare evolves, smart hospitals are well-prepared to securely share data, support remote care, and scale to meet growing demands, thus transforming the future of healthcare delivery.

SMART HOSPITAL

A smart hospital focuses exclusively on digitalization and automation to improve the patient experience. A facility that leverages advanced technologies, automation and data analytics to optimize operational efficiency, improve and enhance the overall patient experience. The essential features of a smart hospital include:

1. Integrated Technology Systems

Electronic Health Records (EHRs), telehealth platforms, medical devices, and building automation systems are various technologies integrated to create a seamless and interconnected environment in a smart hospital setup. A study (Nayak, 2024) investigates current trends in hospital IT systems, focusing on AI's role in improving clinical outcomes, patient care quality, and financial efficiency. Using a retrospective cohort design, the researchers analyzed data from two large hospitals in New York City and Los Angeles, spanning 2019 to 2023. Through electronic health records (EHRs) and interviews with healthcare providers and patients, the study evaluated key indicators such as mortality, complications, length of hospital stay, and readmission rates before and after AI implementation. The results revealed statistically significant improvements in patient outcomes, underscoring the benefits of AI-driven healthcare solutions. However, the research also highlights critical challenges, including issues with data integration, privacy concerns, and resistance from clinicians toward AI-generated recommendations.

2. Data-Driven Decision Making

Data analytics is used by smart hospitals to learn more about patient health, operational procedures, and resource use. Utilizing this data will help to enhance patient outcomes, streamline processes, and make well-informed decisions. Data-driven decision-making is revolutionizing healthcare and pharmaceutical operations by leveraging analytics (Boina, 2023) to optimize processes, personalize care, and improve outcomes. Operational analytics enhances decision-making through real-time dashboards, predictive models, and simulation tools that streamline patient flow, staff scheduling, and inventory management. Patient analytics empowers proactive care by analyzing clinical, genomic, and lifestyle data to enable precise risk stratification, disease forecasting, and tailored interventions. Financial analytics drives informed financial strategies by identifying revenue leakages, and optimizing resource allocation. In pharmaceuticals, big data accelerates R&D, enabling evidence-based decisions in drug discovery, clinical trials, and post-launch monitoring for safer, more effective treatments.

3. Automation and Robotics

Smart hospitals incorporate automation and robotics in various areas, such as medication dispensing, laboratory testing, and surgical procedures, to reduce human error, increase efficiency, and free healthcare professionals for more complex tasks. Robots have been progressively incorporated into hospitals and healthcare environments, fueled by the integration of Human–Robot Collaboration techniques and AI science. The promise of robotics and AI does not stem from the notion that "robot doctors" (Vallès-Peris et al., 2021) will replace human healthcare providers, but from the classic definition of AI, which encompasses a range of techniques that allow machines to perform tasks in a manner deemed intelligent if carried out by humans.

4. Patient-Centered Care

Smart hospitals prioritize patient-centered care by providing personalized treatment plans, remote monitoring, and patient engagement tools. This method increases patient satisfaction through allowing individuals the power to actively participate in their treatment.

5. Cybersecurity and Data Privacy

Smart hospitals prioritize cybersecurity and data privacy to safeguard confidential medical information and ensure compliance with relevant regulations. Advanced security measures, such as encryption, access controls, and intrusion detection systems, are implemented to safeguard data.

6. Sustainable and Eco-Friendly Practices

Smart hospitals adopt sustainable and eco-friendly practices, such as energy-efficient technologies, waste management systems, and renewable energy sources, to reduce their environmental impact and promote sustainability (Lapão & Viegas, 2024b)

By integrating these essential features, smart hospitals aim to deliver high-quality, cost-effective, patient-centered care while optimizing operational efficiency and promoting innovation in the healthcare sector.

INTELLIGENT HOSPITALS

An intelligent hospital harnesses the application of AI to become more data-driven, adaptable, and clinically intelligent and is a more sophisticated and all-encompassing concept of delivery of healthcare in the future. An intelligent hospital is a healthcare facility that employs advanced technologies and data-driven systems to enhance patient care, streamline operations, and support clinical decision-making. The essential features of an intelligent hospital include:

1. Advanced Decision Support Systems

Intelligent hospitals help medical personnel diagnose and treat patients by using advanced clinical decision support systems that use machine learning and artificial intelligence. Large volumes of data can be analyzed by these systems to produce insights and recommendations that increase the precision of clinical judgments.

2. Real-Time Monitoring and Triage

These hospitals implement systems for real-time patient monitoring and triage, often using wearable biosensors and other technologies to continuously assess vital signs and prioritize patient care based on urgency. This capability enhances the efficiency of emergency departments and improves patient outcomes.

3. Integrated Health Information Systems

Integrated health information systems, found in intelligent hospitals, combine patient data from multiple sources, such as laboratory systems, imaging services, and electronic health records (EHRs). This integration facilitates seamless access to patient information, promoting coordinated care and reducing errors.

4. Data Analytics and Predictive Modeling

By using data analytics, efficient hospitals can forecast patient requirements and results, allocate resources optimally, and spot patterns in patient care. Predictive modeling helps in managing patient flow and anticipating potential health crises, such as surges in demand during pandemics. The role of healthcare data analytics and predictive modeling in improving outcomes such as resource allocation, disease forecasting, and identifying high-risk populations is critically examined. The findings (Nwoke, 2024) reveal that predictive modeling enhances resource optimization, forecasts disease prevalence accurately, and identifies vulnerable populations effectively. This research contributes to theory, informs policymakers on data infrastructure investment, and provides actionable strategies for healthcare organizations.

5. Patient Engagement Tools

By facilitating improved communication between patients and healthcare providers via digital platforms, these hospitals aim to increase patient involvement. Patients are given the ability to actively participate in their healthcare management through resources including mobile applications, telehealth services, and patient portals. It emphasizes the importance of data analysis in improving patient diagnosis (Mehta, 2022), even when doctors are unavailable. This functionality is vital in emergencies, enabling healthcare providers to deliver more efficient and effective patient care.

By incorporating these features, intelligent hospitals aim to provide high-quality, efficient, and personalized healthcare services, ultimately improving patient outcomes and operational efficiency.

The concepts of "smart hospitals" and "intelligent hospitals" both revolve around leveraging advanced technologies to optimize healthcare delivery, yet they emphasize distinct aspects of innovation. Smart hospitals focus on the integration of AI, IoT, and data-driven systems to streamline operations, improve patient outcomes, and reduce costs. For instance, Houston Methodist's "Smart Hospital DNA" framework exemplifies this approach by utilizing predictive AI, ambient intelligence, and robotics for enhanced care delivery (Sukin et al., 2024). Similarly, the integration of AI in smart hospitals, as shown in studies from New York and Los Angeles, improves patient outcomes by reducing mortality, complications, and readmissions (Nayak, 2024). On the other hand, intelligent hospitals extend this framework by embedding deep-learning algorithms and IoT to create self-adaptive healthcare environments. For example, (Zhang et al., 2023) IoT systems not only enhance data acquisition efficiency but also optimize medical processes to resolve challenges in accessing care. Furthermore, the synergy (Ahmad, 2024) between IoT and AI, emphasizing predictive analytics and resource optimization as critical enablers for intelligent systems. Both paradigms converge in their goal (Jovy-Klein et al., 2024), where hospitals combine AI, sustainability, and human-centered care models. While smart hospitals primarily address operational efficiency, intelligent hospitals prioritize adaptability and decision-making automation. Together, they represent complementary frameworks for modern healthcare transformation, underpinned by shared challenges such as data privacy, infrastructure investment, and workforce training.

CONTRIBUTIONS OF DEVELOPING TECHNOLOGIES IN HEALTHCARE

Real-Time Location Systems (RTLS)

Smart hospitals utilize real-time location systems (RTLS) based on technologies like Bluetooth and RFID to track the location of personnel, patients, and equipment within the hospital facility. These location-based services provide enhanced workflow efficiency (Kataria et al., 2024) where, Patients can be promptly connected to the right healthcare provider by using real-time staff location information. Additionally, finding equipment is simple, which cuts down on search time and maximizes asset usage and by providing individualized treatments, their location data can enhance the general patient experience. RTLS keeps a check on patients who wander, particularly those who suffer from cognitive impairments. It can also be utilized to monitor high-value asset locations and guarantee worker safety promoting improved privacy and safety for patients and personnels. Hospitals can analyze location data to identify bottlenecks, optimize workflows, and decide on staffing levels and the location of equipment after considering all available information. By leveraging Bluetooth and RFID technologies, smart hospitals can create a more efficient, safe, and patient-centric environment through real-time location-tracking solutions (Meka et al., 2024).

RTLS plays a crucial role in infection control by tracing contact points (Kim & Park, 2024) during outbreaks, helping to prevent disease spread. For hospital staff, RTLS ensures safety through wearable devices, allowing them to call for help during emergencies, as shown in a study at the Mayo Clinic (Jones et al., 2023). However, introducing RTLS isn't without its challenges (Waldie et al., 2023) the need to involve healthcare workers in designing and implementing these systems. Without proper training and communication, the benefits of RTLS can be lost. Despite hurdles like privacy concerns and infrastructure costs, RTLS is paving the way for smarter, safer, and more responsive healthcare environments, benefiting everyone involved.

Integration of the Internet of Things (IoT)

The integration of the Internet of Things (IoT) in healthcare involves the use of connected devices and sensors to continuously monitor patient health data and transmit it to hospital systems for evaluation and management. This integration offers numerous benefits and functionalities. IoT devices(J. C. et al., 2024), such as wearables and remote sensors, enable real-time tracking of vital signs and health metrics, including heart rate, blood pressure, and glucose levels. This continuous health monitoring allows for timely interventions and proactive management of patient health conditions. The health data collected by IoT devices is transmitted to hospital systems, such as electronic health records (EHRs), where it can be analyzed by healthcare professionals. This seamless data flow enhances the ability to make informed clinical decisions and improves care coordination. Remote Patient Monitoring is facilitated through use of IoT, allowing healthcare providers to track patients' health from their homes. This capability is particularly beneficial for managing chronic conditions and reducing hospital admissions, as it enables timely responses to changes in a patient's health status.

Integrating IoT data with clinical decision support systems, healthcare providers can access comprehensive patient information, leading to better-informed decisions. This integration helps in identifying potential health risks and implementing appropriate treatment plans promptly. By giving patients health-related insights, IoT devices can empower patients (Peh, 2024). Through improved communication and health metrics monitoring, patients and healthcare providers can work together to provide better treatment. Reducing hospital visits is one way that the use of IoT in healthcare can lower costs. optimizing resource allocation, and improving operational efficiency. Timely interventions facilitated by real-time data can prevent complications and reduce the need for extensive treatments.

By continuously monitoring patient data, healthcare providers can quickly identify any abnormalities or deterioration in health and intervene promptly, potentially preventing complications or hospitalizations. This capability (El-Gayar et al., 2024) leads to improved patient outcomes, as real-time monitoring and early intervention facilitated by wearables and IoT devices ensure that patients receive timely and appropriate care. Additionally, wearable gadgets enhance patient engagement by enabling patients to actively participate in their healthcare, providing real-time feedback, and improving communication with their healthcare professionals. However, some challenges need to be addressed, such as data security and privacy concerns, device reliability, and user acceptance. Healthcare organizations must ensure that these technologies are implemented in a secure and user-friendly manner to maximize their potential benefits.

Mobile Health Services (mHealth)

Mobile health services, often referred to as mHealth, leverage technology such as wearables, tablets, and smartphones to provide doctors and patients with instant access to medical data and options for remote care. Mobile health services provide quick access to Health Information. Heart rate, blood pressure, glucose levels, and other health parameters can be continually tracked by wearable devices. This data is communicated in real-time to healthcare professionals in order that they can assess and treat patients as soon as needed. Data Integration is done through mobile health services and electronic health records (EHRs), medical professionals can obtain complete patient records while they're on the road. This integration improves care coordination and facilitates well-informed decision-making. Mobile health services facilitate telemedicine capabilities and remote care, allowing patients to consult with healthcare providers via video calls or messaging. This approach is particularly useful for patients in remote areas or those with mobility issues, ensuring they receive timely care without the need to travel to a facility.

Patient Empowerment is one benefit of mHealth (Neravetla et al., 2024). Patients can actively engage in their healthcare by using mobile applications to monitor their health, schedule appointments, and communicate with their healthcare teams. This empowerment leads to increased adherence to treatment plans and better health outcomes. Reduced hospital admissions are possible by enabling continuous monitoring and early interventions, mobile health services might assist avert issues that might otherwise lead to hospital admissions. Cost-effectiveness is a key success of mHealth as it can reduce healthcare expenses by eliminating the need for in-person visits and optimizing resource allocation within healthcare systems. There is convenience in accessing health information and care options through mobile devices improves the overall patient experience, fostering a more collaborative relationship between patients and providers. These services significantly enhance the accessibility and quality of healthcare by providing instant access to medical data and facilitating remote care through advanced technology.

In countries like Pakistan (Arshad Nawaz Malik et al., 2024) and Zambia (Halwiindi et al., 2022) Mobile health (mHealth) services have emerged as transformative tools in healthcare delivery, where access to healthcare is often constrained by geographic and resource limitations. In Pakistan, mHealth applications have been instrumental in improving stroke rehabilitation through wearable devices, gamified therapies, and tele-rehabilitation services, bridging the gap between patients, caregivers, and healthcare providers. Similarly, in Zambia (Halwiindi et al., 2022), mHealth initiatives have played a critical role in raising awareness about cervical cancer and increasing screening rates. For instance, mass text messaging campaigns have significantly encouraged first-time and follow-up screenings by educating women about the importance of early detection. Despite challenges like delivery rates and high transmission costs, these interventions have demonstrated the potential of mobile technology to empower individuals and improve health outcomes in underserved communities Together, these examples highlight how mHealth can be a game-changer in countries with resource-constrained health systems, improving access, awareness, and the overall quality of care for vulnerable populations.

Artificial Intelligence (AI)

Artificial intelligence (AI)-)-enabled services in healthcare are transforming the way conditions are diagnosed, treatments are planned, and outcomes are forecasted. Here are the key aspects of how AI is utilized in these areas:

1. Diagnosis of Conditions
    a. Multi-Modal Data Integration: AI technologies, including machine learning and deep learning, are capable of analyzing diverse medical data types—such as imaging, genetic information, and physiological signals—to provide comprehensive diagnostic insights. This multi-modal approach enhances the accuracy of disease diagnosis, particularly for complex conditions like Alzheimer's disease, breast cancer, and heart disease.
    b. Image Recognition: AI applications, particularly those using Convolutional Neural Networks (CNNs), have shown significant promise in medical image analysis. For instance, AI can effectively diagnose breast cancer through image recognition systems that analyze mammograms with high accuracy, achieving performancc metrics such as 0.88 in detection rates.
2. Treatment Planning
    a. Clinical Decision Support Systems (CDSS): AI-powered CDSS can process massive volumes of patient data and produce useful insights for healthcare providers. These systems help with treatment decisions by examining patient-specific criteria and recommending the best treatment options, hence improving care personalization.
    b. Predictive Analytics: AI can anticipate treatment outcomes using past data and patient attributes. By examining previous cases, AI models can anticipate how patients will react to specific therapies, allowing healthcare providers to modify interventions accordingly.
3. Forecasting Results
    a. Outcome Prediction Models: Artificial intelligence algorithms can identify trends and patterns in patient data to forecast future health outcomes. This skill is critical for proactive healthcare management, allowing doctors to intervene early and modify treatment programs as needed.

b. Comparative Effectiveness Research: AI facilitates the evaluation of AI-assisted care against conventional methods through well-designed studies. This research helps confirm the benefits of AI in clinical settings, guiding healthcare providers in adopting AI technologies based on solid evidence of their effectiveness.

Multi-modal AI systems, which combine data such as imaging, genetic profiles, and physiological signals, have shown significant potential in diagnosing complex conditions. For instance (Shilaskar, 2024) integrating EEG, MRI, and retinal scans enhances early detection of neurological disorders. The use of AI with advanced (Yuan et al., 2024) 7T MRI for brain tumor detection, while (Yang & Yang, 2024) achieved 91% accuracy in diagnosing skin conditions using patient narratives and images. These advancements underline AI's capability to deliver precise and timely healthcare solutions.

AI-enabled services are transforming healthcare by increasing diagnosis accuracy, improving treatment planning, and delivering trustworthy patient outcome estimates. These innovations not only help healthcare professionals make better judgments, but they also lead to more personalized and effective patient care. Robotic and extended reality (XR) services are increasingly being used in healthcare to help medical practitioners improve accuracy, efficacy, and safety in a variety of clinical situations.

Clinical Decision Support Systems (CDSS)

Workflow optimization and efficient resource management in healthcare settings are greatly aided by the integration of clinical decision support systems (CDSS), electronic health records (EHR), and linked medical devices. Integration makes these goals possible by providing improved Quality and Safety of Patient Care. CDSS can boost patient safety and quality of treatment by giving doctors personalized, evidence-based suggestions in real time for each patient. By analyzing large datasets and detecting early warning signs of health issues, CDSS can help prevent or mitigate serious medical events. There is enhanced diagnostic accuracy and treatment effectiveness, by providing clinicians with personalized therapy recommendations based on patient data. CDSS can minimize the probability of unfavorable occurrences and find the best treatment strategies by utilizing deep learning algorithms and predictive analytics. A significant reduction in the cognitive load is witnessed among healthcare providers. CDSS can alleviate the cognitive burden on healthcare providers by providing evidence-based advice and assisting them in reaching well-informed judgments about patient care. In complex or high-risk settings, this can result in more effective and efficient care delivery. However, the adoption and long-term use of CDSS remain limited due to various challenges, such as data quality issues, interoperability barriers, and stakeholder resistance to change. Accessing the full potential of CDSS in enhancing healthcare outcomes requires addressing these issues through focused interventions and stakeholder involvement.

Artificial Intelligence (AI) is increasingly utilized in clinical decision support systems (CDSS) to provide individualized therapy recommendations and enhance patient care. By analyzing data from wearables over time, AI-powered analytics can detect early warning signs of health issues, enabling healthcare providers to take proactive steps to prevent or mitigate serious medical events. Key features of AI in clinical decision support include personalized recommendations, where AI-CDSS leverages algorithms to analyze patient data, including information collected from wearable devices, to offer tailored treatment suggestions based on individual health metrics and historical data. Predictive analytics is another crucial aspect, as these systems identify potential health risks before they escalate by continuously monitoring vital signs and other health parameters, allowing for timely interventions. Real-time monitoring, facilitated by the integration of wearables with AI, enhances the ability of healthcare professionals to monitor patients remotely and respond quickly to changes in their condition. AI systems also benefit from continuous learning, improving over time through machine learning and refining their recommendations based on new data and outcomes. This helps adapt to the evolving needs of patients and healthcare environments. Enhanced decision-making is another significant advantage, as AI-driven CDSS provides evidence-based insights, reducing the cognitive load on healthcare providers and supporting them in making informed choices regarding patient care.

However, challenges such as data privacy, ethical considerations, and the need for rigorous validation of AI models must be addressed. Ensuring that AI systems are transparent and explainable is crucial for building trust among healthcare providers and patients alike. In summary, the use of AI in clinical decision support systems, particularly in conjunction with wearable technology, offers a promising avenue for improving patient outcomes through personalized therapy recommendations and proactive health monitoring. By harnessing the power of AI, healthcare providers can enhance their ability to intervene early and effectively, ultimately leading to better health management and reduced risk of serious medical events.

Robotic Services

Robots are playing an increasingly important role in the healthcare sector by assisting healthcare workers and enhancing patient care in various ways. Studies were conducted to assess the success of inclusion of robotics in the healthcare industry which demonstrated a 25% reduction in operating expenses and a 30% increase in production efficiency. The method (Shalini et al., 2024) achieved a precision rate of approximately 99% in the healthcare industry, surpassing the current systems' average accuracy of 93% by a significant margin.

These robots perform common logistical duties such as delivering prescriptions, supplies, and linens throughout hospitals, operating autonomously and notifying staff when the task is completed, thereby improving clinical processes and lowering the physical demands on human workers. Medication Dispensing Robots: Automated medication dispensing systems enhance safety and accuracy in medication administration. By reducing human error, these robots ensure that patients receive the correct dosages at the right times. Autonomous mobile robots can also quickly sterilize and disinfect hospital rooms, lowering hospital-acquired infections and allowing staff to focus on patient care. Surgical robots, like the da Vinci Surgical System, provide surgeons with enhanced precision, control, and visualization during procedures, enabling less invasive surgery and faster patient recovery times. Robotic-assisted surgery allows for minimally invasive procedures with greater precision. Surgeons can perform complex operations using robotic systems that provide enhanced dexterity and visualization, leading to reduced recovery times and lower risk of complications.

Additionally, service robots assist patients with limited mobility, helping bariatric patients move and providing mobility aids to the elderly or disabled, which helps maintain patient independence and reduces strain on healthcare workers. Telepresence robots allow healthcare workers to remotely interact with and monitor patients, reducing pathogen exposure, especially during isolation situations like the COVID-19 pandemic. Therapeutic robots, such as the PARO therapeutic robot, offer companionship and emotional support to patients with dementia or mental health conditions, helping to reduce loneliness and stress. Rehabilitation Robots assist patient in rehabilitation by providing support and guidance during physical therapy. They help patients regain mobility and strength through tailored exercises, ensuring adherence to rehabilitation protocols.

Robots are transforming healthcare by automating repetitive tasks, assisting with complex procedures, and providing physical and emotional support to both patients and staff. As technology continues to advance, the role of robotics in healthcare is expected to grow significantly.

Extended Reality Services

Extended Reality (XR) technologies, encompassing Virtual Reality (VR), Augmented Reality (AR), and Mixed Reality (MR), are increasingly being integrated into various aspects of healthcare (Garg et al., 2024), revolutionizing education, surgical practices, patient care, and therapeutic interventions. XR technologies are enhancing medical education by providing immersive learning experiences, allowing medical and nursing students to engage in realistic simulations that enable them to visualize anatomical structures and practice clinical skills without the risks associated with real-life procedures. For instance, VR simulations can depict medical emergencies, enabling students to practice diagnosis and treatment in a controlled environment. In surgical settings, XR facilitates preoperative planning and intraoperative navigation, allowing surgeons to visualize patient-specific anatomical models and overlay virtual images onto the surgical field, which improves precision during procedures, shortens operating times, and enhances surgeon confidence. XR tools are also beneficial for patient education, as they allow healthcare providers to explain complex medical procedures and conditions in an engaging manner, enabling patients to interact with 3D models of their anatomy or visualize the effects of treatments, thus enhancing their understanding and involvement in their healthcare.

Additionally, XR (Greener, 2024) is being explored for therapeutic uses, particularly in mental health, including VR applications for pain management and anxiety reduction. Immersive environments can distract patients during painful procedures or help manage conditions such as phobias and PTSD, with studies indicating that VR can effectively reduce anxiety and improve patient experiences in various healthcare settings. The COVID-19 pandemic accelerated the adoption of XR technologies for remote healthcare delivery, facilitating remote consultations and training, allowing healthcare professionals to engage with patients and students from multiple locations while maintaining safety protocols. The potential market for XR (*Virtual Reality In Healthcare Market*, 2023) in healthcare is projected to grow significantly, with estimates suggesting it could reach $19.6 billion by 2030, driven by ongoing research and the development of new XR applications across various medical specialties, including primary care and mental health.

Augmented Reality (Ma, 2023) (AR) applications provide surgeons with real-time overlays of patient data and anatomical structures during procedures. This enhanced visualization aids in surgical planning and execution, improving accuracy and outcomes. Virtual Reality (VR) can be used to train healthcare providers by allowing them to practice procedures in a simulated environment that is safe for patients. It has additionally been employed in patient education to help patients comprehend their diseases and treatments through immersive experiences.

The integration of robotic and extended reality services in healthcare (Salvetti et al., 2023)significantly enhances the abilities of medical professionals, leading to improved accuracy, effectiveness, and safety in patient care. There is significant increase in accuracy. Both robotic and Virtual services improve the precision of medical treatments, resulting in better patient outcomes and fewer complications. Efficiency is enhanced as automation and increased visualization simplify workflows, allowing healthcare workers to concentrate on patient care rather than administrative responsibilities. Safety is enhanced by reducing human error and delivering real-time data, these technologies help to create safer healthcare environments for both patients and professionals. XR technologies are transforming healthcare by enhancing educational outcomes, improving surgical precision, facilitating patient engagement, and offering innovative therapeutic solutions. As the field continues to evolve, further integration of XR into healthcare practices is expected, promising substantial improvements in patient care and medical training.

Simulation Modeling

Simulation modeling is an effective approach for optimizing resource allocation in healthcare supply chains before actual deployment. By simulating different scenarios (Demir et al., 2024), organizations can evaluate the effects of various resource allocation schemes and determine the ideal staffing levels, bed capacity, inventory stocking, and other operational considerations to enhance efficiency. Scenario Testing allows healthcare organizations to test multiple scenarios without disrupting actual operations. This allows to experiment with various resource allocation strategies and evaluate their effects on patient flow, staff usage, and inventory levels and to experiment with various resource allocation strategies and evaluate their effects on patient flow, staff usage, and inventory levels.

Bottleneck Identification in the supply chain process is feasible while simulation model is adopted as the organizations can identify potential bottlenecks and pinpoint areas where resources are underutilized or overloaded. This information aids in making informed resource allocation decisions that improve overall efficiency. It in turn leads to effective capacity planning. Simulation modeling assists in determining the optimal bed capacity, staffing levels, and equipment requirements based on projected patient volumes and demand patterns. This ensures that resources are aligned with anticipated needs, minimizing the risk of overcrowding or underutilization and inventory optimization. Simulation can assist healthcare businesses in optimizing their inventory levels by studying demand patterns, lead times, and storage limits. This reduces waste, improves stock management, and aligns supply and demand. By detecting and addressing inefficiencies through simulation, healthcare businesses can save money by optimizing resource use, eliminating waste, and enhancing overall supply chain efficiency.

While simulation (De Oliveira Almeida & Hinton, 2024) modeling offers significant benefits, its implementation requires careful consideration of factors such as data availability, model complexity, and stakeholder engagement. Healthcare organizations must ensure that simulation models accurately reflect real-world conditions and that the insights generated are effectively communicated to decision-makers for implementation. Simulation modeling is a valuable tool for healthcare supply chain optimization, enabling organizations to test resource allocation strategies, identify bottlenecks, plan capacity, optimize inventory, and achieve cost savings before actual deployment. By leveraging simulation, healthcare organizations can enhance efficiency, improve patient outcomes, and ensure the optimal use of resources.

Digital Twin

Digital twin integration is a powerful tool in healthcare for modeling and improving care plans, enhancing accessibility, and facilitating remote care delivery and telehealth. By creating virtual replicas of physical entities, digital twins enable healthcare organizations to simulate scenarios and optimize procedures such as supply chain management, staff scheduling, and bed management. The key benefits of digital twin integration in healthcare include the development of personalized care plans using real-time patient data from various sources, including wearable devices, to tailor treatment plans to individual requirements and preferences. Integrating digital twins with telehealth technologies allows healthcare providers to deliver care remotely, improving accessibility and convenience for patients. Digital twins (Singh, 2024) enable hospital managers to simulate different scenarios, such as changes in patient volume or resource allocation, to optimize procedures and identify potential bottlenecks. They also help in supply chain optimization by simulating processes to maintain optimal inventory levels, reduce waste, and ensure the availability of necessary supplies. In staff scheduling, digital twins analyze historical data and predict future staffing needs, allowing healthcare organizations to create efficient schedules that match demand and minimize overtime costs. For bed management, digital twins can simulate patient flow and identify opportunities to optimize bed utilization, reducing wait times and improving patient satisfaction. However, challenges such as data privacy, security, and interoperability must be addressed to fully leverage digital twin integration. Healthcare organizations must ensure that digital twin systems comply with data protection regulations and maintain the confidentiality of patient information. In conclusion, digital twin integration is a transformative technology that can significantly improve care delivery, optimize operations, and reduce costs in healthcare settings. By leveraging the power of simulation and data analytics, digital twins enable healthcare organizations to make informed decisions and deliver high-quality, personalized care to patients.

SHIFT IN HOSPITAL DELIVERY MODELS

The traditional healthcare delivery model, which is based on in-person visits and hospital-based care, is shifting toward more distributed and accessible approaches. This includes a greater use of telehealth, home-based treatment, and community health programs. These changes are aided by technological improvements and changing patient preferences, which promote a shift to more flexible and accessible healthcare delivery. Several factors contribute to the transition towards greater integration of technology, patient-centric care, and regulatory compliance in healthcare.

1. Patient Care and Operational Efficiency

The integration of smart technologies improves the quality of patient care by enabling more efficient and preventive healthcare. Technologies such as remote monitoring and telehealth allow for timely interventions, which improve patient outcomes and satisfaction. Smart hospitals streamline workflows and optimize resource management through automation and data analytics. This leads to reduced wait times, better staff allocation, and overall improved operational performance, making healthcare delivery more effective. Mobile health applications and wearables, empower patients to take an active role in their healthcare. This engagement leads to better adherence to treatment plans and improved health outcomes. Linked medical devices facilitate continuous patient monitoring, allowing for real-time adjustments to care plans based on patient conditions.

2. Data-driven decision-making and Technological Advancements

The use of advanced analytics and artificial intelligence in smart hospitals allows healthcare providers to make informed decisions based on real-time data. This capability enhances clinical decision support, leading to better treatment plans and outcomes. The rapid development and availability of IoT devices, AI, and other smart technologies are driving hospitals to adopt these innovations. As technology becomes more accessible and affordable, healthcare facilities are more inclined to integrate smart solutions into their operations.

3. Optimization and Cost Reduction

By improving operational efficiency and reducing unnecessary hospital admissions through proactive care, smart hospital models can lead to significant cost savings for healthcare systems. This financial incentive drives the adoption of smart technologies. Optimized Resource Allocation in healthcare setups can spot trends in patient flow and resource usage by examining data from EHRs and connected devices. By maximizing workforce numbers and equipment availability, this data helps to make sure that resources are deployed where they are most required.

In the subsequent section, a comprehensive overview of the shift in hospital models are outlined.

Model I - Automation in Hospital Management

Hospital automation is a transformative approach that leverages technology to streamline operations, enhance patient care, and improve overall efficiency within healthcare settings. This integration of technology encompasses a wide range of functions, from electronic health record (EHR) management to billing and inventory control, aiming to reduce manual workloads, minimize errors, and enhance the quality of patient care. Key applications of hospital automation include administrative efficiency, where automated systems expedite processes such as patient admissions, billing, and insurance claims, leading to reduced waiting times and improved patient satisfaction. In clinical workflows, automation facilitates tasks like medication administration and vital signs monitoring, thereby reducing the burden on nursing staff and minimizing the risk of human error. Inventory and supply chain management are also enhanced through automation, as systems track medical supplies and medications to maintain optimal stock levels, reduce waste, and prevent shortages. Patient engagement and monitoring benefit from technologies that allow patients to control their environment through voice commands or mobile applications, while real-time monitoring systems alert healthcare providers to changes in patient conditions, enabling timely interventions.

Robotic Process Automation (RPA) is being increasingly adopted in healthcare to automate repetitive tasks such as appointment scheduling, claims processing, and invoice management. By eliminating mundane tasks, RPA reduces the workload on administrative staff, allowing them to focus on more complex tasks that require human interaction.

Data management and analytics are significantly improved through automation, with systems aggregating and analyzing patient data to inform clinical decisions and optimize treatment plans. The benefits of hospital automation include increased efficiency, improved accuracy, enhanced patient experience, and cost reduction, as automation allows healthcare professionals to focus on patient care, minimizes human errors, streamlines processes, and optimizes resource use. As technology continues to evolve, the potential for further automation in hospitals will likely expand, leading to even greater improvements in healthcare delivery. Automating hospital management duties and optimizing procedures in healthcare administration is transforming the way hospitals operate. This shift reduces errors, streamlines processes, and allows medical professionals to focus more on patient care.

ILLUSTRATIVE CASE OF MAYO CLINIC – AUTOMATION AND ROBOTICS

The **Mayo Clinic** (Allison, 2024) in the United States is a leader in integrating automation into hospital operations, improving both efficiency and patient care. The hospital has incorporated robotic systems and automated workflows in various departments. For instance, in its surgical units, robotic-assisted surgeries allow for more precise procedures with quicker recovery times. Automated pharmacy systems ensure the accurate dispensing of medications, reducing human error and improving patient safety. Additionally, Mayo Clinic uses automated patient scheduling and electronic health records (EHR) management, streamlining administrative tasks and minimizing delays. The clinic's use of AI-driven diagnostic tools also speeds up decision-making, allowing for faster diagnosis and treatment plans. By automating routine processes, Mayo Clinic has enhanced operational efficiency, reduced costs, and freed up healthcare professionals to focus more on patient interaction. This commitment to automation is helping the clinic maintain high-quality care while optimizing its resources.

Model II - Artificial Intelligence (AI) and Adopting Smart Devices

AI technologies are revolutionizing healthcare management by automating administrative processes and enhancing decision-making. AI-powered platforms can optimize appointment bookings, monitor patient conditions, and provide virtual assistance, thereby reducing administrative burdens, and enhancing the overall efficiency of healthcare services. Equipping healthcare staff with smart devices can significantly improve productivity and accelerate workflows, leading to better patient care outcomes. Smart devices, such as smartphones and tablets, enable instant communication and collaboration among healthcare teams. Secure messaging apps allow staff to quickly share updates, coordinate care plans, and consult with specialists, reducing delays and improving care continuity. Real-time access to information related to patients. Clinicians can use smart devices to access electronic health records (EHRs) and view patient information in real time, including at the point of care. This rapid access to detailed data enables speedier decision-making and decreases the need for manual data entry, hence streamlining workflows. Smart devices provide healthcare workers with mobility and flexibility, allowing them to perform tasks and access information from anywhere in the hospital. This mobility enables staff to respond quickly to patient needs, conduct bedside rounds, and provide timely updates to families. Smart devices automate various administrative tasks such as appointment scheduling, inventory management and billing which streamlines workflows and reduces errors, eliminating manual, repetitive processes, freeing up staff time for direct patient care. This leads to increase in staff satisfaction and retention. Giving healthcare professionals current, user-friendly smart devices can boost job satisfaction by eliminating aggravation with antiquated technology and streamlining daily chores. This increased satisfaction can help to improve staff retention and engagement, which are critical for providing high-quality patient care. Equipping healthcare staff with smart devices, hospitals can foster better communication, access to data, mobility, and workflow optimization. These improvements ultimately lead to increased productivity, enhanced teamwork, and improved patient outcomes.

CASE STUDY OF CLEVELAND CLINIC

AI Powered Diagnostics

A great example of the shift to a smarter, more intelligent healthcare model is the **Cleveland Clinic** in the United States mentioned in Forbes (Bean, 2024). Traditionally, hospitals operated with in-person consultations, paper-based patient records, and basic diagnostic tools. However, Cleveland Clinic has embraced cutting-edge technologies like AI-powered diagnostics, remote patient monitoring, and robotic systems to transform its approach to patient care. With the help of Internet of Things (IoT) devices, electronic health records (EHR), and advanced data analytics, they can now make quicker, more accurate decisions in real-time. AI applications in radiology and predictive analytics are helping to identify health risks early, leading to fewer readmissions and more personalized treatment plans. Virtual consultations and remote monitoring have also made healthcare more accessible, ensuring patients can receive care from the comfort of their homes. This intelligent model not only enhances patient care but also streamlines operations, cutting costs and improving overall outcomes for both patients and providers.

Model III - Predictive Analytics

Predictive analytics is transforming hospital management by enabling data-driven decision-making and optimizing operations. Patient data can be analyzed from electronic health records, insurance claims, and other sources, predictive models can identify high-risk patients and predict the likelihood of adverse outcomes such as hospital readmissions. This allows hospitals to proactively intervene and provide targeted care to prevent complications. Additionally, predictive analytics can forecast patient volume, length of stay, and resource needs, helping hospitals efficiently allocate staff, beds, and supplies, thereby improving operational efficiency and reducing costs associated with over or understaffing. By analyzing data on patient demographics, past appointment attendance, and other factors, predictive models can also identify patients likely to miss appointments, enabling hospitals to take proactive measures like sending reminders to reduce no-shows and improve access to care. Furthermore, predictive analytics can enhance cybersecurity by monitoring hospital transactions and assigning risk scores to detect potential cyberattacks like ransomware before they occur, helping hospitals prevent data breaches and avoid costly downtime. It also plays a crucial role in improving population health by analyzing community health data to identify emerging health trends and high-risk populations, allowing hospitals to develop targeted prevention programs and allocate resources to address the most pressing population health needs. While predictive analytics offers significant benefits, hospitals face challenges in fully leveraging its potential, including lack of data integration, limited analytical expertise, and resistance to change. However, as the technology continues to advance and more hospitals adopt predictive analytics, it will play an increasingly critical role in optimizing hospital operations and improving patient outcomes.

CASE STUDY OF MOUNT SINAI HEALTH SYSTEM

The **Mount Sinai Health System** in New York has embraced predictive analytics to transform patient care and enhance hospital operations. By harnessing the power of data, the hospital uses machine learning algorithms to predict patient outcomes, such as the risk of readmission, sepsis, and other serious complications. With real-time data from patient records, lab results, and medical histories, these predictive tools help doctors spot high-risk patients early, allowing them to take action before problems escalate. For instance, the hospital's predictive system has successfully lowered readmission rates by identifying patients who are at greater risk, giving healthcare teams the opportunity to provide proactive care. It also helps spot signs of deterioration, like the onset of sepsis, so doctors can intervene quickly, preventing life-threatening situations. This innovative approach not only keeps patients safer but also makes the hospital more efficient, reducing costs and ensuring that resources are used where they're needed most. Mount Sinai's success story shows how data can be used to create a more responsive, patient-centered healthcare environment.

Model IV - Scalable Blockchain Technology

Implementing scalable blockchain technology in healthcare systems significantly enhances data security, privacy (Azaria et al., 2016), and interoperability within electronic health records (EHRs). Blockchain's decentralized and immutable nature ensures secure and transparent data exchanges, addressing key challenges in interoperability while safeguarding sensitive patient information. Advanced encryption techniques, such as the Advanced Encryption Standard (AES) and Zero-Knowledge Proof Protocol (ZKPP), bolster these security measures, ensuring compliance with regulatory standards and minimizing risks of data breaches. For instance, the Security Protocol and Data Model (SPDM) provides a standardized framework for securing communications and enabling device attestation, maintaining data integrity across platforms. A zero-trust security approach further enhances protection by verifying all access requests, regardless of their origin, effectively minimizing the risk of unauthorized access. Similarly, integrating AI-enabled frameworks in healthcare facilitates (Radanovic & Likic, 2018) automated management transactions while complying with regulations, thereby improving data security and operational efficiency. These frameworks also streamline communication between healthcare providers and patients through chatbots and virtual assistants, enhancing appointment scheduling and reducing patient wait times. Automation enables healthcare professionals to shift their focus from administrative tasks to direct patient care, improving both patient outcomes and job satisfaction among healthcare workers.

CASE STUDY OF ESTONIA - SCALABLE BLOCKCHAIN TECHNOLOGY IN HEALTHCARE

Starting in 2011, the Estonian government partnered with Guard time to secure over a million citizens' health records using blockchain-based Keyless Signature Infrastructure (El-Gayar et al., 2024). This initiative enables seamless data sharing while maintaining privacy and accountability, demonstrating how blockchain can bridge interoperability gaps in electronic health records. By automating administrative tasks, including claims processing and patient management, healthcare professionals can focus more on patient care, improving outcomes and efficiency. Estonia's success highlights the transformative potential of blockchain when integrated with national e-health strategies to address global challenges like rising healthcare costs and aging populations. The system's success highlights the potential of blockchain in achieving scalable, secure, and efficient healthcare solutions globally.

Model V - Lean Hospital Management

Lean hospital management emphasizes five core principles: value creation, waste reduction, continuous improvement, respect for people, and visual management. Value creation ensures all processes are aligned to deliver what patients perceive as valuable. The waste reduction principle identifies and addresses eight types of waste in healthcare—defects, waiting, transportation, overproduction, over-processing, inventory, motion, and human potential. Through continuous improvement often using Kaizen (Bhamu & Singh Sangwan, 2014), Lean encourages staff at all levels to identify inefficiencies and suggest solutions. Respect for people fosters a culture where everyone's insights are valued, and visual management uses visual tools to identify problems and track progress, making communication about improvement opportunities clear. On the other hand, Intelligent Asset Management integrates clinical and medical data across various systems, optimizing resource allocation and operational efficiency. The system starts with assessing the quality of clinical data to ensure accurate decision-making. Key technologies like machine learning, IoT sensors, and analytics platforms enhance asset visibility and utilization. Machine learning models can predict asset needs, while IoT sensors provide real-time tracking of medical equipment, helping to minimize downtime and waste. When combined, Lean Thinking and Intelligent Asset Management work in harmony to reduce waste, improve processes, and enhance patient care. Lean principles identify areas where assets may be underused or inefficient, while intelligent asset management ensures real-time monitoring and data-driven decisions. This synergy not only streamlines hospital operations but also leads to cost savings and improved patient outcomes, creating a more efficient, responsive healthcare environment.

CASE STUDY ON VIRGINIA MASON INSTITUTE'S IMPACT

Lean Hospital Management

Lean management has transformed healthcare by fostering patient-centered systems that enhance safety, efficiency, and satisfaction. At the University of Maryland St. Joseph Medical Center (UM SJMC), collaboration with Virginia Mason Institute led to a unified management system that halved annual harm incidents within three years, surpassed patient experience targets, and reduced employee injuries. These achievements earned UM SJMC accolades, including a five-star CMS rating and recognition as Maryland's top community hospital. Similarly, WakeMed Health and Hospitals optimized patient flow in primary care clinics by adopting Lean tools like shared vision alignment and 5S agreements. These efforts improved scheduling, accommodated walk-ins, and ensured staff completed work on time. Virginia Mason's own surgical teams used root cause analysis to streamline instrument setup, reducing prep time and errors while enabling more procedures. These cases showcase Lean's power to improve healthcare quality and operational efficiency.

Model VI - Sustainability and Environmental Stewardship

The healthcare sector has a significant impact on climate change, greenhouse gas emissions, and solid waste creation. Hospitals are among the most energy-intensive facilities, consuming large amounts of electricity for heating, lighting, and medical equipment. Additionally, the production, transportation, and disposal processes in the healthcare supply chain contribute to a substantial carbon footprint. To address these environmental issues, the implementation of energy-efficient smart building technologies in hospitals is crucial. Key strategies include optimizing energy consumption by analyzing needs from both micro (single spaces) and macro scales, quantifying and monitoring energy performance indicators, and identifying critical indicators that can be optimized for efficient energy management. Additionally, reducing greenhouse gas emissions involves quantifying and analyzing CO2 emissions from hospital energy consumption, establishing benchmarks for hospital management, and setting targets for limiting emissions. It also requires investigating the determinants of electrical and thermal energy costs, considering factors such as hospital size, work intensity, and climate zones.

Implementing smart building technologies involves leveraging digital twin integration to model and improve care plans, enhance accessibility and convenience with remote care delivery, and optimize procedures such as supply chain management, staff scheduling, and bed management. Utilizing artificial intelligence (AI) in clinical decision support systems can provide individualized therapy recommendations and detect early warning signs of health issues. Employing wearables and IoT devices for real-time patient monitoring enables early intervention and improved healthcare outcomes. By adopting these strategies and technologies, healthcare organizations can significantly reduce their environmental impact, lower energy costs, and improve patient outcomes. However, challenges such as data privacy, security, and interoperability must be addressed to ensure successful implementation. The healthcare industry significantly impacts the environment through its resource consumption, waste generation, and greenhouse gas emissions. Addressing these issues is critical for reducing the sector's ecological footprint and promoting sustainability.

ILLUSTRATIVE CASE: SUSTAINABILITY AND ENVIRONMENTAL STEWARDSHIP IN HEALTHCARE

Sustainability and environmental stewardship are increasingly prioritized in healthcare to reduce environmental impacts while delivering quality care. Hospitals worldwide are adopting eco-friendly practices, including energy-efficient infrastructure, waste management reforms, and sustainable resource utilization. For example, the National Health Service (NHS. England, 2020) in England has implemented the *Net Zero Strategy* to achieve carbon neutrality by 2045, incorporating renewable energy sources, electric vehicles, and waste reduction programs. Similarly, Cleveland Clinic (Mihaljevic, 2022) in the United States has committed to achieving carbon neutrality by 2027 by transitioning to energy-efficient systems and renewable energy solutions. Another example is the Karolinska University Hospital (Bellander, 2024) in Sweden, which focuses on sustainable construction and water conservation, with its buildings meeting stringent environmental standards. Additionally, Singapore's Khoo Teck Puat Hospital (Jin, 2024) has designed a "hospital in a garden," integrating green spaces to reduce energy use and promote healing. These institutions demonstrate how sustainable practices can benefit both healthcare delivery and the environment, setting global benchmarks for environmental stewardship.

Challenges and Strategies in Smart Hospital Implementation

The adoption of smart hospitals brings transformative potential to healthcare but also presents significant challenges across various domains. A lack of comprehensive data on environmental impacts limits effective decision-making and policy development. Institutional commitment and regulatory frameworks are critical for driving sustainability initiatives. By adopting renewable energy sources like solar and wind within microgrids, hospitals can reduce emissions, enhance efficiency, and ensure reliable operations through energy storage systems. These innovations not only reduce environmental footprints but also strengthen resilience and operational reliability.

Interoperability, data security, and privacy remain critical hurdles. Seamless integration of health information systems allows better care coordination and patient-centered practices. Standards like FHIR enable real-time data sharing, improving patient engagement and reducing data fragmentation. However, implementing these standards demands robust security measures, such as blockchain and zero-trust frameworks, to protect patient information. Addressing these challenges is essential for improving healthcare delivery while maintaining patient trust. Promoting a culture of innovation and digital transformation is crucial for integrating smart technologies. Strong leadership, adaptable organizational culture, and human resource development are key. Leaders must drive change by fostering collaboration, providing training in digital skills, and supporting continuous learning. Addressing resistance to change and ensuring scalability of new systems are also vital.

Effective collaboration between healthcare professionals, policymakers, and technology experts is critical to implementing smart hospital strategies that align with regulatory requirements and community needs. Understanding policy frameworks, such as those governing data privacy and interoperability, is essential. Investing in education and interdisciplinary collaboration ensures healthcare professionals are equipped to manage smart technologies effectively. Ultimately, overcoming challenges and fostering innovation requires a multifaceted approach. By aligning leadership, training, collaboration, and policy advocacy, healthcare organizations can improve operational efficiency, enhance patient care, and create resilient, eco-friendly smart hospital systems.

REFERENCES

Ahmad, A. (2024). Enhancing Hospital Efficiency through IoT and AI: A Smart Healthcare System. [JOSAPEN]. *Journal of Computer Science Application and Engineering*, *2*(2), 2. Advance online publication. DOI: 10.70356/josapen.v2i2.36

Allison, B. (2024). Exploring Intelligent Automation at Mayo Clinic: An Interview with Dr. Anjali Bhagra. *Mayo Clinic Innovation Exchange*. https://innovationexchange.mayoclinic.org/exploring-intelligent-automation-at-mayo-clinic-an-interview-with-dr-anjali-bhagra/

Azaria, A., Ekblaw, A., Vieira, T., & Lippman, A. (2016). MedRec: Using Blockchain for Medical Data Access and Permission Management. *2016 2nd International Conference on Open and Big Data (OBD)*, 25–30. DOI: 10.1109/OBD.2016.11

Bean, R. (2024). *How Cleveland Clinic Is Innovating in Healthcare with Data, Analytics, And AI*. Forbes. https://www.forbes.com/sites/randybean/2024/10/06/how-cleveland-clinic-is-innovating-in-healthcare-with-data-analytics-and-ai/

Bellander, E. (2024, August 21). *IoT in hemmet för jämlik hälsa*. https://www.karolinska.se/forskning-och-utbildning/innovation/aktuell-innovation/iot-hemmonitorering/

Bhamu, J., & Singh Sangwan, K. (2014). Lean manufacturing: Literature review and research issues. *International Journal of Operations & Production Management*, *34*(7), 876–940. DOI: 10.1108/IJOPM-08-2012-0315

Boina, R. (2023). Revolutionizing Healthcare: Unleashing the Power of Data Analytics for Enhanced Clinical Decisions, Operational Efficiency, and Patient Empowerment. [IJSR]. *International Journal of Science and Research (Raipur, India)*, *12*(8), 1–4. DOI: 10.21275/SR23827045322

De Oliveira Almeida, G., & Hinton, J. E. (2024). Simulation and Healthcare Simulation. In *Reference Module in Social Sciences* (p. B9780443137013003042). Elsevier., DOI: 10.1016/B978-0-443-13701-3.00304-2

Demir, E., Yakutcan, U., & Page, S. (2024). Using simulation modelling to transform hospital planning and management to address health inequalities. *Social Science & Medicine*, *347*, 116786. DOI: 10.1016/j.socscimed.2024.116786 PMID: 38493680

El-Gayar, O. F., Bojja, G. R., Ambati, L. S., Boit, J., & Nawar, N. (2024). The Impact of the Internet of Things in Healthcare Delivery: A Systematic Literature Review. In Wickramasinghe, N. (Ed.), (pp. 35–100). Advances in Medical Technologies and Clinical Practice. IGI Global., DOI: 10.4018/979-8-3693-5237-3.ch002

Garg, D., Dubey, N., Goel, P., Ramoliya, D., Ganatra, A., & Kotecha, K. (2024). Improvisation in Spinal Surgery Using AR (Augmented Reality), MR (Mixed Reality), and VR (Virtual Reality). *RAiSE, 2023*, 186. DOI: 10.3390/engproc2023059186

Greener, R. (2024, May 21). XR Healthcare Market will be Worth $19.6 billion by 2033. *XR Today*. https://www.xrtoday.com/mixed-reality/xr-healthcare-market-will-be-worth-19-6-billion-by-2033/

Halwiindi, H., Muliokela, R., Songolo, P., Simanga, T., Joshi, S., Msadabwe, S., Mwaba, C. K., & Kapambwe, S. (2022). Utilizing Mhealth (Mobile Health) Messaging To Increase Uptake Of Cervical Cancer Screening Services: Impact, Perceptions, And Experiences From Lusaka Province, Zambia. *Journal of Disease and Global Health*, •••, 54–65. DOI: 10.56557/jodagh/2022/v15i38061

Jin, O. W. (2024). Garden by the bed: Bringing nature and healing to hospital patients. *The Straits Times*. https://www.straitstimes.com/multimedia/graphics/2024/04/horticulture-therapy-khoo-teck-puat-hospital-singapore/index.html?shell

Jones, D. D., Heaton, H. A., Wallerich, T. J., Riekmann, L. A., Handmacher, B. H., & Hatton, R. L. (2023). Wearable Real Time Location Services Technology for Staff Duress in Healthcare. *2023 IEEE 13th International Conference on RFID Technology and Applications (RFID-TA)*, 127–129. DOI: 10.1109/RFID-TA58140.2023.10290330

Jovy-Klein, F., Stead, S., Salge, T. O., Sander, J., Diehl, A., & Antons, D. (2024). Forecasting the future of smart hospitals: Findings from a real-time delphi study. *BMC Health Services Research*, *24*(1), 1421. DOI: 10.1186/s12913-024-11895-z PMID: 39558347

Kataria, S., Sharma, P., Kataria, S., Saharan, M., & Sikka, R. (2024). Real-Time Location Systems: Revolutionizing Porter Services for Improving Patient Care Efficiency. *Cureus*. Advance online publication. DOI: 10.7759/cureus.69922 PMID: 39439611

Kim, M. H., & Park, Y. S. (2024). Use of a Real-Time Locating System in Infection Control. *Infection & Chemotherapy*, *56*(4), e45. DOI: 10.3947/ic.2024.0043 PMID: 39431344

Lapão, L., & Viegas, S. (2024a). Leveraging digital platforms to improve Public Health in hospital smart buildings. *European Journal of Public Health, 34*(Supplement_3), ckae144.492. DOI: 10.1093/eurpub/ckae144.492

Lapão, L., & Viegas, S. (2024b). Leveraging digital platforms to improve Public Health in hospital smart buildings. *European Journal of Public Health, 34*(Supplement_3), ckae144.492. DOI: 10.1093/eurpub/ckae144.492

Li, J., & Carayon, P. (2021). Health Care 4.0: A Vision for Smart and Connected Health Care. *IISE Transactions on Healthcare Systems Engineering, 11*(3), 171–180. DOI: 10.1080/24725579.2021.1884627 PMID: 34497970

Ma, K. S.-K. (2023). Extended Reality-Augmented Technologies in Healthcare. In Keikhosrokiani, P. (Ed.), (pp. 23–39). Advances in Marketing, Customer Relationship Management, and E-Services. IGI Global., DOI: 10.4018/978-1-6684-7029-9.ch002

Malik, A. N., Afridi, A., & Rathore, F. A. (2024). Mobile health (mHealth) applications for stroke rehabilitation: A mini review. *JPMA. The Journal of the Pakistan Medical Association, 74*(9), 1723–1726. DOI: 10.47391/JPMA.24-74 PMID: 39279090

Mehta, J. K. (2022). Smart Healthcare System Using Data Analysis. *International Journal for Research in Applied Science and Engineering Technology, 10*(1), 1253–1257. DOI: 10.22214/ijraset.2022.40020

Meka, S. C., Achan, S., & Pettit, R. G. (2024). Real-Time Embedded Monitoring Technologies in Modern Healthcare Systems: A Survey. *2024 IEEE 27th International Symposium on Real-Time Distributed Computing (ISORC)*, 1–6. DOI: 10.1109/ISORC61049.2024.10551333

Mihaljevic, T. (2022). *Sustainability & Global Citizenship Report 2022.*

Nayak, S. (2024). Smart Hospitals: Integrating AI for Enhanced Patient Outcomes. *Journal of Electrical Systems, 20*(10s), 1812–1819. DOI: 10.52783/jes.5446

Neravetla, A. R., Nomula, V. K., Mohammed, A. S., & Dhanasekaran, S. (2024). Implementing AI-driven Diagnostic Decision Support Systems for Smart Healthcare. *2024 15th International Conference on Computing Communication and Networking Technologies (ICCCNT)*, 1–6. DOI: 10.1109/ICCCNT61001.2024.10725323

Nwoke, J. (2024). Healthcare Data Analytics and Predictive Modelling: Enhancing Outcomes in Resource Allocation, Disease Prevalence and High-Risk Populations. *International Journal of Health Sciences, 7*(7), 1–35. DOI: 10.47941/ijhs.2245

Odirichukwu, J. C., Eze, E. O., Eze, V. C., Eze, E. I., Njoku, O. A., Chika-Ugada, P. K., ... & Nwoke, J. C. Internet of Things (IoT) Based Patient Information and Heart Beat Monitoring System for Health Information System.

Peh, A. C. (2024). The Evolution of Internet of Things (IoT) in Global Healthcare. *International Journal of Innovative Science and Research Technology (IJISRT)*, 659–666. DOI: 10.38124/ijisrt/IJISRT24SEP294

Radanovic, I., & Likic, R. (2018). Opportunities for Use of Blockchain Technology in Medicine. *Applied Health Economics and Health Policy*, *16*(5), 583–590. DOI: 10.1007/s40258-018-0412-8 PMID: 30022440

Salvetti, F., Gardner, R., Minehart, R., & Bertagni, B. (2023). Intelligent Avatars, Holographic Tools, Digitized Objects: An Extended Reality Simulation Demonstration. [iJAC]. *International Journal of Advanced Corporate Learning*, *16*(3), 73–81. DOI: 10.3991/ijac.v16i3.35739

Shalini, T. G., Ganeshabu, L., Chemudugunta, P., Yamsani, N., Kumar, Ch. A., & Athiraja, A. (2024). Exploring Innovations in Autonomous Robotics and Mechatronics: Application in Manufacturing and Healthcare. *2024 5th International Conference on Smart Electronics and Communication (ICOSEC)*, 336–342. DOI: 10.1109/ICOSEC61587.2024.10722417

Shilaskar, P. (2024). Multi Modal AI-Driven System for Enhanced Neurological Detection Using EEG, Retinal, and Brain Imaging Data. *International Journal for Research in Applied Science and Engineering Technology*, *12*(11), 876–882. DOI: 10.22214/ijraset.2024.65229

Singh, B. (2024). Digital Twins as New Paradigm for Bridging the Gap from Personalized Medicine to Specific Rural Public Health. In P. K. Dutta, P. Raj, B. Sundaravadivazhagan, & C. P. Selvan, *Artificial Intelligence Solutions for Cyber-Physical Systems* (1st ed., pp. 286–309). Auerbach Publications. DOI: 10.1201/9781032694375-16

Vallès-Peris, N., Barat-Auleda, O., & Domènech, M. (2021). Robots in Healthcare? What Patients Say. *International Journal of Environmental Research and Public Health*, *18*(18), 9933. DOI: 10.3390/ijerph18189933 PMID: 34574861

Virtual Reality In Healthcare Market. (2023). Grand View Research. https://www.grandviewresearch.com/press-release/global-virtual-reality-vr-healthcare-market#

Waldie, P., Attef, M., Trudel, C., Chan, A. D. C., & Wallace, B. (2023). Implementation and Use of Real-Time Location Systems in Hospital Environments – Rapid Scoping Review of Human Factors Considerations. *Proceedings of the International Symposium on Human Factors and Ergonomics in Health Care, 12*(1), 164–168. DOI: 10.1177/2327857923121038

Yang, A., & Yang, E. (2024). *A Multimodal Approach to The Detection and Classification of Skin Diseases* (Version 1). arXiv. DOI: 10.48550/ARXIV.2411.13855

Yuan, Y., Chen, K., Zhu, Y., Yu, Y., Hu, M., Chu, Y., Hsu, Y., Hu, J., Yue, Q., & Liu, M. (2024). Exploring the feasibility of integrating ultra-high field magnetic resonance imaging neuroimaging with multimodal artificial intelligence for clinical diagnostics. *iRadiology*, *2*(5), 498–509. DOI: 10.1002/ird3.102

Zhang, N., Feng, Y., Huo, R., & Zhao, Y. (2023). Design of Intelligent Hospital Information Service System Based on Intelligent Internet of Things. *2023 International Conference on Industrial IoT, Big Data and Supply Chain (IIoTBDSC)*, 16–22. DOI: 10.1109/IIoTBDSC60298.2023.00013

Chapter 3
Industry-Specific Fuzzy Front-End Innovation: A Multiple-Case Study of Medical Devices

Jesper Johansson
https://orcid.org/0009-0000-7636-7333
Halmstad University, Sweden

David Rosendal
https://orcid.org/0009-0000-9383-209X
Halmstad University, Sweden

Henrik Barth
Halmstad University, Sweden

ABSTRACT

New product development (NPD) exists at the fuzzy front end (FFE) of innovation – the time when companies must make often ill-defined decisions based on limited information. Many industry-generic studies focus on the causes of this fuzziness: uncertainty, complexity, and equivocality — also identified as ambiguity. In this paper we explore the FFE of innovation in the Swedish medical devices industry where the public sector is a prominent player. Based on our empirical data from the interviews, we constructed a conceptual FFE framework Our findings reveal when public sector organisations purchase medical devices, the fuzziness in the FFE increases for the medical devices industry. Uncertainty and complexity in the FFE increase when medical devices companies must consider the degree of product risk as well as the laws, regulations, and practices involved in sales to the public sector. In addition, equivocality (ambiguity) increases when industry actors and

DOI: 10.4018/979-8-3693-7210-4.ch003

public sector actors have different interpretations of product costs.

INTRODUCTION

The healthcare sector has undergone significant transformation in recent decades, evolving from basic practices to advanced, technology-driven systems, exemplified by innovations like electronic health records, telemedicine, and personalized medicine.

The early stages of the innovation process called the fuzzy front end of new product development, is a critical phase characterised by uncertainty, during which ideas are generated, opportunities are identified, and initial concepts are defined. Successfully managing the fuzzy front end is essential for setting the trajectory of the development process, fostering innovation, and minimising costly errors later. In the healthcare sector, however, the FFE presents unique challenges due to the industry's regulatory complexity, ethical considerations, and multifaceted stakeholder landscape (Tschumi et al, 2024). The rapidly changing medical device market in the European Union makes it even more complex as regulatory aspects also need to be considered. While manufacturers and innovators express concerns over readiness, legislative clarity, and resource availability, critics view the regulation as overly complex, costly, and hindered by a shortage of notified bodies (Maresova, 2023). However, to ensure the sustainability of healthcare systems and transformation towards Healthcare 6.0, it is critical to address the early phases of the innovation process. Only then can we reveal gaps where new solutions could have a major impact.

In this chapter, we focus on the innovation aspect of the Swedish medical devices industry by examining the fussy front end of the innovation process from a theoretical perspective. We describe the early innovation process as presented in the literature: the emergence of the "fussy front end" concept with its definitions, activities, attributes, and critical aspects. With this background, we present an industry-generic theoretical framework that we can compare to an industry-specific conceptual framework.

Many other companies, including medical device companies, systematically work with new product development (NPD). Because of the many crucial activities and decisions involved in NPD, a work environment in NPD is characterized by uncertainty and complexity (Florén & Frishammar, 2012; Kim & Wilemon, 2002a; Mendes & Toledo, 2011). In this innovative environment, companies engage in idea search, conduct marketing analyses, and make technology evaluations (Gassmann & Schweitzer, 2014; Hoonsopon & Puriwat, 2021b). Although the failure of NPD projects often becomes visible only in the development stages, many reasons for project failure can be traced to the pre-development stage, also referred to as the front end of NPD (Florén et al., 2018).

Because the success of NPD depends on whether a company's product delivers value to all its downstream stakeholders (e.g., customers, users, purchasers, and regulators; Vaquero Martín et al., 2021), researchers look for ways to understand and improve the front end of NPD which is also referred to as the fuzzy front end (FFE) of innovation (Rizova et al., 2018; Robbins et al., 2021; Zhang et al., 2019). The fuzziness is typically associated with information shortage, information overload, or different interpretations of the available information with respect to the needs of stakeholders (Hamdani, 2020; Hoonsopon & Puriwat, 2021a; Kornish & Jones, 2021).

Medical Devices Companies: Customers and Products

Private and public hospitals are the primary customers for medical devices companies (Harland et al., 2021; Scala & Lindsay, 2021). More than private sector hospitals, public sector hospitals share purchasing decision responsibility with various internal stakeholders (e.g., physicians and nurses) and with various external stakeholders such as management and procurement teams (Abdulsalam & Schneller, 2021; Pereno & Eriksson, 2020; Tavana et al., 2021; Vaquero Martín et al., 2016). This shared purchasing decision responsibility can have economic and technical implications for medical devices companies in their NPD (Harland et al., 2021; Miller & Lehoux, 2020; Tavana et al., 2021). An example of such an external stakeholder in Sweden is Medicinsk Teknik Halland that assists all hospitals in Halland County, Sweden, with their procurement of medical devices (Tornhagen & Ekstén, 2020).

Medical devices companies in the European Union (EU) classify their products into four risk categories: Class 1, Class 2a, Class 2b, and Class 3. Class 1 is the lowest risk category; Class 3 is the highest risk category. The factors that determine a device's risk category include its degree of invasiveness, its effect on body parts, the duration of device use, and the activity or passivity of the device. In addition, various national health products regulatory authorities (e.g., HPRA, 2014) have issued a Medical Device Regulation (MDR) that regulates the sale of medical devices for specific products such as contraceptives, substance-based products, products containing nanoparticles, and products containing pharmaceuticals.

In addition to the MDRs, companies that supply public sector hospitals with medical devices must comply with various healthcare laws and regulations (Miller & Lehoux, 2020; Wagrell & Baraldi, 2019). For example, the EU issued the 2014/24/EU Directive that regulates public procurement for any public organisation in all member states (European Union, 2014; Siciliani et al., 2021). This Directive also specifies when a public organisation (e.g., a hospital in any member state) need not comply with the Directive such as, for instance, when the procurement cost is less than a certain price threshold (Siciliani et al., 2021; Töyrä et al., 2020).

The FFE of Innovation

Understanding the essential drivers of and obstacles to NPD is crucial to the successful cost- and time-effective development of innovative products (Brun, 2011; Vaquero Martín et al., 2021). A commonly expressed opinion in the NPD literature is that the FFE of innovation is the most challenging stage in NPD (Florén et al., 2018; Florén & Frishammar, 2012; Kim & Wilemon, 2002a; Mendes & Toledo, 2011; Rizova et al., 2018; Russell & Tippett, 2008; Zhang et al., 2019). Thus, a company at the FFE of innovation must "thin-slice" its decision-making process so that its NPD activities prioritize the customers' needs (S.-L. Chang et al., 2007; Kim & Wilemon, 2002b; Russell & Tippett, 2008; Zhang et al., 2019).

A gap exists in the NPD literature, regardless of whether the FFE of innovation is viewed as a cause of potential failure or as a solution for potential failure. Researchers have made Insufficient comparisons between the FFE of innovation and specific industries (Park et al., 2021). Because the fuzziness in the FFE of innovation may link to external demands for NPD, such as customers' needs, it is worthwhile to study the stakeholders in different industries where their needs and demands may differ (Annosi et al., 2022; Pereno & Eriksson, 2019; Vaquero Martín et al., 2016, 2021) and where their governing rules and regulations may differ (Wagrell & Baraldi, 2019). The resulting fuzziness may also relate to how public sector customers (e.g., public hospitals) interact with the private sector producers (i.e., manufacturers) in their different responses to information shortage on product variety, interpretation, and value (Hamdani, 2020; Hoonsopon & Puriwat, 2021a; Kornish & Jones, 2021; Larsen et al., 2022).

One notable exception to this gap in the literature is Wagrell and Barakdi's (2019) case study of an unidentified Swedish medical devices company. The study describes "the joys and sorrows" of the private sphere with the public sphere. In the early 1990s, the company was successful in selling its products to hospitals in Sweden. However, after the 2014/24/EU Directive (European Union, 2014) was issued, and the Swedish public procurement law (Riksdag, 2016) was enacted, the company experienced financial difficulties. A result of the Swedish legislation, Swedish hospitals – which now had the three roles of development partner, financer, and customer – had to engage in a co-development process with private companies when purchasing medical devices that exceeded a specified cost (Töyrä et al., 2020). Problems arose with the co-development of new customers, with complex decision-processes, and with evaluations of products.

More positively, the enforcement of public procurement laws may help companies increase market share when these laws foster competition and create opportunities to win government contracts, provided approved products are the most economical (Hoekman & Taş, 2022). Yet these Swedish laws apply only when companies have already developed their products; they do not apply to pre-development products. To foster and boost Healthcare 6.0, it is important to understand the early phases of product development as more technologies are introduced and evaluated.

In Section 2, we establish the foundational context for our empirical investigation of the FFE within the Swedish medical devices industry by first examining the FFE from a theoretical standpoint. Our discussion begins with a review of the existing literature on the FFE concept, highlighting its origins, definitions, key activities, attributes, and critical components. Drawing upon this theoretical foundation, we then propose an industry-generic theoretical framework for the FFE. This framework serves as a basis for comparison with a more specific, industry-focused conceptual framework for the FFE in the medical devices sector.

THEORETICAL BACKGROUND

The Emergence of the Fuzzy Front End of Innovation

Cooper (1990) proposed a new tool for managing new products: stage-gate systems. Cooper developed this tool from his earlier co-authored research (Cooper & Kleinschmidt, 1988). The stage-gate systems tool divides the NPD process into stages, separated by gates. The first and second stages are in the pre-development phase (Cooper, 1990, 2006). Reinertsen and Smith (1991) named the pre-development phase the "fuzzy front end" (FFE). In a subsequent paper, Reinertsen (1994) noted that the FFE is the phase in which companies, in an economically favourable manner, can alter the direction of the NPD process because it is in the FFE that the first development expenditure is made. Most of the FFE literature draws on Cooper's work (e.g., Kim & Wilemon, 2002b; Park et al., 2021).

Definition of the FFE of Innovation

Most definitions of the FFE of innovation link to Reinertsen and Smith's (1991) original terminology. In this stage, new product or process ideas are proposed (Murphy & Kumar, 1997), strategies are formulated (Khurana & Rosenthal, 1997), marketing analyses are conducted, technical evaluations are made (Hoonsopon & Puriwat, 2021b), and decisions about whether to continue with the product or process are confirmed (Moenaert et al., 1995). The FFE, which is often an unstructured and dynamic stage (Florén et al., 2018; Murphy & Kumar, 1997), precedes the more formal development stage (Frishammar et al., 2011), and ranges from idea generation and screening (Kim & Wilemon, 2002a, 2002b; Murphy & Kumar, 1997) to initial team formation (Parida et al., 2017; Reid & de Brentani, 2004; Reinertsen

& Smith, 1991.) A significant amount of time and other resources are invested in the development of the idea in the FFE stage (Kim & Wilemon, 2002a, 2002b; Moenaert et al., 1995).

Researchers agree on the importance of the FFE of innovation because this is the stage when decisions are taken that may often determine the success or failure of the proposed product or process (Florén & Frishammar, 2012; Frishammar et al.,2011; Hoonsopon & Puriwat, 2021b; Kim & Wilemon, 2002a, 2002b; Khurana & Rosenthal, 1997). Early decision-making strategies applied in the FFE can enormously benefit innovation work by helping companies select good ideas and weed out bad ideas (Florén & Frishammar, 2012; Reinertsen & Smith, 1991; Vettorello et al., 2022). Researchers generally agree on when the FFE starts and when it ends as well as which activities are included in the FFE.

Table 1. Definition of the fuzzy front end (FFE).

Author(s)	Definition
Reinertsen and Smith (1991)	The FFE refers to the earliest stage of NPD in which activities begin before the start of team alignment. The activities in this stage save the most time and incur the least expense.
Moenaert et al. (1995)	During the FFE, the company decides whether it will invest resources in activities that may decrease the uncertainties created by market conditions, technological development, and competitive dynamics.
Murphy and Kumar (1997)	The FFE extends from product idea generation to product idea approval or termination. Because the FFE is unstructured and dynamic, investigation of and generalization about the findings are problematic. The FFE is highly influenced by a company's creativity.
Khurana and Rosenthal (1997)	Although many companies formulate and implement NPD strategies, regularly conduct NPD evaluations, and create NPD plans, they regard the FFE as the weakest stage. The complex information processing conducted in this stage can be linked to product failure.
Kim and Wilemon (2002A, 2002B)	The FFE begins when an opportunity is first considered and ends when that opportunity is ready to be developed.
Reid and de Brentani (2004)	The FFE refers to the time in which activities take place prior to a company's first consideration of the NPD. The FFE activities occur in two stages, regardless of the kind of product innovation: the early stage and the late stage. Early stage FFE activities are based on opportunity analysis, the strategic direction of new product projects, market research, and preliminary evaluations. Late stage FFE activities are based on new product concept definitions, commercial and technical feasibility analysis, and project planning.
Frishammar et al. (2011)	The FFE is the stage prior to the time in which the product concept enters the more formal development process. A successful FFE is critical to the success of the whole NPD process because success or failure of the project is determined in this stage.

continued on following page

Table 1. Continued

Author(s)	Definition
Florén and Frishammar (2012)	The activities conducted in the FFE of NPD are very influential as far as the success or failure of the project. It is here that companies create, structure, and test NPD ideas.
Hoonsopon and Puriwat (2021B)	The FFE, which is the pre-development stage in NPD, has a fundamental effect on the chance of NPD success. In this stage, ideas are identified and screened, and marketing analyses and technical evaluations are conducted.

The FFE Activities in the Literature

Koen et al. (2001) created a model called the New Concept Development (NCD) model that identifies the main activities that occur during the FFE: opportunity identification, opportunity analysis, idea generation, idea selection, and concept definition. The NCD model, which is linked to the FFE research (Bertels et al., 2020; Kutvonen & Torkkeli, 2010), has influenced some FFE researchers in their development of an FFE framework (Da Silva et al., 2020; Millson & Wilemon, 2010). The two activities in the NCD model that many FFE studies typically discuss are idea generation and idea selection (Erat, 2017; O'Brien, 2020). However, despite this focus, FFE researchers generally take an overall activity approach to the FFE of innovation (Juntunen et al., 2019; Roy et al., 2019; Tran et al., 2018; von Geibler et al., 2019; Zhang et al., 2019). [An exception to this holistic focus is O'Brien's (2020) study of an idea search with two strategies. He found an interaction effect between search strategies and innovation performance.]

Table 2. The FFE activities in the literature.

Activity	Author(s)
Idea search/generation	Bollinger (2019); Da Silva et al. (2020); O'Brien (2020)
Idea selection/ screening /validation	Da Silva et al. (2020); Bertels et al. (2020); Erat (2017); Froehlich et al. (2016)
FFE Process	Alblas and Jayaram (2015); Christiansen and Gasparin (2016); Green et al. (2020); Haasee and Laurseen (2018); Hoonsopon and Puriwat (2021a, 2021b); Juntunen et al. (2019); Khan et al. (2021); Neukam (2017); Rizova et al. (2018); Roy et al. (2019); Schweitzer et al. (2018); Thanasopon et al. (2016); Tran et al. (2018); von Gebler et al. (2019); Zhang et al. (2019)

When the FFE literature addresses activities holistically, the focus is seldom on which FFE activity is most essential. For example, when Rizova et al. (2018) examined the importance of social networks in NPD, they found that technical advice networks promote success because they reduce equivocality. They do not point to any FFE activity as a contributing success factor. Similarly, Schweitzer et al. (2018) avoided focusing on FFE activities. They found that R&D employees' proactive customer orientation in the FFE positively moderated the interaction between them and marketing employees. Haase and Laursen (2018) agreed that other aspects (besides the FFE activities) provide better explanations of and solutions to the fuzziness in the FFE.

The FFE Attributes in the Literature

In addition to FFE definitions and FFE activities, the FFE literature examines the FFE attributes: the causes of the fuzziness in the FFE. Some researchers suggest possible solutions for the fuzziness. There is more disagreement among researchers about the FFE attributes than about the FFE definitions and activities or even about the success factors. Three FFE attributes are commonly identified: uncertainty, complexity, and equivocality (ambiguity) (Brun et al., 2009). Vettorello et al. (2022) propose that an innovation system roadmap can help managers make sound decisions, thus reducing the uncertainty caused by fuzziness. Hoonsopon and Puriwat (2021a) conclude uncertainty can be reduced by certain leadership behaviours such as directive path-goal behaviours for incremental innovations and achievement-oriented behaviours for radical innovations. Hoonsopon and Puriwat (2021b), who also point to complexity as a cause of fuzziness, argue that improvements in organisational agility can make the FFE process simpler and more effective. Khan et al. (2021) found that an AI audit tool could increase effectiveness and reduce the complexity in internal auditing in the FFE.

Although uncertainty is often cited as the main cause of fuzziness in the literature, recently some researchers point to equivocality (ambiguity) as the dominant cause. Zhang et al. (2019) claim that team vision can reduce the equivocality resulting from different interpretations of the same information. Schweitzer et al. (2020) state that an intuitive information processing approach by actors can help them deal with ambiguous (i.e., equivocal) information in the idea evaluation. Green et al. (2020) agree that ambiguity (i.e., equivocality) is a cause of the fuzziness in the FFE. They propose that a mobile market research application that collects customers' needs can reduce this ambiguity.

Table 3. The FFE attributes in the literature.

The FFE Attributes	Author(s)
Uncertainty	Bertels et al. (2020); Bollinger (2019); Da Silva et al. (2020); Frishammar et al. (2011); Hoonsopon and Puriwat (2021a, 2021b); Moenaert et al. (1995); Schoonmaker et al. (2013); Schweitzer et al. (2020); Vettorello et al. (2022); Wagner (2012); Zahay et al. (2011); Zhang et al. (2019)
Complexity	Da Silva et al. (2020); Hoonsopon and Puriwat (2021b); Juntunen et al. (2019); Khan et al. (2021); von Geibler et al. (2019); Zahay et al. (2011)
Equivocality /ambiguity	Frishammar et al. (2011); Green et al. (2020); Schweitzer et al. (2020); von Geibler et al. (2019); Wagner (2012); Zhang et al. (2019)

Zack (2001, 2007) takes a knowledge-based perspective to describe these FFE attributes. He differentiates among four distinct knowledge-problems. Uncertainty is described as insufficient information; certification is required to resolve the insufficiency. Ambiguity is described as inadequate knowledge; clarification is required to resolve the inadequacy. Complexity is described as too many situational elements; simplification is required to reduce the information overload. Equivocality is described as multiple interpretations; unification is required to refine the interpretation.

Uncertainty

Uncertainty in the FFE results from the shortage/absence of the internal and external information needed to formulate and evaluate product scenarios (S.-L. Chang et al., 2007; Hong et al., 2022; Rizova et al., 2018). Companies need to know customer wants/needs and to make competitor analyses if they are to make rational technological and other decisions (Alam, 2006; Frishammar et al., 2011; Sætre & Brun, 2012; Zhang et al., 2019). Uncertainty, for example, about targeted markets (Frishammar et al., 2011) can create disagreement among project members (Christiansen & Gasparin, 2016) and can cause disruption in project execution (Verworn, 2009).

Researchers have offered numerous solutions to the uncertainty problem in the FFE of innovation (e.g., Bendavid & Bourgault, 2010; Hoonsopon & Puriwat, 2021b; Koen et al., 2001; Stuer et al., 2010). Solutions vary according to the industry in focus (Backman et al., 2007; Verworn, 2009). Moenaert et al. (1995) propose the creation of information systems between departments for improved communication flows. Koen et al. (2001) propose the creation of opportunity identification methods (such as "what-if" scenarios) that explore and gather information from external sources through inter-organisational partnerships. Thanasopon et al. (2016) propose educating employees in a customer-oriented approach. Schweitzer et al. (2018) propose implementing directive path-goal behaviours for managers working with incremental innovations, and achievement-oriented behaviours for managers working with radical innovations.

Complexity

Researchers have studied complexity in the FFE of innovation from a variety of perspectives. Khan et al. (2021) find that complexity occurs when there is a multiplicity of data. Kornish and Jones (2021) conclude that complexity results from the composition of several interconnected parts. Tran et al. (2018) highlight how the transferability and the use of knowledge are heightened in the FFE. Gupta and Maltz (2015) investigated knowledge diffusion in the FFE. Zack (2001) argues that it is necessary to limit the number of information sources. Adding to the discussion, Da Silva et al. (2020) favour the problem-solving tool "Design Thinking" that companies can use to develop their products closer to end-users, thus, limiting the number of information sources. Juntunen et al. (2019) and von Geibler et al. (2019) encourage greater stakeholder integration that can increase companies' information processing capabilities. Zack (2001, 2007) supports this solution.

Equivocality (Ambiguity)

Although some researchers have emphasized the importance of equivocality (ambiguity) in the FFE of innovation (Florén & Frishammar, 2012; Frishammar et al., 2011; Rizova et al., 2018; Zhang et al., 2021), this FFE attribute has received less attention than uncertainty and complexity. Frishammar et al. (2011) explain this inattention by the fact that most FFE researchers have defined most unclear variables as an uncertainty. However, there is a difference between equivocality (ambiguity) and uncertainty. Equivocality (ambiguity) often occurs when actors offer various interpretations of the same facts, data, or information whereas uncertainty occurs when the insufficiency of information available to the actors means they must acquire new data (Frishammar et al., 2011; Gupta & Maltz, 2015).

Zack (2001) differentiates between equivocality (the existence of multiple interpretations) and ambiguity (the inability to interpret). Therefore, equivocality and ambiguity require different solutions. Equivocality is reduced by iteration among team members; ambiguity is reduced by the acquisition of knowledge (Zack, 2007). Despite these proposed solutions to different problems, researchers generally continue to view equivocality and ambiguity as the same phenomenon, requiring the same solutions (e.g., Chang & Tien, 2006; Daft et al., 1987). Collection of additional information is unlikely to clarify the difference. Stevens (2014) proposes a solution: actors should join in socially interactive and iterative processes where they share, debate, clarify, and align their subjective meanings and interpretations.

Critical Aspects of the FFE Attributes

In comparing the FFE attributes, (uncertainty, complexity, and equivocality (ambiguity), it is possible to distinguish their critical aspects.

Uncertainty: Critical Aspects

To reduce uncertainty in the FFE, Moenaert et al. (1995) propose the creation of information systems between departments. Thanasopon et al. (2016) propose exploration and collection of information from external sources. Zack's (2007) position is consistent with these proposals when he argues that more information is needed in times of uncertainty. Van Aken and Weggeman (2000) agree that informal information networks are most suitable for the reduction of uncertainty in the FFE. Rice et al. (2001) created a framework intended to bridge the internal knowledge communication gap between idea generators and research managers by facilitating the exchange of information internally. Herstatt et al. (2004) found that the integration of corporate functions early in the FFE can reduce uncertainty. Magnusson (2009) proposes the use of ordinary users in the FFE of innovation, confirming that the acquisition of additional information (externally) reduces uncertainty.

Complexity: Critical Aspects

To reduce the complexity in the FFE, Da Silva et al. (2020) and Zack (2001) argue that the number of information sources should be limited. Juntunen et al. (2019) argue in favour of increasing companies' information processing capabilities, which requires richer knowledge (e.g., experiential knowledge). Massey et al. (2002) developed a performance-centred design methodology that features a holistic view of the FFE that addresses the interdependency among the organisation, its processes, and its individual performers. In turn, this interdependency offers a problem-solving approach for the FFE that is characterised by multilevel interactions. Massey et al. (2002) emphasize that the process associated with the generation of new knowledge is often more valuable than the knowledge it produces. This observation correlates with the need to enhance companies' information processing capabilities for managing complex tasks (Zack, 2007).

Equivocality (Ambiguity): Critical Aspects

Some degree of equivocality (ambiguity) can trigger more knowledge transfer and increased team creativity while blocking premature termination of projects with unexplored potential (Eriksson et al., 2016; Stetler & Magnusson, 2015; Zack, 2001). However, if the degree of equivocality (ambiguity) is too great, various obstacles may delay, even prevent, the development of strong and trustworthy ideas (Frishammar et al., 2011). The resolution of the equivocality (ambiguity) balance is a somewhat tricky endeavour. It often involves a combination of various processes including technical advice networks (Rizova et al., 2018), simplification of the company's problem-solving procedures (Rönnberg Sjödin et al., 2016), creation and organisation of improved communication flows between project members (Zhang et al., 2019), and support for the possibility of creating a uniform agreement on internal organisational cooperation (Kim & Wilemon, 2002b).

The FFE Theoretical Framework (Based on the Literature)

Figure 1 is our FFE theoretical framework based on our review of the FFE literature. In the framework, the "Definition" column lists the general activities that Cooper (1990) defined with his stage-gates systems tool that is now referred to as "the fuzzy front end" (FFE) after research by Reinertsen and Smith (1991). Further research has led to the identification of the three main attributes that cause the fuzziness in the front-end activities: uncertainty, complexity, and equivocality (ambiguity). The FFE is divided into activities that can be categorised as idea search/generation and idea selection/screening/validation. The critical aspects of the FFE are listed under these two columns.

Figure 1. The FFE theoretical framework

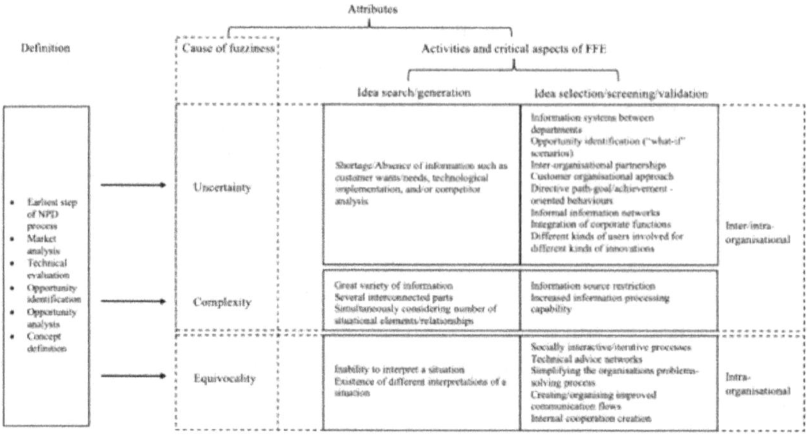

(based on the literature).

Our review of the FFE literature led to our observation that critical aspects of the FFE that create and solve fuzziness for uncertainty and complexity are inter– and intra-organisational options, but only the equivocality (ambiguity) attribute has an intra-organisational option.

RESEARCH METHODOLOGY

Research Design

A qualitative research approach (Bryman & Bell, 2011) and the case study methodology (Yin, 2018) were used in this study to explore the FFE of innovation in the Swedish medical devices industry. Qualitative data were collected from four Swedish companies (identified as A, B, C, and D) that manufacture medical devices that they market to Swedish and international healthcare providers. We interviewed five company respondents: one person from each of three companies and two people from a fourth company. We used a combination of snowball sampling and self-selection sampling within the framework of heterogenous purposive sampling (Saunders et al., 2019).

*Table 4. Medical devices companies in the study. *SEK = Swedish crowns.*

Company	Product type/Risk category	Turn-over/Potential market	Number of employees	Respondent
(A)	Class 3	10 Bn SEK*	9	(A) CEO
(B)	Class 1 & 2	9 Bn SEK	6 500	(B) Program Manager
(C)	Class 1	190 Mn SEK	40	(C) Managing Director
(D)	Class 1 & 2	30.8 Bn SEK	10 795	(D.1) Director – Product Launch (D.2) Chief Project Manager

Company A specializes in wound-care. It sells its Class 3 products worldwide. Company B manufactures and sells Class 1 and Class 2 products worldwide. Company C manufactures and sells Class 1 products mainly in the Swedish market. Company D manufactures and sells Class 1 and Class 2 products world-wide. The four companies' products are marked "CE," which means they meet the safety requirements specified in the *European Medical Devices Regulation*. The risk classification system is explained in Sub-section 1.1.

We also interviewed two respondents (identified as E and F) from two Swedish public sector organisations: *Region Halland* and *Vastra Gotalands Region*. We also collected secondary data from selected audit reports on the examination and acquisition of medical technical equipment for *Region Halland* (Tornhagen et al., 2019; Tornhagen & Ekstén, 2020; Tornhagen & Fornstedt, 2019; Tornhagen & Horstmann, 2020; Tornhagen & Norén, 2018).

Table 5. Public sector organisations in the study

Public sector organisation	Respondent
Halland Region	(E) Operations Manager – Medical Technologies
Vastra Gotalands Region	(F) Project Manager – Group Purchases

Data Collection

We conducted semi-structured, online audio interviews using the platform Microsoft Teams. Table 6. We used our theoretical framework to create an interview guide that allowed for additional open -ended questions and the opportunity for respondents and interviewers to discuss ideas and themes. The questions in the interview guide were based on the FFE attributes, activities, and critical aspects that we had identified in the construction of our FFE theoretical framework.

Table 6. Interviews with company and organisation respondents.

Company	Respondent	Date	Platform	Duration
(A)	*(A)*	2022-04-28	Teams	00:46:21
(B)	*(B)*	2022-05-06	Teams	01:06:00
(C)	*(C)*	2022-05-06	Teams	01:01:32
(D)	*(D1)*	2022-04-25	Teams	01:01:52
(D)	*(D2)*	2022-05-09	Teams	01:06:04
(E)	*(E)*	2022-02-16	Teams	01:06:14
(F)	*(F)*	2022-02-17	Teams	01:17:52

Data Analysis

The interviews were audio-recorded, transcribed, translated from Swedish to English, and grammatically corrected when transferred to text-based data. We used thematic analyses with the interview data (Saunders et al., 2019) to identify 2nd order themes that derived from 1st order concepts (respondent quotations). The 2nd order themes were then further categorised according to the FFE attributes of uncertainty, complexity, and equivocality (ambiguity). This thematic analysis in combination with our use of the adapted data analysis method (Gioia et al., 2013) helped us link the three FFE attributes to respondents' comments as well as structure and visualise our empirical data. Figure 3-1 presents an example of this data analysis methodology.

Figure 2. Interview data analysis

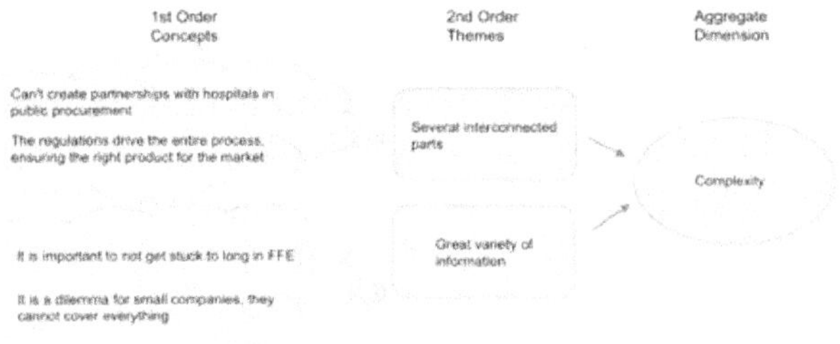

(Adapted from Gioia et al., 2013).

We used the online software tool Atlas.ti (2024), a qualitative research tool, to code and analyse the interview data from the company respondents. Using Atlas.ti, the authors individually read the interview data and assigned codes to various text sections as 2nd order themes. After comparing their results, they decided on the 24 final 2nd order themes, which were then assigned to the FFE attributes.

We used a similar analytical procedure for the interview data from the Swedish regional government employees. Our analysis resulted in the same 24 2nd order themes, which were again assigned to the FFE attributes.

FINDINGS

In Sub-sections 4.1 through 4.3, we present our findings from the interviews conducted with the five respondents at the medical devices companies. The critical aspects of the two FFE activities (idea search/generation; idea selection/screening/validation) are summarized in these sub-sections. In Sub-section 4.4, we present our findings on the relationship between public sector organisations and the medical devices industry. We conclude our findings in Sub-section 4.5 with a conceptual framework of the FFE in the Swedish medical devices industry.

Uncertainty

Idea Search/Generation

The uncertainty attribute for the idea search/generation activity in the FFE is defined in our FFE theoretical framework by the critical aspect of the absence or shortage of necessary information needed to form and evaluate well-defined products.

These scenarios include, for example, customer wants/needs, required technology, and/or competitor analysis.

We conclude that uncertainty is a recurring attribute in the FFE of innovation at medical devices companies. To generate NPD ideas, information gathering is essential. Among many other things, such companies need to identify their potential customers and their actual competitors, to determine if their products meet required safety regulations, to ascertain their product risk classifications, and, obviously, their capacity and ability to manufacture and deliver their products. The difficulties often encountered in gathering this information add to the uncertainty.

The company respondents revealed that the amount of time and other resources they can invest in idea search/generation varies, company to company. The companies that operate in a global market require (and use) considerably more resources for this effort than companies that operate in a domestic market. Companies that market their products both nationally and internationally are much more likely to employ people with the creativity and curiosity needed to imagine new ideas and to solve problems. The ingenuity of such ideas and solutions may add to the uncertainty when practical implementation is in focus.

Idea Selection/Screening/Validation

The uncertainty attribute for the idea selection/screening/validation activity in the FFE of innovation is defined in our FFE theoretical framework by such critical aspects as creating inter-departmental information systems, identifying opportunities, creating inter-organisational partnerships, integrating corporate functions, and involving different users for different innovations.

The company respondents agreed on the importance of internal information for reducing uncertainty. Continual communications between the company and its customers are also important for reducing the uncertainty about customer needs/wants. Respondents emphasized the value of customer involvement in NPD. The needs/wants of the many different stakeholders in the healthcare sector creates uncertainty about which customers to prioritize, which products to develop, and which markets to focus on. Company respondents agreed that some of this uncertainty could be reduced by the formation of inter-organisational relationships (especially for smaller companies) that would provide better access to technologies and other resources.

Complexity

Idea Search/Generation

The complexity attribute for the idea search/generation activity in the FFE of innovation is defined in our FFE theoretical framework by such critical aspects as the great variety of information, the several interconnected parts, and the simultaneous consideration of numerous situational elements/relationships.

The company respondents described how an innovation team, supported by clinical specialists and an advisory board composed of key opinion leaders, is tasked with identifying numerous and varied information sources. With this many actors involved in the collection of information, the complexity of idea search/generation increases. The importance of meeting all stakeholders' needs and satisfying purchasers' tender specifications adds to the complexity.

Idea Selection/Screening/Validation

The complexity attribute for the idea selection/screening/validation activity in the FFE of innovation is defined in our FFE theoretical framework by such critical aspects as informational source restriction and increased information capability.

The company respondents described the importance of knowing the sources of their information. A few key opinion leaders can provide more valuable information than a 1000-person survey can. It is equally important to be sure of the information's reliability and validity. Given these information requirements, selecting, screening, and validating ideas is a complex process. The respondents said that larger staffs, especially on cross-functional teams, could increase the information-processing capability of idea groups.

Smaller medical devices companies have yet another complexity issue. Because such companies in Sweden have regional customers, a problem arises in the idea selection process. Until the product is developed, small companies cannot be certain that regions will enter purchase contracts. Also, typically the regions compete on price, which adds to the small companies' complexity of idea selection. With their larger international markets, the larger companies have more customer alternatives.

Equivocality (Ambiguity)

Idea Search/Generation

The equivocality (ambiguity) attribute for the idea search/generation activity in the FFE of innovation is defined in our FFE theoretical framework by such critical aspects as the difficulty in interpreting a situation and the multiplicity of different interpretations.

Owing to the uncertainty and complexity in generating, selecting, and validating NPD ideas, the possibility of equivocality (ambiguity) is always present. The company respondents emphasized the need to balance too much/too little information. In addition, equivocality about task responsibilities increases when employees are abruptly assigned new roles when NPDs with new FFEs are introduced. Some employees may find the transition difficult.

Idea Selection/Screening/Validation

The equivocality (ambiguity) attribute for the idea selection/screening/validation activity in the FFE of innovation is defined in our FFE theoretical framework by such critical aspects as the introduction of socially interactive/iterative processes and technical advice networks, by simplifying the organisation's problem-solving processes, and by creating/organising improved communication flows and internal cooperation.

The company respondents agreed that internal cooperation creation and technical advice networks can be created by improved internal communication flows. The extensive amount of information that their companies gather when selecting, screening, and validating new product ideas must be swiftly and accurately communicated to all relevant actors. Good communications reduce the equivocality in interpretations and support efficient problem-solving processes.

Public Sector Procurement and the Medical Devices Industry

In this Sub-section, we present our findings from the interviews conducted with the two respondents working in the Swedish public sector: an Operations Manager in Medical Technologies at Halland Region and a Project Manager for Group Purchases at Vastra Gotalands Region. These respondents presented the customer view of NPD development and purchase.

The Swedish Public Procurement Act, based on EU Directives, usually requires that the Swedish public sector purchase goods, services, or construction work through a public procurement process. This process is intended to ensure fair competition for public sector purchases. Thus, it is illegal for medical devices companies to enter pre-development product arrangements with public sector organisations or for these organisations to exert influence on product development. Regulators enforce compliance with the Act.

Both the company employees and the public sector managers are fully aware of the procurement legalities. However, we identified a fundamental misunderstanding between them. While the company respondents understand that product cost is a critical factor in competitive public procurement. they seem not to understand that the cost – from the purchaser's perspective – includes operational costs (e.g., operation-time, staff expenses, and complementary products or consumables associated with the product). This misunderstanding is an example of different interpretations (i.e., equivocality) of the same critical factor by separate seller and buyer.

The Conceptual Framework of the FFE in the Swedish Medical Devices Industry

Our findings generally support the theoretical framework we presented in Figure 2 that is based on our literature review. Interviews with company respondents reveal their understanding that the FFE attributes of uncertainty, complexity, and equivocality (ambiguity) are fundamental problems in NPD in the Swedish medical devices industry. The critical aspects of the FFE activities (idea search/generation and idea selection/screening/validation) are also confirmed by the interviews with the company respondents.

However, although our findings generally validate our theoretical framework, we conclude it is incomplete in some respects. The public sector respondents contributed additional observations to the company respondents' observations. We also identified new dimensions in our theoretical framework that were prompted by comments from company respondents. As a result of these new comments, we modified our theoretical framework.

The primary new dimension of the FFE concerns the importance of local government decentralisation in the Swedish public sector that impacts how purchasing decisions are conducted and regulated. Healthcare in Sweden is decentralized to the county councils and regions although regulated by the national Health and Medical Service Act. This governance structure contributes to the uncertainty and complexity in the FFE for companies that market their products to county councils and regions in Sweden. The second new dimension of the FFE concerns equivocality that, like uncertainty and complexity, occurs inter-organisationally as well as intra-organizationally. The third new dimension of the FFE is the observation that extent of the fuzziness in the FFE broadly depends on industry specifications:

product type and geographic markets. Figure 3 presents our conceptual framework of the FFE in the Swedish medical devices industry.

Figure 3. The conceptual framework of the FFE in the Swedish medical devices industry.

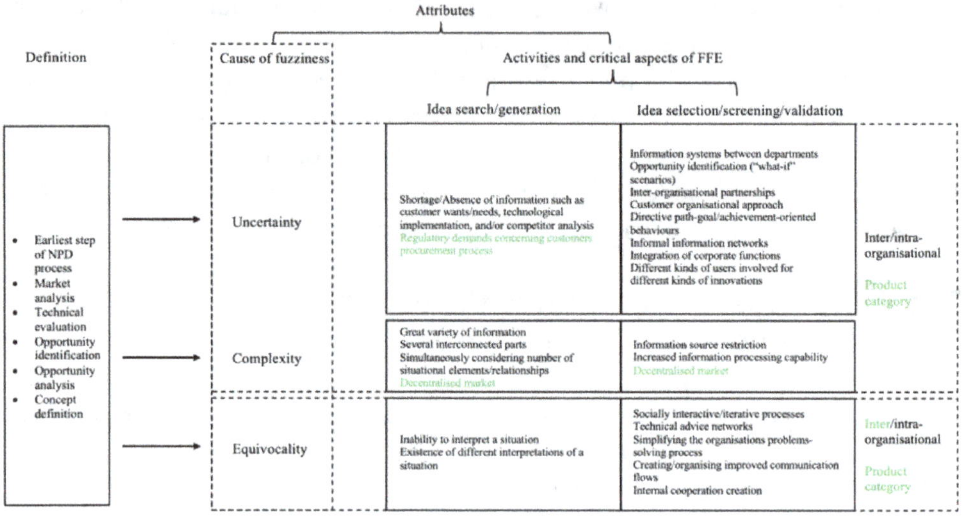

CONCLUSIONS AND DISCUSSION

The aim of this study was to explore the front part of the innovation process – the Fuzzy Front End (FFE) – in the medical devices industry in Sweden where the public sector, as a major customer, plays a prominent role. It is argued that this is one of the most important aspects to address to boost the development of Healthcare 6.0, where new technologies will need to be introduced at a faster pace. One important aspect addresses the added value in the early phases of the innovation process.

Based on a literature review of the FFE in innovation, a theoretical framework was constructed that identified FFE attributes, activities, and critical aspects. Given the breadth of the FFE literature, this framework was generic in its perspective. Based on empirical data acquired from industry actors (manufacturers/sellers) and public sector actors (buyers/users) on their experiences and relationships in the FFE process, a conceptual framework was then constructed. This second framework, which is industry-specific, built on the original framework supplemented with additions.

This study concludes that the causes of fuzziness in the FFE of innovation are uncertainty, complexity, and equivocality (ambiguity). The extent and mixture of these attributes in New Product Development (NPD) vary because of industry-specific factors. In the Swedish medical devices industry, the principal factors are product classification by degree of risk, by functional use, by intricacy, and by market (national or international; private or public sector; a centralised or decentralised purchaser structure). Among our findings, we identified the following recommended actions for medical devices innovators. To better manage uncertainty, they should gather as much information as possible from relevant stakeholders, including recognition of regulatory demands on purchasers. To better manage complexity – especially complexity caused by local government decentralisation – they should exercise informational source restriction and increase their information processing capability. To better manage equivocality (ambiguity), they should pay greater attention to inter- as well as intra-organisational relationships.

The study contributes to the FFE research in two ways. First, its comparison of the theoretical FFE framework (based on the literature) with the conceptual FFE framework (based on empirical data) is a novel methodological research approach. Second, the refined exploration of equivocality (ambiguity) as a cause of FFE adds a new explanatory dimension to the FFE research. Different actors can have different interpretations of the same phenomenon – intra-organisationally and inter-organisationally.

Theoretical Implications

This study of the FFE of innovation in the Swedish medical devices industry has theoretical implications for the FFE research. Although this study of the FFE process in this industry-specific context is similar in some ways to industry-generic studies of the FFE process, differences exist as described previously in this section. We conclude that the fuzziness characteristics of the FFE process may be industry-specific because of the variations in products, customers, and market location and structure. Furthermore, this study amplifies the FFE equivocality (ambiguity) attribute from misunderstandings between an organisation's team members/departments to misunderstandings between organisations.

Managerial Implications

This study reveals that while the FFE of innovation is an inevitable stage in NPD, companies can benefit from a clear-eyed understanding, not only of its inevitability, but also of its principal causes and its two main activities with their critical aspects. Product innovators can use our two FFE frameworks (industry-generic and industry-specific) as information references for the FFE process. This study is directed especially at managers in the Swedish medical devices industry so that they can better understand and manage the initial fuzziness of idea search/generation and idea selection/screening/validation.

Healthcare innovations, especially medical devices, involve a complex ecosystem of stakeholders with varying needs and expectations. To tackle this issue from a managerial point of view, at least three aspects need to be focused on.

Firstly, uncertainty in the FFE of innovation often stems from inadequate or incomplete information regarding customer needs, regulatory requirements, and competitive landscapes. This uncertainty hampers effective decision-making and can lead to misaligned product development efforts. To address this, medical device companies should implement advanced information systems that enable systematic data collection and analysis across departments and organisations. Developing inter-departmental communication channels and establishing collaborations with regulatory bodies and key stakeholders can ensure access to comprehensive and reliable information. By adopting co-creation strategies, companies can potentially reduce uncertainty, align product development with market and regulatory demands, and minimise the risk of costly adjustments in later stages (Tschumi et al, 2024).

Secondly, the complexity inherent in the FFE arises from the need to reconcile diverse stakeholder expectations, manage intricate procurement processes, and process a vast array of information from multiple sources. This complexity is compounded by the involvement of clinical specialists and advisory boards, which, while beneficial, increases the difficulty of decision-making. To mitigate this, companies as well as healthcare professionals should employ frameworks such as "Design Thinking" to streamline problem-solving based on interdisciplinary and human-centered approaches to healthcare management and practice (Roberts et al, 2016). These measures will help companies navigate the complexities of the FFE more effectively, enabling them to meet stakeholder requirements while maintaining clarity and focus in decision-making.

Thirdly, equivocality in the FFE is driven by the multiple interpretations of information and unclear task responsibilities, which are often exacerbated when employees are assigned new roles in novel product development initiatives. The tension between private-sector innovators and public-sector buyers further complicates this issue, particularly around divergent interpretations of cost-effectiveness and product value. To address these challenges, companies should foster iterative and transparent communication practices, both internally and externally, to ensure clarity of roles and alignment of objectives. Training programmes designed to build adaptability and collaboration skills among employees can also mitigate the impacts of role transitions (Houssaini et al, 2024). These efforts could potentially reduce ambiguities, enhance internal coordination, and foster stronger relationships with public procurement officials, ultimately facilitating smoother innovation processes and market success.

Limitations and Future Research Directions

Because our study is industry-specific, it does not increase our understanding of the FFE in innovation in other industries beyond what the literature has already described. However, our study points to the need for more industry-specific studies in the context of the FFE of innovation. Further, our study may serve as a guide for researchers and managers in the medical devices industry in other countries. Additionally, it would be of interest to make an international comparison of the procurement processes and regulatory dynamics in regions such as the EU, the US, and Asia. It would also be of value to address the FFE challenges in other highly regulated industries to learn and stimulate ways of developing more innovative solutions.

REFERENCES

Abdulsalam, Y. J., & Schneller, E. S. (2021). Of barriers and bridges: Buyer-supplier relationships in health care. *Health Care Management Review*, *46*(4), 358–366. DOI: 10.1097/HMR.0000000000000278 PMID: 32167964

Alam, I. (2006). Removing the fuzziness from the fuzzy front-end of service innovations through customer interactions. *Industrial Marketing Management*, *35*(4), 468–480. DOI: 10.1016/j.indmarman.2005.04.004

Alblas, A., & Jayaram, J. (2015). Design resilience in the fuzzy front end (FFE) context: An empirical examination. *International Journal of Production Research*, *53*(22), 6820–6838. DOI: 10.1080/00207543.2014.899718

Annosi, M. C., Marzi, G., Ciampi, F., & Rialti, R. (2022). An ambidextrous approach to practice-based innovation for social product development: Lessons from a Dutch company. *IEEE Transactions on Engineering Management*, *69*(2), 376–387. DOI: 10.1109/TEM.2020.2977976

Atlas.ti. (2024). *ATLAS.ti Web for browsers*. Webpage accessed 241202: https://atlasti.com/

Backman, M., Börjesson, S., & Setterberg, S. (2007). Working with concepts in the fuzzy front end: Exploring the context for innovation for different types of concepts at Volvo Cars. *R & D Management*, *37*(1), 17–28. Advance online publication. DOI: 10.1111/j.1467-9310.2007.00455.x

Bendavid, Y., & Bourgault, M. (2010). A living laboratory for managing the front-end phase of innovation adoption: The case of RFID implementation. *International Journal of Project Organisation and Management*, *2*(1), 84. DOI: 10.1504/IJPOM.2010.031883

Bertels, H. M. J., Mithani, M., Zhu, S., & Koen, P. A. (2020). Corporate champions of early-stage project proposals and the institutionalisation of organisational inertia. *International Journal of Innovation Management*, *24*(03), 2050028. DOI: 10.1142/S1363919620500280

Bollinger, S. R. (2019). Creativity and forms of managerial control in innovation processes: Tools, viewpoints and practices. *European Journal of Innovation Management*, *23*(2), 214–229. DOI: 10.1108/EJIM-07-2018-0153

Brun, E. (2011). Ambiguity: A useful component of "fuzziness" in innovation. In Frick, J., & Laugen, B. T. (Eds.), *Advances in Production Management Systems. Value Networks: Innovation, Technologies, and Management* (Vol. 384, pp. 412–424). Springer Berlin Heidelberg., DOI: 10.1007/978-3-642-33980-6_46

Brun, E., Steinar Saetre, A., & Gjelsvik, M. (2009). Classification of ambiguity in new product development projects. *European Journal of Innovation Management, 12*(1), 62–85. DOI: 10.1108/14601060910928175

Bryman, A., & Bell, E. (2011). *Business Research Methods* (3rd ed.). Oxford University Press.

Chang, A. S., & Tien, C. (2006). Quantifying uncertainty and equivocality in engineering projects. *Construction Management and Economics, 24*(2), 171–184. DOI: 10.1080/01446190500310353

Chang, S.-L., Chen, C.-Y., & Wey, S.-C. (2007). Conceptualizing, assessing, and managing front-end fuzziness in innovation/NPD projects. *R & D Management, 37*(5), 469–478. DOI: 10.1111/j.1467-9310.2007.00489.x

Christiansen, J. K., & Gasparin, M. (2016). Managing controversies in the fuzzy front end. *Creativity and Innovation Management, 25*(4), 500–514. DOI: 10.1111/caim.12174

Cooper, R. G. (1990). Stage-gate systems: A new tool for managing new products. *Business Horizons, 33*(3), 44–54. DOI: 10.1016/0007-6813(90)90040-I

Cooper, R. G. (2006). Managing technology development projects. *Research Technology Management, 49*(6), 23–31. DOI: 10.1080/08956308.2006.11657405

Cooper, R. G., & Kleinschmidt, E. J. (1988). Resource allocation in the new product process. *Industrial Marketing Management, 17*(3), 249–262. DOI: 10.1016/0019-8501(88)90008-9

Da Silva, R. H., Kaminski, P. C., & Armellini, F. (2020). Improving new product development innovation effectiveness by using problem solving tools during the conceptual development phase: Integrating Design Thinking and TRIZ. *Creativity and Innovation Management, 29*(4), 685–700. DOI: 10.1111/caim.12399

Daft, R. L., Lengel, R. H., & Trevino, L. K. (1987). Message equivocality, media selection, and manager performance: Implications for information systems. *Management Information Systems Quarterly, 11*(3), 355. DOI: 10.2307/248682

Erat, S. (2017). Making the best idea better: The role of idea pool structure. *Production and Operations Management, 26*(10), 1946–1959. DOI: 10.1111/poms.12734

Eriksson, P. E., Patel, P. C., Sjödin, D. R., Frishammar, J., & Parida, V. (2016). Managing interorganizational innovation projects: Mitigating the negative effects of equivocality through knowledge search strategies. *Long Range Planning*, *49*(6), 691–705. DOI: 10.1016/j.lrp.2016.05.006

European Union, E. (2014). Directive 2014/24/EU of the European Parliament and of the Council of 26 February 2014 on Public Procurement and Repealing Directive 2004/18/EC (1). *Official Journal of the European Union, 57*(28 March 2014), 65–242. https://doi.org/doi:10.3000/19770677.L_2014.094.eng

Florén, H., & Frishammar, J. (2012). From preliminary ideas to corroborated product definitions: Managing the front end of new product development. *California Management Review*, *54*(4), 20–43. DOI: 10.1525/cmr.2012.54.4.20

Florén, H., Frishammar, J., Parida, V., & Wincent, J. (2018). Critical success factors in early new product development: A review and a conceptual model. *The International Entrepreneurship and Management Journal*, *14*(2), 411–427. DOI: 10.1007/s11365-017-0458-3

Frishammar, J., Floren, H., & Wincent, J. (2011). Beyond managing uncertainty: Insights from studying equivocality in the fuzzy front end of product and process innovation projects. *IEEE Transactions on Engineering Management*, *58*(3), 551–563. DOI: 10.1109/TEM.2010.2095017

Froehlich, J. K., Hoegl, M., & Gibbert, M. (2016). Idea selection in suggestion systems: A thematic similarity perspective. *R & D Management*, *46*(5), 887–899. DOI: 10.1111/radm.12154

Gassmann, O., & Schweitzer, F. (Eds.). (2014). *Management of the Fuzzy Front End of Innovation*. Springer International Publishing., DOI: 10.1007/978-3-319-01056-4

Gioia, D. A., Corley, K. G., & Hamilton, A. L. (2013). Seeking qualitative rigor in inductive research: Notes on the Gioia Methodology. *Organizational Research Methods*, *16*(1), 15–31. DOI: 10.1177/1094428112452151

Green, W., Cluley, R., & Gasparin, M. (2020). Mobile market research Applications as a new voice of customer method: Implications for innovation and design management. *Research Technology Management*, *63*(1), 49–55. DOI: 10.1080/08956308.2020.1686297

Gupta, S., & Maltz, E. (2015). Interdependency, dynamism, and variety (IDV) network modeling to explain knowledge diffusion at the fuzzy front-end of innovation. *Journal of Business Research*, *68*(11), 2434–2442. DOI: 10.1016/j.jbusres.2015.02.018

Haase, L. M., & Laursen, L. N. (2018). Reasoning in the fuzzy front end of innovation: Framing the product DNA. *International Journal of Innovation Management, 22*(05), 1840001. DOI: 10.1142/S1363919618400017

Hamdani, F. E. (2020). Innovation stories platform: A holistic framework for innovation case studies. *Towards the Digital World and Industry X.0 - Proceedings of the 29th International Conference of the International Association for Management of Technology, IAMOT 2020*, 175–186.

Harland, C. M., Knight, L., Patrucco, A. S., Lynch, J., Telgen, J., Peters, E., Tátrai, T., & Ferk, P. (2021). Practitioners' learning about healthcare supply chain management in the COVID-19 pandemic: A public procurement perspective. *International Journal of Operations & Production Management, 41*(13), 178–189. DOI: 10.1108/IJOPM-05-2021-0348

Herstatt, C., Verworn, B., & Nagahira, A. (2004). Reducing project related uncertainty in the 'fuzzy front end' of innovation: A comparison of German and Japanese product innovation projects. *International Journal of Product Development, 1*(1), 23. DOI: 10.1504/IJPD.2004.004890

Hoekman, B., & Taş, B. K. O. (2022). Procurement policy and SME participation in public purchasing. *Small Business Economics, 58*(1), 383–402. DOI: 10.1007/s11187-020-00414-z

Hong, P. C., Park, Y. S., Deng, X., & Hwang, D. W. (2022). Marketing platform products for successful customer outcomes: An empirical investigation of project process integration. *International Journal of Quality and Service Sciences, 14*(3), 349–367. Advance online publication. DOI: 10.1108/IJQSS-09-2021-0130

Hoonsopon, D., & Puriwat, W. (2021a). The role of leadership behaviour of project manager in managing the fuzzy front end in the development of radical and incremental innovation. *International Journal of Innovation Management, 25*(2), 2150022. DOI: 10.1142/S1363919621500225

Hoonsopon, D., & Puriwat, W. (2021b). Organizational agility: Key to the success of new product development. *IEEE Transactions on Engineering Management, 68*(6), 1722–1733. DOI: 10.1109/TEM.2019.2929500

Houssaini, M. S., Aboutajeddine, A., & Toughrai, I. (2024). Development of a Data-Centric Design Thinking Process for Innovative Care Delivery. *HERD, 17*(2), 146–165. DOI: 10.1177/19375867231215071 PMID: 38062743

HPRA. (2014). *Qualification and classification of medical devices and in-vitro diagnostic medical devices (IVDs)*. http://www. hpra.ie/homepage/medical-devices/regulatory-information/classification

Juntunen, J. K., Halme, M., Korsunova, A., & Rajala, R. (2019). Strategies for integrating stakeholders into sustainability innovation: A configurational perspective. *Journal of Product Innovation Management*, *36*(3), 331–355. DOI: 10.1111/jpim.12481

Khan, R., Adi, E., & Hussain, O. (2021). AI-based audit of fuzzy front end innovation using ISO56002. *Managerial Auditing Journal*, *36*(4), 564–590. DOI: 10.1108/MAJ-03-2020-2588

Khurana, A., & Rosenthal, S. R. (1997). Integrating the fuzzy front end of new product development. *Sloan Management Review*, *38*, 19.

Kim, J., & Wilemon, D. (2002a). Strategic issues in managing innovation's fuzzy front-end. *European Journal of Innovation Management*, *5*(1), 27–39. DOI: 10.1108/14601060210415153

Kim, J., & Wilemon, D. (2002b). Focusing the fuzzy front–end in new product development. *R & D Management*, *32*(4), 269–279. DOI: 10.1111/1467-9310.00259

Koen, P., Ajamian, G., Burkart, R., Clamen, A., Davidson, J., D'Amore, R., Elkins, C., Herald, K., Incorvia, M., Johnson, A., Karol, R., Seibert, R., Slavejkov, A., & Wagner, K. (2001). Providing clarity and a common language to the "fuzzy front end". *Research Technology Management*, *44*(2), 46–55. DOI: 10.1080/08956308.2001.11671418

Kornish, L. J., & Jones, S. M. (2021). Raw Iideas in the fuzzy front end: Verbosity increases perceived creativity. *Marketing Science*, *40*(6), 1106–1122. DOI: 10.1287/mksc.2021.1300

Kutvonen, A., & Torkkeli, M. T. (2010). Opening the fuzzy front-end of new product development: A synthesis of two theories. *International Journal of Business Excellence*, *3*(4), 415. DOI: 10.1504/IJBEX.2010.035443

Larsen, A. S. A., Karlsen, A. T., Lund, J.-Å., & Andersen, B. S. (2022). Assessment of early warning signs in hospital projects' front-end phase. *International Journal of Managing Projects in Business*, *15*(2), 299–323. DOI: 10.1108/IJMPB-06-2021-0156

Magnusson, P. R. (2009). Exploring the contributions of involving ordinary users in ideation of technology-based services. *Journal of Product Innovation Management*, *26*(5), 578–593. DOI: 10.1111/j.1540-5885.2009.00684.x

Maresova, P. (2023). Impact of Regulatory Changes on Innovations in the Medical Device Industry Comment on "Clinical Decision Support and New Regulatory Frameworks for Medical Devices: Are We Ready for It? - A Viewpoint Paper.". *International Journal of Health Policy and Management*, *12*(1), 7262–7262. DOI: 10.34172/ijhpm.2022.7262 PMID: 35942961

Massey, A. P., Montoya-Weiss, M. M., & O'Driscoll, T. M. (2002). Performance-centered design of knowledge-intensive processes. *Journal of Management Information Systems*, *18*(4), 37–58. DOI: 10.1080/07421222.2002.11045700

Mendes, G. H. S., & Toledo, J. C. (2011). The fuzzy front end of new product development for Brazilian technology-based companies in the medical device industry: A causal model. *Brazilian Journal of Operations & Production Management*, *8*(1), 83–102. DOI: 10.4322/bjopm.2011.005

Miller, F. A., & Lehoux, P. (2020). The innovation impacts of public procurement offices: The case of healthcare procurement. *Research Policy*, *49*(7), 104075. DOI: 10.1016/j.respol.2020.104075

Millson, M. R., & Wilemon, D. (2010). The impact of changing markets and competition on the NPD speed/market success relationship. *International Journal of Innovation Management*, *14*(05), 841–870. DOI: 10.1142/S1363919610002908

Moenaert, R. K., De Meyer, A., Souder, W. E., & Deschoolmeester, D. (1995). R&D/marketing communication during the fuzzy front-end. *IEEE Transactions on Engineering Management*, *42*(3), 243–258. DOI: 10.1109/17.403743

Murphy, S. A., & Kumar, V. (1997). The front end of new product development: A Canadian survey. *R & D Management*, *27*(1), 5–15. DOI: 10.1111/1467-9310.00038

Neukam, M. N. (2017). Managing the fuzzy front-end in multicultural teams. *European Journal of Innovation Management*, *20*(4), 578–598. DOI: 10.1108/EJIM-11-2016-0112

O'Brien, K. (2020). Innovation types and the search for new ideas at the fuzzy front end: Where to look and how often? *Journal of Business Research*, *107*, 13–24. DOI: 10.1016/j.jbusres.2019.09.007

Parida, V., Patel, P. C., Frishammar, J., & Wincent, J. (2017). Managing the front-end phase of process innovation under conditions of high uncertainty. *Quality & Quantity*, *51*(5), 1983–2000. DOI: 10.1007/s11135-016-0376-4

Park, D., Han, J., & Childs, P. R. N. (2021). 266 Fuzzy front-end studies: Current state and future directions for new product development. *Research in Engineering Design*, *32*(3), 377–409. DOI: 10.1007/s00163-021-00365-w

Pereno, A., & Eriksson, D. (2020). A multi-stakeholder perspective on sustainable healthcare: From 2030 onwards. *Futures, 122*, 102605. DOI: 10.1016/j.futures.2020.102605 PMID: 32834076

Reid, S. E., & de Brentani, U. (2004). The fuzzy front end ofnew product development for discontinuous innovations: A theoretical model. *Journal of Product Innovation Management, 21*(3), 170–184. DOI: 10.1111/j.0737-6782.2004.00068.x

Reinertsen, D. (1994). Streamlining the fuzzy front-end. *World Class Design to Manufacture, 1*(5), 4–8. DOI: 10.1108/09642369210069751

Reinertsen, D. G., & Smith, P. G. (1991). The strategist's role in shortening product development. *The Journal of Business Strategy, 12*(4), 18–22. DOI: 10.1108/eb039425 PMID: 10113668

Rice, M., Kelley, D., Peters, L., & Colarelli O'Connor, G. (2001). Radical innovation: Triggering initiation of opportunity recognition and evaluation. *R & D Management, 31*(4), 409–420. DOI: 10.1111/1467-9310.00228

Riksdag, S. (2016). *Lag (2016:1145) om offentlig upphandling*. https://www.riksdagen.se/sv/dokument-lagar/dokument/svensk-forfattningssamling/lag-20161145-om-offentlig-upphandling_sfs-2016-1145

Rizova, P. S., Gupta, S., Maltz, E. N., & Walker, R. W. (2018). Overcoming equivocality on projects in the fuzzy front end: Bringing social networks back in. *Technovation, 78*, 40–55. DOI: 10.1016/j.technovation.2018.05.006

Robbins, P., O'Gorman, C., & Huff, A. S. (2021). The impact of team goal orientation in the fuzzy front end of the innovation process. *International Journal of Innovation Management, 25*(6), 2150071. DOI: 10.1142/S1363919621500717

Roberts, J. P., Fisher, T. R., Trowbridge, M. J., & Bent, C. (2016). A design thinking framework for healthcare management and innovation. *Healthcare (Amsterdam, Netherlands), 4*(1), 11–14. DOI: 10.1016/j.hjdsi.2015.12.002 PMID: 27001093

Rönnberg Sjödin, D., Frishammar, J., & Eriksson, P. E. (2016). Managing uncertainty and equivocality in joint process development projects. *Journal of Engineering and Technology Management, 39*, 13–25. DOI: 10.1016/j.jengtecman.2015.12.001

Roy, S., Dan, P. K., & Modak, N. (2019). Leveraging new product innovation through R&D practices in engineering manufacturing sector: A study in Indian context. *International Journal of Innovation and Sustainable Development, 13*(3–4), 275–295. DOI: 10.1504/IJISD.2019.100418

Russell, R. K., & Tippett, D. D. (2008). Critical success factors for the fuzzy front end of innovation in the medical devices device industry. *Engineering Management Journal, 20*(3), 36–43. DOI: 10.1080/10429247.2008.11431775

Sætre, A. S., & Brun, E. (2012). Strategic management of innovation: Managing exploitation by balancing creativity and constraint. *International Journal on Management of Innovation & Technology, 09*(04), 1250025. DOI: 10.1142/S0219877012500253

Saunders, M. N. K., Lewis, P., & Thornhill, A. (2019). *Research Methods for Business Students* (8th ed.). Pearson.

Scala, B., & Lindsay, C. F. (2021). Supply chain resilience during pandemic disruption: Evidence from healthcare. *Supply Chain Management, 26*(6), 672–688. DOI: 10.1108/SCM-09-2020-0434

Schoonmaker, M., Carayannis, E., & Rau, P. (2013). The role of marketing activities in the fuzzy front end of innovation: A study of the biotech industry. *The Journal of Technology Transfer, 38*(6), 850–872. DOI: 10.1007/s10961-012-9296-1

Schweitzer, F., Palmié, M., & Gassmann, O. (2018). Beyond listening: The distinct effects of proactive versus responsive customer orientation on the reduction of uncertainties at the fuzzy front end of innovation. *R & D Management, 48*(5), 534–551. DOI: 10.1111/radm.12252

Schweitzer, F., Roeth, T., & Gillier, T. (2020). The eye of the beholder: The influence of intuition, rationality, and leeway on the assessment of an Idea's market-creation potential. *Industrial Marketing Management, 91*, 274–284. DOI: 10.1016/j.indmarman.2020.09.018

Siciliani, L., McKee, M., Garcia-Altes, A., De Maeseneer, J., Gruson, D., Kringos, D., Lehtonen, L., Lionis, C., Murauskiene, L., Nuti, S., Pita Barros, P., Rogers, H.-L., Wieczorowska-Tobis, K., Zacharov, S., Zaletel, J., & Stahl, D. (2021). Public Procurement in Healthcare Systems; Opinion of the Expert Panel on Effective Ways of Investing in Health (EXPH). *European Union.*

Stetler, K. L., & Magnusson, M. (2015). Exploring the tension between clarity and ambiguity in goal setting for innovation: Clarity and ambiguity in goal setting for i Dnnovation. *Creativity and Innovation Management, 24*(2), 231–246. DOI: 10.1111/caim.12102

Stevens, E. (2014). Fuzzy front-end learning strategies: Exploration of a high-tech company. *Technovation, 34*(8), 431–440. DOI: 10.1016/j.technovation.2013.12.006

Stuer, C., Husig, S., & Biala, S. (2010). How to create and sustain an open and radical innovation capability in the fuzzy front end: The case of Vodafone Group R&D Germany and selected ongoing radical innovation projects. *International Journal of Product Development, 11*(3/4), 196. DOI: 10.1504/IJPD.2010.033958

Tavana, M., Nazari-Shirkouhi, S., & Farzaneh Kholghabad, H. (2021). An integrated quality and resilience engineering framework in healthcare with Z-number data envelopment analysis. *Health Care Management Science, 24*(4), 768–785. DOI: 10.1007/s10729-021-09550-8 PMID: 33834321

Thanasopon, B., Papadopoulos, T., & Vidgen, R. (2016). The role of openness in the fuzzy front-end of service innovation. *Technovation, 47*, 32–46. DOI: 10.1016/j.technovation.2015.11.007

Tornhagen, L., & Ekstén, E. (2020). *Revisionsrapport: Granskning av anskaffning av medicinteknisk utrustning: Region Halland* [Audit Report]. PWC.

Tornhagen, L., & Fornstedt, C. (2019). *Revisionsrapport: Granskning av anskaffning av medicinteknisk utrustning: Region Gävleborg*. PWC. [Audit Report]

Tornhagen, L., Fornstedt, C., & Olausson, C. (2019). *Revisionsrapport: Anskaffning av medicinteknisk utrustning: Region Norrbotten* [Audit Report]. PWC.

Tornhagen, L., & Horstmann, H. (2020). *Granskning av anskaffning av medicinteknisk utrustning: Region Örebro* [Audit Report]. PWC.

Tornhagen, L., & Norén, S. (2018). *Revisionsrapport: Granskning av anskaffning av medicinteknisk utrustning: Region Västmanland* [Audit Report]. PWC.

Töyrä, A., Monfors, J., & Bern, A.-B. (2020). Upphandlingsmyndigheten och Konkurrensverket December 2020. *Swedish Competition Authority*, 216.

Tran, M. K., Goulding, C., & Shiu, E. (2018). The orchestra of ideas: Using music to enhance the 'fuzzy front end' phase of product innovation. *Journal of Business Research, 85*, 504–513. DOI: 10.1016/j.jbusres.2017.10.029

Tschumi, P., & Mayer, H. (2024). How does co-creation influence healthcare regulations? An analysis of co-creation in social innovation. *Innovation (Abingdon), 37*(1), 85–117. DOI: 10.1080/13511610.2023.2296380

Van Aken, J. E., & Weggeman, M. P. (2000). Managing learning in informal innovation networks: Overcoming the Daphne-dilemma. *R & D Management, 30*(2), 139–150. DOI: 10.1111/1467-9310.00164

Vaquero Martín, M., Reinhardt, R., & Gurtner, S. (2016). Stakeholder integration in new product development: A systematic analysis of drivers and firm capabilities: Stakeholder integration in NPD. *R & D Management*, *46*(S3), 1095–1112. DOI: 10.1111/radm.12220

Vaquero Martín, M., Reinhardt, R., & Gurtner, S. (2021). The dilemma of downstream market stakeholder involvement in NPD: Untangling the effects of involvement and capabilities on performance. *Journal of Business Research*, *124*, 136–151. DOI: 10.1016/j.jbusres.2020.11.040

Verworn, B. (2009). A structural equation model of the impact of the "fuzzy front end" on the success of new product development. *Research Policy*, *38*(10), 1571–1581. DOI: 10.1016/j.respol.2009.09.006

Vettorello, M., Eisenbart, B., & Ranscombe, C. (2022). The innovation system roadmap: A novel approach to instil futures-oriented reasoning in strategic decision making. *Creativity and Innovation Management*, *31*(1), 5–18. DOI: 10.1111/caim.12472

von Geibler, J., Piwowar, J., & Greven, A. (2019). The SDG-Check: Guiding open innovation towards sustainable development goals. *Technology Innovation Management Review*, *9*(3), 20–37. DOI: 10.22215/timreview/1222

Wagner, S. M. (2012). Tapping supplier innovation. *The Journal of Supply Chain Management*, *48*(2), 37–52. DOI: 10.1111/j.1745-493X.2011.03258.x

Wagrell, S., & Baraldi, E. (2019). The joys and sorrows of a start-up's interactions with the public sphere: A case from medical technology. *Journal of Business and Industrial Marketing*, *34*(1), 267–283. DOI: 10.1108/JBIM-11-2018-0326

Yin, R. K. (2018). *Case Study Research and Applications: Design and Methods* (6th ed.). SAGE.

Zack, M. H. (2001). If managing knowledge is the solution, then what's the åroblem? *Knowledge Management and Business Model Innovaiton, IGI Global*, 16–36.

Zack, M. H. (2007). The role of decision support systems in an indeterminate world. *Decision Support Systems*, *43*(4), 1664–1674. DOI: 10.1016/j.dss.2006.09.003

Zahay, D., Griffin, A., & Fredericks, E. (2011). Information use in new product development: An initial exploratory empirical investigation in the chemical industry. *Journal of Product Innovation Management*, *28*(4), 485–502. DOI: 10.1111/j.1540-5885.2011.00821.x

Zhang, Q., Cao, M., & Doll, W. (2019). Fuzzy front end of innovation: A dual theoretical rationale. *Journal of Business and Industrial Marketing*, *34*(1), 176–191. DOI: 10.1108/JBIM-06-2017-0144

Zhang, W., Jiang, Y., & Zhang, W. (2021). Capabilities for collaborative innovation of technological alliance: A knowledge-based view. *IEEE Transactions on Engineering Management*, *68*(6), 1734–1744. DOI: 10.1109/TEM.2019.2936678

Chapter 4
Motivational Digital Health App Design for Behavioral Change:
Harnessing Gamification to Drive Engagement and Behavioral Change Through Digital Health Apps

Niladri Neel Majumder
University of Toronto, Canada

ABSTRACT

This chapter examines how gamification enhances digital health apps by integrating game design elements to drive and sustain behavioral change. It highlights how mechanics like points and badges improve user engagement and adherence to health interventions, aligning with Healthcare 6.0 focus on patient-centered care. Key topics include the evolution of gamification, foundational psychological theories, and the connection between gamification, design thinking, and user-centric design. The chapter covers core and advanced design elements, future trends, challenges, and strategies for effective gamified interventions. It outlines metrics for evaluating effectiveness and provides insights from case studies of successful gamified health apps, offering best practices for sustaining engagement and adherence while reflecting on future advancements in the field.

DOI: 10.4018/979-8-3693-7210-4.ch004

1.INTRODUCTION: THE CRITICAL ROLE OF GAMIFICATION IN DIGITAL HEALTH APPS

In the digital age, healthcare innovation has become synonymous with leveraging technology to enhance patient outcomes, foster engagement, and promote behavioral change. Gamification, the application of game design elements in non-game contexts, has emerged as a powerful tool to address persistent challenges in healthcare, such as low patient adherence, lack of motivation, and engagement gaps. The chapter examines the transformative potential of gamification in context of digital health and clinical informatics solution development.

Gamification not only introduces an element of fun into serious health tasks but also harnesses psychological principles to sustain user motivation. This chapter delves into the concept through theoretical underpinnings, real-world case studies, challenges, and future trends.

1.1 The Engagement Conundrum in Digital Health

Digital health apps face a daunting engagement conundrum. Many studies (Ozaki, 2019; Krebs, 2015) found that a significant portion of health app users stop using the app after a short period and many users disengaged from health apps due to a lack of perceived relevance and personalisation. This underscores a critical issue: without engaging and retaining users, the potential benefits of digital health interventions cannot be realized.

Consider the analogy of a gym membership. Just having access to a gym does not guarantee improved fitness; regular attendance and active participation are necessary. Similarly, the mere availability of digital health tools is insufficient without active and ongoing user engagement. As noted by Dr. Joseph Kvedar, a prominent digital health expert, "The value of digital health lies not in the technology itself but in its use". (Garett, 2019)

1.2 The Importance of Design in Digital Health Apps

Designing for engagement involves a multitude of decisions, each impacting how users interact with the app. These decisions range from the obvious, such as user interface (UI) and user experience (UX) design, to the more subtle, such as font choice and color schemes. For instance, the readability of text blocks, the cultural sensitivity of content, and the difficulty level of activities all play a role in how users perceive and interact with the app.

Moreover, the frequency and length of interactions, the relationship of trust built through the app, and data and device interoperability are crucial for sustained engagement. Every design element, no matter how small, can influence user behavior. For example, a study by B.J. Fogg at Stanford University highlights that even minor changes in font size and color can significantly affect user trust and engagement (Aseel Berglund, 2022).

Gamification: A Strategic Design Consideration

Gamification, the application of game design elements in non-game contexts, emerges as a powerful tool to enhance user engagement. By integrating game mechanics such as points, badges, leaderboards, and rewards, digital health apps can make the user experience more interactive and enjoyable. These elements tap into intrinsic motivators, such as the desire for achievement, competition, and social interaction.

Jane McGonigal, a leading advocate of gamification, argues that "games are the most elevated form of investigation," providing structured environments that motivate and engage users (Damaševičius, 2023). This principle applies to digital health apps, where gamification can transform mundane health tasks into compelling challenges.

Evidence-Based Benefits of Gamification

Empirical evidence supports the efficacy of gamification in health behavior change. A meta-review of serious games and gamification in healthcare found that gamified interventions significantly improve user engagement and health outcomes (Damaševičius, 2023). For instance, the "Zamzee" activity tracker for children uses gamification to encourage physical activity, resulting in a 59% increase in physical activity levels among users compared to a control group (Garett, 2019).

Similarly, a study published in the Journal of Medical Internet Research found that a gamified mobile app for diabetes management improved medication adherence and glycemic control among users (Garett, 2019). These examples illustrate how gamification can lead to meaningful and sustained behavior change, a critical goal for digital health apps.

1.3 The Secret Sauce of Engagement: Ten Critical Factors

Drawing from extensive research and practical experience, we have identified ten critical factors that constitute the "Secret Sauce of Engagement" for digital health apps:

1. **UI/UX Design:** Creating an intuitive and aesthetically pleasing interface.
2. **Outreach Optimization:** Ensuring effective communication and engagement strategies.
3. **Intrinsic Motivators:** Leveraging internal drivers such as curiosity and achievement.
4. **Clinical Relevance:** Ensuring the app addresses real clinical needs and provides valuable health insights.
5. **Activity Variety:** Offering diverse and dynamic activities to keep users engaged.
6. **Personalization:** Customizing experiences to meet individual user preferences and needs.
7. **Social Interaction:** Facilitating social connections and community support.
8. **Accountability Anchors:** Incorporating mechanisms for accountability, such as reminders and progress tracking.
9. **Effective Storytelling:** Using narratives to create engaging and relatable content.
10. **Immersive Experiences:** Creating immersive and engaging experiences through advanced technologies like virtual reality.

Each of these factors contributes to the overall user experience, making the app not just a tool but a companion in the user's health journey. By optimizing these elements, digital health apps can achieve higher levels of activation, engagement, and desired behavior change.

The challenge of engaging users in digital health apps is multifaceted, involving numerous design considerations and strategies. Gamification stands out as a pivotal design consideration, offering a robust framework to enhance user engagement and drive behavioral change. By integrating gamification with the ten critical factors of engagement, digital health apps can transcend traditional boundaries, creating experiences that are not only effective but also enjoyable and meaningful for users. As we move forward in the digital health revolution, understanding and applying these principles will be key to unlocking the full potential of digital health technologies.

2. EVOLUTION AND SIGNIFICANCE OF GAMIFICATION

Gamification refers to the application of game-design elements and principles in non-game contexts to engage users, enhance learning, and solve problems. This approach leverages the human predisposition for competition, achievement, and social interaction by incorporating elements such as points, badges, leaderboards, and challenges into everyday tasks and activities. The goal is to transform mundane or complex tasks into enjoyable and motivating experiences.

In the context of technology design, gamification has been effectively employed in various industries to drive user engagement and behavior change. A prime example is **Duolingo**, a language-learning app that uses gamified elements to make learning a new language fun and engaging. Duolingo incorporates points, levels, and streaks to motivate users to continue their learning journey, showcasing how gamification can significantly enhance user retention and satisfaction.

2.1 Historical Context and Evolution of Gamification

The concept of gamification is not new; it has its roots in the fields of education and psychology. The term itself was coined in the early 2000s, but the practice dates back to the use of game-like elements in education to motivate and engage students. The introduction of game mechanics into business processes began in earnest in the late 2000s, driven by advancements in technology and a growing understanding of human motivation.

One of the earliest and most successful implementations of gamification was in the realm of marketing and customer loyalty programs. For example, airline frequent flyer programs, which reward customers with points for each flight taken, can be seen as a form of gamification. These programs use elements like points, levels, and rewards to encourage repeat business and customer loyalty.

The integration of gamification into digital platforms gained momentum with the rise of smartphones and mobile apps. The accessibility and interactive nature of mobile technology made it an ideal medium for gamification. Apps across various sectors, including education, fitness, and finance, began incorporating game-design elements to improve user engagement and outcomes,

2.2 Application of Gamification in Healthcare

The healthcare industry has been relatively slow to adopt gamification compared to other sectors. However, the potential benefits of gamification in healthcare are immense, ranging from improved patient adherence to treatment plans to enhanced health education and behavior change. The application of gamification in healthcare can be categorized into three main areas: patient engagement, health education, and behavior modification.

Patient Engagement

One of the significant challenges in healthcare is ensuring patient adherence to treatment plans and medication regimens. Non-adherence can lead to poor health outcomes and increased healthcare costs. Gamification can address this issue by making the process of following treatment plans more engaging and rewarding.

For instance, the mobile app "MySugr" is designed for diabetes management. It uses gamified elements such as points, challenges, and rewards to encourage users to regularly log their blood sugar levels, track their medication, and maintain a healthy lifestyle. By making the management of diabetes more interactive and enjoyable, MySugr helps improve patient adherence and outcomes,

Health Education

Gamification can also play a crucial role in health education by making learning more interactive and enjoyable. Educational games and apps can help patients understand complex medical information, learn about their conditions, and make informed decisions about their health.

"Re-Mission," developed by HopeLab, is a notable example of a gamified health education tool. It is a video game designed for young cancer patients, where players control a character that fights cancer cells within the body. The game educates patients about their condition and the importance of adhering to their treatment plans while providing a sense of empowerment and control.

Behavior Modification

Behavior change is another critical area where gamification can have a profound impact. Encouraging individuals to adopt healthier behaviors, such as regular exercise, healthy eating, and smoking cessation, can be challenging. Gamified health apps can provide the motivation and support needed to make these changes.

The app "Zombies, Run!" is an innovative example of gamification for behavior change. It turns running into an immersive game where users complete missions and escape from zombies. The app uses narrative storytelling, challenges, and rewards to motivate users to run regularly, making exercise fun and engaging.

Significance of Gamification in Healthcare

The significance of gamification in healthcare lies in its ability to address some of the industry's most pressing challenges. By making health-related tasks more enjoyable and motivating, gamification can enhance patient engagement, improve health outcomes, and reduce healthcare costs. It offers a promising solution to the problem of patient non-adherence and provides innovative ways to educate patients and promote healthy behaviors.

Gamification also aligns with the broader trend towards patient-centered care. It empowers patients to take an active role in managing their health, leading to greater satisfaction and better health outcomes. Moreover, as healthcare systems increasingly embrace digital health solutions, the integration of gamification can help maximize the effectiveness of these technologies.

3. FOUNDATIONS & CONCEPTS OF GAMIFICATION FOR BEHAVIORAL CHANGE

Gamification, the integration of game-like elements into non-game contexts, has become a prominent strategy for encouraging behavioral change. This approach is particularly relevant in digital platforms for healthcare and social services. The efficacy of gamification is deeply rooted in several psychological and motivational theories, as well as principles from behavioral economics. Additionally, gamification intersects with design thinking and user-centric design, further enhancing its impact. This chapter explores these theoretical foundations and their application in creating effective gamification strategies.

3.1 Psychological and Motivational Theories Underpinning Gamification

1. Self-Determination Theory (SDT)

Self-Determination Theory, formulated by Edward Deci and Richard Ryan, underscores the importance of intrinsic motivation. According to SDT, people are most motivated when their actions align with their personal values and when their psychological needs are met. The theory identifies three core needs:

- **Autonomy:** The need to feel in control of one's actions and decisions.
- **Competence:** The need to feel effective and capable in one's activities.

- **Relatedness:** The need to feel connected to others and valued within a community.

In gamification, these needs are addressed by providing users with choices (autonomy), challenges and feedback (competence), and opportunities for social interaction (relatedness). For example, health and wellness apps that allow users to set personal goals and track their progress fulfill these psychological needs, enhancing user engagement and motivation.

Case Study: MyFitnessPal

MyFitnessPal is a prime example of SDT in practice. The app allows users to set personal fitness and nutritional goals, track their progress, and engage with friends. By giving users autonomy over their goals, providing feedback on their progress, and fostering social connections, MyFitnessPal aligns with the principles of SDT and effectively encourages healthy behavior.

2. Behaviorism

Behaviorism, particularly B.F. Skinner's theory of operant conditioning, emphasizes the role of external rewards and punishments in shaping behavior. Skinner's theory posits that behavior can be modified through reinforcement—positive or negative. In gamification, this translates into using rewards (e.g., points, badges) to reinforce desired behaviors.

Case Study: Fitbit

Fitbit incorporates behaviorist principles by offering users tangible rewards, such as badges for achieving milestones. These rewards serve as positive reinforcement, encouraging users to maintain their physical activity levels. The app's gamified elements, including goal-setting features and progress tracking, help to keep users engaged and motivated.

3. Expectancy Theory

Expectancy Theory, proposed by Victor Vroom, asserts that individuals are motivated to act based on their expectations of outcomes. Motivation is influenced by the belief that effort will lead to desired performance and that this performance will result in rewards.

In gamification, Expectancy Theory is applied by designing systems where users believe their efforts will lead to success and rewards. For instance, digital health platforms that clearly outline pathways to rewards for completing tasks leverage Expectancy Theory to motivate users.

Case Study: Duolingo

Duolingo exemplifies Expectancy Theory through its goal setting and feedback mechanisms. Users earn points and advance through levels, which creates a clear link between their efforts and rewards. This structure enhances user motivation by making the connection between effort and success explicit.

3.2 Behavioral Economics and Its Application to Health Behavior Change

Behavioral economics integrates psychological insights with economic theory to understand decision-making. It challenges the notion of rationality in traditional economics, highlighting how cognitive biases and heuristics influence behavior. Key concepts from behavioral economics relevant to gamification include:

1. Loss Aversion

Loss aversion, a principle from behavioral economics, posits that losses are felt more intensely than gains of the same magnitude. This concept can be utilized in gamification by creating a sense of urgency or potential loss to motivate behavior.

Case Study: StickK

StickK employs loss aversion by allowing users to set personal goals with financial stakes. Users commit money to a goal, and if they fail to meet it, their money is donated to an undesired cause. This approach leverages the fear of losing money to drive adherence to goals, demonstrating the power of loss aversion in behavior change.

2. Nudge Theory

Nudge Theory, developed by Richard Thaler and Cass Sunstein, involves guiding people towards desirable behaviors without restricting their freedom of choice. Nudges can be implemented in gamification to subtly influence user behavior.

Case Study: Healthful

Healthful uses nudging techniques by sending personalized reminders and suggestions based on user behavior. By making healthy choices more visible and accessible, the platform nudges users towards better health practices without coercing them, thereby facilitating behavior change through subtle guidance.

3. Social Proof

Social proof refers to the influence of others' behaviors on individual choices. In gamification, social proof can be leveraged by showcasing user achievements and promoting social interaction.

Case Study: Charity Miles

Charity Miles uses social proof by displaying the total number of miles run or walked by users and their friends. This visibility encourages users to participate and contribute to charitable causes, driven by the desire to be part of a collective effort and to compare their achievements with others.

3.3 Linking Gamification to Design Thinking and User-Centric Design

1. Design Thinking

Design thinking is a problem-solving approach that emphasizes empathy, creativity, and iterative testing. It involves understanding users' needs, brainstorming solutions, prototyping, and testing. Gamification aligns with design thinking by focusing on creating engaging and effective experiences based on user insights.

Empathy and User Understanding

Incorporating empathy into gamification design involves understanding users' motivations, challenges, and preferences. By employing design thinking principles, gamification strategies can be tailored to address users' specific needs and enhance their experience.

Case Study: Zocdoc

Zocdoc, a medical appointment booking platform, uses design thinking to improve user experience. The platform's gamified features, such as reminders and incentives for booking and attending appointments, are designed based on user feedback and behavior analysis, demonstrating how empathy-driven design can enhance gamification effectiveness.

2. User-Centric Design

User-centric design focuses on creating products and experiences that prioritize users' needs and preferences. In gamification, this involves designing systems that are intuitive, engaging, and aligned with users' goals.

Personalization and Customization

Personalization is a key aspect of user-centric gamification. By tailoring experiences and rewards to individual preferences, gamification can become more relevant and motivating.

Case Study: Fitbit

Fitbit's user-centric design approach includes personalization features such as customizable goals, progress tracking, and social interactions. The platform allows users to set goals based on their fitness levels and preferences, enhancing motivation through a tailored experience.

3. Iterative Testing and Feedback

Design thinking advocates for iterative testing and feedback to refine solutions. In gamification, this means continuously evaluating and improving gamified elements based on user feedback and performance data.

Case Study: Habitica

Habitica employs iterative testing by regularly updating its features and gamified elements based on user feedback. This approach ensures that the platform remains engaging and effective in motivating users to complete tasks and achieve their goals.

The theoretical foundations of gamification for behavioral change are deeply rooted in psychological and motivational theories, as well as principles from behavioral economics. By understanding and applying concepts from Self-Determination Theory, behaviorism, Expectancy Theory, loss aversion, nudge theory, and social proof, designers can create effective gamification strategies that drive meaningful behavior change.

4. DESIGN ELEMENTS OF GAMIFIED HEALTH APPS

Gamified health apps are becoming increasingly important in the landscape of digital health, offering innovative ways to engage users and promote healthier behaviors. The design elements of these apps play a crucial role in their effectiveness. By integrating core game mechanics such as points, badges, leaderboards, and rewards, alongside advanced features like narratives, challenges, avatars, and social interaction, these apps can significantly enhance user engagement and motivation.

In this section, we'll delve into the various gamification features, how they influence positive user engagement and behavioral change, and the role of notifications in maintaining user involvement.

4.1 Core Game Mechanics: Points, Badges, Leaderboards, and Rewards

1. **Points**
   - **Concept**: Points are a fundamental game mechanic used to quantify users' achievements and progress. They serve as instant feedback for completing tasks or reaching milestones, providing a clear indicator of success.
   - **Influence on Engagement**: Points create a sense of accomplishment and motivation. Users are more likely to continue engaging with an app when they see tangible rewards for their efforts. This is particularly effective in health apps where consistent engagement is necessary for achieving long-term health goals. For example, apps like Fitbit use points to encourage daily physical activity, rewarding users for steps taken, calories burned, and active minutes.
   - **Behavioral Change**: The accumulation of points can trigger positive reinforcement, encouraging users to maintain or increase their efforts. This aligns with behavioral theories such as Operant Conditioning, where rewards reinforce desired behavior.
2. **Badges**
   - **Concept**: Badges are visual representations of achievements, earned by completing specific tasks or reaching certain milestones. They often symbolize mastery, progress, or expertise in a particular area.

- o **Influence on Engagement**: Badges provide users with a sense of pride and accomplishment. They cater to the human desire for recognition and status. Apps like Duolingo utilize badges to mark language-learning milestones, which keeps users motivated to continue their lessons.
- o **Behavioral Change**: By setting specific goals that users must achieve to earn badges, apps can encourage consistent behavior. Badges also tap into the social aspect of gamification, as users often share their achievements within their community, further reinforcing the desired behavior through social recognition.

3. **Leaderboards**
   - o **Concept**: Leaderboards rank users based on their performance, often comparing them to their peers. They introduce a competitive element, encouraging users to outperform others to achieve a higher rank.
   - o **Influence on Engagement**: Leaderboards leverage the competitive nature of users, driving them to engage more frequently with the app to maintain or improve their ranking. This mechanic is particularly effective in social fitness apps like Strava, where users compete on running or cycling segments.
   - o **Behavioral Change**: Competition can be a strong motivator for behavior change. The desire to outperform others can push users to set higher personal goals, thus driving more significant behavioral improvements. However, it is essential to balance competitiveness with inclusivity to avoid discouraging lower-ranking users.
4. **Rewards**
   - o **Concept**: Rewards can take many forms, including tangible rewards (e.g., discounts, vouchers) and intangible rewards (e.g., virtual goods, access to premium features). They are given in recognition of user achievements or consistent engagement.
   - o **Influence on Engagement**: Rewards are powerful motivators, providing users with an incentive to continue using the app. The prospect of earning rewards can drive initial engagement, while the ongoing accumulation of rewards can sustain long-term usage. Health apps like Sweatcoin convert physical activity into digital currency, which can be redeemed for goods and services.
   - o **Behavioral Change**: Rewards can promote consistent engagement and help establish new habits. According to Self-Determination Theory (SDT), rewards can satisfy intrinsic motivators such as autonomy, competence, and relatedness, which are crucial for long-term behavior change.

4.2 Advanced Features: Narratives, Challenges, Avatars, and Social Interaction

1. **Narratives**
   - **Concept**: Narratives are stories or scenarios that provide context and meaning to users' actions within the app. They create a storyline that users can follow, making the experience more immersive and engaging.
   - **Influence on Engagement**: A compelling narrative can draw users into the app and keep them invested in their progress. For instance, apps like Zombies, Run! use a narrative of surviving a zombie apocalypse to motivate users to run, turning exercise into an exciting adventure.
   - **Behavioral Change**: Narratives can make mundane tasks more exciting, thereby increasing the likelihood of user engagement. They can also provide emotional resonance, making users feel more connected to their goals. This emotional connection can be crucial for sustaining long-term behavior change.
2. **Challenges**
   - **Concept**: Challenges are specific tasks or objectives that users must complete within a set timeframe. They can be individual or group-based, often involving a competitive element.
   - **Influence on Engagement**: Challenges introduce variety and a sense of urgency, keeping users engaged and motivated to meet the objectives. Apps like Nike Run Club use challenges to encourage users to achieve specific running goals within a community setting.
   - **Behavioral Change**: Challenges can help users push beyond their usual limits, leading to more significant health improvements. They can also foster a sense of accomplishment and boost self-efficacy, which is critical for maintaining long-term behavior change.
3. **Avatars**
   - **Concept**: Avatars are digital representations of the user, often customizable to reflect personal preferences. They serve as the user's identity within the app, providing a visual and interactive element to the experience.
   - **Influence on Engagement**: Avatars allow users to personalize their experience, making the app feel more tailored to their needs. This personalization can increase emotional investment in the app. For example, Habitica uses avatars to represent users in a gamified productivity app, where completing tasks helps the avatar grow stronger.
   - **Behavioral Change**: Avatars can help users visualize their progress and achievements, making the experience more tangible. They can also

promote a sense of responsibility and accountability, as users are often motivated to care for and improve their avatars by engaging with the app consistently.

4. **Social Interaction**
   - **Concept**: Social interaction features include the ability to connect with other users, share progress, and participate in group activities. These features leverage the social aspects of human behavior to enhance engagement.
   - **Influence on Engagement**: Social interaction can create a sense of community and support, which can be a powerful motivator for continued engagement. Apps like MyFitnessPal incorporate social features, allowing users to share their progress, encourage each other, and participate in community challenges.
   - **Behavioral Change**: Social support is a well-documented factor in behavior change, providing users with encouragement, accountability, and validation. The ability to connect with others on a similar journey can enhance motivation and increase the likelihood of sustained behavior change.

4.3 The Role of Notifications

- **Concept**: Notifications are alerts or messages sent to users to prompt interaction with the app. They can remind users of upcoming tasks, celebrate achievements, or provide encouragement.
- **Influence on Engagement**: Notifications serve as gentle nudges, bringing users back to the app and reminding them of their goals. When timed appropriately and crafted carefully, notifications can significantly boost engagement. However, excessive or poorly timed notifications can lead to user fatigue and disengagement.
- **Behavioral Change**: Notifications can help reinforce habits by providing timely reminders and encouraging consistent engagement. They can also provide real-time feedback and encouragement, which can be crucial for maintaining motivation. Apps like Headspace use notifications to remind users to meditate, offering tips and encouragement to help them stay on track with their mindfulness practice.

5. FUTURE TRENDS IN GAMIFICATION IN HEALTH APPS

As technology continues to evolve, so too will the gamification strategies employed in health apps. Here are some key future trends:

1. **Integration of Artificial Intelligence (AI)**: AI is set to play a crucial role in enhancing gamified health apps. By analyzing user behavior and preferences, AI can personalize the gamification experience, ensuring that the challenges, rewards, and feedback are tailored to the individual's needs. For instance, an AI-driven health app might adjust the difficulty level of a task based on the user's previous performance, or it might recommend specific activities that align with the user's health goals. The adaptive nature of AI can keep users engaged by providing a continuously evolving experience that feels both relevant and rewarding.
2. **Augmented Reality (AR) and Virtual Reality (VR) Experiences**: AR and VR have the potential to revolutionize the way users interact with gamified health apps. Imagine a fitness app that uses AR to turn your daily run into a treasure hunt, where you collect virtual rewards in real-world environments. VR, on the other hand, can create immersive environments for activities like meditation or therapy, making the experience more engaging and effective. These technologies can transform mundane health tasks into exciting and interactive experiences, significantly boosting user engagement.
3. **Wearable Technology Integration**: As wearable technology becomes more sophisticated, its integration with gamified health apps will become more seamless. Wearables like smartwatches and fitness trackers can provide real-time data that enhances the gamification experience. For example, a health app might use heart rate data from a smartwatch to adjust the intensity of a workout or to trigger in-app rewards when the user reaches a certain milestone. This integration can make the gamified experience more immediate and impactful, driving better health outcomes.
4. **Social and Community-Based Gamification**: Social interaction has always been a powerful motivator in gamification, and this trend is likely to grow. Future health apps might incorporate more community-based challenges, where users can collaborate or compete with others in real-time. This could include group fitness challenges, shared health goals, or even virtual support groups that offer both accountability and encouragement. The social aspect of gamification can foster a sense of belonging and motivate users to stay committed to their health goals.

5. **Behavioral Data Analytics**: As health apps gather more data on user behavior, they will be able to refine their gamification strategies to be more effective. Data analytics can identify which gamification elements work best for different types of users, allowing app developers to optimize the user experience. This data-driven approach can lead to more personalized and engaging gamification, ultimately improving user retention and health outcomes.

6. CHALLENGES AND PITFALLS OF GAMIFICATION IN HEALTH APPS

While gamification offers significant potential for enhancing user engagement in health apps, it also comes with its own set of challenges and ethical considerations.

1. **Risk of Disengagement**: One of the primary risks of gamification is the potential for user disengagement if the gamified elements are not carefully designed. For example, if the challenges are too difficult or the rewards are not perceived as valuable, users may lose interest and stop using the app.
2. **Overemphasis on Rewards**: While rewards can be a powerful motivator, an overemphasis on extrinsic rewards (such as points, badges, or tangible incentives) can undermine intrinsic motivation. Users might become more focused on earning rewards than on achieving their actual health goals, leading to short-term engagement but long-term disengagement once the rewards are no longer compelling. Gamification in health apps, while motivational, poses safety risks such as overexertion, as highlighted by (Barratt, 2017) where users may push beyond their limits for rewards
3. **Ethical Considerations**: Gamification in health apps raises several ethical concerns, particularly around user data and privacy. For example, health apps that collect and analyze user data to personalize the gamification experience must ensure that this data is handled securely and transparently.
4. **Cultural Sensitivity**: Gamification elements that work well in one cultural context may not be effective or appropriate in another. For example, competitive leaderboards might motivate users in some cultures but could be seen as discouraging or alienating in others.
5. **Sustainability of Engagement**: Gamified health apps need to ensure that user engagement is sustainable over the long term. This involves continuously updating the content, challenges, and rewards to keep the experience fresh and engaging. However, this can be resource-intensive, requiring ongoing investment in content development and technology upgrades. Developers must plan for the

long-term sustainability of their gamification strategies to avoid user burnout and disengagement.

6. **Legal and Regulatory Compliance**: As health apps become more sophisticated in their use of gamification, they must navigate a complex landscape of legal and regulatory requirements. This includes ensuring that the gamified elements comply with healthcare regulations, such as those related to patient consent, data protection, and medical advice. Failure to comply with these regulations can result in legal repercussions and damage the app's reputation.

In conclusion, while gamification offers exciting opportunities for enhancing user engagement in health apps, it is not without its challenges. Developers must carefully consider the design, ethical, and regulatory aspects of gamification to create experiences that are both effective and responsible. As technology continues to advance, the future of gamification in health apps looks promising, with AI, AR, and data analytics poised to take user engagement to new heights. However, the success of these innovations will depend on their ability to address the complex needs and preferences of users in a sustainable and ethical manner.

7. STRATEGIES FOR DESIGNING EFFECTIVE GAMIFIED HEALTH INTERVENTIONS

Designing effective gamified health interventions requires a careful balance between engaging users and promoting healthy behaviors. From an app developer or UI/UX designer standpoint, the process involves not only integrating gamification elements but also ensuring that these elements are user-centered, customizable, and aligned with the overall health goals of the app. This section will explore critical success factors, decision-making criteria, and a template plan for incorporating these features into health apps.

7.1 User-Centered Design Principles

User-centered design (UCD) is at the heart of successful gamified health interventions. UCD is a design philosophy that prioritizes the needs, preferences, and limitations of the end-users throughout the development process. For health apps, this means creating an experience that is both engaging and accessible, encouraging sustained use and promoting positive health outcomes.

1. **Understanding the User's Needs and Context**: The first step in UCD is understanding the user's needs, motivations, and the context in which they will use the app. This involves conducting thorough user research, including surveys, interviews, and observational studies. For instance, a weight loss app might target users who are motivated by social interaction and competition. In this case, features like leaderboards and social challenges would be appropriate. However, if the app is targeting individuals with chronic conditions who may be more focused on long-term health outcomes, features like progress tracking and personalized feedback would be more relevant.
2. **Iterative Design and Testing**: UCD is an iterative process, meaning that designers should continuously test and refine their designs based on user feedback. This can be done through usability testing, where users interact with prototypes of the app, allowing designers to identify and address any usability issues. For example, if users find a particular gamification feature confusing or unengaging, designers can modify or replace it to better meet user needs.
3. **Accessibility and Inclusivity**: Health apps must be accessible to a wide range of users, including those with disabilities or limited technological literacy. This involves designing the app to be compatible with assistive technologies, such as screen readers, and ensuring that the interface is intuitive and easy to navigate. Inclusivity also means considering the cultural and linguistic diversity of users, ensuring that the app is relevant and engaging for all target demographics.

7.2 Customization and Personalization of Gamified Experiences

Customization and personalization are key to creating engaging and effective gamified health interventions. These strategies involve tailoring the app's content and features to individual users, making the experience more relevant and motivating.

1. **Personalized Content and Challenges**: Personalized content is essential for maintaining user engagement over time. This could include personalized health goals, tailored challenges, and individualized feedback. For instance, a fitness app might offer personalized workout plans based on the user's fitness level, goals, and preferences. As the user progresses, the app could adjust the difficulty level of the challenges to keep them motivated and prevent burnout.
2. **Adaptive Gamification**: Adaptive gamification involves dynamically adjusting the gamification elements based on the user's behavior and preferences. For example, if a user consistently completes challenges early in the day, the app could introduce morning-specific rewards or challenges. Similarly, if a user struggles with a particular type of task, the app could offer alternative activi-

ties that are more aligned with their strengths. This approach ensures that the gamification experience remains engaging and aligned with the user's abilities and motivations.

3. **User-Generated Content and Social Features**: Allowing users to customize and create content can significantly enhance engagement. For example, a mental health app might allow users to create their own mindfulness challenges or share their progress with a community of users. Social features, such as peer support and competition, can also be customized to align with the user's preferences. For instance, some users might prefer collaborative challenges, while others might be more motivated by competition.
4. **Notifications and Reminders**: Notifications play a crucial role in keeping users engaged with the app. However, they must be carefully designed to avoid being intrusive or annoying. Personalized notifications, such as reminders to complete a challenge or updates on progress, can be effective in maintaining user engagement. The timing and frequency of notifications should also be customizable, allowing users to choose how and when they want to receive updates.

7.3 Plan for Incorporating Gamification Features

To effectively incorporate gamification features into health apps, developers and designers can follow a structured plan. Below is a template plan that outlines the key steps in this process:

1. **Define the Target Audience and Health Goals**: Begin by clearly defining the target audience for the app and the specific health goals the app aims to achieve. This could include goals like increasing physical activity, improving mental health, or managing chronic conditions. Understanding the user's motivations and barriers to achieving these goals is crucial for designing effective gamification features.
2. **Conduct User Research**: Conduct user research to gather insights into the target audience's needs, preferences, and behaviors. This could involve surveys, interviews, and focus groups. The findings from this research will inform the design of the gamification features, ensuring that they are aligned with the user's needs.
3. **Select Gamification Features**: Based on the user research, select the gamification features that are most likely to engage and motivate the target audience. For example, if the research indicates that users are motivated by social interaction, features like leaderboards and social challenges might be appropriate. If users are more focused on personal growth, features like progress tracking and personalized feedback could be more effective.

4. **Design and Prototype**: Design the user interface (UI) and user experience (UX) of the app, incorporating the selected gamification features. Create prototypes of the app and conduct usability testing with real users to identify any issues or areas for improvement.
5. **Implement Adaptive Gamification**: Develop the app with adaptive gamification in mind, allowing the gamification features to adjust based on the user's behavior and preferences. This could involve using AI to analyze user data and dynamically adjust the challenges, rewards, and feedback.
6. **Incorporate Personalization and Customization**: Ensure that the app allows for a high degree of personalization and customization. This could include personalized health goals, tailored challenges, and customizable notifications. Allow users to adjust the gamification features to suit their preferences and needs.
7. **Test and Iterate**: Continuously test the app with real users, gathering feedback and making adjustments as needed. This iterative process is crucial for ensuring that the app remains engaging and effective over time.
8. **Launch and Monitor**: Once the app is launched, monitor user engagement and health outcomes. Use data analytics to track how users are interacting with the gamification features and make adjustments as needed to optimize the experience.
9. **Refine and Update**: Based on user feedback and data analytics, continue to refine and update the gamification features. This could involve adding new challenges, updating the UI, or introducing new personalization options.

8. METRICS AND METHODS FOR EVALUATING THE EFFECTIVENESS OF GAMIFIED INTERVENTIONS

Gamification, when applied effectively, can significantly enhance user engagement, motivation, and ultimately, health outcomes. However, to ensure that these interventions are indeed producing the desired effects, it's crucial to establish robust metrics and methods for evaluating their effectiveness. This section will explore the key performance indicators (KPIs) that should be considered when assessing the impact of gamification in health apps, outline industry benchmarks for these metrics, and provide an evaluation strategy for continuous improvement.

1. User Engagement Metrics:

User engagement is one of the primary indicators of the success of a gamified health app. Metrics in this category help determine how often users interact with the app and the duration of these interactions.

- **Active Users:** Track the number of daily active users (DAU) and monthly active users (MAU). These metrics indicate how many users are consistently engaging with the app.
- **Session Duration:** Measure the average time spent per session, which can reflect how engaging the content and activities are.
- **Frequency of Use:** Assess how frequently users return to the app over a specific period, such as daily or weekly.
- **Retention Rate:** Calculate the percentage of users who continue to use the app over time. High retention rates typically indicate that the app provides sustained value to its users.

2. Behavioral Change Metrics:

The ultimate goal of many gamified health apps is to drive positive behavioral change. Metrics in this category help assess whether the gamified elements lead to the desired actions.

- **Goal Achievement:** Monitor the percentage of users who achieve their health-related goals, such as weight loss, increased physical activity, or improved medication adherence.
- **Completion Rates:** Evaluate the percentage of users who complete specific tasks or challenges within the app. High completion rates often indicate that the tasks are appropriately challenging and rewarding.
- **Behavioral Adherence:** Track the consistency with which users follow recommended behaviors, such as taking medication on time or following a prescribed exercise routine.

3. Health Outcomes Metrics:

To measure the direct impact of gamification on health outcomes, it’s important to track changes in users' health status over time.

- **Biometric Data:** Collect data on key health indicators such as blood pressure, blood glucose levels, or body weight. Improvements in these metrics can suggest that the app is effectively supporting users in managing their health.
- **Self-Reported Health Status:** Utilize surveys or self-assessment tools within the app to gather users' perceptions of their health and well-being.

- **Clinical Outcomes:** If the app is integrated with healthcare providers, track clinical outcomes such as reduced hospital visits or improved disease management.

4. User Satisfaction Metrics:

User satisfaction is a crucial determinant of the app's long-term success. Metrics in this category assess how satisfied users are with the app's features and overall experience.

- **Net Promoter Score (NPS):** Measure users' likelihood to recommend the app to others. A high NPS indicates strong user satisfaction and loyalty.
- **User Feedback:** Collect qualitative feedback through surveys, reviews, or in-app messaging to gain insights into users' likes, dislikes, and suggestions for improvement.
- **App Store Ratings:** Monitor ratings and reviews in app stores as an external measure of user satisfaction.

8.1 Data-Driven Insights and Feedback Loops

To continually enhance the effectiveness of gamified health interventions, it's essential to leverage data-driven insights and establish feedback loops. This process involves collecting and analyzing data, applying the insights to improve the app, and then reassessing the impact of those improvements.

1. Data Collection:
    - **Automated Tracking:** Implement automated tracking tools to gather data on user interactions, health outcomes, and satisfaction in real-time. This allows for continuous monitoring and quick identification of issues.
    - **Surveys and Polls:** Use surveys and polls to gather additional qualitative data from users. This can provide deeper insights into user motivations and experiences that may not be captured through automated tracking.
2. Data Analysis:
    - **Predictive Analytics:** Apply predictive analytics to identify patterns and trends in user behavior. This can help anticipate which users might be at risk of disengagement and which gamification strategies are most effective.

- **A/B Testing:** Conduct A/B testing to compare the effectiveness of different gamification features. For example, test the impact of different reward systems (e.g., points versus badges) on user engagement.

3. Feedback Loops:
   - **Iterative Design:** Use the insights gained from data analysis to make iterative improvements to the app. For example, if a certain challenge is found to be too difficult, it can be adjusted to better match user abilities.
   - **Personalization:** Apply feedback loops to enhance the personalization of the app. For instance, if users consistently skip certain types of activities, the app can offer alternative challenges that better align with their preferences.

8.2 Industry Benchmarks for Measuring Effectiveness

When evaluating the effectiveness of gamified health interventions, it can be helpful to compare your metrics against industry benchmarks. These benchmarks provide a standard for assessing whether your app's performance is on par with, or exceeds, industry norms.

1. Engagement Benchmarks:
   - **Retention Rates:** According to popular industry reports, the average retention rate for mobile apps is about 25% after 30 days. Health apps should aim to meet or exceed this benchmark, with a target retention rate of at least 30-35% after one month.
   - **Session Duration:** The average session duration for health apps varies widely depending on the type of app, but a benchmark of 5-10 minutes per session is often cited as a reasonable target.
2. Behavioral Change Benchmarks:
   - **Goal Achievement:** Studies have shown that well-designed gamified interventions can lead to a 20-30% increase in goal achievement rates. Apps should aim to match or exceed this benchmark.
   - **Adherence Rates:** In clinical contexts, adherence rates of 50-60% are often considered acceptable. However, gamified apps should strive for adherence rates of 70% or higher.
3. User Satisfaction Benchmarks:
   - **NPS:** A Net Promoter Score of 30 or higher is generally considered good for health apps. However, leading apps often achieve NPS scores of 50 or above.
   - **App Store Ratings:** Aim for an average app store rating of 4.5 stars or higher, as this indicates strong user satisfaction.

9. CASE STUDIES OF SUCCESSFUL GAMIFIED APPS (INCLUDING HEALTH & WELLNESS)

This section analyzes few successful gamified health apps, exploring their impact on user behavior and the lessons learned from their implementations.

Table 1. Comparison of Gamified Apps

App Name	Core Features	Impact on Engagement	Behavioral Change Outcomes	Key Takeaways
Fitbit	Step tracking, leaderboards	Increased daily activity by 20%	Sustained physical activity habits	Gamification enhances social motivation
MyFitnessPal	Points for logging meals	Boosted meal tracking adherence by 25%	Improved diet quality	Rewards-based systems drive adherence
Zombies, Run!	Narrative-based exercise gamification	Doubled weekly running consistency	Enhanced cardiovascular health	Narratives create immersive engagement
Mango Health	Medication adherence rewards	Reduced missed doses by 35%	Improved chronic condition management	Reward systems improve adherence
Headspace	Meditation streaks, badges	Increased daily usage by 30%	Improved mental health outcomes	Habit formation through streaks
Strava	Community challenges, leaderboards	Boosted exercise frequency among users	Improved fitness levels	Social competition fosters consistency
Pact	Financial incentives for fitness	Increased activity compliance	Positive health behavior change	Financial stakes motivate commitment
Happify	Positive psychology games	Improved mood metrics among users	Reduced symptoms of depression	Games support mental health outcomes
SuperBetter	Gamified mental resilience tasks	Increased completion rates for mental health goals	Strengthened coping mechanisms	Gamification aids emotional well-being
Sweatcoin	Rewards for steps	Boosted step count by 25%	Increased daily activity	Tangible rewards drive engagement

By understanding the successes and challenges of these apps, future gamified health applications can build on established strategies while addressing potential limitations.

10. BEST PRACTICES FOR FOSTERING ENGAGEMENT AND LONG-TERM ADHERENCE IN GAMIFIED HEALTH APPS

As we conclude this chapter on gamification in healthcare, it's essential to reflect on the best practices that can foster user engagement and promote long-term adherence. The ultimate goal of gamified health apps is not only to captivate users in the short term but also to drive sustained behavioral change that leads to improved health outcomes. Achieving this requires a careful balance of motivational design, human-centered principles, and a deep understanding of the factors that influence user behavior in digital health.

10.1 Motivational Design: The Key to Sustained Engagement

At the heart of any successful gamified health app is a robust motivational design. This design should tap into intrinsic motivators—such as the desire for mastery, autonomy, and relatedness—while also leveraging extrinsic motivators like rewards and recognition.

1. **Personalized Rewards:** One of the most effective ways to maintain user interest is through personalized rewards that are meaningful and relevant to each user. These can range from digital badges and points to tangible incentives like discounts on health services. However, it's crucial that these rewards align with the user's personal goals and values. For instance, a fitness app might offer different rewards based on whether the user is motivated by competition, self-improvement, or social interaction.
2. **Balanced Challenge and Skill:** The challenge-skill balance is another critical element of motivational design. To keep users engaged, the app must present challenges that are neither too easy nor too difficult. This balance ensures that users remain in a state of "flow," where they are fully immersed and motivated by the task at hand. Regularly updating and adjusting the difficulty of tasks based on user progress is essential for maintaining this state.
3. **Progress Feedback:** Immediate and clear feedback is vital in gamification. Providing users with real-time insights into their progress reinforces positive behavior and helps them understand the impact of their actions. This feedback can be visualized through progress bars, achievements, or even narrative elements that evolve as the user progresses.

10.2 Human Factors in Digital Health Design

Human factors play a crucial role in the design of gamified health apps. Understanding the psychological, cognitive, and emotional needs of users is essential for creating an experience that is not only engaging but also supportive of long-term behavior change.

1. **User-Centered Design:** A user-centered approach ensures that the app is designed with the end-user's needs, preferences, and limitations in mind. This involves conducting thorough user research, including interviews, surveys, and usability testing, to gather insights into what motivates and frustrates users.
2. **Customization and Flexibility:** Offering customization options allows users to tailor the app to their specific needs and preferences. This can include the ability to choose from different types of challenges, set personal goals, and adjust the frequency of notifications. Flexibility in how users interact with the app—such as through different devices or in various environments—also enhances the user experience and supports long-term adherence.
3. **Emotional Engagement:** Incorporating elements that evoke positive emotions—such as humor, storytelling, and community—can strengthen the user's connection to the app. For example, incorporating avatars or narratives that users can relate to or that evolve with their progress can create a sense of companionship and emotional investment. This emotional engagement is critical for sustaining motivation over time.

11. FINAL THOUGHTS: THE FUTURE OF GAMIFICATION IN DIGITAL HEALTH

Gamification in healthcare represents a convergence of behavioral psychology, technology, and patient-centered design. By leveraging game mechanics to drive engagement and adherence, gamified health apps have the potential to transform health outcomes at both individual and population levels. However, successful implementation requires careful consideration of user diversity, ethical concerns, and ongoing innovation.

As healthcare evolves into its next phase, integrating gamification with AI, AR, and machine learning will define the future of digital health. Developers and policymakers must collaborate to ensure these tools are accessible, effective, and equitable. The chapter concludes by urging stakeholders to embrace gamification as a key strategy in the journey toward Healthcare 6.0—an era defined by personalized, engaging, and impactful health solutions.

REFERENCES

Aseel Berglund, T. J. (2022). Understanding and assessing gamification in digital healthcare interventions for patients with cardiovascular disease. *European Journal of Cardiovascular Nursing*, *21*(6), 630–638. DOI: 10.1093/eurjcn/zvac048 PMID: 35709297

Barratt, P. (2017). A qualitative study investigating persuasive technologies and the gamification of cycling. *Health & Place*, *46*, 328–336. DOI: 10.1016/j.healthplace.2016.09.009 PMID: 28029434

Brown, T. (2008). Design thinking. *Harvard Business Review*, *86*(6), 84–92. https://hbr.org/2008/06/design-thinking PMID: 18605031

Charity Miles. (n.d.). Social proof in action. Retrieved from https://www.charitymiles.org

Deci, E. L., & Ryan, R. M. (2000). The "what" and "why" of goal pursuits: Human needs and the self-determination of behavior. *Psychological Inquiry*, *11*(4), 227–268. DOI: 10.1207/S15327965PLI1104_01

Deterding, S., Dixon, D., Khaled, R., & Nacke, L. (2011). From game design elements to gamefulness: Defining "gamification." *Proceedings of the 15th International Academic MindTrek Conference: Envisioning Future Media Environments* (pp. 9–15). ACM. https://doi.org/DOI: 10.1145/2181037.2181040

Duolingo, Inc. (n.d.). Duolingo: Learn languages for free. Retrieved from https://www.duolingo.com

Fast Company. (2016, January 12). This app turns exercise into charitable donations. *Fast Company*. Retrieved from https://www.fastcompany.com/3064854/this-app-turns-exercise-into-charitable-donations

Forbes. (2021, September 16). How Noom's gamification strategy is revolutionizing weight loss. *Forbes*. Retrieved from https://www.forbes.com/sites/forbestechcouncil/2021/09/16/how-nooms-gamification-strategy-is-revolutionizing-weight-loss

Garett, R. Y., & Young, S. D. (2019, September 1). Health Care Gamification: A Study of Game Mechanics and Elements. *Tech Know Learn*, *24*(3), 341–353. DOI: 10.1007/s10758-018-9353-4

Habitica. (n.d.). Gamification for daily tasks. Retrieved from https://habitica.com

Hamari, J., Koivisto, J., & Sarsa, H. (2014). Does gamification work? – A literature review of empirical studies on gamification. *Proceedings of the 47th Hawaii International Conference on System Sciences* (pp. 3025–3034). IEEE. https://doi.org/DOI: 10.1109/HICSS.2014.377

Healthful. (n.d.). Nudging towards better health. Retrieved from https://www.healthfulapp.com

Healthline. (n.d.). Gamification in wellness apps. *Healthline*. Retrieved from https://www.healthline.com/health/gamification-in-wellness-apps

Johnson, D., Deterding, S., Kuhn, K.-A., Staneva, A., Stoyanov, S., & Hides, L. (2016). Gamification for health and wellbeing: A systematic review of the literature. *Internet Interventions : the Application of Information Technology in Mental and Behavioural Health*, *6*, 89–106. DOI: 10.1016/j.invent.2016.10.002 PMID: 30135818

Maguire, M. (2001). Methods to support human-centered design. *International Journal of Human-Computer Studies*, *55*(4), 587–634. DOI: 10.1006/ijhc.2001.0503

McGonigal, J. (2012). The game that can give you 10 extra years of life. *TED*. Retrieved from https://www.ted.com/talks/jane_mcgonigal_the_game_that_can_give_you_10_extra_years_of_life

Damaševičius, R., & M. R. 2023. Serious Games and Gamification in Healthcare:Meta-Review, A. (•••).. . *Information (Basel)*, *14*(2), 105. DOI: 10.3390/info14020105

MySugr. (n.d.). Rewards in diabetes management. Retrieved from https://www.mysugr.com

Norman, D. A. (2013). *The design of everyday things: Revised and expanded edition*. Basic Books.

Open, A. I. (2024). ChatGPT (Aug 2024 version) [Large language model]. Retrieved from https://chat.openai.com

Psychology Today. (2018, March). The impact of gamification on mental health. *Psychology Today*. Retrieved from https://www.psychologytoday.com/us/blog/mindful-anger/201803/the-impact-gamification-mental-health

Skinner, B. F. (1953). *Science and human behavior*. Macmillan.

Stick, K. (n.d.). Behavioral economics in action. Retrieved from https://www.stickk.com

Strava. (n.d.). Social interaction in fitness. Retrieved from https://www.strava.com

Sundar, S. S., & Marathe, S. S. (2010). Personalization vs. customization: The importance of agency, privacy, and power usage. *Human Communication Research, 36*(3), 298–322. DOI: 10.1111/j.1468-2958.2010.01377.x

Thaler, R. H., & Sunstein, C. R. (2008). *Nudge: Improving decisions about health, wealth, and happiness*. Yale University Press.

Vroom, V. H. (1964). *Work and motivation*. Wiley.

Werbach, K., & Hunter, D. (2012). *For the win: How game thinking can revolutionize your business*. Wharton Digital Press. Retrieved from https://books.google.com/books?hl=en&lr=&id=ywxq_c4XSHMC

Chapter 5
Adoption of Innovative Digital Technologies for Enhancing Health Financing

Jayathra Datla
https://orcid.org/0009-0002-9442-7680
IQVIA, India

Parul Goela
https://orcid.org/0009-0004-4699-4087
IQVIA, India

Tatjana Prenđa Trupec
https://orcid.org/0000-0003-1122-5443
Maastricht University, The Netherlands

ABSTRACT

Innovative technologies such as mobile applications, web platforms, digital payments, blockchain, big data analytics, and artificial intelligence can significantly enhance health financing functions like revenue raising, pooling, and service purchasing. Transformative impact of digital solutions include Kenya's M-TIBA platform, India's Ayushman Bharat Pradhan Mantri Jan Arogya Yojana, which uses a digital Transaction Management System to support the entire patient journey from registration to claims payment, and Estonia's e-invoicing system. Successful implementation requires a robust digital ecosystem encompassing governance, infrastructure, and skilled human resources. This involves establishing dedicated digital health departments, developing regulatory frameworks, and ensuring data

DOI: 10.4018/979-8-3693-7210-4.ch005

security and interoperability. Moreover, it is crucial to address challenges such as technology access inequities and weak health systems to maximize the benefits of digital health financing.

INTRODUCTION

Universal health coverage (UHC) integrates equitable service utilization, high-quality care, and financial protection for those in need. It represents the ideal scenario where everyone can access necessary health services of adequate quality without facing financial hardship (WHO, 2019). Emphasizing the various financial risks and trade-offs individuals encounter when planning and seeking health services, financial protection is a critical component of UHC. Despite its importance, UHC remains out of reach for many as half of the global population lacks access to essential health services. Annually, 800 million people allocate at least 10 percent of their household budget to healthcare expenses, and 100 million people are driven into extreme poverty due to these costs (World Bank and WHO: Half the World Lacks Access to Essential Health Services, 100 Million Still Pushed Into Extreme Poverty Because of Health Expenses, 2017). There is an urgent need for solutions that can enhance population health coverage, improve the efficiency of health service delivery, and reduce healthcare costs. Gaps in existing social health protection schemes due to insufficient funding, lack of awareness, and difficulties in identifying eligible beneficiaries impede access to quality care services.

Advancements in digital technology and the widespread adoption of mobile phones and the Internet worldwide present significant opportunities to accelerate progress towards UHC. By 2025, the global unique mobile subscriber penetration rate is projected to increase from 67 to 70 percent, with a compound annual growth rate of 1.9 percent (The Mobile Economy, GSMA, 2020). Even more notable is the anticipated 4.6 percent growth rate among mobile Internet users, expected to rise from 49 percent to 61 percent of the global population (The Mobile Economy, GSMA, 2020). This rapid expansion in technology access and use has facilitated greater inclusion in the global economy and highlights individuals' readiness to adopt digital technologies. The potential of digital financing tools in healthcare was particularly evident during the COVID-19 pandemic. Now is the time to build on this momentum to strengthen digital health financing strategies and adopt innovative models. These efforts will address existing gaps and advance towards UHC by enabling efficient health financing, beneficiary identification, and improved access to quality healthcare. As healthcare 6.0 is focused on delivering value-based care through emerging and innovative technologies, it is essential for those who are part of healthcare industry to have an overview of various digital health financing models and innovative practices that are currently in place. Hence this chapter explores the arena of digital health financing, presenting global examples of innovative practices adopted by various countries and its significance in future.

DIGITAL HEALTH FINANCING ARENA

Digital health financing applies the technologies and business models of financial inclusion to achieve UHC goals, resulting in increased access to and affordability of high-quality care for everyone. These technologies include a wide range of data analysis tools, mobile applications, web platforms, digital payments, blockchain, big data analytics, and artificial intelligence (including machine learning). Such technologies can be used in supporting and optimizing core health financing functions, i.e. revenue raising, pooling, and the purchasing of services (Stahl et al., 2021). Figure 1 illustrates the integration of various aspects of health financing & digital technology.

Figure 1. Integration of Health Financing & Digital Technology

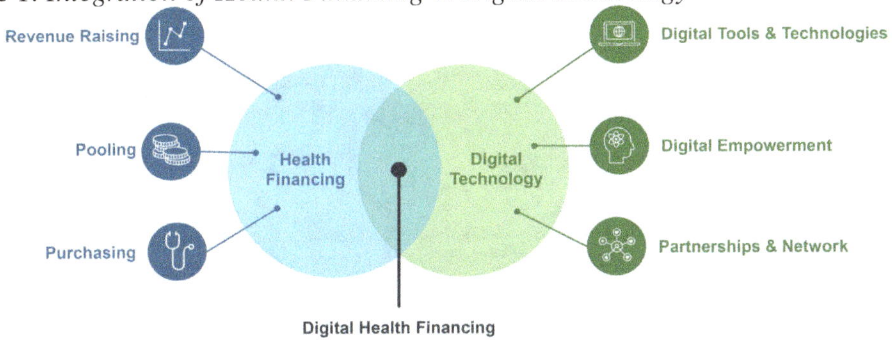

Source: (Stahl et al., 2021)

For each of these core functions there are several scenarios where digital technologies can make considerable impact. For instance, revenue-raising through mobile applications for health insurance payments, as part of mobile wallet services can significantly increase revenue collection, particularly in rural areas, while reducing transaction, opportunity, and administrative costs. Also, the pooling function in health financing can greatly benefit from interoperable information management systems across different health coverage schemes. This interoperability allows for seamless data exchange and integration among various health insurance programs, creating a unified and comprehensive view of health financing. Furthermore, innovations in purchasing, including analytics supporting innovative payments in schemes for targeted incentives, automatic claims management, business intelligence, fraud detection and intelligent dashboards, transform purchasing into strategic purchasing. Maximum benefits of such emerging technologies can be reaped with the help of a robust digital health financing ecosystem. This ecosystem encompasses efficient digital services and involves key stakeholders, including beneficiaries, service providers and payers. It relies on strong infrastructure and stringent regulations to function effectively (Development Asia, 2022). Figure 2 illustrates various components of digital health financing ecosystem.

Figure 2. Digital health financing ecosystem

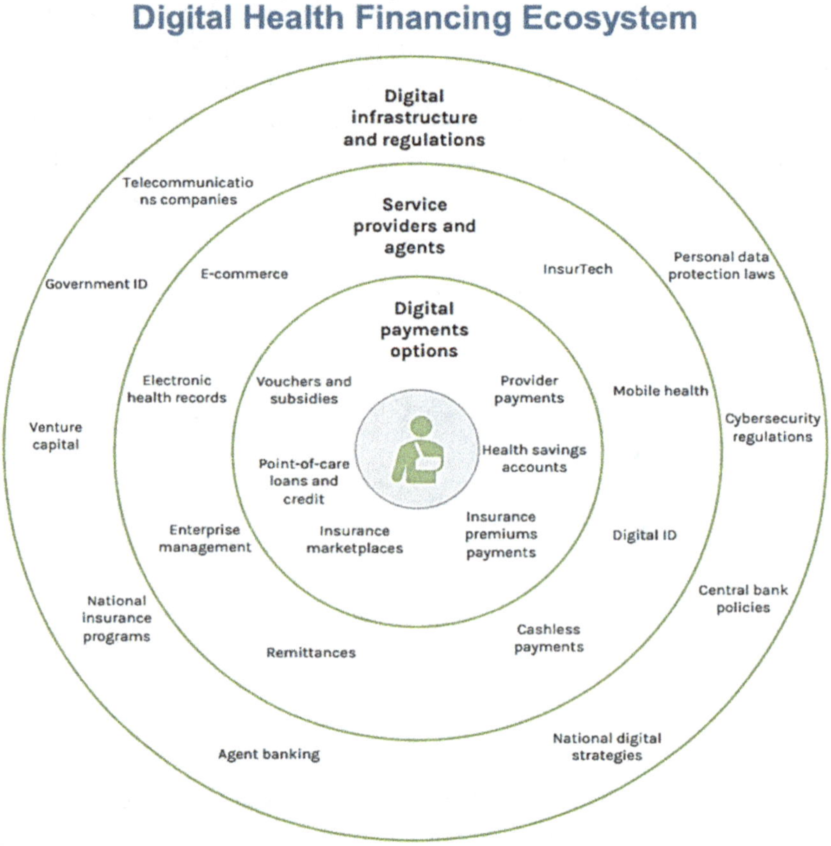

Source: (Development Asia, 2022)

ADVANTAGES OF ADOPTING DIGITAL TECHNOLOGIES IN HEALTH FINANCING

Digital technologies offer significant benefits in strengthening key aspects of health financing:

Improved Revenue Raising

Mobile applications and online platforms streamline easier payments, thereby encouraging greater participation in healthcare funding.

Enhanced Pooling

Digital technologies support managing and merging of pools, enhance risk equalization and adjustment mechanisms like "cherry picking", and harmonize benefits and payment rates through improved linkages and interoperability across various schemes.

Efficient Service Purchasing

Intelligent dashboards provide advanced visualization and analysis of financial data, facilitating better public financial management, budget allocation, and targeted budget execution by enabling informed decision-making pertaining to type the of services, providers, and costs/incentives.

Informed Decisions Making

Digital technologies enable the integration of diverse data sources, significantly enhancing decision-making. By unifying electronic health records, financial systems, and demographic databases, these technologies create a comprehensive data ecosystem that supports sophisticated analytics and real-time insights. This integration improves resource allocation, risk management, and policy making by providing a holistic view of healthcare information. Additionally, it fosters better communication among stakeholders and facilitates evidence-based decision-making, leading to more effective and efficient health financing systems as well as improved management of health systems and public health interventions (Aijli, 2021). Figure 3 illustrates the efficiency of digital technologies in enabling the integration of diverse data sources to promote informed decision making.

Figure 3. Integration of data sources to promote informed decision making

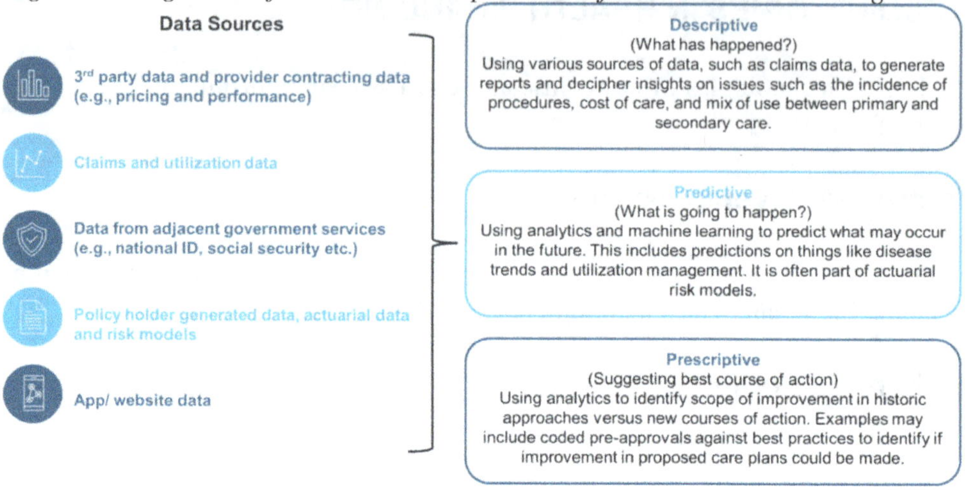

Source: (Aijli, 2021)

ADDED VALUE OF DIGITAL TECHNOLOGIES IN HEALTH FINANCING

There are many opportunities for digitization at almost every point in the health financing value chain. Social protection schemes/ public health insurance schemes are crucial aspects of health financing that ensure financial protection of the population by safeguarding them from catastrophic health expenditures. Few of such initiatives include:

E- Wallets

Digital savings wallets that facilitate easy healthcare payments between patient, payer and provider. They also facilitate aggregated payments from multiple payers and subsidization of healthcare expenses (co-payments).

Digital Lending

Loans that are dispersed and managed through digital channels for healthcare expenditure are considered as part of digital lending process. Digital systems adopt alternative risk scoring methods that allow patients, clinics, and pharmacies to access advanced loans without credits.

Direct Benefits Transfer

Payments made directly from the government or donor to beneficiaries. E-vouchers are issued or accessed to pay for specific healthcare services. Digital technologies enable efficient identification of beneficiaries and their coverage schemes or applied benefits packages for prompt disbursement of payments.

Insurtech

Insurtech uses technological innovations to enhance savings and efficiency within the insurance industry. The term combines "insurance" and "technology," referring to any insurance product that is applied for, purchased, claimed against, or reimbursed digitally. Insurtech plays a crucial role in the end-to-end digitalization of the beneficiary journey under social health insurance schemes.

For example, digital technologies can strengthen beneficiary databases by enabling the interoperability of data sources during the beneficiary identification process. To facilitate beneficiary eligibility verification, these technologies can link with unique national IDs or use advanced techniques such as biometric authentication. In claims management, AI-based digital platforms with built-in mechanisms can identify and flag suspicious claims, improving verification efficiency and reducing human error. Interoperability across systems also enables faster turnaround times and prompt payments. Real-time analytical dashboards enable stringent monitoring. Adopting digital technologies enhances operational efficiency and ensures transparency throughout the process.

CHALLENGES TO OVERCOME

Implementing digital health technologies in developing regions encounters several challenges, stemming from various factors such as limited access and experience with technology, inadequate internet connectivity, insufficient training and literacy, cultural and trust issues, integration with existing systems (including health literacy and digital health literacy), concerns about long-term viability and alignment with Universal Health Coverage (UHC) objectives, and dependency on external support.

Limited Access and Experience with Technology

While high mobile phone coverage can facilitate the implementation of digital health initiatives, limited access to mobile phones/digital platforms in certain areas remains a significant barrier. For example, in Madagascar, the rollout of mobile health wallets was slowed because only few users had prior experience with mobile payment technologies (Muller et al., 2019). This lack of familiarity with mobile technologies and low digital literacy levels can hinder successful implementation and uptake of new digital health solutions.

Internet Connectivity

Inadequate internet infrastructure is another major impediment to the use of digital health technologies. For instance, users of the Accredited Social Health Activists (ASHAs)-soft system in India often had to travel long distances to access internet services necessary for data entry (Meena et al., 2020). This lack of easy internet access can lead to delays and decreased efficiency in implementing digital health systems.

Training and Literacy

The successful adoption of digital health technologies requires adequate training for users, including health workers, pharmacists, and patients. Insufficient orientation and training can lead to confusion and slow adoption rates. For example, some ASHA in India struggled to use the ASHA-soft system even after receiving training (Meena et al., 2020). Moreover, high illiteracy rates among target populations can further prevent the effective use of digital health solutions, as seen with the mobile health wallets in Madagascar, where low literacy levels hindered user engagement (Muller et al., 2019).

Integration with Existing Systems

Interoperability challenges often arise when trying to integrate digital solutions with existing health system structures and data systems. These difficulties can impede the seamless implementation of new technologies, leading to inefficiencies and reduced effectiveness of health interventions. Ensuring that new digital health systems can work smoothly with existing infrastructure is essential for their success.

Data Security and Privacy Concerns

These challenges include data breaches, unauthorized access, ransomware attacks, and the potential misuse of sensitive patient information on digital platforms. Identifying and understanding these threats is vital for developing effective strategies to protect patient privacy and ensure data integrity.

Long-Term Viability and Alignment with UHC Objectives

For digital health technologies to support UHC effectively, they need to align with the goals of equity and efficiency. Digitally supported financing projects that focus on individual mobilization and purchasing may not align with UHC objectives, which require prepayment mechanisms and pooled funds for cross-subsidization. A lack of focus on population-level efforts may limit the potential of digital solutions to support UHC comprehensively.

Dependency on External Support

The sustainability of digital health initiatives can be compromised if they are overly reliant on donor support rather than being locally driven. For instance, in Tanzania's novel purchasing approach, success was threatened due to heavy dependency on external support (Hamad, 2019). Locally driven initiatives tend to be more sustainable and better aligned with the needs and capacities of the communities they serve.

Cultural and Trust Issues

Cultural barriers and trust issues also play a significant role in the acceptance of digital health technologies. In Madagascar, cultural reluctance towards new technologies and financial services limited the adoption of mobile health wallets (Muller et al., 2019). Additionally, issues such as mismanagement and corruption, including demands for bribes to enter data, can undermine trust and hinder the implementation of digital health initiatives. Building trust within communities is crucial for the successful deployment of these technologies.

In nut-shell, while digital health technologies hold great potential for improving health outcomes, especially in developing regions, numerous challenges must be addressed to ensure their successful implementation and sustainability. These include improving access to technology, enhancing internet connectivity, providing adequate training, improving awareness & communication, overcoming cultural and trust barriers, ensuring interoperability with existing systems and establishing stringent regulation for data privacy & security, aligning with UHC objectives, and reducing dependency on external support.

COUNTRY CASE STUDIES

Several countries have successfully adopted innovative digital technologies to enhance their health financing ecosystems. For instance, Kenya utilizes mobile applications for efficient healthcare fund management, while Estonia has implemented e- invoicing systems. In India, online platforms ensure the efficiency of scheme operations and transparency throughout the patient journey. Tonga has created an enabling environment to leverage digital technologies. Detailed examples of these practices are provided below, serving as best practices for other countries facing similar challenges or requirements.

M-TIBA-Kenya

A major challenge for many countries in Africa—and globally—is attracting capital and resources to meet healthcare needs. In nations with large formal sectors, healthcare financing often includes employer-based insurance schemes. However, in countries with significant informal sectors, these approaches are inadequate. Such countries need to develop community-based strategies for raising and utilizing health funds and promoting timely healthcare utilization.

An exemplary innovation is M-TIBA in Kenya, implemented nationally in 2015, has transformed the health financing landscape through community-driven health funding and utilization. FinTech and payments administrator CarePay, in partnership with Safaricom, and PharmAccess, developed M-TIBA (M-TIBA Is Truly Leapfrogging Healthcare in Kenya, n.d.).

M-TIBA (where "M" stands for 'Mobile' and "Tiba" means 'Care' in Swahili) allows users to enroll in the NHIF (National Health Insurance Fund), the national health scheme in Kenya. Governments and donors can use M-TIBA to top up individuals' health savings accounts, allowing for the identification of vulnerable groups and enabling payers to allocate money or entitlements for treatment directly to users' mobile phones. In countries like Kenya, where out-of-pocket healthcare payments are significant (both formal and informal), M-TIBA serves as a reliable digital health financing tool and financial protector. Donors, employers, and insurers can also use M-TIBA to offer healthcare financing products, such as vouchers, managed funds, and low-cost hospital cash insurance, directly to specific segments of the Kenyan population (M-TIBA Is Truly Leapfrogging Healthcare in Kenya, n.d.).

Clinics can register healthcare claims and invoice patients on a tablet connected to the mobile platform, enabling quick claims payments. The collected data allows clinics to track patients, manage diseases, and monitor the quality of healthcare services and their financial income. The digital platform connects patients, payers, and healthcare providers at minimal transaction costs, benefiting all stakeholders.

Additional benefits include enhanced efficiency, transparency, and access to digitally generated data (Morgan, n.d.). Figure 4 illustrates the salient features of M-Tiba application.

Figure 4. Overview of M-TIBA

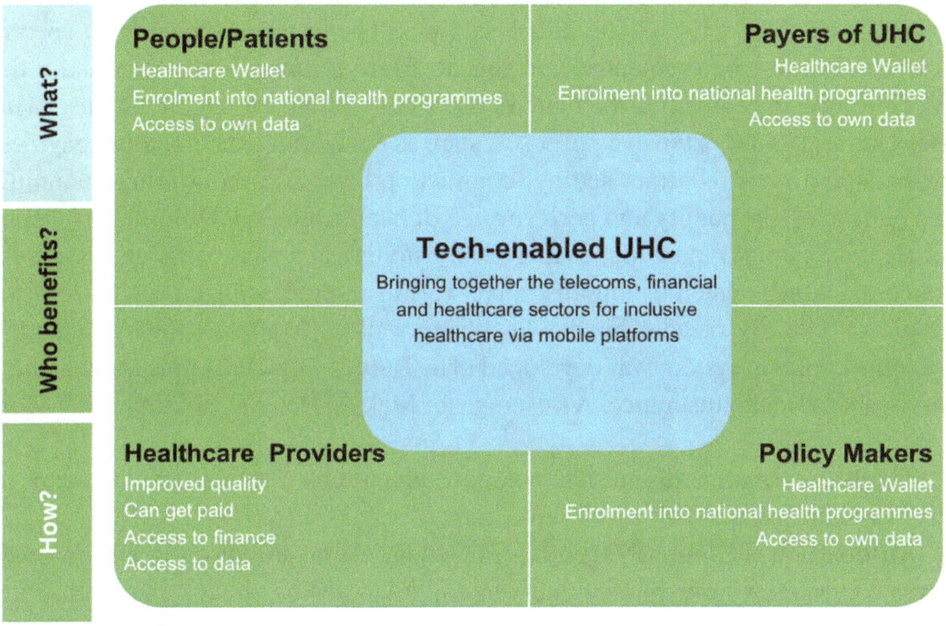

Source: (Morgan, n.d.)

Additionally, M-TIBA offers a variety of digital health services, including telemedicine consultations, medication reminders, and access to health information resources. M-tiba has more than 4.7 million registered users, 4,552 connected healthcare facilities, and over half a million medical treatments were provided to Kenyans. By leveraging technology and fostering collaboration, M-TIBA effectively addresses healthcare challenges in Kenya, leading to improved health outcomes, greater affordability, and enhanced access to healthcare services (Onkundi, 2023).

E-Invoicing System- Estonia

Estonia is a global leader in digital innovation, having made significant strides in digital health over the last 20 years. The country offers a wide range of online health tools and services, including electronic health records, national image archiving, e-consultations, e-prescriptions, and e-referrals. Estonia continuously improves and upgrades its digital health system, setting a benchmark for others to follow.

The Estonian Health Insurance Fund (EHIF) serves as the central entity for pooling public funds and procuring health services. The EHIF and healthcare providers have a contractual arrangement that governs purchasing of health services. Health insurance claims data base is primary source of information about essential functions involved in providing health services. The terms of the contract specify how claims must be completed and sent to EHIF (EInvoicing in Estonia, n.d.). While receiving payment is the main reason health providers submit claims, EHIF uses claims data for extensive purposes, such as developing and updating payment methods and rates, contract setting, contract/performance monitoring, planning, and enhancing the quality and performance of healthcare (WHO Barcelona Office for Health Systems Financing, 2023/2023). Estonia's claims processing system encountered issues related to administrative workload, processing errors, and delays, despite the country's leadership in e-health innovation. To address these challenges, a digital invoicing system was developed (The Role of Digital Claims Management for Estonia's Health Insurance: A Leverage for Making Healthcare Purchasing More Strategic, 2023).

The transformative digital technologies adopted by Estonia for enhancing its EHIF system are detailed below

Automation of Claims Processing. In Estonia, claims are automatically reviewed in the e-channel without human intervention before the payment stage. Claims undergo a life cycle that begins with submission via an e-channel, where automated checks are conducted. Throughout this cycle, various errors may occur, such as coding issues, billing compliance discrepancies, and patient eligibility problems. Automated controls help identify many of these errors before payment. Claims with errors are rejected, while error-free claims proceed to payment. Errors requiring further examination are addressed in the post-payment phase, where additional undetected errors may also be resolved. The automated controls are divided into format and content checks. Format controls ensure data fields are filled correctly, while content controls verify the claim's compliance with contract terms and legislation, such as checking diagnosis codes and service coverage. Approximately 300 of the controls focus on content verification. Accepted claims receive a unique identifier, and a log is sent to the provider for tracking. The e-channel also detects duplicate claims, preventing unnecessary resubmissions.

Claims are grouped into Diagnosis-Related Groups (DRGs) and checked by system for outliers. Non-outlier claims receive reimbursement based on a combination of DRG payments, per diem, and Fee-For-Service (FFS), while outliers are reimbursed through FFS only. Providers can submit test claims for evaluation without them being stored for contract monitoring. The payment phase involves compensating providers once claims pass all controls. Various payment methods are used, including key performance and quality indicators in primary and hospital care, while dental and outpatient specialist care are reimbursed through FFS. Payment methods and tariffs are regulated by a government-approved benefits package, ensuring equal compensation for the same service across all providers, which is supported by claims management system. This approach maintains fairness and consistency in reimbursements while promoting quality care throughout the healthcare system. Figure 5 illustrates the automated controls used in Estonia's e-invoicing system.

Figure 5. Process of automated controls and DRG assignment of inpatient claims

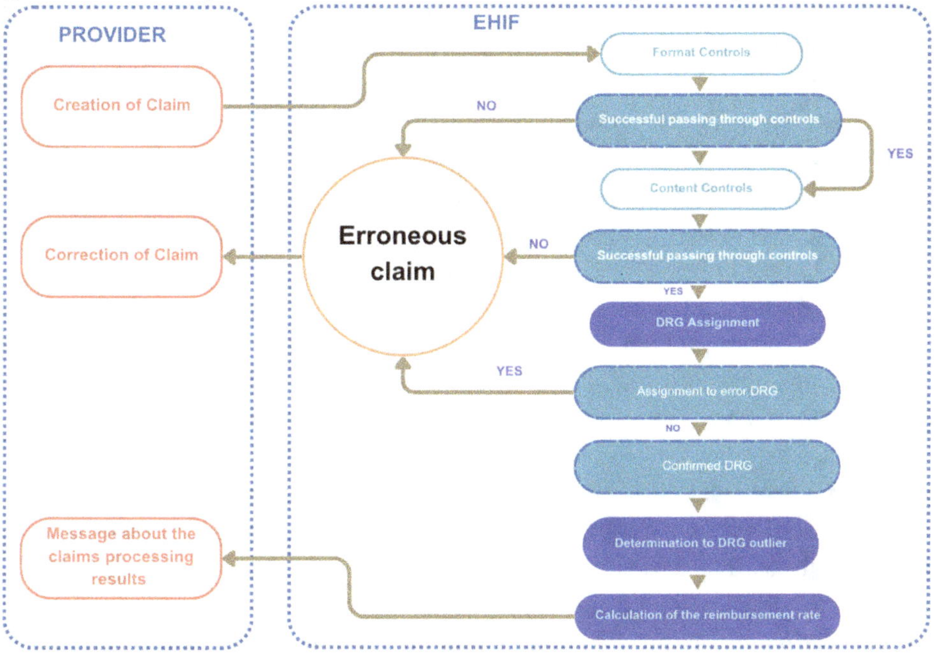

Source: (The Role of Digital Claims Management for Estonia's Health Insurance: A Leverage for Making Healthcare Purchasing More Strategic, 2023)

Machine Learning in EHIF. EHIF implemented Machine Learning (ML) in 2019 to automate the verification of claims, prescriptions, sick leave certificates, and other digital documents submitted for reimbursement (WHO Barcelona Office for Health Systems Financing, 2023/2023). Both supervised and unsupervised ML models are applied to all documents processed through the e-channel. Supervised learning detects predefined errors and fraud patterns, while unsupervised learning identifies outliers for further investigation. Prior to ML, only a fraction of claims underwent manual fraud checks, potentially missing some fraudulent claims. ML has reduced the number of claims needing manual review and aims to ensure no more than 5% of flawed claims are missed. Suspicious claims are flagged for targeted manual inspection by EHIF experts. ML has expedited post-payment processing, replaced time-consuming manual data queries, and improved fraud detection speed. Additionally, monthly controls enhance communication with hospitals, while ML aids in identifying new errors and managing provider payments efficiently. Overall, ML has revolutionized EHIF's ability to optimize the claim process and fraud detection mechanisms, ensuring the effective and purposeful use of health insurance resources.

Automated Monitoring of Contract Execution. The implementation of automated contract monitoring in Estonia has transformed healthcare contract management. By linking real-time claims data with actual contract volumes per provider, categorized by specialty and care setting, the system allows seamless comparison with planned volumes. This automation enables continuous and real-time monitoring of contract execution, ensuring adherence to agreed-upon terms. Before 2020, EHIF systems already allowed some flexibility in managing contract volumes. However, automation further enhances this by allowing providers to autonomously reallocate contract volumes within established conditions based on the real needs without EHIF intervention. This streamlines the reallocation process, making it more efficient and agile, and improves overall healthcare contract management.

Power BI in EHIF. EHIF uses Power Business Intelligence (Power BI) to visualize data through interactive dashboards and reports. This platform provides actionable insights into claims data, enabling EHIF to identify deviations from planned contract volumes and highlight discrepancies in average reimbursement per case across medical specialties, for instance change in the price of healthcare services. By leveraging Power BI, EHIF can monitor reimbursement patterns, make informed decisions, and optimize resource allocation to ensure efficient utilization of healthcare funds. The dashboards also promote transparency by allowing healthcare providers to view contract information and compare themselves with their peers.

Digitalizing invoicing through streamlined e-channels introduced automated controls to ensure accuracy and compliance with established criteria. Leveraging machine learning technologies facilitated automated claim verification and effective monitoring. This automation has significantly reduced manual workload, improved payment processes, minimized patient waiting times, and streamlined beneficiary operations. Furthermore, it ensures fairness and consistency in provider reimbursement while aligning incentives with quality patient care across the healthcare system (Rtc, 2023).

IT Ecosystem under Ayushman Bharat Pradhan Mantri - Jan Arogya Yojana (AB PM-JAY) - India

Ayushman Bharat Pradhan Mantri - Jan Arogya Yojana (AB PM-JAY) launched in 2018 stands as the largest health assurance program globally, providing an annual health cover of INR 5 lakhs (5970.49 USD) per family for secondary and tertiary care hospitalization. The primary objectives of PM-JAY include ensuring comprehensive coverage for secondary & tertiary care, reducing out-of-pocket expenses for catastrophic events, enhancing access to hospitalization services, addressing unmet healthcare needs, and integrating various state-level health insurance schemes. This scheme targets over 12 Crore (120 million) economically disadvantaged and vulnerable families, which equates to approximately 55 Crore (550 million) beneficiaries representing the bottom 40% of the Indian population (About Pradhan Mantri Jan Arogya Yojana (PM-JAY), n.d.).

The key stand-out feature of PM-JAY is its IT ecosystem which facilitates digitalization of scheme operations, enables interoperability, provides a hosting environment to applications for fraud detection and deterrence etc., making the scheme implementation paperless.

There are three main pillars of this IT ecosystem:

Beneficiary Identification System (BIS). It is an online portal for registration of beneficiaries. Since it is an entitlement-based scheme, the beneficiary base is provided at the backend of the portal and identification process is undertaken at the empaneled hospitals where they furnish the required details as provided by the eligible beneficiaries and is followed by two step authentications process that involves biometric verification and cross-verification using national ID.

Hospital Empanelment Management (HEM). It facilitates empanelment (onboarding) of hospitals (both public & private), it captures details on infrastructure, human capital, facilities, and services provided etc. along with accreditation status of a facility in terms of quality of care. Applications received from hospitals in HEM are reviewed by State Health Agency (SHA) through an on-line process, whereas District Implementation Unit (DIU) undertakes in-person audit to these facilities for verification.

Transaction Management System (TMS). It is multi-user online platform, for patient's entire journey during care delivery and claims processing, that includes modules for patient registration, pre-authorization, claim submission, document verification, and discharge. The system incorporates built-in check mechanisms, known as "triggers," designed for fraud detection and mitigation. Interlinked through Application Program Interface (API) for data exchange, these platforms populate data to dynamic dashboards, allowing real-time monitoring of the entire scheme process. Figure 6 illustrates the implementation process of AB PM-JAY scheme.

Figure 6. Process flow under AB PM-JAY

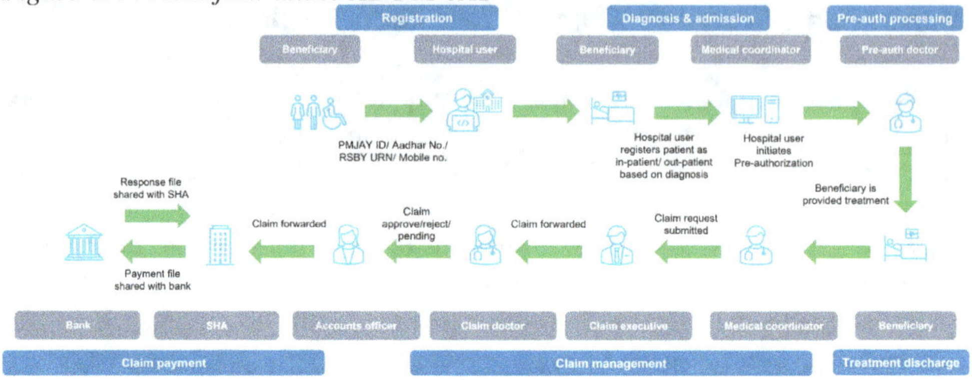

Source: (Claim Adjudication Manual AB PM-JAY, National Health Authority n.d.)

The system employs real-time analytics and tracking dashboards known as RADAR (Risk Assessment, Detection, and Analytical Reporting) and FACTS (Fraud Analytics Control and Tracking System),

The key features of these dashboards include –

Risk Assessment, Detection, and Analytical Reporting (RADAR). Monitors the key indicators under Transaction Management System (TMS) such as hospitals showing abrupt pattern of utilization and Country-wide health benefit package utilization/ patient demographics etc. and key indicators under Beneficiary Identification System (BIS) such as suspicious beneficiary cards created, claims submitted on suspicious cards, hospitals and correlation between approver, creator, and beneficiary.

Fraud Analytics Control and Tracking System (FACTS). This dashboard enables risk scoring of entities in Ayushman Bharat ecosystem. Enables the tracking of transparency of actions, management, and verification across administrative levels. Furthermore, it provides insights on fraudulent or suspicious cases taking place in a state, drilling down to the lowest level of granularity.

The digitalization and IT integration of the scheme processes are significantly enhancing monitoring and evaluation, facilitating timely payments to empaneled healthcare providers, and streamlining claims processing. System-based triggers help prevent duplication and double billing, while real-time dashboards enable effective data visualization and analysis. These technological advancements implement robust anti-fraud measures by identifying outliers and suspicious claims, thus enhancing the scheme's effectiveness in preventing and detecting fraudulent activities. Additionally, they ensure effective and timely grievance redressal. Overall, these improvements contribute to a more efficient, transparent, and reliable healthcare financing system.

Mobile JKN Application in Indonesia

Indonesia is working to establish one of the world's largest single-payer social health insurance systems to cover its population of over 260 million. Historically, Indonesia faced a fragmented health insurance landscape, with OOP payments accounting for about 50% of total health expenditures between 2002 and 2013, highlighting the need for reform towards UHC (Wasir et al., 2020).

In 2014, Indonesia launched Jaminan Kesehatan Nasional (JKN) to address these issues. JKN unified all existing insurance schemes and over 300 risk pools into a national program, offering all Indonesians the same benefit package and standardizing regulations for healthcare providers. The goal was to integrate members of previous health insurance schemes and achieve 100% coverage (Suryanto et al., 2016; Mahendradhata et al., 2017). The program provides free healthcare for the poorest citizens, while wealthier individuals pay monthly premiums to help finance it. To manage JKN, the government established Badan Penyelenggara Jaminan Sosial (BPJS) Kesehatan. Despite progress, challenges like inefficient service delivery, complex administrative procedures, and limited access to health information persisted, prompting the need for digital solutions.

In 2017, Indonesia launched the JKN mobile application to address these challenges. The app simplifies payments, allows for membership data updates, reduces patient waiting times, provides information about health facilities, and enhances overall operations for beneficiaries. The JKN mobile application is tailored for smartphones and mobile devices operating on iOS or Android systems, emphasizing its mobile-centric design. It features chat technology and artificial intelligence to deliver the "JKN chat assistant," which provides users with information. An internet connection is likely required for its operation, as it is intended to be an online service accessible "anytime and anywhere without having to visit the office physically." The app appears to integrate with the JKN (Jaminan Kesehatan Nasional) website, as evidenced by the availability of website visitor statistics. Additionally, it utilizes screening algorithms or questionnaires for features like "COVID-19 self-screening" and "Medical History screening" (Satriana, 2019).

The technology stack supporting the JKN mobile app includes advanced tools for seamless cross-platform development, ensuring a robust and user-friendly mobile healthcare experience (Vayed et al., 2022; Technologies used on Mobile JKN -Fork.ai, n.d.). Figure 7 illustrates the technology stack supplementing JKN Mobile application. Regarding data integration, the plan involves adopting international/national standards to facilitate seamless data interoperability and outlines the expected storage needs and architecture as data volume, variety, and scope increase over time. For the JKN mobile app, data will be collected from internal sources within the organization (such as Litbangkes, Ministry of Health (MOH), BPJS-K) and potentially from external sources. Organizations like Litbangkes, MOH, or BPJS-K might be responsible for data cleaning, integration, and quality assurance. Overall, the plan aims to create a cohesive system where data from various sources is collected, standardized, stored, managed, and made accessible to meet the needs of the JKN mobile app and its stakeholders ("International Bank for Reconstruction and Development Program Appraisal Document on a proposed loan in the amount of US$400 million to the republic of Indonesia for a National Health Insurance (JKN) reforms and results program program-for-results," 2021).

Figure 7. Technology stack supplementing JKN - Mobile app

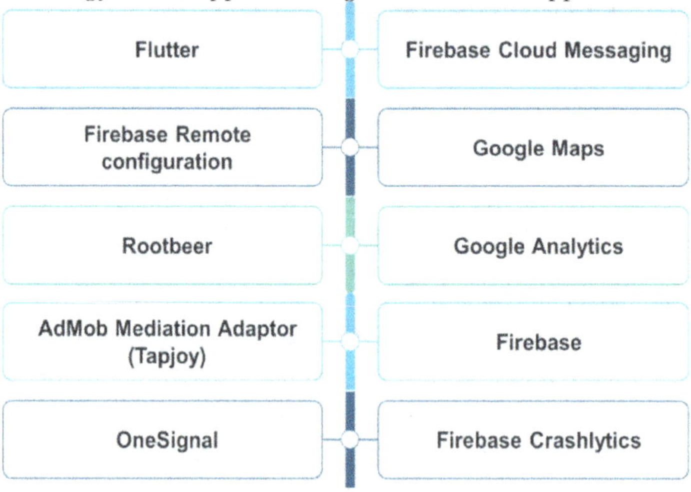

Source: (Technologies used on Mobile JKN - Fork.ai, n.d.)

The JKN app has undergone several updates to enhance the user experience and improve healthcare accessibility for its beneficiaries. Following are few examples

Queue Management. One notable feature of JKN application is the online queue management system, which allows users to obtain their queue numbers via smartphone before arriving at the hospital. This eliminates the need for beneficiaries to manually provide their JKN card number and identification number, as these details are automatically filled in by the app. Additionally, beneficiaries can select their preferred polyclinic at the hospital without needing a referral letter, as this functionality is integrated into the application (Uns, 2022).

i-Care JKN and JKN Mobile App Collaboration. The i-Care JKN app provides healthcare professionals with easy access to view the health service history of National Health Insurance (JKN) participants over the past year. This feature enables doctors to plan appropriate treatments based on more real-time, accurate, and factual data. i-Care JKN also facilitates communication and collaboration between doctors, especially when patients are referred to other doctors or specialists. This application interacts with the P-Care and SIM RS applications through a bridging scheme, enabling a smoother exchange of information between various healthcare service providers.

JKN participants can access the i-Care JKN features directly via the JKN mobile application. This integration allows users to easily view the history of services provided at First Level Health Facilities (FKTP) and Advanced Level Referral Health Facilities (FKRTL) in Indonesia. The information available includes details of diagnosis, medical treatment, the health facility providing the service, and the date of service (Reporter, 2023).

REHAB Program in JKN Mobile App. BPJS Health has launched a significant health financing initiative known as the Phased Contribution Payment Plan (REHAB) program, designed to assist participants of the National Health Insurance Program (JKN), especially Non-Wage-Earning Workers (PBPU), in settling outstanding contributions through installments. Participants with arrears ranging from 4 to 24 months can register via the JKN mobile app or by contacting BPJS Health Care Center at 165, with a maximum repayment period of 12 months per cycle. This initiative aims to alleviate financial burdens and reactivate membership status upon full payment completion. Additionally, the JKN mobile app, updated to version 4.5.1, provides easy access to the REHAB program and offers features such as Digital KIS, participant information, health facility navigation, and premium management, thereby enhancing the accessibility and utilization of health services (Ayo Manfaatkan Program REHAB BPJS Kesehatan, n.d.). Figure 8 illustrates the user interface of Mobile JKN application.

Figure 8. User interface of Mobile JKN app

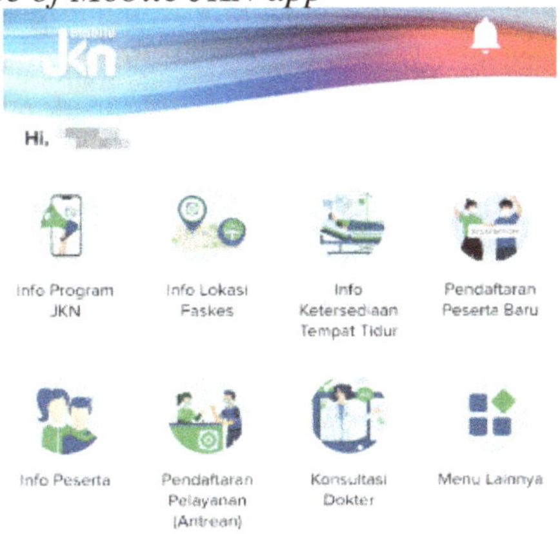

Source: (Mobile JKN, 2017)

The Mobile JKN app has had a significant impact on Indonesia's National Health Insurance system by improving access to healthcare services and enhancing the user experience. Since its introduction, there have been notable improvements in various metrics, including increased user satisfaction and a significant reduction in the number of users visiting BPJS Kesehatan offices, which has helped reduce crowding. The app's continuous development has expanded its service offerings, leading to over 2.6 million downloads and registrations and nearly 2 million active users. Additionally, the responsiveness to user complaints has improved, with more complaints being handled promptly, reflecting a proactive approach to user feedback (Mobile JKN, Health Insurance Services in Your Hand - Observatory of Public Sector Innovation, 2019).

Optical Character Recognition (OCR) Technology in Nordic Regions

Nordic insurance companies encountered several challenges in processing claims due to the high volume of unstructured data coming from various sources that required careful examination and categorization. This data was diverse, including bills, invoices, cash receipts from pharmacies and local clinics, as well as medical treatment diagnoses with accompanying documentation. The claim processing system relied heavily on manual labor, leading to time-consuming processes as insurance agents were required to perform repetitive tasks. Each document needed thorough analysis to extract essential data, which was then categorized based on its relevance to the claim process. This manual system resulted in reduced customer service efficiency, as teams found it difficult to process claims quickly. Their technology infrastructure was not equipped to handle end-to-end automation, further exacerbating the issue.

To improve operational efficiency and address challenges in claims management, these insurance companies have implemented Optical Character Recognition (OCR) technology. This technology allows agents to upload documents—such as PDFs, images, or scanned handwritten documents—into a digital platform. The OCR software then converts this unstructured data from various sources and formats into structured data, enhancing claims verification and decision-making capabilities (How a Nordic Insurance Company Automated Claims Processing, 2024). Figure 9 illustrates the adoption of OCR technology for effective claims management.

Figure 9. Use of OCR to enhance claim verification process

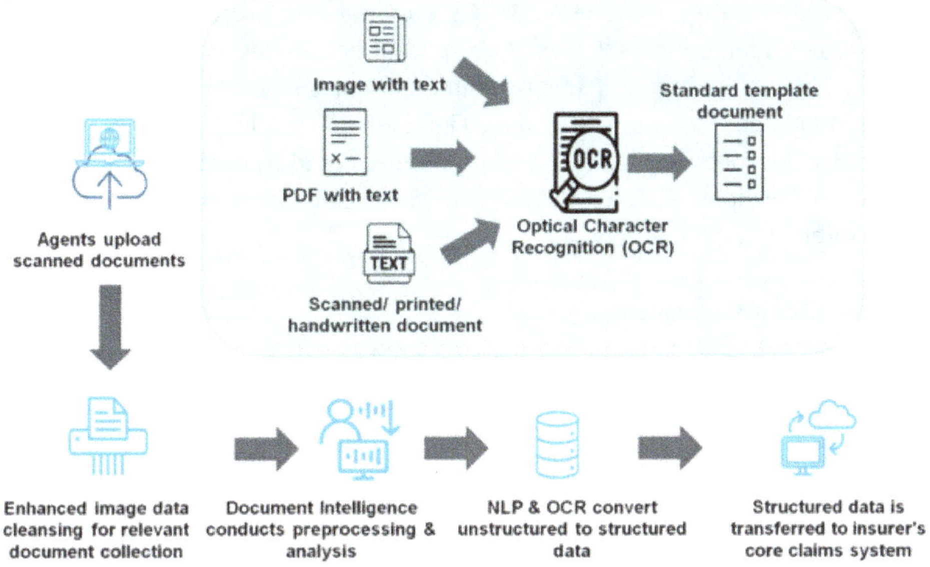

Source: (How a Nordic Insurance Company Automated Claims Processing, 2024), (Using OCR to Search and Edit Scanned Documents, 2022)

OCR technology automates data entry, reducing errors and increasing efficiency for insurance companies. The process involves several key phases: data capture, scanning and data extraction, character recognition, data integration and classification, and output (Kulkarni, 2024).

Data Capture. Documents like claim forms, invoices, and identification papers are collected and prepared for scanning.

Scanning and Data Extraction. High-resolution scanners create digital images, which the OCR software analyzes. This step involves separating text from the background, correcting document rotation, and reducing noise to improve the quality of the scanned images.

Character Recognition: Using advanced algorithms, machine learning and natural language processing (NLP) techniques, the software converts the scanned images into accurate digital text, ensuring precise data extraction.

Data Integration and Classification. The extracted data is organized into predefined categories, such as customer information and policy details, and integrated into the company's databases.

Output. The final stage ensures that the data is correctly formatted for use in various applications, such as updating records or generating reports, thereby enhancing decision-making and operational processes.

Thus, OCR technology provides significant benefits not only to insurance companies but also to their customers. By streamlining claim resolutions and enhancing customer interactions, OCR enables quicker processing times. It also reduces operational costs, minimizes manual intervention, and improves data accuracy, making fraud detection more effective. These advantages lead to better regulatory compliance, a reduction in paper-based processes, and more competitive product offerings for customers. Overall, OCR creates a mutually beneficial situation for both insurers and their clients.

E-Governance-Tonga

A robust e-governance system in healthcare is essential for creating effective interdepartmental linkages and enabling access to comprehensive data. This connectivity enhances informed decision-making and efficient monitoring of health allocations and expenditures by policymakers, thereby improving the overall effectiveness of health financing.

Tonga exemplifies a small country, with a population of less than 1.5 million, that is successfully establishing a resilient e-governance system. The Government of Tonga launched the Tonga Digital Government Strategic Framework 2019-2024 (Digital Transformation Department: Prime Minister's Office, n.d.), a strategic plan envisioning a digitally enabled government where ministries and agencies use information and communication technologies (ICT) to promote inter-governmental collaboration, transition from a paper-based system, and deliver efficient government services to citizens. As part of this initiative, Tonga has launched the first Integrated National Health Information System (INHIS) in the Pacific region in 2021 (Tonga Launches Pacific Islands First Integrated National Health Information System, 2021).

To create an enabling environment to strengthen health data, the country has undertaken several initiatives, including setting up digital health governance mechanisms, developing health ICT architecture linked to the Digital Government Strategic Framework (DGSF), and revising health-specific legal and regulatory frameworks. Tonga has also established a project management unit (PMU) and defined national health standards and updated terminology services (ADB, 2019).

Furthermore, the country has customized and strengthened its Digital Health Information System (DHIS), incorporating patient, facility, and workforce registries, as well as adopting health information standards and disease classification systems. Importantly, change management workshops were held across Tonga, focusing on people change rather than technology change, to address concerns, resistance, or fear of change within the health workforce. A strong emphasis has been placed on data security and privacy, with the implementation of systems featuring unique health identifiers, clear user permissions, and well-established role-based access (ADB, 2024).

These focused initiatives have led to the adoption of a comprehensive digital health strategy, the establishment of effective interoperable systems, the adoption of stringent data privacy and security laws, and enhanced digital literacy among the human resources and population. All these efforts have contributed to Tonga's progress towards a more integrated and efficient digital health governance system. Figure 10 illustrates the key initiatives taken up by Tonga.

Figure 10. Key initiatives undertaken by Tonga

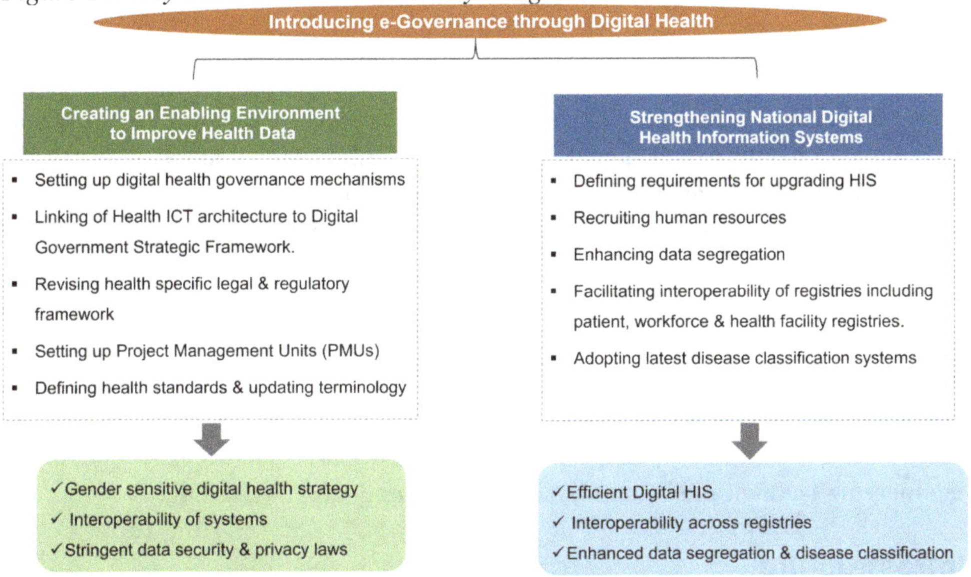

Source: (ADB,2019; ADB, 2024)

COUNTRY ROADMAP FOR ADOPTION OF DIGITAL HEALTH FINANCING TECHNOLOGIES

The examples above clearly demonstrate that countries need to strengthen various aspects of their digital ecosystems to promote the adoption of innovative technologies in health financing. To create an enabling environment for the adoption of innovative digital health financing technologies, emphasis should be placed on strategic planning, governance, infrastructure, skilled human resources, ease of use for key stakeholders, and robust health analytics systems.

Strategic Planning

The journey toward digital health financing is multifaceted and requires a comprehensive approach. Strategic planning is essential to align digital health initiatives with national health priorities and ensure that the implemented technologies meet the specific needs of the healthcare system. This planning should involve setting clear goals, defining measurable objectives, and outlining the steps needed to achieve them along with a framework for efficient monitoring & evaluation. By taking a strategic approach, countries can ensure that digital health financing initiatives are sustainable and scalable.

Governance

A conducive governance system is essential for progress toward digitalization. This includes having a dedicated department for digital health under the Ministry of Health with clear roles and responsibilities for implementation of digital transformation and a comprehensive national digital health strategy. Strong emphasis should be placed on a robust regulatory framework for digital health, including stringent data protection and security laws. Compliance with global benchmarks for digital health standards is crucial. Additionally, establishing an independent authority or institution for complaint resolution will ensure transparency. An effective governance system also ensures continuous and dedicated funding for digital health initiatives. Moreover, institutions that support digital health research can drive advancements in emerging technologies like AI, machine learning, and blockchain.

Infrastructure

Countries should ensure robust access to the internet and network infrastructure, including mobile devices, tablets, and computers. Establishing data centers, whether on-premise or cloud-based, is necessary, along with data backup and disaster recovery systems to ensure data safety. Efficient data exchange systems must be in place to enable interoperability and secure exchange of health data.

Skilled Human Resources

Building a skilled workforce is critical for the successful implementation of digital health technologies. Training programs should be developed to enhance the digital literacy of healthcare professionals, health literacy and digital health literacy of patients, ensuring they are equipped to leverage new technologies effectively.

Adoption Across Key Stakeholders

In the health financing ecosystem, key stakeholders include 4Ps: payers, providers, policy makers and patients (beneficiaries). For the successful adoption and utilization of digital health financing technologies, it is crucial to address the specific needs of each stakeholder group and ensure systems are designed for ease of use and efficiency.

For payers and insurers, systems must be developed to ensure efficient operations and effective monitoring. Key components include the implementation of a unique ID system for citizens to improve beneficiary identification, standardized clinical coding and costing software for accurate coding and costing of medical services, automated claim management systems for processing and managing claims efficiently, advanced analytics for fraud and abuse detection to identify and prevent fraudulent activities, and real-time income and expenditure dashboards for tracking financial flows, enabling effective financial management and oversight.

Healthcare providers require robust digital systems to streamline operations and improve service delivery. This includes the implementation of standardized electronic health records (EHRs) and patient health records (PHRs) to ensure uniformity and ease of access, integration of various systems to facilitate seamless data exchange and interoperability, and the establishment of reimbursement review and payment tracking systems to ensure prompt reimbursement and payment tracking, encouraging provider participation and reducing financial barriers.

For beneficiaries, user-friendly platforms are essential to enhance access to healthcare services and information. This involves the development of a digital e-marketplace (one-stop-shop) for healthcare services that enables easy discovery and access, the availability of mobile health (mHealth) services for convenient access to care and health management, secure access to personal health records with advanced features offering personalized health information and services, and an efficient digital grievance redressal system for handling complaints and ensuring prompt resolution, building trust and satisfaction among the population.

For policy makers it is important to improve evidence-based decision making and to enable sustainable health system in times when resources are limited and demand unlimited.

To ensure successful adoption and utilization of digital health financing technologies, awareness & capacity building across all key stakeholders is essential. This includes developing training programs to enhance digital literacy and technical skills among healthcare providers, payers, and beneficiaries, ongoing education initiatives to keep stakeholders informed about new technologies and best practices and establishing support systems to assist stakeholders in navigating and utilizing digital health platforms effectively. By addressing the specific needs of each stakeholder group and investing in capacity building, countries can foster an environment conducive to the adoption and integration of digital health financing technologies, ultimately improving health outcomes and financial sustainability.

Robust Health Analytics Systems

Health analytics plays a crucial role in digital health financing by transforming vast amounts of health data into actionable insights, driving improvements that enhance decision-making, efficiency, and patient care. By leveraging data and analytics tools, healthcare organizations and policymakers can optimize financial resources, improve healthcare delivery, and achieve better health outcomes for individuals and populations.

To fully realize these benefits, it is essential for countries to have robust health analytical systems in place. This includes implementing population-level Health Management & Information Systems (HMIS), developing analytical dashboards for effective monitoring and evaluation of key performance indicators (KPIs), and establishing population health risk stratification systems for preventive care. Additionally, integrating health big data and AI analytics with non-health sectors can promote deeper insights and foster more comprehensive strategies.

To assess progress, countries should regularly evaluate their strategies, systems, and processes, documenting their findings in comprehensive reports. These reports can serve as valuable sources of insight for policymakers and the public, guiding future improvements in health policy and practice.

CONCLUSION

In conclusion, the adoption of innovative digital technologies in health financing holds transformative potential for healthcare systems worldwide. As the examples of Kenya, Estonia, and Tonga illustrate, embracing digital advancements can lead to substantial improvements in efficiency, transparency, and access to care. These technologies not only streamline administrative processes but also empower healthcare providers and patients, ultimately leading to better health outcomes for individuals and populations.

Moreover, digital health financing can significantly contribute to improving health equity. By reducing administrative burdens and facilitating access to financial resources, digital technologies can help address disparities in healthcare access and quality. In underserved regions, mobile health platforms and telemedicine services can extend the reach of healthcare services, ensuring that even remote populations receive timely and appropriate care. Additionally, digital health technologies can empower individuals to take a more active role in managing their health, promoting preventive care and encouraging healthier lifestyles.

Digital health financing can drive economic growth and development. By increasing efficiency in healthcare delivery and reducing waste, these technologies can lower healthcare costs and improve resource allocation. As a result, countries can invest more in other critical areas, such as orphan drugs and highly specialized treatments, leading to broader economic benefits. Furthermore, the digital health sector itself can become a significant contributor to economic growth, creating new jobs and fostering innovation.

In summary, the adoption of innovative digital technologies in health financing has the potential to revolutionize healthcare systems by enhancing efficiency, quality, safety, transparency, and access to care. However, realizing this potential requires strategic planning, robust governance, stakeholder engagement, and continuous evaluation. By addressing these key elements, countries can ensure that digital innovations translate into tangible benefits for healthcare systems and the communities they serve, ultimately leading to improved health outcomes and greater health equity.

By understanding the various strategies, challenges, and essential aspects of implementing digital health financing models, health care professionals and health industry experts will be better equipped to adopt the best suitable model tailored to their requirements and contexts. This will enable them to leverage emerging technologies more efficiently.

REFERENCES

About Pradhan Mantri Jan Arogya Yojana (PM-JAY). (n.d.). National Health Authority. Retrieved August 5, 2024, from https://pmjay.gov.in/about/pmjay

ADB. (2019, August 23). ADB-Supported Digital Health Information System to Help Manage Patient Care in Tonga. Asian Development Bank. https://www.adb.org/news/adb-supported-digital-health-information-system-help-manage-patient-care-tonga

ADB. (2024, June 28). Introducing eGovernment through Digital Health. Asian Development Bank. https://www.adb.org/projects/50281-001/main

Aijli. (2021, December 14). Key takeaway from practicum - Aijli - Medium. Medium. https://medium.com/@aijli/key-takeaway-from-practicum-612adf0389e7

Ayo Manfaatkan Program REHAB BPJS Kesehatan. (n.d.). https://www-bekasikab-go-id.translate.goog/ayo-manfaatkan-program-rehab-bpjs-kesehatan?_x_tr_sl=id&_x_tr_tl=en&_x_tr_hl=en&_x_tr_pto=sc

Claim Adjudication Manual. (n.d.). National Health Authority. Retrieved August 5, 2024, from https://pmjay.gov.in/sites/default/files/2021-01/Claims-Adjudication-Manual-2_0-final.pdf

Development Asia. (2022, May 4). Training on Successful Implementation of a Digital Financial Services for Health Project [Video]. YouTube. https://www.youtube.com/watch?v=ZiAuqu3

Digital Government Strategic Framework 2019-2024. (2019). Finance.Govt. Tonga. https://finance.gov.to/sites/default/files/2021-07/Digital%20Strategic%20Framework.pdf

Digital Transformation Department. Prime Minister's Office. (n.d.). https://digitaltransformation.gov.to/?page_id=154

EInvoicing in Estonia. (1424, August). Language selection | European Commission. https://ec.europa.eu/digital-building-blocks/wikis/display/DIGITAL/eInvoicing+in+Estonia

Hamad, W. B. (2019). CURRENT Position and Challenges of E-health in Tanzania: A review of literature Master of Science in... ResearchGate. https://www.researchgate.net/publication/357901194_current_position_and_challenges_of_e-health_in_tanzania_a_review_of_literature_master_of_science_in_information_system

How a Nordic insurance company automated claims processing. (2024, January 22). https://www.ey.com/en_in/financial-services-emeia/how-a-nordic-insurance-company-automated-claims-processing

International Bank For Reconstruction And Development Program Appraisal Document On A Proposed Loan In The Amount Of Us$400 Million To The Republic Of Indonesia For A National Health Insurance (Jkn) Reforms And Results Program Program-For-Results. (2021). In International Bank For Reconstruction And Development. https://documents1.worldbank.org/curated/en/780101641932861182/pdf/Indonesia-National-Health-Insurance-JKN-Reforms-and-Results-Program.pdf

Kulkarni, P. (2024, June 7). How OCR Is Transforming The Insurance Industry. Hyperverge. Retrieved August 4, 2024, from https://hyperverge.co/blog/ocr-insurance/

M-TIBA is truly leapfrogging healthcare in Kenya. (n.d.). PharmAccess. https://www.pharmaccess.org/update/M-Tiba-is-truly-leapfrogging-healthcare-in-kenya/#:~:text=M%2DTIBA%2C%20whereby%20the%20M,healthcare%20at%20very%20low%20costs

Mahendradhata, Y., Trisnantoro, L., Listyadewi, S., Soewondo, P., Marthias, T., Harimurti, P., Prawira, J., & Hort, K. (2017). The Republic of Indonesia Health System Review. Health Systems in Transition, 7–7(1). https://iris.who.int/bitstream/handle/10665/254716/9789290225164-eng.pdf

Meena, S., Rathore, M., Kumawat, P., & Singh, A. (2020). Challenges Faced by ASHAs during their Field Works: A Cross Sectional Observational Study in Rural Area of Jaipur, Rajasthan. *International Journal of Medicine and Public Health, 10*(3), 97–99. DOI: 10.5530/ijmedph.2020.3.20

Mobile, J. K. N. (2017, June 15). App Store. https://apps.apple.com/sg/app/JKN%20-%20mobile/id1237601115

Mobile, J. K. N. Health Insurance Services in Your Hand - Observatory of Public Sector Innovation. (2019, February 5). Observatory of Public Sector Innovation. https://oecd-opsi.org/innovations/mobile-jkn-health-insurance-services-in-your-hand/

Morgan, L. (n.d.). M-TIBA DIGITAL HEALTH PLATFORM. In PharmAccess. https://www.ilo.org/sites/default/files/wcmsp5/groups/public/@ed_emp/documents/publication/wcms_749427.pdf

Muller, N., Emmrich, P., Rajemison, E., De Neve, J., Bärnighausen, T., Knauss, S., & Emmrich, J. (2019). A Mobile Health Wallet for Pregnancy-Related Health Care in Madagascar: Mixed-Methods Study on Opportunities and Challenges. *JMIR mHealth and uHealth*, *7*(3), e11420. https://mhealth.jmir.org/2019/3/e11420. DOI: 10.2196/11420 PMID: 30457972

Onkundi, C. (2023, August 4). M-TIBA: Top 25 Most Customer-Obsessed Brands Impacting Lives in 2023. Simplify Your Health Insurance Journey. https://mtiba.com/m-tiba-top-25-most-customer-obsessed-brands-impacting-lives-in-2023/#:~:text=With%20over%204.7%20million%20registered,in%20the%20nation's%20health%20sector

Reporter, S. (2023, September 20). BPJS Kesehatan wins big at the Asian Technology Excellence Awards. Asian Business Review. https://asianbusinessreview.com/event-news/bpjs-kesehatan-wins-big-asian-technology-excellence-awards

Rtc. (2023, December 25). Digital Transformation in Action: e-Invoicing in Estonia - RTC Suite. RTC Suite. https://rtcsuite.com/digital-transformation-in-action-e-invoicing-in-estonia/

Satriana, S. (2019). Easing Access to the National Health Insurance through a Mobile Application. In ILO Social Protection Department. ILO. Retrieved August 5, 2024, from https://www.social-protection.org/gimi/Media.action?id=16856

Stahl, M., Srivastava, S., Majakari, D., Dutta, A., Liu, R., & Chin, B. (2021). *Digital technologies for government-supported health insurance systems in Asia and the Pacific*. Asian development bank., DOI: 10.22617/TCS210526

Suryanto, S., Plummer, V., & Boyle, M. (2016). Financing Healthcare in Indonesia. *Asia Pacific Journal of Health Management*, *11*(2), 33–38. DOI: 10.24083/apjhm.v11i2.185

Technologies used on Mobile JKN - Fork.ai, https://fork.ai/lookup/ai-doc-7960137

The Mobile Economy. (2020). GSMA. https://www.gsma.com/solutions-and-impact/connectivity-for-good/mobile-economy/wp-content/uploads/2020/03/GSMA_MobileEconomy2020_Global

The role of digital claims management for Estonia's health insurance: A leverage for making healthcare purchasing more strategic. (2023, February 14). World Health Organization (WHO). https://www.who.int/publications/i/item/9789240066687

Tonga launches Pacific Islands first integrated national health information system. (2021, December 17). Matangi Tonga. https://matangitonga.to/2021/11/30/tonga-launches-pacific-islands-first-integrated-national-health-information-system

Tonga's experience in implementing national digital health. (2023). Pacific Health Information Network.

Uns, H. (2022, March 11). UNS Hospital-BPJS Kesehatan Launched JKN Mobile-Connected Online Queue System. Universitas Sebelas Maret. https://uns.ac.id/en/uns-hospital-bpjs-kesehatan-launched-jkn-mobile-connected-online-queue-system/

Using OCR to Search and Edit Scanned Documents. (2022, September 28). Foxit PDF Blog. https://www.foxit.com/blog/search-and-edit-scanned-documents-with-ocr/

Vayed, D. A., Nurmandi, A., Muallidin, I., & Loilatu, M. J. (2022). Utilization of the JAKI Application in Realizing Smart Living in the COVID-19 Pandemic Era (Case Study of DKI Jakarta Government, Indonesia). In Lecture notes in networks and systems (pp. 399–410). https://doi.org/DOI: 10.1007/978-981-19-2397-5_38

Wasir, R., Bahar, M. A., Irawati, S., & Wasir, R. (2020). Moving forward to achieve universal health coverage in Indonesia. https://doi.org/DOI: 10.33612/diss.124431881

WHO, Barcelona Office for Health Systems Financing. (2023). How can digital technologies be used to enhance health financing? Claims management in Estonia. In Health Financing Policy Papers (Report WHO/EURO:2023-7340-47106-68912). World Health Organization. https://iris.who.int/bitstream/handle/10665/367965/WHO-EURO-2023-7340-47106-68912-eng.pdf?sequence=1 (Original work published 2023)

WHO, Universal Health Coverage. (2019, July 16). https://www.who.int/health-topics/universal-health-coverage#tab=tab_1

World Bank and WHO. Half the world lacks access to essential health services, 100 million still pushed into extreme poverty because of health expenses. (2017, December 13). World Health Organization (WHO). https://www.who.int/news/item/13-12-2017-world-bank-and-who-half-the-world-lacks-access-to-essential-health-services-100-million-still-pushed-into-extreme-poverty-because-of-health-expenses

Chapter 6
Machine Learning in Medicine:
Enhancing Diagnosis, Treatment, and Healthcare Delivery

Pooja Dehankar
Ajeenkya D.Y. Patil School of Engineering, India

Susanta Das
https://orcid.org/0000-0002-9314-3988
Ajeenkya D.Y. Patil University, India

ABSTRACT

ML is a game-changing technology for improving diagnosis, customizing therapy, & streamlining healthcare delivery because of its capacity to handle & learn from enormous volumes of data. ML-based big data analysis has many benefits for assimilating & assessing vast volumes of intricate health care data. Early diagnosis & monitoring of drug-related safety issues were facilitated by ML algorithms that discovered hidden correlations between medications, medical products, & adverse events. This chapter highlights the benefits of ML in Medicine. To achieve the best possible results, it will be essential to improve clinical decision support, sickness diagnosis, & individualized treatment techniques. The chapter discusses important issues to keep in mind when applying ML in the medical field, e.g., data privacy, model interpretability, bias reduction, & regulatory compliance. Lastly it discusses the future of ML in medicine. Through responsible & ethical adoption of new technology, medical community can provide more individualized, efficient, & effective care to improve patient outcomes.

DOI: 10.4018/979-8-3693-7210-4.ch006

1. INTRODUCTION

Machine learning (ML) automatically identify patterns in data and use those patterns to forecast future data or facilitate decision-making in unpredictable situations. ML falls within the category of "artificial intelligence" (AI). Symbolism (rule-based, like IBM Watson), connectionism (network and connection-based, like deep learning or artificial neural net), and Bayesian (based on the Bayesian theorem) are the three general approaches to AI. The most defining feature of machine learning is that it is data-driven and makes decisions with little assistance from humans. Training data analysis allows the computer to learn, and when new data is added, it can predict. The use of deep learning with large healthcare data is currently receiving a lot of interest. Its ability to address actual problems was severely limited. However, with the advent of large data, improved processing power through graphics processing units, and new deep neural network training techniques, these constraints have now been overcome. In the world of medical imaging, these deep learning techniques have demonstrated remarkable results in simulating humans. Finding structural anomalies and categorizing them into disease groups is the practice of radiography. Many machine learning algorithms with various implementations, mathematical foundations, and logical frameworks have been used to carry out these categorization tasks since the 1980s. As a result, in the early 2000s, a number of computer-aided detection (CAD) systems were created and used into clinical workflow (Fenton et al., 2007; Lehman et al., 2015).

Medical datasets were analyzed using machine learning methods from the start. Several essential techniques for intelligent data analysis are now made possible by machine learning. The digital revolution, particularly in recent years, has made it possible to gather and store data in a reasonably accessible and affordable manner. Large information systems are used to capture and distribute data, and modern hospitals are well-equipped with monitoring and other data collection tools. Nowadays, machine learning technology is ideally suited for evaluating medical data. In particular, a lot of effort has been done in medical diagnostics for small, specialized diagnostic difficulties. In specialty hospitals or their departments, information regarding accurate diagnoses is frequently available in the form of medical records. Entering patient records with a confirmed correct diagnosis into a computer software to execute a learning algorithm is all that is required. Although this is obviously oversimplified, in theory, medical diagnostic information can be automatically extracted from the descriptions of previously resolved cases. After then, the generated classifier can be used to help doctors identify new patients more quickly, accurately, and/or reliably, or it can be used to teach non-specialist doctors or students how to diagnosis patients with unique diagnostic problems (Kononenko, 2001).

The goal of the chapter is to understand benefits, applications and challenges of Machine Learning in Medicine. The chapter gives overview of Medical Machine Learning. At the end of this chapter Future of Machine Learning in Medicine is discussed. Lastly, we draw some conclusion on how Machine Learning in Medicine is Enhancing Diagnosis, Treatment, and Healthcare Delivery.

2. BENEFITS OF MACHINE LEARNING IN MEDICINE

One of the most revolutionary uses in contemporary healthcare is the use of AI to improve diagnostic precision. AI and ML technologies use large data sets and complex algorithms to increase diagnostic accuracy, lower human error, and facilitate early disease diagnosis. Medical imaging is among the most notable fields where artificial intelligence has advanced significantly. Conventional diagnostic techniques, which mostly depend on human interpretation of imaging data, are constrained by the intrinsic complexity of medical images and the variation in radiologists' levels of skill. Imaging technologies powered by AI, especially those that use deep learning algorithms, have demonstrated impressive abilities in analyzing computed tomography (CT), magnetic resonance imaging (MRI), and X-ray images (Susarla et al., 2023).

A subset of artificial intelligence called deep learning models analyzes imaging data using neural networks. Large datasets of tagged medical images are used to train these models, which gives them the ability to accurately recognize and categorize patterns. AI algorithms, for instance, can now identify and diagnose diseases like tumors, fractures, and other abnormalities in medical images at a level that is on par with or even better than that of skilled radiologists.

In addition to increasing diagnostic precision, these developments drastically cut down on image analysis time, facilitating quicker treatment start and decision-making. By predicting disease development and patient risk factors using historical and current data, predictive analytics—another crucial AI application—improves diagnostic accuracy. To estimate the chance of a disease developing, machine learning models use a wide range of data from electronic health records (EHRs), such as laboratory findings, medical histories, and patient demographics.

In order to enable earlier intervention and preventive actions, AI algorithms, for example, can forecast the likelihood of acquiring disorders like diabetes, cardiovascular diseases, and even some types of cancer. AI is also quite good at pattern detection, particularly when it comes to processing complicated and multidimensional data. Traditional diagnostic techniques might overlook tiny trends in patient data that AI systems can spot. By identifying these trends, AI can recommend more diagnostic tests, offer early disease warnings, and assist physicians in making better decisions (Lin et al., 2023).

Genomic medicine is a paradigm shift in healthcare that uses advances in genetic and genomic data to improve illness prevention, diagnosis, and treatment. Precision medicine is made possible by this science, which combines the thorough analysis of genomes to comprehend the complex interaction between genetics and health. Next-generation sequencing (NGS) and other high-throughput sequencing technologies have made it easier to quickly compile enormous genomic datasets. A vast range of genetic data, such as structural variations, epigenetic changes, and single nucleotide polymorphisms (SNPs), are included in these databases. Among the advanced computational techniques required for the understanding of such vast and intricate data, ML has become a crucial instrument. The need for effective analysis and interpretation of massive amounts of genomic data is what led to the development of machine learning in genomics. As a branch of AI, ML includes methods that let computers recognize patterns in data and anticipate or decide without explicit task programming. ML algorithms are used in genomics to find genetic variations linked to illnesses, forecast disease risk, and create individualized treatment regimens based on each patient's unique genetic profile. By enabling more precise, effective, and individualized medical interventions, the combination of machine learning and genomic medicine has the potential to completely transform healthcare (Prabhod, 2022).

3. APPLICATIONS OF MACHINE LEARNING IN MEDICINE

Some applications of ML in Medicine are Disease diagnosis, Personalized medicine, Medical Imaging, Early detection of diseases, Assisting clinical research and Drug discovery.

Figure 1. Applications of machine learning in medicine

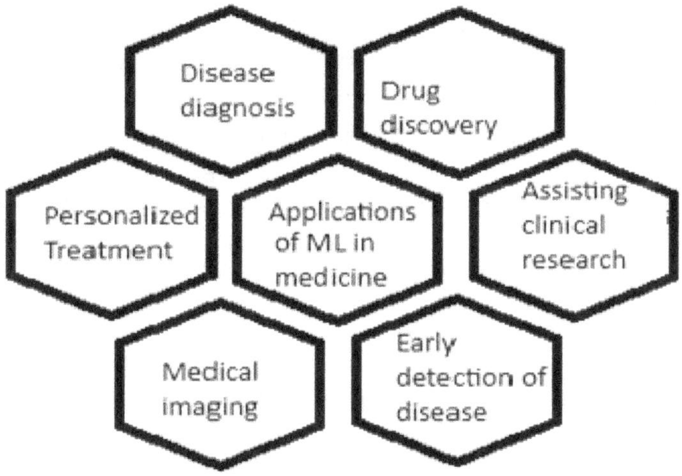

3.1 Disease diagnosis

Computer-aided diagnosis (CAD) is a vibrant field of study in medical imaging that is expanding quickly. Errors in medical diagnostic systems can lead to seriously misleading medical treatments, which is why big efforts have been undertaken in recent years to improve computer-aided diagnostics applications. A key component of computer-aided diagnosis is machine learning. Using a simple equation may result in inaccurate indications of organs. Learning from examples is therefore a vital aspect of pattern recognition. Pattern recognition and machine learning have promise in the biomedical industry for better perception and disease diagnosis. Additionally, they support the impartiality of the decision-making process. Creating sophisticated and automated methods for the analysis of high-dimensional and multimodal biomedical data is made possible by machine learning. Hepatitis, diabetes, liver, dengue, and heart disease are among the illnesses that can be diagnosed using machine learning algorithms (Fatima & Pasha, 2017).

3.2 Personalized medicine

New technologies have the potential to help the customized medical industry by utilizing big data in omics, such as individualizing and speeding up cancer tests and treatments. With several underlying molecular etiologies and each subtype exhibiting a range of clinical outcomes, breast cancer is one of the most prevalent cancers in the world. Therefore, the effective and customized clinical management of breast cancer depends on disease stratification. A new machine learning technique called the support vector machine (SVM) provides reliable categorization of large, high-dimensional data into a small number of data points, or support vectors, and quickly distinguishes between subgroups. With the speed at which the majority of aggressive malignancies must be diagnosed and treated, this new machine learning technique has significant clinical and public applications as well as implications for contextualization and high-throughput data analysis (Ozer et al., 2020).

3.3 Medical Imaging

Deep learning and machine learning methods are expanding quickly in the dynamic field of medical imaging research. In order to identify flaws in illness detection systems that could lead to very ambiguous medical treatments, significant efforts are currently being made to improve medical imaging applications employing these algorithms. In medical imaging, machine learning and deep learning algorithms are crucial tools for predicting early illness symptoms. In particular convolutional networks, deep learning techniques have quickly produced a unique methodology for analyzing medical images. It indicates predictions using supervised or unsupervised algorithms on a particular standard dataset. Concepts in medical imaging include object identification, pattern recognition, image classification, reasoning, and more. By identifying the relevant patterns for the particular condition in medical imaging, these are used to increase accuracy (Latif et al., 2019).

3.4 Early detection of diseases

Chronic illnesses have been one of the main issues in the medical sector since they can negatively impact quality of life and place a significant strain on healthcare resources. a new framework that uses classification modeling and sequential rules mining to mine sequential risk patterns using time interval data from diagnostic clinical records in order to detect chronic diseases early. The four stages of the framework's full workflow are post-analysis, classification modeling, risk pattern mining, and data preprocessing (Cheng et al., 2017).

3.5 Assisting clinical research

The field of clinical research is broad; preclinical research and observational analysis result in both traditional and pragmatic trials, which in turn lead to clinical registries and additional implementation work. Although clinical research as it is now carried out is essential to enhancing healthcare and results, it is complicated, time-consuming, costly, and subject to biases and unforeseen errors that can jeopardize its successful application, implementation, and acceptance.

Clinical trials may become more successful, generalizable, patient-centered, and efficient with the aid of machine learning. For managing vast and diverse data sources, seeing subtle and complex patterns, and forecasting complicated outcomes, a variety of machine learning techniques are available. " Consequently, ML can be useful in a variety of clinical trial processes, including preclinical drug discovery, pre-trial planning, study execution, data management, and analysis. The abundance of established and start-up companies investing substantial resources in the field suggests a high level of interest in, and growing attempts to use, ML application to clinical research, and specifically clinical trials, despite the relative dearth of academic and lay publications devoted to ML-enabled clinical research (Weissler et al., 2021).

3.6 Drug discovery

Pipelines for drug discovery and development are drawn out, intricate, and reliant on many variables. When considering well-defined issues with a wealth of high-quality data, ML techniques offer a collection of tools that can enhance discovery and decision-making. ML can be used at every stage of the drug discovery process. Examples include analyzing digital pathology data in clinical trials, finding prognostic biomarkers, and validating targets. Context and methodology have varied in applications, with some strategies producing precise forecasts and insights. The primary obstacle to using machine learning is the inability of ML-generated findings to be consistently interpreted, which may restrict their use. It is still necessary to generate thorough and organized high-dimensional data in every field. The use of ML can encourage data-driven decision making and has the potential to expedite and lower failure rates in drug discovery and development if these problems are continuously addressed and the criteria required to verify ML approaches are well understood (Vamathevan et al., 2019).

4. CHALLENGES OF USE OF MACHINE LEARNING IN MEDICINE

The ethical and regulatory implications of health data have been discussed for a while, and laws like the GDPR are a prime example of the legislative drive to address new digital issues. Nonetheless, other jurisdictions have arrived at and are likely to arrive at distinct outcomes. For instance, the GDPR and the US's Health

Insurance Portability and Accountability Act (HIPAA) are different in that the former focuses on healthcare data from patient records while excluding data from other sources, such as data generated by entities other than covered entities and business associates, such as life insurance companies or smartphone apps that monitor blood sugar (Cohen & Mello, 2018).

The saying “garbage in, garbage out” is used in computer science. This is particularly true for ML in medicine, as the ethical use of predictive algorithms depends on the data sets used to train and evaluate ML in medicine models. ML in medicine -trained algorithms may be biased by training data sets that are not very representative. With at least two paradigms prevalent in medical data, the term “bias” is loaded with connotations. For example, population data skewed by the long-standing overdiagnosis of schizophrenia among African Americans are examples of situations where the data sources themselves do not accurately represent the true epidemiology within a particular group (Neighbors et al., 1989).

The situations where an algorithm is taught on data that does not include enough members of a certain demographic, such as when an algorithm is based primarily on data from older white men. An algorithm like that would forecast poorly, for instance, among younger Black women. Algorithms developed on data sets with these features could make health inequities worse if they are used in healthcare (Braveman, 2006).

5. FUTURE OF MACHINE LEARNING IN MEDICINE

Future difficulties lie in creating increasingly complex algorithms, like DL, to address intricate issues, but the goal is also to have more individualized medicine. With vast resources, machine learning (ML) is a rapidly developing area of medicine that combines statistics and computer science to solve medical issues. Supporters of ML rave about its capacity to handle vast amounts of complicated and divergent data, which are frequently encountered in the medical field. They believe that ML will play a major role in the advancement of computer-aided diagnostics, customized treatment, and biomedical research in the future. However, many medical practitioners are not conversant with the ideas of ML, and the potential of using ML as a research tool remains unrealized (Handelman et al., 2018).

6. HEALTHCARE 6.0

In the past, local healers, herbal cures, and traditional medical techniques were used to treat medical conditions. Significant advances in medical science, such as the creation of vaccinations, antibiotics, and surgical methods, occurred during the 19th and 20th centuries. It resulted in the development of contemporary hospitals, healthcare systems, and pharmaceutical businesses. With the widespread use of wearable technology, telemedicine, electronic health records, and health apps, the digital era has caused a paradigm shift in the way healthcare is delivered. It enabled people to remotely consult healthcare providers, monitor their health, and receive medical information, resulting in more convenient and individualized treatment. It stands for a comprehensive method of providing healthcare that prioritizes patient involvement, preventive care, and group decision-making. It improves health outcomes by customizing treatments to each patient's needs through the use of genetics, AI, and predictive analytics (Tyagi et al., 2024).

An era of unparalleled innovation is being ushered in by the swift development of new technologies in the healthcare industry, which are changing patient outcomes and medical procedures. Virtual reality (VR), augmented reality (AR), the internet of medical things (IoMT), remote patient monitoring (RPM), financial technology (fintech) integration, cloud migration, and the critical role of ML are just a few of the technologies changing the healthcare industry. RPM enables proactive care, IoMT expands healthcare borders, fintech integration improves financial operations, and virtual reality and augmented reality transform medical education. While ML uses algorithms for precise diagnosis and individualized care, cloud migration guarantees scalable and effective data management (Yadav, 2024).

Resilient health systems necessitate ongoing innovation and advancement in the face of global health issues. Stakeholders emphasize how important digital technologies are to quickening this advancement. The sensitivity of health data, the lack of evidence-based standards, data governance concerns, and the paucity of data on the effectiveness of digital health tactics are just a few of the major obstacles facing the digital health industry. To fully realize the potential of digital health technologies in improving healthcare outcomes and delivery, several obstacles must be overcome. Making security and privacy a top priority is crucial to creating transparent, usable, and efficient digital health systems. Non-fungible tokens (NFTs) have drawn a lot of interest, particularly in the healthcare industry, where they use blockchain technology to solve problems and provide creative solutions (Nunes et al., 2024).

7. CUTTING-EDGE ADVANCEMENTS

Machine learning is one of the most promising technologies to transform healthcare in the age of intelligent algorithms. Up until recently, the main sectors where machine learning algorithms had a big influence were manufacturing, transportation, and administration. However, these algorithms are already having an impact on previously unaffected sectors like healthcare. Even though machine learning has been around for a while, its application in the medical field is growing steadily as data becomes more accessible. Through the use of statistics, computers can learn from historical data. Based on the information that is provided to them, they are able to recognize patterns and create opinions. There are several potential uses for machine learning (ML) in the healthcare sector. They cover everything from clinical diagnostics and decision-making to medication discovery. Petabytes of data pertaining to healthcare need to be analyzed. Additionally, a lot of data is produced by carry-and-wear devices, such as heart rate, blood pressure, and gait. Therefore, ML approaches can be used to forecast diseases and create customized treatments based on these facts. Additionally, an ML algorithm for possible disease diagnosis can be built using X-ray and MRI image classification techniques, which will lessen the workload for clinicians. Similarly, machine learning algorithms have been used in medication research and discovery to forecast drug toxicity, create new drug candidates, and find novel therapeutic targets. Predictive models for patient outcomes such as mortality, readmission, and disease progression can be developed using machine learning techniques. Clinical decision-making, such as predicting readmission rates or identifying patients who would benefit from a particular treatment, can be facilitated by applying machine learning (ML) algorithms to analyze data from electronic health records (EHRs). Therefore, by offering techniques to group, categorize, forecast, and help physicians make well-informed judgments, machine learning (ML) holds the potential to completely transform the healthcare sector (Shaik et al., 2024).

7.1 ML's integration with emerging technologies in healthcare

In order to solve issues like data interoperability, security, and scalability, the healthcare industry has profited immensely from the integration of AI/ML with distributed technologies like edge computing, blockchain, and the IoT. Patient care, medical research, and the effectiveness of the healthcare system are all significantly impacted by this synergy. Drug research, medical imaging interpretation, image identification, predictive analytics, and illness prediction are just a few of the domains that employ AI/ML techniques. It discusses the connection between AI/ML and distributed technologies, including edge computing for low-latency processing, blockchain for data integrity and privacy, and decentralized architectures for secure access to real-time data sources. The healthcare industry encounters trends and difficulties pertaining to interoperability, legal compliance, and ethical considerations when integrating AI/ML with distributed technologies (Gopi et al., 2024).

The Internet of Things (IoT) has enabled connectivity technologies that have revolutionized several fields, including health monitoring systems. Machine learning and advanced artificial intelligence techniques can be used to find patterns linked to illnesses and medical issues. Scientific efforts are being focused on improving IoT-enabled applications including the administration of medical reports, prescription traceability, and infectious disease surveillance by combining blockchain technology (BCT) with machine learning (ML) models. Even while recent developments have tried to make blockchain (BC) and machine learning (ML) more flexible for Internet of Things applications, several important factors still need to be taken into account for better results (Vaigandla et al., 2024).

7.2 Progression of ML in healthcare over the past decade

Precision medicine could be accelerated by technological advancements like artificial intelligence (AI) and machine learning (ML), particularly when paired with expanded therapeutic modalities and a greater capacity for large amounts of data from various sources. Nevertheless, these advancements also come with a number of drawbacks. The objectives of precision medicine and put the use of AI in precision medicine into context by demonstrating creative uses (e.g., predicting tumor development and overall survival, identifying biomarkers using biomedical pictures, and identifying patient populations for clinical practice). The interdisciplinary character of AI, emphasizing in particular the necessity of AI's reliability. Differential privacy, synthetic data generation, and federated learning are some useful strategies to overcome these issues (Naik et al., 2024).

7.3 ML's role in IoT, blockchain, and telemedicine

The combination of Artificial Intelligence (AI), Machine Learning (ML), and Distributed Ledger Technology (DLT), sometimes known as blockchain, is a groundbreaking development in psychology and healthcare at an era of rapid technological advancement. It is investigated how combining these technologies can revolutionize conventional methods and open up new avenues for therapy, mental health management, diagnostics, and patient care. The distinct and complementary functions that AI, ML, and DLT can play in psychology and healthcare, offering a thorough road map for stakeholders, practitioners, and researchers. Together, blockchain's safe, decentralized data management and AI and ML's sophisticated analytical and predictive powers can improve administrative operations, optimize resource allocation, customize treatment regimens, and improve diagnostic accuracy (de Filippis & Al Foysal, 2024).

7.4 ML integration with technologies like robotics

The goal of the robot-based method is to solve the problem of promptly giving medical support to those who are unable to commit to prolonged hospitalization. For thorough health monitoring, the main goal is to create low-cost, low-power integrated circuits with intelligent systems that make use of wireless communication technologies, sensors, and machine learning methods. Developments in medical technology to carefully identify, quantify, and evaluate vital health indicators, such as body temperature, heart rate, electrocardiogram (ECG), and blood oxygen saturation level (SpO2). Smooth data transfer is made possible by real-time data processing and Wi-Fi connection capabilities. UV sanitization, haptic video communication, and the delivery of food and medications are all improved by integration with robotic platforms (Gowri et al., 2024).

7.5 Cost-effectiveness and accessibility of ML in low-resource healthcare systems

AI has shown significant promise in a number of medical domains. It helps with risk assessment, automated picture interpretation, and the treatment of cardiovascular disorders in cardiology. AI in oncology improves tailored medication selection, treatment planning, and cancer diagnosis. While improvements in patient triage and resource efficiency are seen in critical care, radiology gains from enhanced image analysis and diagnostic precision. AI has also demonstrated notable gains in diagnostic accuracy, individualized treatment, and overall patient care in the fields of pediatrics, surgery, public health, neurology, pathology, and mental health. AI's application in low-resource environments has had a particularly significant impact, improving access to cutting-edge diagnostic and therapeutic tools. AI is drastically boosting patient outcomes across a range of medical specialties, expediting treatment plans, and improving diagnosis accuracy, all of which are transforming the healthcare sector. This paper highlights AI's revolutionary potential, from tailored treatment plans to early disease detection, and its capacity to enhance healthcare delivery, especially in environments with limited resources (Dangi et al., 2024).

Low physician-to-patient ratios, a lack of top-notch medical knowledge, and inadequate infrastructure are all problems in low-resource clinical settings. When combined, these factors result in healthcare systems that are overworked and under-responsive to community demands. The implementation of clinical decision support systems (CDSSs), which assist clinical stakeholders (from doctors to patients) in their daily tasks, can help alleviate this strain. Despite their success in the industrialized world, these systems are still not well understood in environments with limited resources (Kiyasseh et al., 2020).

The main factors promoting comparative effectiveness research (CER) worldwide are the need to concentrate healthcare spending on creative, sustainable health systems that effectively employ currently available, effective treatments. In many nations, the high cost of key medications and technology, coupled with inadequate access, leads to increased morbidity and mortality rates as well as care costs that push individuals and families into poverty owing to out-of-pocket spending and disabilities. Value-added global health care comparative effectiveness research's capacity to influence health systems and paradigms for health care delivery in the "global south."

Because CER encourages the sharing of vital assets, resources, skills, and capabilities as well as the creation of collaborative multi-sectoral frameworks to improve health outcomes and metrics globally, facilitating the development of successful CER systems around the world opens the door for concrete local and regional definitions of equity in health care (Balkrishnan et al., 2013).

7.6 ML role in global health equity

Large academic medical facilities have made significant strides in utilizing artificial intelligence (AI) to support clinical decision-making in secondary and tertiary care. The uneven utilization of preventative care and gaps in chronic care management are two further issues that need to be resolved if such innovations are to have an effect across the range of care. up order to fill up these gaps, it may be essential to integrate additional data, such as genomics and wearable data, but there are ethical, legal, and technical obstacles. There is a need for technical methods for combining complicated and disorganized data. Confounding, missing data, and selection bias are examples of data and design flaws that need to be fixed (Wiens et al., 2024).

The Sustainable Development Goals (SDGs) emphasize how crucial it is to take inequality into account while developing, putting into practice, and running sustainable intelligent healthcare systems. When promoting healthcare, these systems frequently address health inequalities. Unfortunately, developing economies and vulnerable communities are constantly impacted by the intricacy of these disparities. This is mostly explained by the differences in social determinants brought about by social inequality between social groupings in the general population and the social factors that overlap with them. To solve the problem of equitable access to healthcare, a variety of technologies, such as mobile health, have been developed. Unfortunately, several of the disruptive, cutting-edge technologies that underpin mobile health—

like artificial intelligence (AI) and machine learning (ML)—continue to display algorithmic unfairness. The primary cause of this is the unequal healthcare datasets that result from the contextual and intersectional variations among the people who get mobile health services. Furthermore, despite the slow adoption of contextually appealing research paradigms for the responsible creation of inclusive AI and ML training datasets for Intelligent Healthcare Technologies, AI and ML are now widely used in the establishment of sustainable intelligent predictive and preventive Mobile Healthcare systems (Marvin et al., 2023).

8. INTERDISCIPLINARY COLLABORATION

Studying complicated phenomena requires the use of collaborative methods. In order to guarantee support and foster trust and understanding among participating practitioners at various levels in the healthcare system, research collaboration requires time allotted, interaction spaces, and project management and communication skills. The scientific method requires time and effort from researchers to handle this complexity. This places pressure on practitioners to comprehend the research process, how it aligns with ongoing organizational agendas and activities, and how to allocate time. Funders and other stakeholders may fail to consider some of the factors that have been highlighted when planning, carrying out, and assessing multidisciplinary, collaborative, and partnership research (Nyström et al., 2018).

There are many obstacles in creating interpretable models for medical settings as artificial intelligence (AI) becomes more integrated into the fields of computational biology and healthcare. In image-based specialties like pathology and radiology, where supplementary AI solutions for diagnostic image analysis are being used more and more, explainable AI (XAI) is essential for building trust and facilitating the efficient use of AI in healthcare. Interdisciplinary cooperation is necessary to overcome these obstacles and advance XAI to improve patient care. The importance of interdisciplinary conferences in fostering the cross-disciplinary interaction required for XAI innovation is highlighted by this commentary. To find important issues, best practices, and case studies pertaining to interdisciplinary cooperation for XAI in healthcare, a survey of the literature was done. The unique ways that specialist conferences promote discussion, stimulate creativity, and impact research paths were examined. The literature was used to develop best practices and suggestions for promoting teamwork, planning conferences, and obtaining specific XAI solutions. In order to develop new ideas, discover knowledge gaps, crystallize solutions, and foster long-term relationships that yield high-impact research, interdisciplinary conferences facilitate critical collaborative junctures that propel XAI growth. The key to focusing diverse expertise on solving fundamental problems is the careful planning of these events, which includes sessions on theoretical underpinnings, practical implementations, and standardized evaluation in addition to plenty of networking opportunities. Building mutual respect and understanding, communicating clearly, defining roles, and having a shared commitment to the moral creation of reliable, interpretable models are all necessary for successful collaborations. In order to influence explainable AI and computational biology in the future and support better patient outcomes and advancements in healthcare, specialized conferences are crucial. Accelerating the development and application of interpretable AI in medicine requires an understanding of the collaborative model's catalytic potential (Patel et al., 2024).

8.1 Collaboration frameworks for clinicians and data scientists

Big data analytics is a revolutionary method for managing large, intricate datasets that are impossible to handle with conventional data processing methods. It entails utilizing sophisticated analytical methods and algorithms to discover significant trends, patterns, and insights from massive amounts of data. Big data can be used to analyze the complex nature of epidemic data because of its volume, velocity, variety, and truthfulness (Ghosh et al., 2023; Mittal, 2020).

Big data analytics has grown in importance in the fields of epidemiology and health. An enormous amount of data about health is produced by the emergence of digital health records, wearable technology, social media, mobile health apps, and other digital platforms. Big data analytics can forecast disease outbreaks, provide real-time surveillance, and provide insights into the efficacy of public health initiatives by utilizing these many data sources. The ability to identify and address new infectious diseases more quickly and precisely is improved by this data-driven strategy (Jayaraman et al., 2020; Li et al., 2021).

There is a unique chance to improve public health responses by incorporating big data analytics into epidemic predictions. However, only a strong policy framework that takes ethical, strategic, and regulatory factors into account can make this potential a reality. Good policy frameworks guarantee that the advantages of big data analytics are optimized while lowering the dangers associated with data security, privacy, and ethical issues (Pramanik et al., 2021).

9. REGULATORY FRAMEWORKS

By utilizing current diversity, equality, and inclusion strategies, the FDA intends to assist projects that take into account health disparities related to AI use in medical product development. By using representative and varied datasets, this method supports industry efforts to lessen biases in AI applications. The FDA also stresses how crucial it is to continuously evaluate AI tools used in the creation of medicinal products. The need of ongoing attention in tackling AI hazards in healthcare is shown by this focus on guaranteeing standard adherence and preserving performance and dependability throughout the AI lifespan. As demonstrated by the lessons learnt from medical device recalls, it emphasizes the necessity of thorough testing standards and rapid reaction procedures to handle unforeseen challenges (Santra et al., 2024).

There are many ethical and legal concerns with using big data in public health that need to be properly considered. The privacy of the people whose data is being gathered and examined is one of the main issues. Health information is very delicate, and abuse or illegal access can have serious consequences. Strict guidelines on data protection are provided by legal frameworks such as the Health Insurance Portability and Accountability Act (HIPAA) in the US and the General Data Protection Regulation (GDPR) in Europe. These rules require that personal health information be handled openly, with individuals' express agreement, and protected from security breaches (Bakare et al., 2024).

9.1 Frameworks for bias reduction or privacy safeguards

Artificial intelligence's explosive growth has transformed several industries and presented previously unheard-of chances for efficiency and creativity. But this advancement has a price: in order for AI systems to work well, enormous volumes of personal data are frequently needed, which raises serious privacy and security issues. The nuances of data privacy, permission, transparency, and security in this dynamic environment as it dives into the complex problems of protecting personal data in the AI era is explored. We look at the particular dangers that AI presents, such as algorithmic decision-making, data bias, and the possibility of sensitive data being misused. The problem is made more difficult by the absence of clear regulatory frameworks, which leaves people and organizations in the dark (Daniel, 2023).

10. TOOLS TO IMPLEMENT ML SOLUTIONS EFFECTIVELY IN HEALTHCARE

Deep learning has been applied extensively in a variety of research domains in recent years, including natural language processing, autonomous driving, image classification, and speech recognition. In challenging classification and regression issues, where it is challenging to identify the complicated structure in high-dimensional data using traditional machine learning methods, deep learning has demonstrated noticeably better performance. Deep learning applications in biology are becoming more and more well-liked for forecasting the composition and capabilities of genomic components including enhancers, promoters, and gene expression levels (Liu et al., 2020).

The goal is to develop a medical chatbot that can diagnose illnesses and offer helpful information about them before a patient visits a doctor using artificial intelligence. By using medical chatbots, this will lower medical expenses and improve access to medical information. Python-based solution connects patients with chatbots to assist them deliver accurate answers to questions and prevent. The Health Bot chatbot will try to address or respond to users' inquiries or concerns about their health. Chatbots are improved by the application of NLP and ML. In an emergency, the system will also assist users in locating hospitals, clinics, and physicians in their area (Sharma et al., 2023).

High energy physics, nuclear physics, accelerator physics, medicine, and space science have all made extensive use of radiation simulations. For Monte Carlo radiation simulations, Geant4 is a potent radiation simulator. It creates physical quantities in detectors, machinery, or the human body by simulating particle movements via matter. Particle trajectories, scored physical quantities in a patient volume, radiation delivery equipment in simulation, and DICOM dataset captured in CT can all be drawn by the visualization program gMocren for Geant4-based radiotherapy simulations. A software tool for modifying regions of interest (RoI) has been developed utilizing NVIDIA Clara. It allows for the manipulation of ROIs for radiotherapy simulation and the use of artificial intelligence to extract tumor or organ regions from medical picture data, such as the DICOM dataset. DVHs (dose volume histogram) and ROIs are helpful for Geant4-based radiation modeling (Kimura & Nadege, 2020).

Reliability, transparency, quality assurance, and interorganizational compatibility are the four facets of trust. Both procedural and substantive criteria apply to these elements. The process of building acceptable levels of trust in AI in healthcare is intricate and involves a number of different considerations. To meet these needs, a variety of stakeholders will need to be involved in the development of AI solutions for radiology and healthcare. AI must be given the chance to supplement human expertise rather than replace it if it is to enhance radiology. Finding the elements and prerequisites for trust enables the creation of AI implementation plans that promote the field's advancement. The involvement of multiple stakeholders is necessary to create the conditions for trust to arise; they must find and promote well-defined solutions to offset the inherent complexity of the situation (Bergquist et al., 2024).

The development of eHealth has progressed from stand-alone technologies to all-encompassing digital health settings, encouraging data sharing between various systems and stakeholders. However, current research and implementation frameworks have mostly focused on the organizational and technological aspects of eHealth deployment, ignoring the complex financial, ethical, and regulatory factors.

To guarantee the successful and long-lasting deployment of eHealth, it is crucial to identify the legal, ethical, economical, and technological issues that need to be taken into account. In order to successfully adopt complex eHealth technologies that affect many levels and stakeholders, the authors hope to shed light on the legal, ethical, financial, and technological obstacles and enablers (Bente et al., 2024).

10.1 AI-Assisted Medicine

In assisted reproductive medicine, AI-aided ChatGPT consultations present a viable substitute for conventional in-person consultations. Even while ChatGPT improved patient happiness and shortened consultation times, further research is needed to fully comprehend the long-term effects and clinical results of AI-powered medical consultations (Cheng et al., 2024).

The Internet of Medical Things (IoMT) makes it possible to provide patients with healthcare and conduct widespread surveillance in the era of smart devices and linked communities. The quantity and complexity of biological data are growing as more implanted electronic devices that can be remotely monitored are added. In order to improve the quality of treatment given, the gathered data may provide useful diagnostic information that may be utilized to quickly intervene and maintain implanted devices. Device diagnostics are not being fully utilized in current remote monitoring procedures due to incompatibilities and data integration across DHR platforms and proprietary apps. Remote monitoring could be strengthened by establishing a technological framework that creates information and improves interoperability (Malathi et al., 2024).

10.2 GPT in clinical decision-making

In the healthcare industry, artificial intelligence—in particular, chatbot systems—is becoming a vital tool that supports patient involvement and clinical decision-making. ChatGPT has the ability to improve diagnosis, treatments, and ethics while also helping doctors with medical problems. Although it could be useful, integration into healthcare operations must enhance human expertise rather than replace it. To guarantee safe and efficient adoption in clinical settings, more research is necessary (Lahat et al., 2024).

11. ML INFECTIOUS DISEASES APPLICATIONS

The introduction and re-emergence of infectious illnesses have been a constant challenge to the global health landscape. The fundamental understanding of disease dynamics has been supplied by conventional epidemiological models. However, more sophisticated predictive algorithms are required due to the complex network of contemporary global contacts and the exponential growth of available data. By incorporating AI into the prediction of infectious diseases, AI for Science (AI4S) presents a revolutionary strategy. Real-time monitoring, complex data integration, and more accurate predictive modeling are made possible by AI4S. A paradigm change in the study of infectious diseases is represented by AI4S. It overcomes the drawbacks of conventional models and opens the door to a more proactive and knowledgeable reaction to outbreaks in the future. The next stage of disease prediction evolution, known as AI4S, is distinguished by improved efficiency, accuracy, and adaptability (Zhao et al., 2024).

11.1 ML applications in mental health

Developments in Natural Language Processing (NLP) and artificial intelligence (AI) in general are opening up new avenues for the automated identification and prognosis of mental health conditions in the general population. By using deep learning techniques, recent research in this field has placed a higher priority on predicting accuracy than model interpretability. Predictive accuracy over model interpretability, however, might lead to a lack of decision-making openness, which is crucial in delicate applications like healthcare. XAI methods for psychiatric diagnosis and prognosis are therefore becoming more and more necessary. A thorough analysis of XAI techniques using textual data from social media in the field of automatic mental disorder detection from language behavior was carried out. Extensive studies were conducted to assess the balance between interpretability and accuracy among predictive mental health models. A wide range of human-interpretable features, including syntactic complexity, lexical sophistication, readability, cohesion, stylistics, topics, and sentiment/emotions gleaned from lexicon-based dictionaries, were used to train BiLSTM models in order to capture various aspects of language production. Extensive feature ablation tests were conducted to identify the most informative feature groups linked to particular mental health disorders. The transformers models were made more interpretable by employing a multi-task fusion learning framework that combined data from two pertinent areas such as personality traits and emotion (Kerz et al., 2023).

12. SUCCESSFUL MODELS IN THE WORLD & INDIA

In the realm of healthcare, namely surgery, India is at the forefront of the global deployment of robots. This trend started in 1998 when a robotic arm helped perform a groundbreaking heart procedure. Since then, hospitals nationwide—both public and private—have been using robots extensively. Beyond merely developing robots, India has made significant strides in the realm of medicine thanks to AI. Hospitals like Manipal use IBM's Watson to help with surgery because of its vast medical knowledge and sophisticated data processing abilities. The surgical robotics sector is anticipated to grow fivefold by 2025, indicating a bright future for medical innovation in India. A 20% compound annual growth rate (CAGR) and an increasing demand for automation will drive this expansion. Voice-activated assistants and chatbots driven by artificial intelligence are revolutionizing patient education and engagement. Chatbots can help with mental health treatment, answer commonly asked questions, and provide patients with advice on a range of health-related topics. By offering information about illnesses, treatment options, and lifestyle advice, these interactive assistants empower users to take charge of their health. Moreover, voice assistants are simple to integrate into daily routines, monitoring health indicators and promptly reminding users to take their medications to encourage improved self-management and reduce prescription error rates (Matheny et al., 2022).

Additionally, by using own vocabulary and expressions, patients can interact with these virtual assistants in a genuine and conversational manner thanks to Natural Language Processing (NLP). In addition to increasing patient participation and overall pleasure, this also makes it easier for patients and medical staff to communicate. By understanding human language, providing targeted responses, prioritizing recommendations, and assisting with appointment scheduling, Natural Language Processing (NLP) assistants ultimately improve the effectiveness and efficiency of healthcare delivery. This ground-breaking technology has the potential to transform the healthcare experience, improve health outcomes, and empower people (Ziqitza, 2023).

Robots and AI are increasingly used in India's healthcare system, which is seen as a way to improve treatment quality. The lack of qualified healthcare workers may be addressed by artificial intelligence (AI), machine learning, and robotics, which could also provide patients with more individualized care. However, there are a number of barriers to the use of AI and robotics in healthcare, including the high cost of these technologies and the requirement for ethical frameworks (Murdoch, 2021).

13. KEY TAKEAWAYS

Numerous AI approaches are available and can be used to address a range of therapeutic issues. Nevertheless, despite early expectations, medical AI technology has not been warmly received. The clinicians' attitudes toward the use of technology in the decision-making process are one factor contributing to this. Ironically, magnetic resonance imaging images and biochemical data from an auto-analyzer are accepted without hesitation. Nonetheless, it is the responsibility of the researchers working in this area to provide proof that these methods are effective in real-world situations. Therefore, it is imperative to conduct additional randomized controlled experiments to demonstrate the effectiveness of AI systems in medicine. There is strong evidence that in the twenty-first century, medical AI can help clinicians provide healthcare more effectively. These methods will undoubtedly help to improve and supplement the future clinician's "medical intelligence" (Holmes et al., 2004).

AI in medicine has a direct impact on the field, but it is also becoming more and more linked to a number of possible ethical issues. To properly prepare aspiring medical professionals for the efficient use of these tools and handle the ethical dilemmas they raise, medical education must also adapt to the growing usage of AI and AI-based apps (Weidener & Fischer, 2024).

14. CONCLUSION

Machine learning techniques can be widely used to solve challenges in the medical field by implementing categorization models and systems that assist medical professionals in diagnosing and predicting diseases. However, because medical data and records are high dimensional, heterogeneous, and disorganized, it is challenging to extract knowledge and information from them. Additionally, this data includes outliers and noise in the gathered data. The primary relevant strategy will be applied by examining several machine learning approaches. Through accuracy verification and validation, the effectiveness of machine learning techniques is examined.

Decision tree algorithms, support vector machines, random forests, evolutionary algorithm-based models, and swarm intelligence-based methods are examples of machine learning approaches that are useful and applicable in the diagnosis and treatment of various illnesses. Through the use of imaging technology, doctors are able to diagnose diseases with more certainty thanks to advanced medical diagnosis criteria. Medical image analysis is a very complicated and challenging undertaking. Using machine learning techniques to analyze images will support and greatly aid in the diagnosis of diseases. Because machine learning techniques demonstrate their ability and ease of use in addressing bioinformatics-related issues, they are used to big data for diagnosis interpretation.

Current healthcare delivery methods may change as a result of the clinical application of machine learning in medicine. Healthcare professionals will employ machine learning in clinical settings, it will be integrated into smart devices via the internet of things, and patients will use it outside of clinical settings for chronic condition self-management. Investment in machine learning is growing exponentially, which suggests that research is speeding up and that more products may soon be aiming for market launch. In order to gain patients' trust and clinicians' adoption, machine learning in medicine needs to be completely compliant with data protection regulations, reduce the impact of bias, be efficiently controlled, and be transparent. Early resolution of these moral and legal concerns is crucial to preventing needless dangers and mistakes that could impede machine learning in medicine's future development.

AI use declaration: AI was used to enhance the readability of sentences/paragraphs. It was not used for content creation/generation, paraphrasing/rephrasing, word spinning, etc.

REFERENCES

Bakare, S. S., Adeniyi, A. O., Akpuokwe, C. U., & Eneh, N. E. (2024). Data privacy laws and compliance: A comparative review of the EU GDPR and USA regulations. *Computer Science & IT Research Journal*, *5*(3), 528–543. DOI: 10.51594/csitrj.v5i3.859

Balkrishnan, R., Chang, J., Patel, I., Yang, F., & Merajver, S. D. (2013). Global comparative healthcare effectiveness research: Evaluating sustainable programmes in low & middle resource settings. *The Indian Journal of Medical Research*, *137*(3), 494–501. DOI: 10.21203/rs.3.pex-2593/v1 PMID: 23640555

Bente, B. E., Van Dongen, A., Verdaasdonk, R., & van Gemert-Pijnen, L. (2024). eHealth implementation in Europe: A scoping review on legal, ethical, financial, and technological aspects. *Frontiers in Digital Health*, *6*, 1332707. DOI: 10.3389/fdgth.2024.1332707 PMID: 38524249

Bergquist, M., Rolandsson, B., Gryska, E., Laesser, M., Hoefling, N., Heckemann, R., Schneiderman, J. F., & Björkman-Burtscher, I. M. (2024). Trust and stakeholder perspectives on the implementation of AI tools in clinical radiology. *European Radiology*, *34*(1), 338–347. DOI: 10.1007/s00330-023-09967-5 PMID: 37505245

Braveman, P. (2006). Health disparities and health equity: Concepts and measurement. *Annual Review of Public Health*, *27*(1), 167–194. DOI: 10.1146/annurev.publhealth.27.021405.102103 PMID: 16533114

Cheng, S., Xiao, Y., Liu, L., & Sun, X. (2024). Comparative outcomes of AI-assisted ChatGPT and face-to-face consultations in infertility patients: A cross-sectional study. *Postgraduate Medical Journal*, *100*(1189), 851–855. DOI: 10.1093/postmj/qgae083 PMID: 38970829

Cheng, Y. T., Lin, Y. F., Chiang, K. H., & Tseng, V. S. (2017). Mining sequential risk patterns from large-scale clinical databases for early assessment of chronic diseases: A case study on chronic obstructive pulmonary disease. *IEEE Journal of Biomedical and Health Informatics*, *21*(2), 303–311. DOI: 10.1109/JBHI.2017.2657802 PMID: 28129195

Cohen, I. G., & Mello, M. M. (2018). HIPAA and protecting health information in the 21st century. *Journal of the American Medical Association*, *320*(3), 231–232. DOI: 10.1001/jama.2018.5630 PMID: 29800120

Dangi, R. R., Sharma, A., & Vageriya, V. (2024). Transforming Healthcare in Low-Resource Settings With Artificial Intelligence: Recent Developments and Outcomes. *Public Health Nursing (Boston, Mass.)*, phn.13500. Advance online publication. DOI: 10.1111/phn.13500 PMID: 39629887

Daniel, J. (2023). Safeguarding Privacy in the Age of AI: Navigating the Complexities of Data Protection. *Revista de Inteligencia Artificial en Medicina*, *14*(1), 693–704.

de Filippis, R., & Al Foysal, A. (2024). Blockchain Brains: Pioneering AI, ML, and DLT Solutions for Healthcare and Psychology. *OAlib*, *11*(12), 1–24. DOI: 10.4236/oalib.1112543

Fatima, M., & Pasha, M. (2017). Survey of machine learning algorithms for disease diagnostic. *Journal of Intelligent Learning Systems and Applications*, *9*(01), 1–16. DOI: 10.4236/jilsa.2017.91001

Fenton, J. J., Taplin, S. H., Carney, P. A., Abraham, L., Sickles, E. A., D'Orsi, C., Berns, E. A., Cutter, G., Hendrick, R. E., Barlow, W. E., & Elmore, J. G. (2007). Influence of computer-aided detection on performance of screening mammography. *The New England Journal of Medicine*, *356*(14), 1399–1409. DOI: 10.1056/NEJMoa066099 PMID: 17409321

Ghosh, P., Biswas, A., & Ghosh, S. (2023). Fundamentals and Technicalities of Big Data and Analytics. In *Intelligent Systems in Healthcare and Disease Identification using Data Science* (pp. 51–106). Chapman and Hall/CRC. DOI: 10.1201/9781003354178-3

Gopi, B., Kokila, M. S., Bibin, C. V., Sasikala, D., Howard, E., & Boopathi, S. (2024). Distributed Technologies Using AI/ML Techniques for Healthcare Applications. In *Social Innovations in Education, Environment, and Healthcare* (pp. 375-396). IGI Global.

Gowri, V., Uma, M., & Sethuramalingam, P. (2024). Machine learning enabled robot-assisted virtual health monitoring system design and development. *Multiscale and Multidisciplinary Modeling, Experiments and Design*, 1-30.

Handelman, G. S., Kok, H. K., Chandra, R. V., Razavi, A. H., Lee, M. J., & Asadi, H. (2018). eD octor: Machine learning and the future of medicine. *Journal of Internal Medicine*, *284*(6), 603–619. DOI: 10.1111/joim.12822 PMID: 30102808

Holmes, J., Sacchi, L., & Bellazzi, R. (2004). Artificial intelligence in medicine. *Annals of the Royal College of Surgeons of England*, *86*(5), 334–338. DOI: 10.1308/147870804290 PMID: 15333167

Jayaraman, P. P., Forkan, A. R. M., Morshed, A., Haghighi, P. D., & Kang, Y. B. (2020). Healthcare 4.0: A review of frontiers in digital health. *Wiley Interdisciplinary Reviews. Data Mining and Knowledge Discovery*, *10*(2), e1350. DOI: 10.1002/widm.1350

Kerz, E., Zanwar, S., Qiao, Y., & Wiechmann, D. (2023). Toward explainable AI (XAI) for mental health detection based on language behavior. *Frontiers in Psychiatry*, *14*, 1219479. DOI: 10.3389/fpsyt.2023.1219479 PMID: 38144474

Kimura, A., & Nadege, M. T. (2020, October). RoI Editing Tool Using AI for Radiotherapy Simulation. In *2020 IEEE Nuclear Science Symposium and Medical Imaging Conference (NSS/MIC)* (pp. 1-3). IEEE. DOI: 10.1109/NSS/MIC42677.2020.9508040

Kiyasseh, D., Zhu, T., & Clifton, D. (2020). The promise of clinical decision support systems targetting low-resource settings. *IEEE Reviews in Biomedical Engineering*, *15*, 354–371. DOI: 10.1109/RBME.2020.3017868 PMID: 32813662

Kononenko, I. (2001). Machine learning for medical diagnosis: History, state of the art and perspective. *Artificial Intelligence in Medicine*, *23*(1), 89–109. DOI: 10.1016/S0933-3657(01)00077-X PMID: 11470218

Lahat, A., Sharif, K., Zoabi, N., Shneor Patt, Y., Sharif, Y., Fisher, L., Shani, U., Arow, M., Levin, R., & Klang, E. (2024). Assessing generative pretrained transformers (GPT) in clinical decision-making: Comparative analysis of GPT-3.5 and GPT-4. *Journal of Medical Internet Research*, *26*, e54571. DOI: 10.2196/54571 PMID: 38935937

Latif, J., Xiao, C., Imran, A., & Tu, S. (2019, January). Medical imaging using machine learning and deep learning algorithms: a review. In *2019 2nd International conference on computing, mathematics and engineering technologies (iCoMET)* (pp. 1-5). IEEE. DOI: 10.1109/ICOMET.2019.8673502

Lehman, C. D., Wellman, R. D., Buist, D. S., Kerlikowske, K., Tosteson, A. N., & Miglioretti, D. L.Breast Cancer Surveillance Consortium. (2015). Diagnostic accuracy of digital screening mammography with and without computer-aided detection. *JAMA Internal Medicine*, *175*(11), 1828–1837. DOI: 10.1001/jamainternmed.2015.5231 PMID: 26414882

Li, L., Novillo-Ortiz, D., Azzopardi-Muscat, N., & Kostkova, P. (2021). Digital data sources and their impact on people's health: A systematic review of systematic reviews. *Frontiers in Public Health*, *9*, 645260. DOI: 10.3389/fpubh.2021.645260 PMID: 34026711

Lin, C. C., Huang, A. Y., & Yang, S. J. (2023). A review of ai-driven conversational chatbots implementation methodologies and challenges (1999–2022). *Sustainability (Basel), 15*(5), 4012. DOI: 10.3390/su15054012

Liu, J., Li, J., Wang, H., & Yan, J. (2020). Application of deep learning in genomics. *Science China. Life Sciences, 63*(12), 1860–1878. DOI: 10.1007/s11427-020-1804-5 PMID: 33051704

Malathi, K., Shruthi, S. N., Madhumitha, N., Sreelakshmi, S., Sathya, U., & Sangeetha, P. M. (2024). Medical Data Integration and Interoperability through Remote Monitoring of Healthcare Devices. [JoWUA]. *Journal of Wireless Mobile Networks, Ubiquitous Computing and Dependable Applications, 15*(2), 60–72. DOI: 10.58346/JOWUA.2024.I2.005

Marvin, G., Hellen, N., & Nakatumba-Nabende, J. (2023, February). Research Paradigms for Health Equity in Intelligent Mobile Healthcare Technologies: A Critical Review. In *International Conference on Intelligent Sustainable Systems* (pp. 365-375). Singapore: Springer Nature Singapore. DOI: 10.1007/978-981-99-1726-6_28

Matheny, M. S., Israni, T. M., & Ahmed, M.. (2022). *Artificial Intelligence in Health Care: The Hope, the Hype, the Promise, the Peril.* National Academy of Medicine., Available from https://nap.nationalacademies.org/read/27111/chapter/3

Mittal, P. (2020). Big data and analytics: A data management perspective in public administration. *International Journal of Big Data Management, 1*(2), 152–165. DOI: 10.1504/IJBDM.2020.112415

Naik, K., Goyal, R. K., Foschini, L., Chak, C. W., Thielscher, C., Zhu, H., Lu, J., Lehár, J., Pacanoswki, M. A., Terranova, N., Mehta, N., Korsbo, N., Fakhouri, T., Liu, Q., & Gobburu, J. (2024). Current status and future directions: The application of artificial intelligence/machine learning for precision medicine. *Clinical Pharmacology and Therapeutics, 115*(4), 673–686. DOI: 10.1002/cpt.3152 PMID: 38103204

Neighbors, H. W., Jackson, J. S., Campbell, L., & Williams, D. (1989). The influence of racial factors on psychiatric diagnosis: A review and suggestions for research. *Community Mental Health Journal, 25*(4), 301–311. DOI: 10.1007/BF00755677 PMID: 2697490

Nunes, T., da Cunha, P. R., de Abreu, J. M., Duarte, J., & Corte-Real, A. (2024). Non-Fungible Tokens (NFTs) in Healthcare: A Systematic Review. *International Journal of Environmental Research and Public Health, 21*(8), 965. DOI: 10.3390/ijerph21080965 PMID: 39200576

Nyström, M. E., Karltun, J., Keller, C., & Andersson Gäre, B. (2018). Collaborative and partnership research for improvement of health and social services: Researcher's experiences from 20 projects. *Health Research Policy and Systems*, *16*(1), 1–17. DOI: 10.1186/s12961-018-0322-0 PMID: 29843735

Ozer, M. E., Sarica, P. O., & Arga, K. Y. (2020). New machine learning applications to accelerate personalized medicine in breast cancer: Rise of the support vector machines. *OMICS: A Journal of Integrative Biology*, *24*(5), 241–246. DOI: 10.1089/omi.2020.0001 PMID: 32228365

Patel, A. U., Gu, Q., Esper, R., Maeser, D., & Maeser, N. (2024). The Crucial Role of Interdisciplinary Conferences in Advancing Explainable AI in Healthcare. *BioMedInformatics*, *4*(2), 1363–1383. DOI: 10.3390/biomedinformatics4020075

Prabhod, K. J. (2022). The Role of Machine Learning in Genomic Medicine: Advancements in Disease Prediction and Treatment. *Journal of Deep Learning in Genomic Data Analysis*, *2*(1), 1–52.

Pramanik, M. I., Lau, R. Y., Hossain, M. S., Rahoman, M. M., Debnath, S. K., Rashed, M. G., & Uddin, M. Z. (2021). Privacy preserving big data analytics: A critical analysis of state- of-the-art. *Wiley Interdisciplinary Reviews. Data Mining and Knowledge Discovery*, *11*(1), e1387. DOI: 10.1002/widm.1387

Santra, S., Kukreja, P., Saxena, K., Gandhi, S., & Singh, O. V. (2024). Navigating regulatory and policy challenges for AI enabled combination devices. *Frontiers in Medical Technology*, *6*, 1473350. DOI: 10.3389/fmedt.2024.1473350 PMID: 39669903

Shaik, F., Yelchuri, R., Gudur, N. A., & Dash, J. K. (2024). ML Applications in Healthcare. *How Machine Learning is Innovating Today's World: A Concise Technical Guide*, 201-220.

Sharma, S., Malakar, S., Yadav, V., & Kak, S. M. (2023).. . *AI-Based Healthcare System.*, *IRSD2024*, 181.

Susarla, A., Gopal, R., Thatcher, J. B., & Sarker, S. (2023). The Janus effect of generative AI: Charting the path for responsible conduct of scholarly activities in information systems. *Information Systems Research*, *34*(2), 399–408. DOI: 10.1287/isre.2023.ed.v34.n2

Tyagi, A. K., Arumugam, S. K., Prasad, P. R., & Sharma, A. (2024). The Position of Digital Society, Healthcare 5.0, and Consumer 5.0 in the Era of Industry 5.0. In *Advancing Software Engineering Through AI, Federated Learning, and Large Language Models* (pp. 262-280). IGI Global. DOI: DOI: 10.4018/979-8-3693-3502-4.ch017

Vaigandla, K. K., Vanteru, M. K., & Siluveru, M. (2024). An Extensive Examination of the IoT and Blockchain Technologies in Relation to their Applications in the Healthcare Industry. *Mesopotamian Journal of Computer Science, 2024*, 1–14. DOI: 10.58496/MJCSC/2024/001

Vamathevan, J., Clark, D., Czodrowski, P., Dunham, I., Ferran, E., Lee, G., Li, B., Madabhushi, A., Shah, P., Spitzer, M., & Zhao, S. (2019). Applications of machine learning in drug discovery and development. *Nature Reviews. Drug Discovery*, *18*(6), 463–477. DOI: 10.1038/s41573-019-0024-5 PMID: 30976107

Weidener, L., & Fischer, M. (2024). Artificial intelligence in medicine: Cross-sectional study among medical students on application, education, and ethical aspects. *JMIR Medical Education*, *10*(1), e51247. DOI: 10.2196/51247 PMID: 38180787

Weissler, E. H., Naumann, T., Andersson, T., Ranganath, R., Elemento, O., Luo, Y., Freitag, D. F., Benoit, J., Hughes, M. C., Khan, F., Slater, P., Shameer, K., Roe, M., Hutchison, E., Kollins, S. H., Broedl, U., Meng, Z., Wong, J. L., Curtis, L., & Ghassemi, M. (2021). The role of machine learning in clinical research: Transforming the future of evidence generation. *Trials*, *22*(1), 1–15. DOI: 10.1186/s13063-021-05489-x PMID: 34399832

Wiens, J., Spector-Bagdady, K., & Mukherjee, B. (2024). Toward Realizing the Promise of AI in Precision Health Across the Spectrum of Care. *Annual Review of Genomics and Human Genetics*, *25*(1), 141–159. Advance online publication. DOI: 10.1146/annurev-genom-010323-010230 PMID: 38724019

Yadav, S. (2024). Transformative frontiers: A comprehensive review of emerging technologies in modern healthcare. *Cureus*, *16*(3). Advance online publication. DOI: 10.7759/cureus.56538 PMID: 38646390

Zhao, A. P., Li, S., Cao, Z., Hu, P. J. H., Wang, J., Xiang, Y., Xie, D., & Lu, X. (2024). AI for science: Predicting infectious diseases. *Journal of Safety Science and Resilience = An Quan Ke Xue Yu Ren Xing (Ying Wen).*

Ziqitza, (2023), https://analyticsindiamag.com/how-surgical-robot-assistants-are-becoming-areality-in-indian-hospitals-and-healthcare-sector/

ADDITIONAL READING:

Ahsan, M., Khan, A., Khan, K. R., Sinha, B. B., & Sharma, A. (2024). Advancements in medical diagnosis and treatment through machine learning: A review. *Expert Systems: International Journal of Knowledge Engineering and Neural Networks*, *41*(3), e13499. DOI: 10.1111/exsy.13499

Ali, M. T., Ali, U., Ali, S., & Tanveer, H. (2024). Transforming cardiac care: AI and machine learning innovations. *International Journal of Multidisciplinary Research and Growth Evaluation.*

Husnain, A., Hussain, H. K., Shahroz, H. M., Ali, M., & Hayat, Y. (2024). Advancements in health through artificial intelligence and machine learning: A focus on brain health. *Revista Española de Documentación Cientifica*, *18*(01), 100–123.

Hussain, I., & Nazir, M. B. (2024). Empowering Healthcare: AI, ML, and Deep Learning Innovations for Brain and Heart Health. *International Journal of Advanced Engineering Technologies and Innovations*, *1*(4), 167–188.

Kasula, B. Y. (2024). Optimizing healthcare delivery: Machine learning applications and innovations for enhanced patient outcomes. *International Journal of Creative Research In Computer Technology and Design*, *6*(6), 1–7.

Olawade, D. B., David-Olawade, A. C., Wada, O. Z., Asaolu, A. J., Adereni, T., & Ling, J. (2024). Artificial intelligence in healthcare delivery: Prospects and pitfalls. *Journal of Medicine, Surgery, and Public Health*, *3*, 100108. DOI: 10.1016/j.glmedi.2024.100108

Shiwlani, A., Khan, M., Sherani, A. M. K., Qayyum, M. U., & Hussain, H. K. (2024). REVOLUTIONIZING HEALTHCARE: THE IMPACT OF ARTIFICIAL INTELLIGENCE ON PATIENT CARE, DIAGNOSIS, AND TREATMENT. *JURIHUM: Jurnal Inovasi dan Humaniora, 1*(5), 779-790.

Singh, P., & Tiwari, S. (2024). Machine learning models for cost-effective healthcare delivery systems. *Digital Transformation in Healthcare 5.0: Volume 1: IoT, AI and Digital Twin*, 245.

Srinivasaiah, B. (2024). The Power of Personalized Healthcare: Harnessing the Potential of Machine Learning in Precision Medicine. *International Journal of Scientific Research*, •••, 426–429.

Zeb, S., Nizamullah, F. N. U., Abbasi, N., & Fahad, M. (2024). AI in Healthcare: Revolutionizing Diagnosis and Therapy. *International Journal of Multidisciplinary Sciences and Arts*, *3*(3), 118–128. DOI: 10.47709/ijmdsa.v3i3.4546

KEYWORDS AND DEFINITIONS

Healthcare 6.0: The combination of cutting-edge technologies, data-driven strategies, and human-centered innovations is known as Healthcare 6.0, and it aims to build a healthcare ecosystem that is more intelligent, effective, and customized. In order to change health and wellbeing, this paradigm embraces emerging disruptive technologies while building on the foundations of Healthcare 4.0 (IoT, AI, and big data) and Healthcare 5.0 (human-centered care).

Healthcare 6.0 Transformative Technologies: Artificial Intelligence (AI) and Machine Learning (ML), Internet of Medical Things (IoMT), Blockchain Technology, Virtual Reality (VR), Augmented Reality (AR), Quantum Computing, Nanotechnology, 5G Connectivity, Precision Medicine and Genomics, Advanced Robotics.

One-dimensional bio signal analysis: Processing and interpreting bio-signals that change over time, such as electrocardiograms (ECGs), electroencephalograms (EEGs), electromyograms (EMGs), and photoplethysmograms (PPGs), is known as one-dimensional (1D) bio-signal analysis. To extract useful physiological and therapeutic information, these signals are processed and displayed as functions of time.

Computer-aided detection: enhances radiologists' ability to identify possible tumors by decreasing false negatives. To determine the location of possible malignancies, CAD systems employ computer vision and image processing.

Computer-aided diagnosis: gives radiologists the probability that a lesion is malignant, which aids in their decision regarding the necessity of a biopsy.

Clinical decision making: Clinical decision making is the process of developing clinical options based on objective clinical data and evidence-based criteria, taking into account a variety of aspects such patient preferences and medical technology improvements. The diagnostic, severity evaluation, and management phases are the three interconnected stages of clinical decision making. Making the right clinical decisions involves taking into account both the necessity of a precise diagnosis and the expenses related to the careless or inappropriate use of diagnostic testing. The costs and potential negative consequences of therapeutic interventions are also evaluated, as is the chance of an unfavorable outcome due to improper management.

Survival analysis: a field of data analysis and statistics that focuses on forecasting when a significant event will take place. This "event" could be any quantifiable result, such as failure, recovery, or death. The social sciences, engineering, and medicine are among the disciplines that frequently use survival analysis.

Drug discovery: the process of finding and creating novel drugs that could be used to treat illnesses. This field is multidisciplinary and encompasses pharmacology, chemistry, and biology.

Chapter 7
Application of Machine Learning in Healthcare IoT:
An Investigation on Disease Diagnosis and Analytic Cases

Ashwini Kumar Pradhan
https://orcid.org/0000-0002-1822-4235
Galgotias University, India

Rudra Kalyan Nayak
https://orcid.org/0000-0003-4447-8391
VIT Bhopal University, India

Arvind Yadav
https://orcid.org/0000-0002-8988-9947
Galgotias University, India

Hitesh Mohapatra
https://orcid.org/0000-0001-8100-4860
KIIT University, India

Nilamadhab Mishra
https://orcid.org/0000-0002-1330-4869
VIT Bhopal University, India

Lambodar Jena
Shiksha 'O' Anusandhan University, India

Akhilesh Kumar Tripathi
Galgotias University, India

ABSTRACT

Machine learning (ML) is the most prominent topic, with many applications in video processing, language processing, visual diagnosis of illnesses, drug development, biochemistry, and biomedical. Healthcare systems and medical science-related applications are rapidly growing among these applications. Large data expansion, the Internet of Things (IoT), networked devices, and high-performance computers with graphics processing units are all contributing to the growing popularity of ML.

DOI: 10.4018/979-8-3693-7210-4.ch007

Healthcare in IoT (HIoT), and electronic health record (EHR) data are the key data resources for neural network (NN) models. Several possible challenges, including security and quality of service improvement, are important to ML. Based on the comprehensive literature survey (CLS), ML for HIoT is examined in this research.

INTRODUCTION

Introducing cutting-edge technology like deep learning (DL) and the Internet of Things (IoT) is causing a radical change in the healthcare sector. The term "healthcare IoT" (HIoT) describes the network of medical equipment, sensors, and systems that are connected and that make it easier to gather, send, and analyze data about health. These tools have made predictions, individualized care delivery, and real-time patient monitoring possible. However, processing, evaluating, and deriving valuable insights have become extremely difficult due to the exponential explosion of data produced by HIoT devices. Deep learning (DL) has become a potent instrument, providing advanced techniques for managing intricate, high-dimensional healthcare data and aiding in crucial decision-making. Early and precise illness identification is essential for successful treatment and better patient outcomes. If identified early, many illnesses, including diabetes, heart disease, and some types of cancer, can be controlled or even cured. However, static testing and physician knowledge are frequently the mainstays of current diagnostic procedures, which might overlook important patterns, especially when dealing with rare or complicated illnesses. By analyzing real-time data streams to identify anomalies that may indicate the early stages of disease, lowering diagnostic errors through consistent and objective analysis, enabling continuous monitoring, and offering a dynamic view of a patient's health status, integrating DL into HIoT systems offers a promising way to get around these limitations.

Deep learning (DL) is a novel topic in machine learning (ML) and a subset of artificial intelligence (AI). Both authors (McCulloch & Pitts, 1943) were the first to suggest artificial neural networks (ANN) in the 1940s. The core idea of NNs for processing information was inspired by biological brain systems (Jain and Mohiuddin, 1996). This article outlines the artificial computational model, the basic biological neuron, and the reasons behind the development of ANNs. Some of the most widely used ANN models and an overview of network designs and learning procedures are presented. ANN has multiple layers, as seen in **Figure 1**. Every layer takes care of extracting and sending data represented by weight to the next layer. The output is the sum of all the values associated with certain inputs. Every layer oversees gathering data, expressed as a score multiplied by a weight, and sending it to the layer behind it. The output is the total of all the values associated with a certain input. The input layer is responsible for gathering the input data, the output layer produces the output results, and hidden layers store the relevant weights.

The widespread availability of the internet, along with improvements in network engineering and hardware sophistication, has brought forth a new era marked by a large amount of data and various data analyzing methods. This combination of variables has made it possible to analyze and validate the signals that sensors have received, opening new possibilities in many fields, including healthcare, transportation, agriculture, and the creation of smart cities. **Figure 2** shows how NNs and the Internet of Things (IoT) are integrated in a futuristic environment. It demonstrates how NNs and networked devices combine to interpret data and make wise decisions.

Figure 1. The architecture of a neural network with 2 Hidden Layer

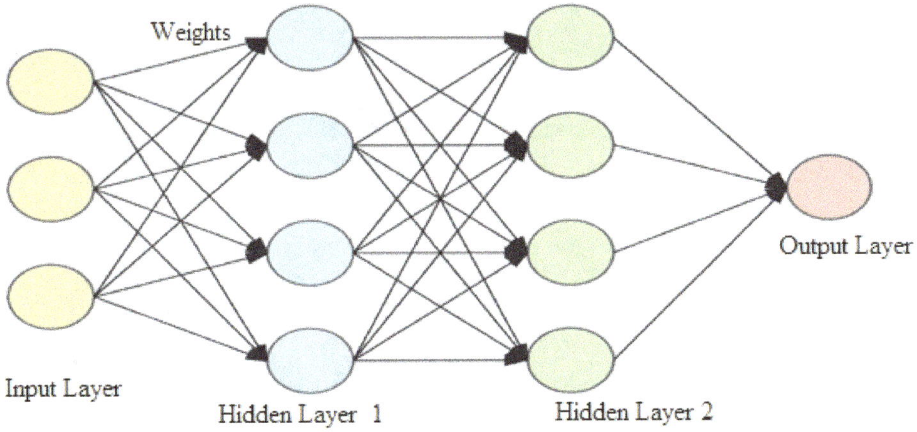

Figure 2. Deep learning using IoT systems

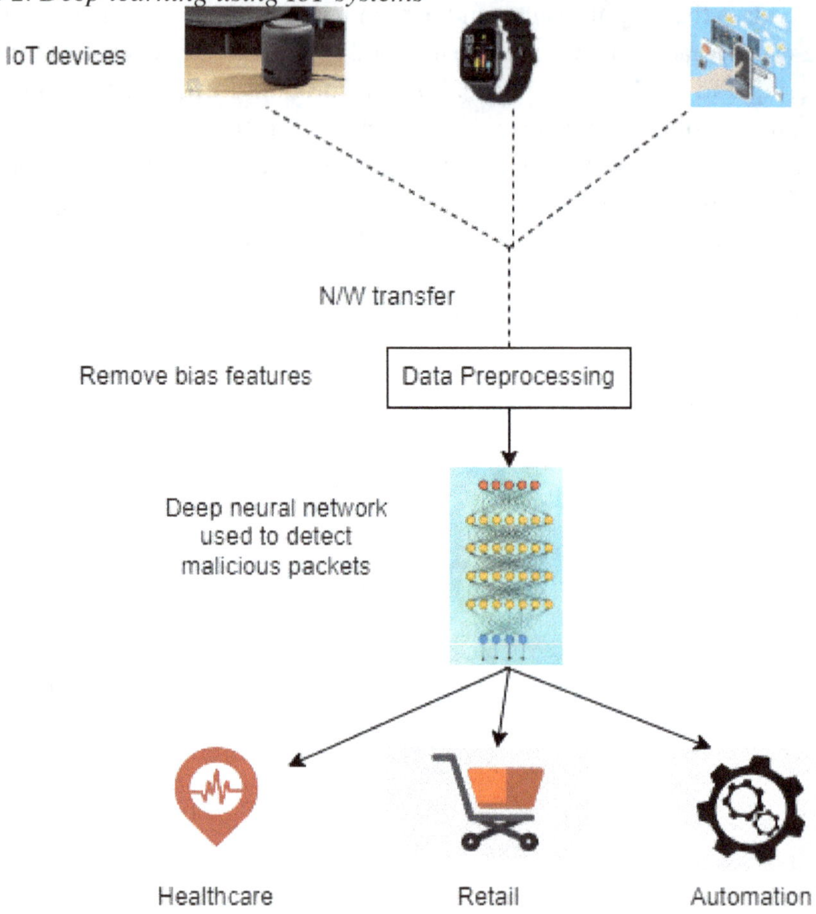

When paired with NNs, IoT devices work as data producers, providing real-time data for the NNs to process. The NNs may then analyze the data, look for trends, anticipate outcomes, and automate decision-making. Applications requiring automation, decision-making, and real-time analytics will find this integration helpful.

Important Uses

Cities: IoT sensors in cities can track energy use, pollution, and traffic in "smart cities." Using data analysis, NNs optimize emergency responses, energy distribution, and traffic signals.

Healthcare: Wearable IoT devices, such as fitness trackers, continuously collect patient data. NNs can analyze this data to identify early illness indicators or health hazards.

Predictive Maintenance: IoT sensors can monitor machinery in an industrial context. Preemptive maintenance is made possible by NNs' ability to examine data and forecast when a machine is going to break.

Smart Homes: To optimize energy usage, improve security, or customize user experiences, NNs can analyze data from IoT devices such as smart thermostats, security cameras, or home assistants.

The IoT integrates the physical and digital worlds (Ray,2018). To facilitate developers' requirements, this paper explored IoT-oriented architectures that can improve the understanding of relevant tools, technology, and techniques. The architectures that are being discussed aim to address real-world issues either directly or indirectly by developing and implementing strong IoT concepts.

There are several methods to explain the IoT, such as ''3 A concept: any time, any place, and any medium, resulting in a constant ratio between the radio and man" (Srivastava, 2006). Medical Internet of Things (MIoT) plays a major role in people's lives because Internet services and electronic apps are crucial parts of healthcare (Hu et al.,2013). Using sensing devices and interconnected medical instruments brings unique medical assistance to clinics, patients, and specialists, referred to as the MIoT. The authors of this study examine how the IoT might be advantageous in terms of information perception, transmission, and application. They also anticipate that the IoT will have a wide range of applications in the medical and healthcare fields. Future development will inevitably lead to the creation of a system that is intelligent, accessible, and interactive. This article focuses on the uses of the IoT in the medical and healthcare industries, such as medical information management, telemedicine and mobile medical care, medical equipment and medication control, personal health management, etc.

IoT devices are currently producing a large amount of data, which is then processed by DL algorithms to produce useful information. DL has several implications and is widespread in our daily lives. Medical and healthcare applications are among the most popular, and they are continually expanding in popularity. Electronic health records (EHRs) and medical databases, digitized photographs, data from mobile apps, IoT medical instruments, and data from browsers are all major sources of DL algorithms that may forecast, diagnose, and assist with clinical decisions (Esteva et al.,2019). This paper intends to examine the most recent research and analyses on various ML and IoT applications in medical sciences. Disease forecasting, detection, treatment, pharmacology, and health informatics are among the important applications examined in this review which separates this study from others. It focuses on the application of ML, IoT, and a combination of the two, whereas previous studies only concentrated on one of these areas. This survey is a comprehensive literature survey (CLS) that covers the following topics:

- Demonstrating a technological nomenclature for various IoT and ML applications in healthcare.
- Examining the difficulties of using the associated application.
- Examining current issues and prospects.

This chapter mainly focuses on 4 things:

- Reviewing research work.
- ML applications for IoT in healthcare.
- Current prospects and challenges.
- Conclusion.

RELATED REVIEWS

This section will go through the research that has been done on ML applications for IoT in healthcare. This study investigates relevant studies that were chosen from 15 published research papers over 5 years, from 2017 to 2021. Conceptual notions and theories of ML are presented first, followed by examining related research on IoT in health care. Each study's basic idea, benefits, drawbacks, and constraints are examined, followed by recommendations for further research. The idea of the Internet of Health Things (IoHT) was discussed by (Da Costa et al., 2018). Shifting objects regulate patients' physical states by aggregating and integrating data on critically important signals in hospitals. Gathering, preserving, interpreting, and visualizing are the four stages of IoHT. As a foundation for creating the IoHT, this review has presented the monitoring and analysis of vital signs to predict patient health concerns. The first section of the review covered the primary physiological measurements that might be tracked, which led to the identification of eight variables: blood pressure, body temperature, heart rate, respiration rate, oxygen saturation, pain threshold, consciousness level, and urine output. The first five vital signs, systolic blood pressure, body temperature, heart rate, respiration rate, and degree of consciousness, were also emphasized in the essay as the most crucial bodily measurements. After that, an analysis was done on the hospital's current methods for assessing health risks based on tracking and triggering systems. IoHT has two advantages: minimising service downtimes and efficiently allocating limited resources. The survey's main shortcomings are connected to the number and complexity of data collected, interpreting a difficult effort for caregivers.

In another research work, (Islam et al., 2015) reviewed many aspects of IoT-based innovations in the health sector and proposed a variety of medical network topologies and interfaces that make the IoT framework available and facilitate data movement. Furthermore, the paper presents comprehensive research efforts related to the potential of IoT in the areas of private health, fitness management, chronic disease supervision, and pediatric cum geriatric care. The paper provides a broad overview of how recent advancements in sensors, devices, internet applications, and other technologies have motivated connected health services and affordable healthcare gadgets to endlessly expand the potential of IoT-based healthcare services for further development. It provides deeper insights into industry trends and enabling technologies. The paper considers various security requirements and obstacles, reveals many research concerns in this field, and proposes a model that can mitigate associated security risks to comprehend IoT healthcare security better. It is anticipated that the conversation on several crucial topics, including standards, network architecture, business models, service quality, and health data security, would help to provide the framework for additional study on IoT-based healthcare solutions. This document presents eHealth and IoT policies and regulations to assist stakeholders interested in evaluating IoT innovations. The benefits of IoT-based healthcare care include cost savings and improved quality of life. IoT healthcare products, on the other hand, are embedded with sluggish processors. Furthermore, these gadgets are incapable of doing computationally intensive tasks.

Digital sensor data monitoring for senior unwell patients is for quick data access and dependable service by a healthcare service provider's proper forecast (Rajan et al., 2019). To handle this difficulty, emphasize a unique IoT application-based biosensors monitoring system to enhance the e-healthcare system using a deep neural network (DNN)-based accurate signal prediction. Using an intelligent sensor for signal measurement and myRIO for smart data capture, the suggested system is prototyped as an advanced electronics component. Four biosensor prediction accuracies for two users were obtained to verify the theoretical Smart-Monitor model. The average accuracy of the prototype experimental set-up was 97.2 percent.

METHODOLOGY

This section presents the CLS approach as a research study evaluation technique for identifying ML applications for IoT in healthcare (Ghomi, E. J. et al., 2017; Effatparvar, M et al.,2016).

This chapter responds to the main Research Questions about the study's objectives:

- Research Question 1: What are the different types of ML applications for IoT in healthcare?
- Research Question 2: Which important scenarios for ML applications in IoT for healthcare are noted?

Figure 3 demonstrates how the research survey assessment guidelines were chosen. Chapters from books, incomplete studies, and non-peer-reviewed surveys are among the sections that have been eliminated. Research published between 2017 and 2021 that received over ten citations are considered. **Figure 4** depicts the propagation of research surveys from major publishers such as IEEE, Google Scholar, ACM, Elsevier, and Springer.

Figure 3. Identification, Refinement, and Selection criteria for analyzing study findings.

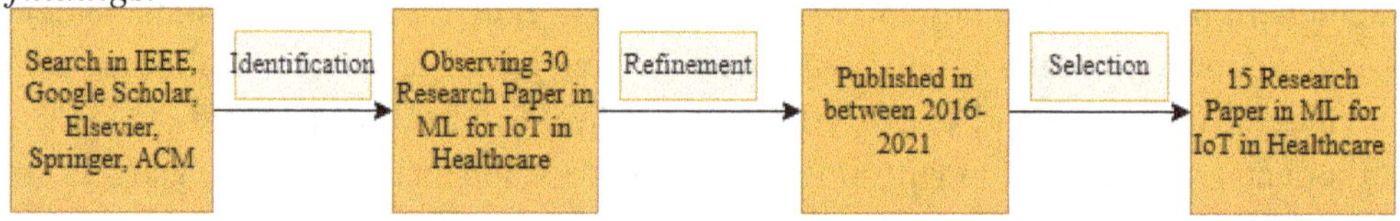

Figure 4. Different publisher research distribution from 2017 to 2021

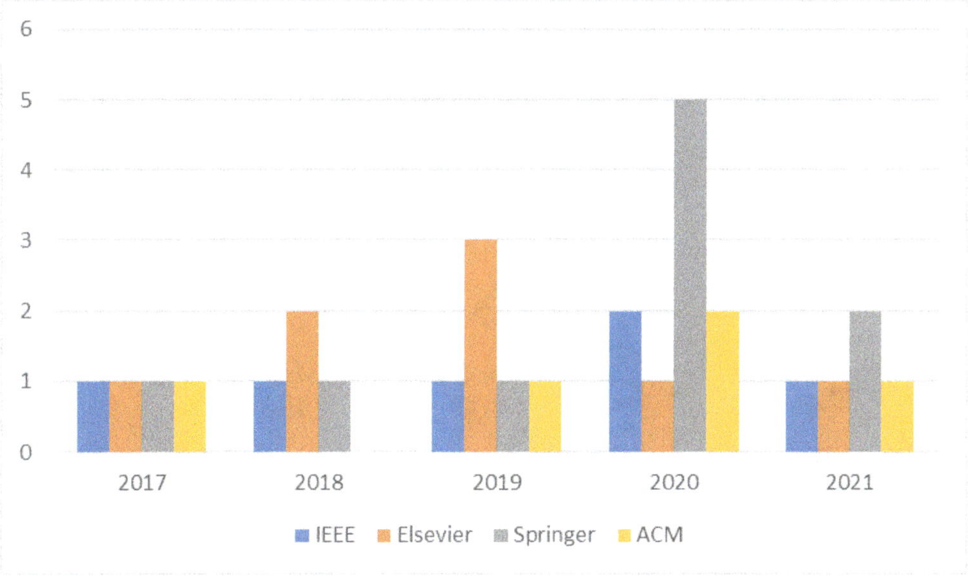

Machine learning applications for IoT in healthcare

According to the literature study, this section gives an overview of selected ML applications for IoT in healthcare for the current surveys. Medical diagnostics, home-based technologies, diagnosis of disease, and human behaviour identification are all included in **Figure 5**. We examine publications that address issues concerning DL applications in healthcare. For example, major topics such as smartphone sensor information, multi-morbidity chronic patients, physiological signals, smart dental Health-IoT systems, fall detection frameworks, injuries, and nutrition monitoring systems were specified.

The following subsections illustrate various strategies for ML applications. We also analyze and compare those publications' major portion, case studies, advantages, shortcomings, and new achievements.

Figure 5. The classification of ML applications for IoT in healthcare.

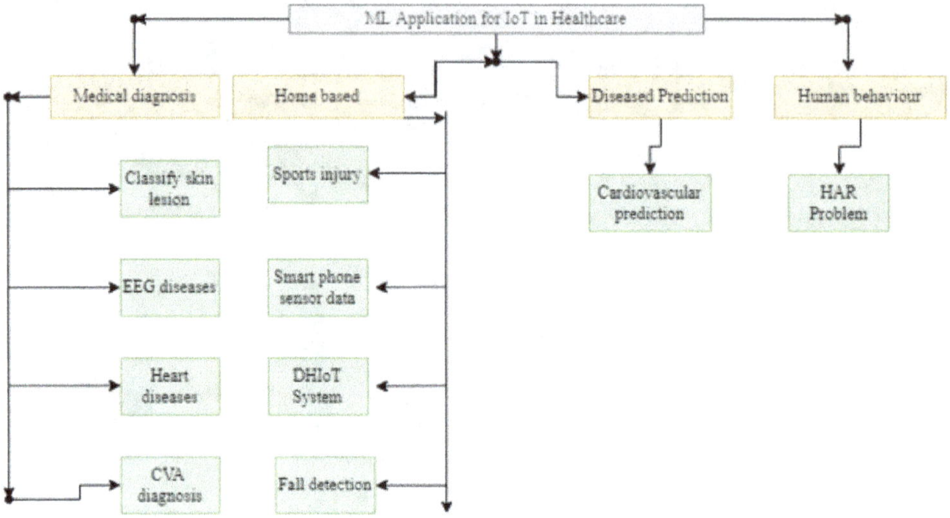

HealthFog was described by (Tuli et al., 2020) for autonomous diagnosis of cardiac problems using ML and IoT, which provides a lightweight fog solution and effective data handling for patients with heart conditions from various IoT devices. The benefits of a new fog and edge computing pattern include energy-saving solutions and low-latency data processing solutions. HealthFog uses IoT devices to deliver healthcare as a fog service and effectively manages patient data upon request. FogBus, a fog-enabled cloud framework, is used to deploy and test the proposed model's performance in terms of power consumption, network bandwidth, latency, jitter, accuracy, and execution time. HealthFog can be configured to operate in various ways that offer the best quality of service or prediction accuracy, depending on the user's needs and different fog computation scenarios. According to (Pradhan et al., 2021), ML algorithms have resulted in neoteric technological improvements in automatic EEG illness diagnosis. The automated feature extraction ability improved EEG decoding performance, one of the survey's favorable aspects. Furthermore, analyzing their EEG allows for diagnosing unique health issues (Kamnitsas et al., 2017; Hossain et al., 2019; Acharya et al., 2018). CVA (cerebral vascular accident) (Filho et al., 2017), often known as stroke, is a condition in which some areas of the brain stop working due to clotting. It can usually result in death. This problem can be solved with prompt diagnosis. Typically, CT and MRI imaging are utilized to detect strokes. The IoT framework can be used to classify stroke using CT images and convolutional neural networks (CNN) to determine whether the brain is normal, the stroke is hypoxic, or the stroke was caused by bleeding. The benefits of using

IoT in healthcare include considerably fewer regions and fewer errors. Melanoma (Ma & Tavares, 2015) is a dangerous form of skin cancer because it is more prone to spread. There are three forms of melanocytic lesions: common nevi, atypical nevi, and melanomas. This study employs a platform based on IoT technology to classify skin lesions. The suggested method used CNN models on the ImageNet dataset to obtain images. The benefits of this method include its versatility and ease of use. The study's drawback is related to internet access.

The work (Mendes et al., 2017) proposed a workshop on smart living spaces for multimorbidity chronic patients receiving home-based treatment. To activate the less differentiated caregiver (LDC), a particular care needs. The environments combine the chronicle patient clinical history semantic representation ICP (Individual Care Process) with the capability of monitoring the living conditions using IoT technologies and events recurring to a fully managed semantic web of things (SWoT) and ML Algorithms. These gadgets make providing healthcare at home feasible, reducing the need for institutionalization. In addition to increasing the generality of health and satisfaction metrics, the ensuing integrated healthcare framework will result in significant cost reductions. The biggest impediment to accumulating sufficient indications of medical knowledge is the "Knowledge Acquisition Bottleneck." Maps from one input to another output are a system component in this technique. This strategy adds to a new wave of caregiving conveniences by improving the quality of life for people with comorbidities and lowering expenditures.

Even though data is kept on cloud servers these days, there is still a chance of hacking and privacy breaches. The security concern of personal information mixed in with raw data gathered from many dispersed and heterogeneous wearable healthcare devices has received little attention (Hongliang et al., 2021). DL-based data analytics and privacy preservation solutions for IoT-enabled healthcare should be created to address this issue. User's private information is segregated in the privacy-isolation zone, and raw data is collected. At the cloud end, the authors build a sensitive security module based on CNN and analyze health-related data without revealing user personal information. In addition, they test and implement the prototype system, demonstrating its robustness and efficacy through numerous trials.

Conventional patient monitoring systems typically consist of vision-based techniques and wearable sensors. Using a DL-based algorithm, an IoT-based, non-invasive, automated patient discomfort monitoring system is presented and put into practice (Hongliang et al., 2021). The system's foundation is an IP camera device, which allows it to detect the patient's posture and movement without any wearable technology. Various critical spots on the patient's body are extracted using the Mask-RCNN approach. The six main bodily organs are created from these identified important sites using data mining association rules. Information about detected key point coordinates is also measured to analyze the patient's discomfort.

Ultimately, the distance and temporal threshold categorize movements as belonging to uncomfortable or typical circumstances. The patient's lying posture on the bed is also ascertained using these important details. Comfort and discomfort levels are differentiated based on the patient's posture and body position, which are continuously monitored. Different video sequences covering the beds of two patients are captured for experimental evaluation. With a true-positive rate of 94% and a false-positive rate of 7%, the testing findings demonstrate the value of the suggested approach.

According to (Ma & Tavares, 2015), the DL-based Internet of Health framework for Alzheimer Patients' Assistance, or DeTrAs, is suggested. In three stages, DeTrAs operates: (1) Using sensory movement data, a recurrent neural network-based Alzheimer prediction system is developed; (2) an ensemble approach consisting of two components is designed for anomaly tracking in Alzheimer patients: The following schemes are also presented: (a) a CNN-based emotion detection strategy; (b) a timestamp window-based natural language processing scheme; and (3) an IoT-based Alzheimer sufferers' help mechanism. DeTrAs's study shows an approximate 10–20% increase in accuracy compared to other ML algorithms already in use.

A vast amount of sensing data is created from various sensing devices due to the increasing demands of the IoT. AI methods are essential for real-time, scalable, and accurate data analysis. However, several obstacles to overcome in designing and developing a practical big data analysis method include resource limitations, centralized architecture, security and privacy issues, and a dearth of sufficient training data. Conversely, the emerging field of blockchain technology provides a decentralized design. It is supported by eliminating centralized control and addressing AI-related issues. It permits the safe transfer of resources and data across the many IoT network nodes. Thus, an optimal DL-based secure blockchain (ODLSB) enabled intelligent IoT, and healthcare diagnosis model was developed by (Veeramakali et al., 2021). Three main procedures are included in the suggested model: secure transaction, hash value encryption, and medical diagnostic. It includes the orthogonal particle swarm optimization (OPSO) algorithm for sharing medical images in secret. Furthermore, the neighborhood indexing sequence (NIS) algorithm is used in hash value encryption. Ultimately, the disorders are diagnosed using the optimum DNN as a classification model. Using the OPSO method for optimal parameter adjustment and secret sharing demonstrates the work's uniqueness. With sensitivity (92.75%), specificity (91.42%), and accuracy (93.68%) during the diagnosis procedure, the OPSO-DNN model has produced excellent results.

A new cloud-based and IoT-based healthcare application that monitors and diagnoses dangerous diseases is being created to provide excellent service to users utilizing online healthcare services (Ganesan & Sivakumar, 2019). To estimate the population's likelihood of having heart disease, a practical framework for the condition is developed in this study using data from the UCI Repository and medical sensors. A series of classifiers, including J48, logistic regression (LR), multilayer perception (MLP), and support vector machines (SVM), are tested on a benchmark dataset to conduct experiments. The simulation's outcomes confirmed that the J48 classifiers perform better across various metrics, including recall, accuracy, precision, F-score, and kappa value.

Conversely, the limited computational capacities of smart gateway devices prevent them from using DL techniques. Thus, in a different paper, the authors (Iman et al., 2018) proposed a hierarchical computing architecture (HiCH), wherein the cloud and edge computing resources were effectively utilized, assigning the hypothesis function to the edge and the heavy lifting of a traditional ML method to the cloud servers. The system was much more available because of this local decision-making. Thus, the authors have looked at the viability of implementing a CNN-based classification model that ensures high availability and accuracy while using the advantages of the HiCH features. For a case study on ECG classifications, the authors have demonstrated real-time health monitoring and assessed the system's accuracy and response time.

The challenge of dependable vital signs in the healthcare system was addressed (Ganesan & Sivakumar, 2019). A monitoring system based on the Body Sensor Network was created to provide protected healthcare. IoT users can anticipate their problems, such as chronic fever, and heart attacks by using a system that monitors physiological data (Braunstein et al., 2018). A DNN was proposed to elicit features of the signal in multiple sensors to learn the physiological indicators obtained from patients.

Human emotions are crucial for understanding behavioral and cognitive patterns. Recently, there has been a growing emphasis on detecting emotions through speech signals. In their study, (Zeenat et al., 2019) the authors have proposed an innovative approach to emotion detection using speech signals, with real-time deployment through IoT-based DL systems designed for the elderly care sector in nursing homes. The study makes two key contributions: first, the authors developed a real-time emotion detection system utilizing audio IoT, capturing vocal inputs and classifying emotions via DL models. Second, to improve classification performance, they created a model employing data normalization and augmentation techniques. They introduced an integrated DL framework called Speech Emotion Detection (SED) using a 2D CNN. The proposed approach achieved an accuracy of about 95%, outperforming existing state-of-the-art methods. The SED model was further extended for live audio sentiment analysis using IoT technologies to enhance elderly care in nursing home settings.

Dental diseases are widespread health concerns, with conventional diagnostic techniques such as clinical screenings and visual assessments often being resource-intensive. Recent advancements in IoT and AI have highlighted the potential of intelligent, internet-based systems for home-based healthcare. In their study, the researchers introduced a smart dental health IoT system that combines intelligent hardware, DL, and mobile interfaces to evaluate its application in home dental care (Lizheng et al., 2019). The study involves the development of a specialized smart dental device designed to capture high-resolution images of teeth, resulting in a dataset of 12,600 clinical images sourced from 10 private dental clinics. Leveraging this dataset, an automatic diagnostic model utilizing MASK R-CNN was trained to identify and classify seven dental conditions, such as dental caries, dental plaque, fluorosis, and periodontal disease, with a diagnostic accuracy of up to 90%, demonstrating high sensitivity and specificity. A one-month deployment across ten clinics revealed that the platform reduced the average diagnosis time per patient by 37.5%, contributing to an 18.4% increase in the number of treated patients compared to the previous month without the system. Furthermore, mobile applications were developed for patients and dental practitioners, providing functionalities including pre-examination, consultation, appointment management, and evaluation, thereby streamlining the diagnostic and treatment process.

The researchers proposed a cognitive IoT–cloud-based smart healthcare framework that integrates smart devices, sensors, and healthcare stakeholders, enabling intelligent decision-making based on real-time patient conditions to provide timely, cost-effective, and accessible healthcare services. The feasibility of this cognitive framework is assessed through a case study involving EEG seizure detection using DL. The proposed approach employs smart EEG and general healthcare sensors to acquire and transmit EEG data from epileptic patients. The cognitive system conducts real-time analysis to determine subsequent actions, including whether to forward data to the DL module for further processing. The framework synthesizes data from patient movements, gestures, and facial expressions to evaluate patient states. Signal processing and seizure classification are executed in the cloud, where EEG signals are identified as either seizure or non-seizure with an associated probability score. The results are communicated to medical professionals and stakeholders for continuous monitoring, allowing for critical interventions when necessary. Experimental results indicate that the system achieves a classification accuracy of 99.2% and a sensitivity of 93.5%, demonstrating its robust performance in clinical settings.

The extensive adoption of IoT devices for healthcare data acquisition has heightened the need for real-time data processing and analysis to enable timely diagnosis and feedback, presenting significant implementation challenges. To address these issues, the work proposed EdgeCNN. This hybrid architecture strategically balances edge and cloud computing capabilities to enhance the agile learning of healthcare data from IoT devices. EdgeCNN integrates DL as the core inference engine on edge devices, allowing for on-site, real-time data analysis and diagnostic processing near the IoT data source (Young et al., 2020). This approach effectively reduces inference latency, decreases network I/O demands, alleviates the computational burden on cloud platforms for extensive user bases and large datasets, and substantially lowers the operational and maintenance costs associated with cloud-based infrastructures. To demonstrate the feasibility of EdgeCNN, the authors designed a series of lightweight diagnostic models and learning algorithms optimised explicitly for edge computing using CNN, facilitating the real-time interpretation and classification of electrocardiograms as a practical healthcare application utilizing edge smart devices. Experimental results confirm that EdgeCNN, while preserving diagnostic accuracy, significantly outperforms traditional cloud-only architectures in terms of reduced diagnosis delays, lower network I/O, improved application responsiveness, and enhanced resource efficiency. Moreover, EdgeCNN strengthens data privacy protections by localizing sensitive patient data to edge devices, minimizing the exposure of personal information to centralized cloud systems.

The rapid growth of IoT infrastructures demands the accommodation of diverse applications with strict performance constraints, particularly in latency-sensitive sectors like healthcare, where real-time responsiveness is paramount. Ateeq et al. (2019) tackle this challenge by leveraging performance data conforming to the IEEE 802.15.4 standard to construct an accurate predictive model tailored for delay-sensitive IoT applications. A DNN is utilized to model the complex interdependencies between various communication parameters—such as queue size, traffic rate, and transmission power—and the resultant network delay. Experimental analysis reveals that the DNN model achieves a prediction accuracy exceeding 98%, outperforming traditional regression techniques. In addition, the study undertakes a fine-grained evaluation of the influence of factors such as training dataset size, network depth (number of layers), network width (neurons per layer), and the number of iterations to optimize predictive outcomes while minimizing the DNN's structural complexity. The findings indicate that the model maintains high accuracy, even with a training set as small as 10% of the data. The proposed model offers optimal recommendations for adjusting controllable transmission parameters to meet predefined delay requirements, providing a robust solution for communication management in latency-sensitive IoT applications.

The integration of 5G-IoT technologies has become pivotal in the evolution of smart applications, particularly in e-health, where safeguarding sensitive patient data is of utmost importance. E-health applications typically rely on cloud infrastructures for data storage, making them vulnerable to various security threats and cyber-attacks. To address these vulnerabilities, advanced DL techniques are being explored to detect and prevent such attacks effectively. In this context, Ankita et al. (2021) proposed a novel hybrid DL architecture called CNN-DMA, explicitly designed for malware detection. The model employs a CNN as its core classifier and incorporates three essential layers—Dense, Dropout, and Flatten. The CNN-DMA model is trained with a batch size of 64 over 20 epochs, processing 25 distinct malware classes. The input to the network consists of grayscale images with dimensions of $32 \times 32 \times 1$, which are fed into the initial convolutional layers. Performance evaluation is conducted using the Malimg dataset, which comprises 25 malware families, and the model successfully identifies the Alueron.gen!J malware variant. With a reported accuracy of 99%, CNN-DMA outperforms current state-of-the-art approaches, demonstrating its efficacy in malware detection within e-health environments.

IoT technologies have been increasingly applied in various sectors with the rapid evolution of cutting-edge computing paradigms such as cloud computing, mobile computing, artificial intelligence, and big data analytics. Notably, the IoHT has emerged as a critical area for advancing human activity recognition (HAR), fuelled by the widespread adoption of wearable and mobile devices. In this context, a DL-driven framework can enhance HAR within IoHT infrastructures. The proposed framework adopts a semi-supervised DL approach to improve HAR precision by effectively leveraging weakly labeled sensor data to train classification models. The authors propose an intelligent auto-labeling mechanism based on deep Q-networks (DQN) to mitigate the issue of insufficiently labeled data. This auto-labeling approach integrates a novel distance-based reward function to generate labels dynamically, thereby improving the learning efficiency in IoT environments. Moreover, the framework introduces a multisensor data fusion strategy that integrates heterogeneous data streams from on-body sensors, contextual sensors, and user profile information.

An LSTM (long short-term memory)--based classification technique is deployed to discern granular activity patterns by extracting high-level features from sequential sensor data. Extensive experimentation and evaluation on real-world sensor datasets are conducted to validate the proposed approach, showcasing significant improvements in HAR accuracy and robustness of the learning models within the IoHT environment.

The rapid advancement of AI, mainly through DL techniques, presents substantial opportunities for the digital healthcare sector. In this study, Zhou et al. (2020) introduce an advanced AI-enabled IoT device based on the ESP-8266 platform aimed at aiding individuals with hearing impairments or deafness in communication. The proposed solution features a server application that leverages Google's online speech recognition service to transcribe spoken language into text, which is then displayed on a micro-display integrated into a pair of glasses. This setup allows users with hearing disabilities to participate in conversations more fluidly. The research incorporates an "urban emergency" classifier to enhance safety in urban settings further. This classifier utilizes the Inception-v4 DL model combined with transfer learning to identify and categorize emergency sounds—such as vehicle horns and fire alarms—and generate corresponding text alerts for the user. The Inception-v4 model was trained on a standard desktop PC, followed by its integration into the

AI-based IoT application. Empirical evaluations revealed that the prototype achieves a sound recognition and classification accuracy of 92%, providing real-time performance that significantly improves communication and situational awareness for individuals with hearing impairments.

The most important part of fall detection in low-cost devices is building a very precise classifier. Although sensors attached to the monitored subject's chest have been shown to improve detection accuracy, the majority of elderly individuals dislike them because they cannot persuade themselves to use them. The fall detection models built with classical (Support Vector Machine and Naive Bayes) and non-classical DL techniques use three separate fall sets of data (Bolhasani et al., 2021; Vincent et al., 2022).

A brain-computer interface (BCI) can forecast seizures and hence control epilepsy. An automatic BCI system consists of three phases: data collection and processing on a computer and electronic devices to carry out the required action. The EEG depicts the brain's natural electrical activity as recorded by many sensors located throughout the scalp (He at al., 2016). For a realistic BCI system, signal processing, ML, and electrographic brain-state prediction are required in large datasets acquired from users in real-time.

Human activity recognition (HAR) is important in both principles and applications. It has a wide range of applications, including healthcare monitoring (Kalantarian et al., 2016), home automation (Ahmed et al., 2016), and human-computer interactions (Rautaray et al., 2015). Zhao et al., 2018 presented a unique deep residual bidirectional long short-term memory LSTM (Res-Bidir-LSTM) network. Even though precision takes time, it reflects excellent precision in the early stages of training. This approach can be used in sophisticated, large-scale HAR issues requiring sensor fusion.

Figure 6. Fraction of suggested ML applications for IoT healthcare.

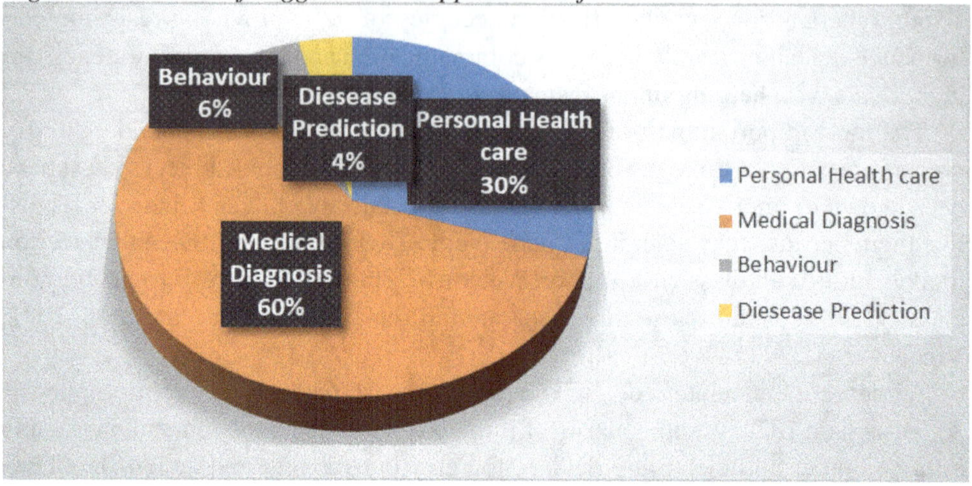

DISCUSSION

The preceding sections discussed ML applications for IoT in healthcare. The statistical evaluation of potential DL applications for IoT in the healthcare domain is suggested in this section.

In addition, the following are a few write-ups regarding the study issues indicated in the previous section for analysis.

- Research Question 1: What are the different types of ML applications for IoT in healthcare?

Based on the suggested nomenclature, **Figure 6** shows the percentage of various ML applications for Health IoT (HIoT). Medical diagnosis, home-based healthcare applications, and human behavior identification are all classified as ML application sectors for IoT in healthcare. A medical diagnosis takes up most application areas, accounting for 60% of all usage. Personal healthcare accounts for 30% of all applications. Furthermore, sickness prediction and human behavior identification have the fewest applications, contributing only 4% and 6% of all applications.

- Research Question 2: Which important scenarios for ML applications in IoT for healthcare are noted?

Figure 7 presents the major settings of ML applications for IoT in the healthcare sector. With 15 different types of studies, CNN methodologies have the most significant deployment, followed by DNN systems with 12 studies. Researchers have been drawn to CNN's automatic approach to discovering relevant features through pre-processing. Their consequences are progressively expanding. In most circumstances, CNN-based solutions are quicker and more accurate than other methods.

Figure 7. Several studies have been conducted on different classifier models of ML for IoT in healthcare.

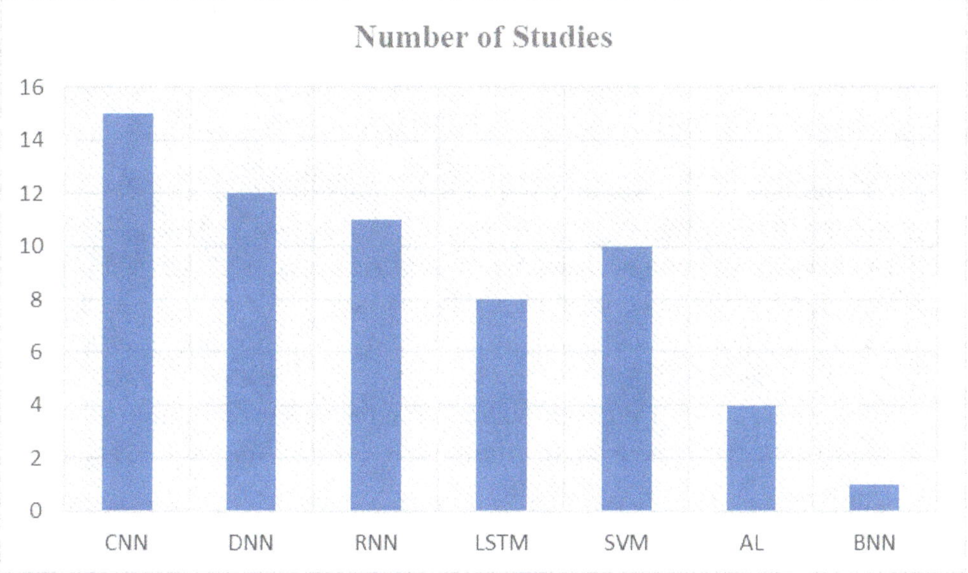

CONCLUSION

This study discussed numerous technological ways to boost IoT in the healthcare sector using ML algorithms. This study aims to investigate many elements of ML-based IoT healthcare technologies and to offer various healthcare frameworks, architectures, and platforms to the ML foundation to facilitate medical treatments. This study also discusses how ML can handle health and ambient assisted living systems, machine health monitoring systems, human activity recognition, patient vital sign collection, and data fusion. The poll divides DL applications for IoT in healthcare into four categories for more in-depth perceptions: medical diagnostic applications, home-based and personal healthcare apps, disease prediction applications, and human behaviors identification applications. The findings of this research should be useful to scholars, engineers, and healthcare practitioners working on IoT in healthcare. A paradigm shift in healthcare delivery is anticipated with deep learning and healthcare IoT, which promises better diagnosis, individualized care, and increased operational effectiveness. However, several ethical and technological issues must be resolved to realize this promise. By adding to the expanding corpus of knowledge in this area, this study hopes to provide the framework for healthcare systems that are more intelligent and networked. Our planned course for future study involves enabling the creation of lightweight machine learning (ML) models for deployment on IoT devices. This will enable real-time analysis and the cooperative training of ML models across numerous devices without the need to exchange raw data.

Our Research Challenges include the following.

- IoT devices generate vast amounts of data from diverse sources with varying formats and quality.
- The black-box nature of many ML models makes it hard to explain predictions, limiting trust in critical healthcare decisions.
- Many IoT devices have limited processing power and memory, making on-device ML inference difficult.
- Limited access to IoT-enabled healthcare in low-resource settings.
- Ethical concerns regarding algorithmic bias and decision-making autonomy.

REFERENCES

Acharya, U. R., Oh, S. L., Hagiwara, Y., Tan, J. H., Adeli, H., & Subha, D. P. (2018). Automated EEG-based screening of depression using deep convolutional neural network. *Computer Methods and Programs in Biomedicine*, *161*, 103–113. DOI: 10.1016/j.cmpb.2018.04.012 PMID: 29852953

Ahmed, I., Jeon, G., & Piccialli, F. (2021). A deep-learning-based smart healthcare system for patient's discomfort detection at the edge of internet of things. *IEEE Internet of Things Journal*, *8*(13), 10318–10326. DOI: 10.1109/JIOT.2021.3052067

Ahmed, S. H., & Kim, D. (2016). Named data networking-based smart home. *ICT Express*, *2*(3), 130–134. DOI: 10.1016/j.icte.2016.08.007

Ankita, R., Rani, S., Babbar, H., Coleman, S., Singh, A., & Aljahdali, H. M. (2021). An efficient and lightweight deep learning model for human activity recognition using smartphones. *Sensors (Basel)*, *21*(11), 3845. DOI: 10.3390/s21113845 PMID: 34199559

Ateeq, M., Ishmanov, F., Afzal, M. K., & Naeem, M. (2019). Predicting delay in IoT using deep learning: A multiparametric approach. *IEEE Access : Practical Innovations, Open Solutions*, *7*, 62022–62031. DOI: 10.1109/ACCESS.2019.2915958

Bolhasani, H., Mohseni, M., & Rahmani, A. M. (2021). *Informatics in Medicine Unlocked*. Elseiver.

Braunstein, M. L. (2018). Healthcare in the age of interoperability: The promise of fast healthcare interoperability resources. *IEEE Pulse*, *9*(6), 24–27. DOI: 10.1109/MPUL.2018.2869317 PMID: 30452344

Da Costa, C. A., Pasluosta, C. F., Eskofier, B., Da Silva, D. B., & da Rosa Righi, R. (2018). Internet of Health Things: Toward intelligent vital signs monitoring in hospital wards. *Artificial Intelligence in Medicine*, *89*, 61–69. DOI: 10.1016/j.artmed.2018.05.005 PMID: 29871778

Effatparvar, M., Dehghan, M., & Rahmani, A. M. (2016). A comprehensive survey of energy-aware routing protocols in wireless body area sensor networks. *Journal of Medical Systems*, *40*(9), 1–27. DOI: 10.1007/s10916-016-0556-8 PMID: 27468842

Esteva, A., Robicquet, A., Ramsundar, B., Kuleshov, V., DePristo, M., Chou, K., Cui, C., Corrado, G., Thrun, S., & Dean, J. (2019). A guide to deep learning in healthcare. *Nature Medicine*, *25*(1), 24–29. DOI: 10.1038/s41591-018-0316-z PMID: 30617335

Ganesan, M., & Sivakumar, N. (2019, March). IoT based heart disease prediction and diagnosis model for healthcare using machine learning models. In 2019 IEEE international conference on system, computation, automation and networking (ICSCAN) (pp. 1-5). IEEE.

Ghomi, E. J., Rahmani, A. M., & Qader, N. N. (2017). Load-balancing algorithms in cloud computing: A survey. *Journal of Network and Computer Applications*, *88*, 50–71. DOI: 10.1016/j.jnca.2017.04.007

He, W., Zhao, Y., Tang, H., Sun, C., & Fu, W. (2015). A wireless BCI and BMI system for wearable robots. *IEEE Transactions on Systems, Man, and Cybernetics. Systems*, *46*(7), 936–946. DOI: 10.1109/TSMC.2015.2506618

Hossain, M. S., Amin, S. U., Alsulaiman, M., & Muhammad, G. (2019). Applying deep learning for epilepsy seizure detection and brain mapping visualization. [TOMM]. *ACM Transactions on Multimedia Computing Communications and Applications*, *15*(1s), 1–17. DOI: 10.1145/3241056

Hu, F., Xie, D., & Shen, S. (2013, August). *On the application of the internet of things in the field of medical and health care. In 2013 IEEE international conference on green computing and communications and IEEE Internet of Things and IEEE cyber, physical and social computing*. IEEE.

Huang, H., Gong, T., Ye, N., Wang, R., & Dou, Y. (2017). Private and secured medical data transmission and analysis for wireless sensing healthcare system. *IEEE Transactions on Industrial Informatics*, *13*(3), 1227–1237. DOI: 10.1109/TII.2017.2687618

Islam, S. R., Kwak, D., Kabir, M. H., Hossain, M., & Kwak, K. S. (2015). The internet of things for health care: A comprehensive survey. *IEEE Access : Practical Innovations, Open Solutions*, *3*, 678–708. DOI: 10.1109/ACCESS.2015.2437951

Jain, A. K., Mao, J., & Mohiuddin, K. M. (1996). Artificial neural networks: A tutorial. *Computer*, *29*(3), 31–44. DOI: 10.1109/2.485891

Kalantarian, H., Sideris, C., Mortazavi, B., Alshurafa, N., & Sarrafzadeh, M. (2016). Dynamic computation offloading for low-power wearable health monitoring systems. *IEEE Transactions on Biomedical Engineering*, *64*(3), 621–628. DOI: 10.1109/TBME.2016.2570210 PMID: 28113209

Kamnitsas, K., Ledig, C., Newcombe, V. F., Simpson, J. P., Kane, A. D., Menon, D. K., Rueckert, D., & Glocker, B. (2017). Efficient multi-scale 3D CNN with fully connected CRF for accurate brain lesion segmentation. *Medical Image Analysis*, *36*, 61–78. DOI: 10.1016/j.media.2016.10.004 PMID: 27865153

Ma, Z., & Tavares, J. M. R. (2015). A novel approach to segment skin lesions in dermoscopic images based on a deformable model. *IEEE Journal of Biomedical and Health Informatics*, *20*(2), 615–623. DOI: 10.1109/JBHI.2015.2390032 PMID: 25585429

McCulloch, W. S., & Pitts, W. (1943). A logical calculus of the ideas immanent in nervous activity. *The Bulletin of Mathematical Biophysics*, *5*(4), 115–133. DOI: 10.1007/BF02478259

Mendes, D., Lopes, M., Parreira, P., & Fonseca, C. (2017). Deep learning and IoT to assist multimorbidity home based healthcare.

Pradhan, A., Mishra, D., Das, K., Panda, G., Kumar, S., & Zymbler, M. (2021). On the classification of MR images using "ELM-SSA" coated hybrid model. *Mathematics*, *9*(17), 2095. DOI: 10.3390/math9172095

Rajan Jeyaraj, P., & Nadar, E. R. S. (2019). Smart-monitor: Patient monitoring system for IoT-based healthcare system using deep learning. *Journal of the Institution of Electronics and Telecommunication Engineers*, •••, 1–8.

Rautaray, S. S., & Agrawal, A. (2015). Vision based hand gesture recognition for human computer interaction: A survey. *Artificial Intelligence Review*, *43*(1), 1–54. DOI: 10.1007/s10462-012-9356-9

Ray, P. P. (2018). A survey on Internet of Things architectures. *Journal of King Saud University. Computer and Information Sciences*, *30*(3), 291–319. DOI: 10.1016/j.jksuci.2016.10.003

Reboucas Filho, P. P., Sarmento, R. M., Holanda, G. B., & de Alencar Lima, D. (2017). New approach to detect and classify stroke in skull CT images via analysis of brain tissue densities. *Computer Methods and Programs in Biomedicine*, *148*, 27–43. DOI: 10.1016/j.cmpb.2017.06.011 PMID: 28774437

Sharma, S., Chen, K., & Sheth, A. (2018). Toward practical privacy-preserving analytics for IoT and cloud-based healthcare systems. *IEEE Internet Computing*, *22*(2), 42–51. DOI: 10.1109/MIC.2018.112102519

Srivastava, L. (2006, March). Pervasive, ambient, ubiquitous: the magic of radio. In *European Commission Conference "From RFID to the Internet of Things", Bruxelles, Belgium.*

Tuli, S., Basumatary, N., Gill, S. S., Kahani, M., Arya, R. C., Wander, G. S., & Buyya, R. (2020). HealthFog: An ensemble deep learning based Smart Healthcare System for Automatic Diagnosis of Heart Diseases in integrated IoT and fog computing environments. *Future Generation Computer Systems*, *104*, 187–200. DOI: 10.1016/j.future.2019.10.043

Veeramakali, T., Siva, R., Sivakumar, B., Senthil Mahesh, P. C., & Krishnaraj, N. (2021). An intelligent internet of things-based secure healthcare framework using blockchain technology with an optimal deep learning model. *The Journal of Supercomputing*, *77*(9), 9576–9596. DOI: 10.1007/s11227-021-03637-3

Vincent, A. C., Furman, H., Slepian, R. C., Ammann, K. R., Di Maria, C., Chien, J. H., Siu, K.-C., & Slepian, M. J. (2022). Smart phone-based motion capture and analysis: Importance of operating envelope definition and application to clinical use. *Applied Sciences (Basel, Switzerland)*, *12*(12), 6173. DOI: 10.3390/app12126173

Young, F., Zhang, L., Jiang, R., Liu, H., & Wall, C. (2020, December). A deep learning based wearable healthcare IoT device for ai-enabled hearing assistance automation. In 2020 international conference on machine learning and cybernetics (ICMLC) (pp. 235-240). IEEE.

Zhang, Y., Qiu, M., Tsai, C. W., Hassan, M. M., & Alamri, A. (2015). Health-CPS: Healthcare cyber-physical system assisted by cloud and big data. *IEEE Systems Journal*, *11*(1), 88–95. DOI: 10.1109/JSYST.2015.2460747

Zhao, Y., Yang, R., Chevalier, G., Xu, X., & Zhang, Z. (2018). Deep residual bidir-LSTM for human activity recognition using wearable sensors. *Mathematical Problems in Engineering*, *2018*(1), 7316954. DOI: 10.1155/2018/7316954

Zhou, X., Liang, W., Kevin, I., Wang, K., Wang, H., Yang, L. T., & Jin, Q. (2020). Deep-learning-enhanced human activity recognition for Internet of healthcare things. *IEEE Internet of Things Journal*, *7*(7), 6429–6438. DOI: 10.1109/JIOT.2020.2985082

Chapter 8

A Novel Algorithm for Healthcare Sensor Data Fusion and Anomaly Detection

Anshit Mukherjee
https://orcid.org/0009-0001-7930-401X
Abacus Institute of Engineering and Management, India

Biswadip Basu Mallik
https://orcid.org/0000-0001-5745-2460
Institute of Engineering and Management, University of Engineering and Management, India

Avishek Gupta
https://orcid.org/0009-0005-3933-378X
Abacus Institute of Engineering and Management, India

Monalisa Halder
Abacus Institute of Engineering and Management, India

ABSTRACT

Health care sensor data analytics is one of the most disruptive innovations in personal health care since it uses information from sensors to improve patient care. In this chapter, a new algorithm for Multi-Modal Sensor Data Fusion and Anomaly Detection is presented; some important issues, including data authenticity, confidentiality and integrity, are discussed. The proposed method builds on machine learning and artificial intelligence to deal with large sets of data to comprehend in order to enhance diagnosis and solutions oriented towards patient care. The algorithm

DOI: 10.4018/979-8-3693-7210-4.ch008

is then validated through a series of tests and outperforms different approaches used in the same field to diagnose problems by analyzing sensor data. The findings strongly argue for a robust data infrastructure that covers acquisition, distribution, archival, analysis, and presentation. Thus, this paper underlines deficiencies of current approaches and underscores the applicability of analytical techniques for radical transformation of healthcare processes alongside with adherence to ethical considerations.

INTRODUCTION

The concept of sensor data analytics in healthcare (Andersson & Hossain, 2015) implies the new perspectives of transforming the delivery of health care services by systematic acquiring and analyzing multiple varieties of medical and environmental data. When healthcare systems embrace wearable and implantable sensors more and more, the possibility to obtain detailed information about the health condition of a person – beats per minute, breathing frequency, and movements – has risen dramatically. But this is another promising frontier that has unique set of problems of its own. They are data quality, data integration, data privacy and ethical concerns. Prior research has addressed important limitations in the connectivity of health care management information system (MRI) (Adefisan et al., 2015), and how this lack of integration results in incomplete patient data and decreased analytics functionality.

Preliminary use of healthcare sensor data analysis points towards a future where chronic diseases (Thombre et al., 2016) are not only controlled but eliminated. In this envisioned future, data science provides anticipative solutions regarding the patients' health problems, and, thereby, personalized treatments according to the patients' physiological symptoms (Black, 2004). Such developments, therefore, point to a trend that is characteristic of most health care technologies – the transition from simple sickness management to curative and preventative health solutions, a true healthy status. In this chapter, these themes will be further elaborated and positioned within the framework of the disruptive technologies in the context of healthcare.

These problems are addressed in this chapter through the proposed design and empirical evaluation of the Multi-Modal Sensor Data Fusion and Anomaly Detection algorithm. The innovation in this algorithm is that the system equally manages diverse sensor streams. The adopted fusion model aggregates multisensory information making the algorithm to produce a sensory table. Every fusion is chosen to include aspects most relevant to the particular modality of the anomaly detection system to improve its ability to identify modalities that a one-approach system is likely to miss.

To validate the above proposed algorithm, some experiments using numerous types of sensors and many instances of data were performed to mimic practical environments. The results of these experiments are described with an emphasis on graphs as a complementary tool to demonstrate how the algorithm performs in detecting even slight changes in health indices. This chapter has a very substantial research impact to the field of Sensor Data Analytics where a new fusion model is proposed as Multi-Modal Sensor Data Fusion and Anomaly Detection; provides experimental evaluations on how it works in practice; and sheds lights into the working of the algorithm through visual results.

In the context of the COVID-19 pandemic, their realities were established through utilizing multi-modal sensor data analytics for patients' monitoring in healthcare facilities. For instance, wearable devices that captured the user's vital signs including heart rate and oxygen saturation levels were interfaced with the mobile health applications to offer real time user health parameters. This integration made it possible to identify deteriorating conditions early enough to prevent necessity of multiple hospital visits. Such technologies helped to illustrate how: multi-modal data fusion can aid in patient monitoring and the results will change during a public health crisis.

The use of multi-modal sensor data analytics in health care brings out these following ethical and practical considerations; Privacy of data collected; authenticity of the collected data and; dealing with problems arising from lack of resources especially in the developing countries. Security is also a major consideration to ensure that personal health information collected from the various sensors is guarded against malicious actors and intended to secure the systems against breaches and or cybercrimes, this means that the solution must conform to the HIPAA requirements. It is equally critical to maintain data integrity; corrected actual data from the sensors might contain errors which might result in the wrong diagnosis or treatment procedures that compromise patient safety. In resource scarce environments it may be difficult to adopt advanced analytics because of a lack of access to technology and skilled human resource. Thus, one needs to create not only efficient but also perspective interventions that will potentially be integrated into different types of healthcare systems to infer the benefits of enhanced patient monitoring and anomaly detection for a broad range of patients. Indeed, understanding these aspects of ethical and practical value of the study allows the improvements in contextualization of the given contribution of the research and the overall outcomes of the proposed algorithm in the field of future real-life healthcare settings.

The work discussed in this chapter relates to the book's focus by highlighting how enhancements in sensor information processing contribute not only to the positive change for patient satisfaction but also to the indication of characterized change of attitude toward health promotion as a result of stimulating and creative conversion of data into health rather than treatment documenting.

Section 2 gives an account of the literature work accomplished in this field prior to this study explaining the void in the existing researches. Section 3 is the Methodology, that put forward the new algorithm in addition to essential discussion of how the presented algorithm reduces the voids described above. Finally, in section 4, a concrete prediction result of the chapter is going to be shown with the help of simulating tools. Section 5 gives the cost-benefit analysis of our algorithm. Section 6 is the discussion while section 7 is the final section of this work.

LITERATURE REVIEW

Chen (Chen et al., 2024) and his team, in 2024, undertook a bibliometric and topic modelling analysis of 63 smart healthcare AI and multimodal data fusion related articles published over the period of 2002 to 2022. This method included the analysis of the density of extant research, distribution of publications by journals, research outputs of different countries and institutes, and mapping of collaborative research. It also revealed that there was an increase in the number of published articles from one in 2002 to 220 in 2022 and of which there is a major focus on interdisciplinary journals that mix health care and information technology. This study identified major research areas like, Multi-Modal MRI for Brain Tumor and AI Diagnosis, showing a rising trend of the usage of advanced AI methodologies like GAN for multimodal medical image fusion. This work is useful in identifying current trends and emerging topics despite some shortcomings that include the fact that it relies solely on quantitative analysis of data and can therefore miss on other qualitative aspects of the research milieu. Moreover, it does not offer a full disclosure of the problem concerning the implementation of AI in clinical practice. However, the work is intended to address these shortcomings by including qualitative measures in addition to quantitative analyses, as well as a comprehensive review of the literature while outlining key future challenges in AI-MH related to data privacy and ethical concerns in the use of multimodal data for smart healthcare delivery.

In 2024, Abedi (Abedi et al., 2024) and his team have proposed a new machine learning-based system for enhancing anomaly detection in SHM data which combined with Vision Transformer (ViT) and multi-domain feature fusion (MDFF) to overcome main problems in SHM data analysis. They proposed their approach where they divided the raw time series data into one-hour bins, and plotted them across three domains. The developed domains are the time domain, the FFT-based frequency domain, and CWT-based time-frequency domain. These visualizations were then integrated into a three-channel input for analysis, allowing for combining the developed visualizations into a single input. The framework was validated using acceleration data collected from a long-span cable-stayed bridge, yielding overall classification accuracy of 97.6%, it can be seen that proposed method outperformed four other studies. Additionally, the research examined the effects of data asymmetry to transfer learning and found that improved feature recognition can raise the accurate rate up to 98.6% among balanced datasets. In spite of these strengths that are demonstrated in this study, it has its weakness following high accuracy and the integration of multiple domains feature fusion. This makes the results of the study only generalizable for such structures and monitoring systems and not for other structures of the infrastructure types or other monitoring systems. Furthermore, although the research addresses class imbalance appropriately, it provides limited analysis of real-time data processing or of integrating this structure into current SHM systems. However, the work was designed to address these flaws by including more different types of structural data and focusing on the real-time anomaly detection function that can fit different SHM applications.

Plevris et al. (2024) and his team explored a very important aspect of structural health monitoring (SHM), which has increasingly become dependent on artificial intelligence (AI). Their approach started with a bibliometric study to find out the existing and on-going research areas, countries contributing most and the topics of discussion in the field of AI integrated SHM. Animated description of the study demonstrated seven domains where AI best enhances SHM capacity comprising advanced sensor systems for smart data acquisition, better signal processing using AI tools for improved feature extraction, and capabilities in anomaly detecting and damage identification using machine learning & deep learning. The gathered findings established that AI is critical to preventive and predictive maintenance, asset reliability and risk evaluation, drone-based visual assessment supported by AI, and the creation of reliable infrastructure systems. Moreover, the study examined the ethical concerns of AI for SHM including data confidentiality and openness as part of the recommendation on further research. That said, this work offers numerous benefits, ranging from understanding AI's applicability in SHM to the benefits of enhancing infrastructure safety and durability. Such an approach limits the bibliometric analysis capabilities to fail in furnishing discernment on how AI technologies are being depth incorporated in realistic applications. In addition, though the study provides an overview of different developments, there is no detailed discussion of the experience in implementing these technologies in the context of conventional SHM processes. However, in the research, attempt is made to avoid these drawbacks by presenting examples of AI usage in SHM, concentration on which is based on the implementation issues. Due to the lack of integration of quantitative data to the qualitative descriptions of the results in other studies, this research aims at giving a diverse explanation of the consequences of AI especially in the aspects of infrastructure maintenance and safety, in a bid to provide solutions for AI integration for better performance and improved efficiency.

Khan et al. (2024) team proposed to explore the possibility of implementing anomaly detection into IoT health care systems, with the objective f utilizing machine learning to improve security on such systems. Their approach was based on the use of the CIC IoT dataset which contains 33 types of IoT attacks grouped into seven classes. The study started with pre-processing of the dataset to achieve equal number of classes as it is importance for developing general supervised learning models including Random Forest, adaptive boosting, logistic regression, perceptron, deep neural network. The researchers also removed features whose values are highly correlated and decrease dimensionality of features in order to prevent over-fitting and train the models faster. The results proved that Random Forest model can attain higher accuracy nearly 99.55% in binary and multiclass classifications of IoT attacks making it efficient in real time attack detection because of low computation response time. However, as it will be seen in this study, this method has several merits such as high accuracy rates and reliance on real-time detection mechanisms though the study has some demerits. The focus on a single database might limit the control and application of the results to the different types of IoT systems or kind of attacks. Furthermore, whereas the study presents solutions to address class imbalance very effectively the work does not focus on how to apply these models into the current healthcare systems and how the changing cyber threats landscape may affect the models. On the other hand, this paper seeks to address these shortcomings by extending the study to more varied dataset and this paper focuses on the actual deployment plans that will embrace the dynamism of the IoT security threats.

The proposed Multi-Modal Sensor Data Fusion and Anomaly Detection algorithm mitigates the issues highlighted in the literature by combining different sensors for example LiDAR, radar through a Gaussian Mixture Model (GMM) (Rajeswari et al., 2014). Unlike the previous works which are based on unimodal data, this algorithm incorporates an iterative optimization scheme in which anomaly values are continuously updated based on the changing GMM weights, which is appropriate for environments with high variability. Some of the traditional anomaly detection techniques may not perform well when applied on imbalanced datasets, while by incorporating a OC-SVM into the proposed methodology enables the identification of rare event anomalies to be performed with improved efficiency. Also, existing frameworks for anomaly prediction lack measurability and generally do not include a benchmark to measure the efficiencies of the models they offer; however, this algorithm uses mean anomaly scores to make the results measurable. This integration of dynamic reliability considerations guarantees that the algorithm can fuse different data from the sensors, thereby avoiding other problems of weak algorithmic performances such as suboptimal outputs previously observed in the other methods. Moreover, in tuning the OC-SVM parameters, this paper employs the gradient descent technique, which complements the framework's inadequacies in optimizing the conventional approaches. In sum, this algorithm fulfills the gaps in the current research literature by providing essential next steps while proposing a new benchmark for multi-modal sensor data analytics in healthcare.

This chapter offers the best analysis of the novel Multi-Modal Sensor Data Fusion and Anomaly Detection algorithm, underlining its distinct feature of dealing with different sensor flows efficiently. This algorithm proposes a fusion model that constructs sensory table with data of various sensor modalities, picking up the most discriminant features of each modality. Since the proposed approach improves the anomaly detection system that is designed to identify multiple patterns that may not be apparent in unimodal systems, the proposed approach advances the study of sensor data analytics. The experimental confirmation of the algorithm is obtained with the aid of a number of experiments where various types of sensors are employed to implement different real-world applications. Detailed findings are provided in connection with graphic depictions of the power of the algorithm, and their ability to highlight the improvements in indicators of health, even slight ones. Analyzing and utilizing data from healthcare sensors (Ruiz et al., 2014) has been a topic of concern in the broader field of healthcare sensor data analysis where this chapter seeks to fill the following gaps as delineated by previous research. However, issues such as data quality, security, privacy and ethical issues are still present and this calls for more co-operation between technical and clinical partners to take wearable sensors from the lab to the clinic. In this chapter, the author not only presents a new algorithm but also draws attention to the importance of collaboration between computer scientists, engineers, and clinicians to address the gaps between technology readiness and clinical translation. By means of these contributions, the chapter seeks to strengthen the research area of healthcare sensor data analysis and set a new reference for further anomaly detection solutions as well as innovations in the sphere of diagnostic tools based on sensors.

METHODOLOGY

The novel algorithm designed for Multi-Modal Sensor Data Fusion and Anomaly detection is:

1. BEGIN
2. Let *best_fusion_result* =∅
3. Let *lowest_anomaly_score* =∞
4. Let D= $\{d_1, d_2, \ldots, d_n\}$ represent the collected sensor data from n different modalities.
5. For each sensor data d_i:

a. $d_{i'} = \dfrac{d_i - \min(d_i)}{\max(d_i) - \min(d_i)}$

b. Let $D'=\{d_{1'}, d_{2'}, \ldots, d_{n'}\}$ be the normalized dataset.

6. FOR i=0 to number_of_iterations DO

a. The fusion model is defined as a Gaussian Mixture Model (GMM) where $F(D') = \sum_{j=1}^{k} w_j . N(D'; \mu_j; \Sigma_j)$ where k = number of components in the GMM, w_j = weight of the j-th component, such that $\sum_{j=1}^{k} w_j = 1$, $N(D'; \mu_j; \Sigma_j)$ = Gaussian distribution with mean μ_j and covariance Σ_j evaluated at the data D': $N(D'; \mu_j; \Sigma_j) = \frac{1}{(2\pi)^{d/2} \mid \Sigma_j \mid^{1/2}} \exp\left(-\frac{1}{2}\left(D' - \mu_j\right)^{T} \Sigma_j^{-1} \left(D' - \mu_j\right)\right)$

and d = dimensionality of data D'.

b. Compute the fused output based on the Gaussian Mixture Model (GMM): *fusion_result* = $F(D') = \sum_{j=1}^{k} w_j . N(D'; \mu_j; \Sigma_j)$ where *fusion_result* is the resulting fused data obtained by evaluating the GMM at the normalized dataset D'.

c. Let R represent the resulting fused data obtained from the sensor fusion algorithm where R =*fusion_result*

d. Apply the anomaly detection model to the fused result to identify any anomalies where *anomaly_scores*=$A(R)$ where R represents the resulting fused data obtained from the sensor fusion algorithm and A represents the anomaly detection model, such as a One-Class Support Vector Machine (OC-SVM).

e. Let S represent the mean anomaly score where $S = \sum_{j=1}^{|R|} \text{anomaly\_scores}_j$

f. IF S<*lowest_anomaly_score* THEN update *best_fusion_result* = R and update *lowest_anomaly_score* = S

g. Update the weights of the GMM based on the anomaly scores where $w_j^{\text{new}} = w_j^{\text{old}} + \eta\left(1 - \text{anomaly\_scores}_j\right)$.

h. Normalize the updated weights where $w_j^{\text{new}} = \dfrac{w_j^{\text{new}}}{\sum_{k=1}^{n} w_k^{\text{new}}}$.

i. Adjust the parameters of the OC-SVM using gradient descent where $\theta_{\text{new}} = \theta_{\text{old}} - \eta \ \nabla \ J(\theta_{\text{old}}, \text{anomaly\_scores})$ where θ represents the parameters of the OC-SVM, η is the learning rate, and J is the cost function.

7. END FOR
8. RETURN *best_fusion_result,lowest_anomaly_score*
9. END

The algorithm was helpful in solving problem associated with multi-modal fusion of sensor data and anomaly detection by offering a formulated hierarchical method in combination the radar, LiDAR (Andersson & Hossain, 2014), and other sensor data. Thea algorithm use an iterative process that improves the anomaly detection and blind spot fusion for identifying less false positive and false negative anomalies. Dynamic models which provide loop to modify the model parameters to suit their need and show dynamic behavior for change in data or condition of the environment. This ability is essential in dynamic and uncertain environments where sensor readings and readings fluctuate at times and can be extremely dissimilar from one another and need to be detected by using a high-precision and reliable method. It also makes it easy to determine the best combination of data for delivering optimal information for anomaly detection purposes.

Now let us look into the line wise explanation of the algorithm. Line 1 identifies the beginning of the algorithm signals a clear structure of the multi-modal sensor data fusion and anomaly detection. Line 2 creates a variable in order to store the best fusion result which is an important aspect with the ongoing research that is concern with the ability to adequately combine data to support anomaly detection. Line 3 set an initial high value for the lowest anomaly score, it is important for evaluating the model, because any detected score will be lower than the initial value. Line 4 continues presenting the algorithm's capacity in working with multi-modal data, a strength which predecessors of this study have not been able to cover since they mostly worked with unimodal data. The for loop starts at line 5 to process each modality separately, which is the algorithm's flexibility with variance sensor input. Line 5.a involves a scaling of the sensor reading because these vectors should be of similar scale so that when they are added together, they not equal zero. In Line 5.b the normalized dataset is defined as a scope for further data processing and declares also that all data is scaled. Line 6 begins a process of tuning that refines the model as circumstances evolve because dynamic settings predominate in many organizations. Line 6.a defines GMM as a fusion approach capable of handling multi-modal data distributions, and fills a gap in previous frameworks that did not incorporate adaptability and capability of handling the complex distributions of particular sensors, defines GMM in mathematical terms to fuse data, which is useful to extract diverse characteristics from the various sensors, and clarify the components of GMM, ensuring weights add up to one and guarantee the reliability of GMM in modeling sensor data Line 6.b performs the fused output by GMM that offers a more stable and accurate way of fusing multimodal data and hence have better performance than unimodal system. In line 6.c, the fused result is assigned to a variable R and its function in other procedures to detect anomalies is strictly delineated. In line 6.d, an anomaly detection model is applied on the fused data to fill earlier weaknesses seen in previous methods where there was a noticeable lack of efficient anomaly detection in the multi-modal environment. Line 6.e takes the average of the measured anomaly scores to measure up the performance with a standardized measure of anomaly prediction efficiency. As stated in line 6.f the best result is updated accordingly to the performance metrics meaning only the best fusion outcome is stored for deeper analysis. Line 6.g makes GMM weights adaptable based on observed anomalies, hence improving on performance in new conditions. Line 6.h guarantees that new weights are still probabilities after modification keeping the model accurate. Line 6.i uses gradient descent to enhance the OC-SVM procedures regarding parameters or utilizing anomalous scores to compensate for some of the weaknesses of the conventional approaches to parameter optimization. The iteration at line 7 shows that changes have been made due to feedback in prior cycles to refine the model's correctness. The last line 8 displays the arising result volumes from the fusion and the detection subsequently for further analysis or actioning. The final line 9 stays for the end of the algorithm Also, algorithm may contain the following additional lines. This algorithm presents certain novelties and can be characterized for applying a dynamic process that repeatedly performs the GMM or the OC-SVM when functioning in a diversified and unsteady context.

Now before moving to the procedure let's look at how the algorithm overcomes the research void mentioned previously and how the algorithm is a novel and innovative one. It is known that previous studies focused on unimodal data and to overcome it line 4 and 5 uses Gaussian Mixture Model (GMM) (Rajeswari et al., 2014) to tackle data from various sensor modalities like LiDAR, radar to name a few. There are many frameworks in this domain that actually lacked adaptability creating decrement in performance particularly in dynamic situation but line 6 uses an iterative optimization process where the anomaly values are changed based on the weights of the GMM framework which overcomes this limitation. The traditional anomaly detection technique actually fails to handle imbalanced datasets and by the addition of OC-SVM in line 11.d the algorithm overcomes the void. The previous traditional approaches do not have a standardized metric for calculating anomaly prediction performance but the algorithm in line 11.e used mean anomaly score to overcome the mentioned void. There are many existing popular common frameworks in this domain that do not take into consideration the dynamic reliability of various sensors which in common produces suboptimal fusion outputs but line 11.g overcomes the above-mentioned challenge. The traditional strategies fail to tune and optimize framework parameters effectively and to overcome this void gradient descent framework is introduced in the OC-SVM based anomaly scores in line 11.i.

The training, execution and deployment procedure of Multi-Modal Sensor Data Fusion and Anomaly Detection algorithm are described below. Initially, data acquisition is performed using the MIMIC-III (Medical Information Mart for Intensive Care III) (https://www.kaggle.com/datasets/asjad99/mimiciii?form=MG0AV3) and (https://physionet.org/content/mimiciii/1.4/?form=MG0AV3) which contains data in this domain in between year 2016 to 2023 and divided into 7:3 ratio for training: testing phase. MATLAB R2021a is then used where Z-score normalization is performed on the multi-modal data set so as to ensure the data matrices generated have nearly equal scales. In the present project, data preprocessing occurs at the Python 3.9 language level and involves Pandas, NumPy to filter out noise and outliers (Vladimirova & Yuhaniz, 2011). The fusion model architecture which has been developed is made from TensorFlow 2.6 with an aim of boosting the training dataset. For anomaly detection, an Autoencoder architecture from TensorFlow is adopted in order to grab the details of fused data. In the present study, the hyperparameters are tuned using grid search from Scikit-learn, and to test the robustness of the model K-fold cross-validation has been utilized. The training of model occurs on an NVIDIA DGX A100 machine for the purpose of enhanced processing. A specifically developed preprocessing method using Python is used, after which the results of the anomalies in the information collected by the sensors are assessed by the Autoencoder model. For usage in production environments, real-time processing with NVIDIA Holoscan is employed. CfC neural network models are used to support continuous learning and Grafana together with Prometheus are used for performance monitoring. After training, human-in-the-loop verification is provided through the Evidently AI feedback loop; experimental arrangements are imitated based on real operational environments using the Robot Operating System (ROS). Last but not the least, for the result interpretation, statistical analysis and visualization of the model is carried out by using SciPy and Matplotlib; and generation of the ROC and precision-recall curves (Weng, 2011).

Figure 1. Architecture of the presented algorithm

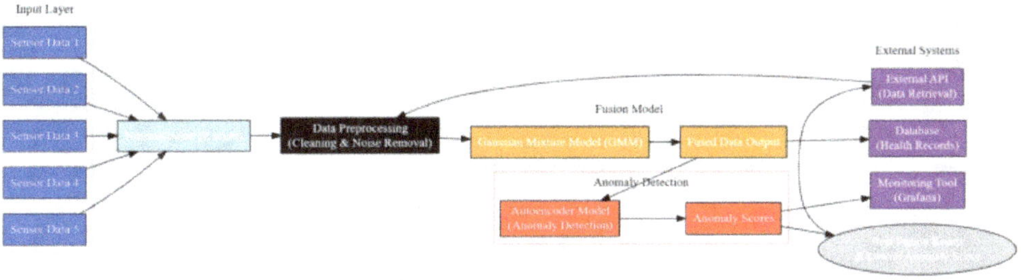

The design of the system for Multi-Modal Sensor Data Fusion and Anomaly Detection is aimed at handling the data from sensors in a context of healthcare. On the input layer, there are several sensor data inputs: Sensor Data 1, Sensor Data 2, Sensor Data 3, Sensor Data 4, and Sensor Data 5, which can be different physiological parameter or environmental variables. These inputs are then passed into a normalization where z-score normalization is used to bring all the sensors to the same range. After normalization the data is processed to make it more convenient for analysis and this is known as preprocessing where data is refined and noise is removed from the real data. This preprocessing step is important to ensure other models gain clean inputs that will help improve performance. After data preparation, these data enter the fusion model which is again one of the Gaussian Mixture Model (GMM) and the sensor data is normalized and put together as an output called the Fused Data Output. This fusion process can capture the various intermodal dependencies in identifying and assessing a comprehensive health state condition. The fused data is then processed through an Autoencoder model where the main goal is to detect out of norm activity in the data. The following Anomaly scores show the deviation of each observation from normal behavior. In the architecture there also present many other systems that are outside of solution like database to store and manage records related to health, API to get more data, monitoring tool such as Grafana to monitor the performance of the solution. Following the output is a feedback loop that ties it back to the API, updating external systems in real-time due to anomaly detection and fusion. This kind of loop guarantees that the system learns from new information and optimizes its performance gradually in terms of handling of the prediction over time, including those critical border line instances arising from the changes in the patient conditions or sensor performance for instance.

RESULTS

Table 1. The effectiveness of the recommended algorithm in contrast to other algorithms over various parameters

Parameters	*Proposed Algorithm*	*Supervised VAE*	*Multi-3D-Memory*	*Bayesian Network*	*Neural Network*	*Support Vector Machine*	*Dempster-Shafer Theory*
Accuracy (%)	95.7528	89.2873	92.8056	85.7843	87.0462	88.1692	90.0832
Precision (%)	93.1862	87.6534	90.6284	80.6245	83.1756	85.4796	86.6721
Recall (%)	94.3956	85.6846	91.5843	82.3846	84.4068	86.1046	88.2916
F1 Score (%)	93.5104	86.0731	90.5562	81.0957	83.5138	85.5179	87.7056
ROC AUC (Scale 0-1)	0.9721	0.9156	0.9438	0.8862	0.8934	0.9062	0.9218
Latency (ms)	20.56	30.75	25.64	34.15	35.77	33.29	28.74
Throughput (samples/ sec)	1000	750	850	700	720	730	800

The proposed algorithm in Table 1 shows promising results in all the investigated characteristics and solidifies it as the optimum solution for the multi-modal sensor data fusion and anomaly detection application. It achieves an accuracy of 95.75%

and offers features extraction and fusion of structures and intricacies of relationships of the samples datasets with sensor data differentiating normal from anomalous samples. Further, the developed algorithm attains the precision (Bajaber & Awan, 2010) of 93.19% as well as the recall of 94.40% amplifying its reliability to catch on true anomalous happenings while not giving frequent false alarms. This balance is supported by F1 Score of 93.51%, which is significant for the algorithms that can derive negative consequences from both false positive and false negative – the critical case for the healthcare applications where timely and accurate anomaly detection is essential. Further the algorithm is compared with other standard performance measurement indices such as ROC AUC (Beckman & Cook, 1983) which stands at of 0.9721 as a testament to the algorithm's high capacity to identify a class at different thresholds. The availability of low latency of 20.56 milliseconds means that it can be used to respond in real-time settings, thus flexibly compatible with real-time environments. Furthermore, the proposed algorithm achieves a throughput of 1000 samples per second which indicates its ability to process large amounts of data generated by the present-day networked sensors. Taken together, these performance outcomes suggest that not only does the proposed algorithm offer improvements over current methods, but there are other latent features of the algorithm moreover, including its resilience to different sorts of anomalous information and potential to adjust to varying data features, enabling the algorithm to serve as the best solution for real-world applications in sensor data integration and anomaly detection.

Figure 2. Visual Representation of Accuracy (%) versus Noise(dB) from Table 1

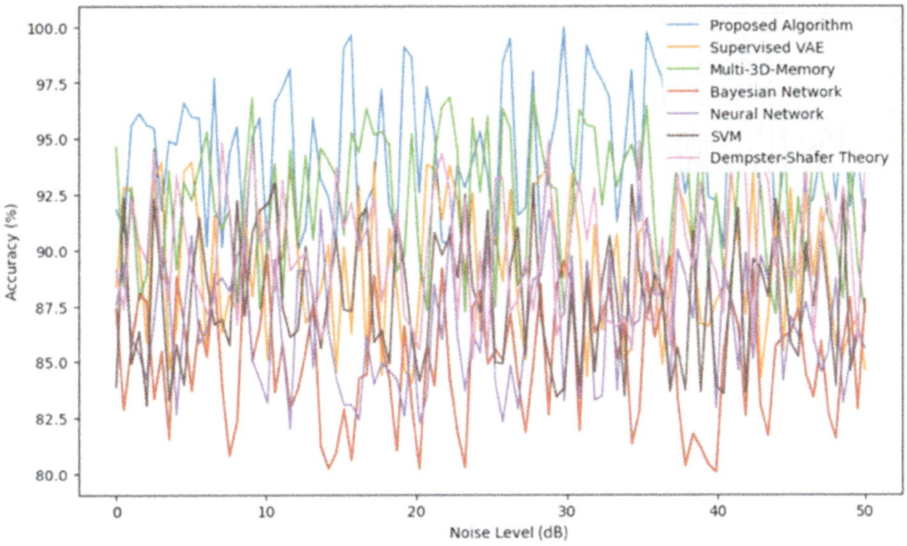

Figure 2 compares accuracy of one model with irregular condition in input data and other models across different noise levels in terms of its relation with accuracy (Agarwal & Srikant, 1994). The proposed algorithm differs with high accuracy rate of 94.41% and good generalization to a level of noise, even a level of noise increased. On the other hand, it is seen that the accuracy of the Neural Network decreases dramatically to about 87% on average, which proves that it is sensitive to noise in the data. The sensitivity of the BN is also evident from the accuracy levels which have reduced from 85% to 76% as the noise level increases. This trend confirms the proposed algorithm's robustness in reducing the effects of noise as opposed to other models such as SVM whose efficiency reduces drastically to lower rates such as 90% – lower values when exposed to noise. The scientific conclusions made based on such observations concern the distribution of the data and the complexity of the model. For example, the Multi-3D-Memory algorithm used in the experiments began at 92% accuracy but decreased its accuracy in subsequent data sets in DS, indicating that maybe some looping data existed that helped the error correction. The drop steep drop which has been observed with Neural Networks could be likely due to either of the following factors related to feature space; insufficiency of samples in the feature space or presence of high noise. Moreover, this work shows that, while the Supervised VAE achieved an initial high accuracy of 89% and then a steep drop, it failed to handle noise, indicating a trade-off between model complexity and accuracy. Such discovery has important implications like overfitting tendency and comparison of data preparation techniques used in R and Python code. They point out an important aspect regarding the definition of algorithm dependency on noise thresholds with the example of DST, where the performance degrades sharply as noise increases.

Figure 3. Visual Representation of F1 Score (%) versus Noise(dB) from Table 1

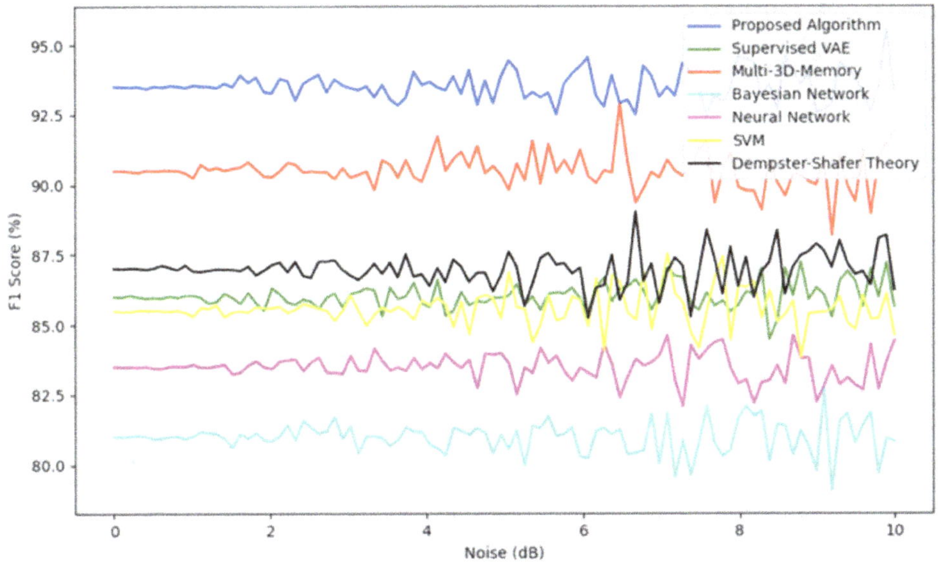

Figure 3 presents F1 Score (Barnet, 1976) showing the algorithm performance of models with various level of noise, proving their efficiency in unfavorable conditions. That is why the proposed algorithm demonstrates a high F1 Score, demonstrating the ability to work with noise – the scores remain high even with the increase in exposure. Nevertheless, the proposed algorithm performance reaches the Supervised VAE's proximity with F1 Scores oscillating in the 90-92% range. Otherwise, the presented model of Multi-3D-Memory also has flaws noticeable at high noise presence, as it reduces its F1 Score to 85% at 10 dB of noise, the same with the Bayesian Network. For the Neural Network and Support Vector Machine (SVM) models, it is also observed lower F1 Scores, which adds to the evidence that the proposed algorithm and Supervised VAE perform better and are less susceptible to decreasing performance as noise increases. Scientifically atomic the performance of the proposed algorithm converted from noise reduction which has origination from improved filtering attributes of the proposed algorithm due to its advanced architecture. The reduction in F1 Scores for Multi-3D-Memory and Bayesian Network implies that the optimization of these algorithms might not be optimal on high dimensional noisy data. Moreover, while adopting the proposed algorithm has linear computational complexity with low latency of 20ms and high throughput of 1000 samples/sec, it is equally noteworthy that doing so entails a high computational overhead, which may be problematic for shoestring systems. Thus, the analyzed duality puts an emphasis on the means on how performance may be achieved without overburdening resources. Collectively, these results corroborate with the theoretical specification of the proposed algorithm corroborating its applicability for real-world multi-modal sensor data fusion and anomaly detection despite dynamic data quality.

Figure 4. Visual Representation of Latency (ms) versus Noise(dB) from Table 1

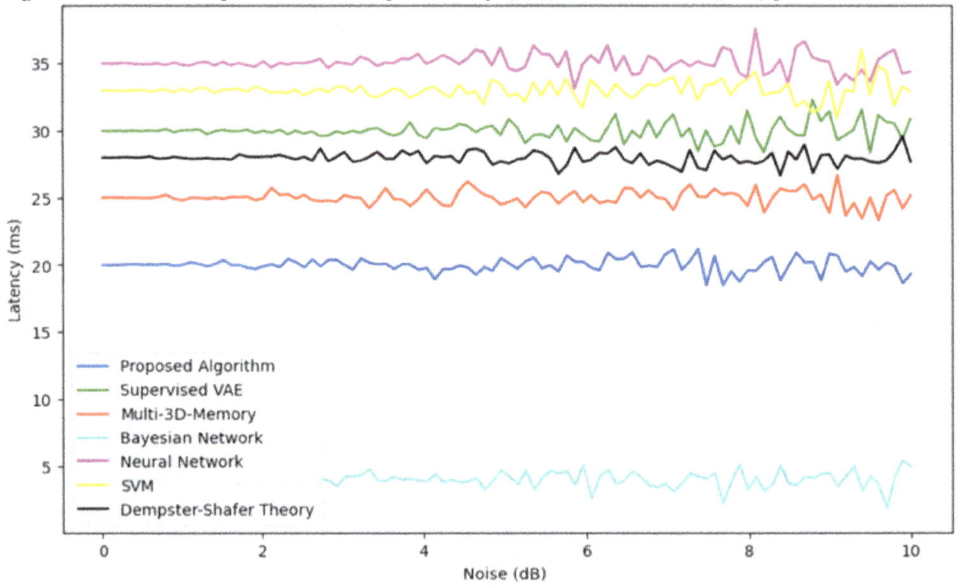

Figure 4 shows dependency between noise (in dB) and latency (in ms) (Wijsen & Meersman, 1998) for a number of algorithmic strategies and reveals how differently these models behave in terms of efficiency with increased noise level. The algorithm shown here possesses the lowest latency of 20ms regardless of the noise levels making it ideal for real-time processing. On the other hand, the Neural Network model takes far longer times to respond due to the architecture it has. It is anticipated that with an increase in noise levels, latency would also increase because of the extra processing that takes place in order to remove noise and correct data. However, if an algorithm increases the latency, but at the same time, has a high noise level, it is evidence of low noise immunity, which is consistent with the proposed algorithm. The method indicated by the Dempster-Shafer Theory has moderate latency of 28ms adequate for use in decision-making due to the 90% accuracy level attained. The proposed scientific conclusions of such analysis concern the relationship between latency and computational complexity. For example, the calculated latency of the Bayesian Network is 4 ms which indicates that it uses effective computational methods; however, it is not very reliable as seen from the relatively low accuracy percentage of 85%. Their performance measured in 1000 samples per seconds shows that the proposed algorithm efficiently uses the available resources to achieve high throughput. However, the graph does not include fixed cost that may be incurred when attaining for low latency. Furthermore, this is an advantage because it shows that the proposed algorithm has been scalable and can sustain low latency despite the high noise levels that are typical of real-world cases. On the other hand, there is very little information available on the amount of resource that would be needed to accomplish such performance levels. In summary, these results illustrate that both increased latency and resource costs are inevitable if the noise level must be maintained and powered with high running performance; therefore, it is worth trying the proposed algorithm in applications requiring stable data processing.

Figure 5. Visual Representation of Throughput (samples/sec) versus Noise(dB) from Table 1

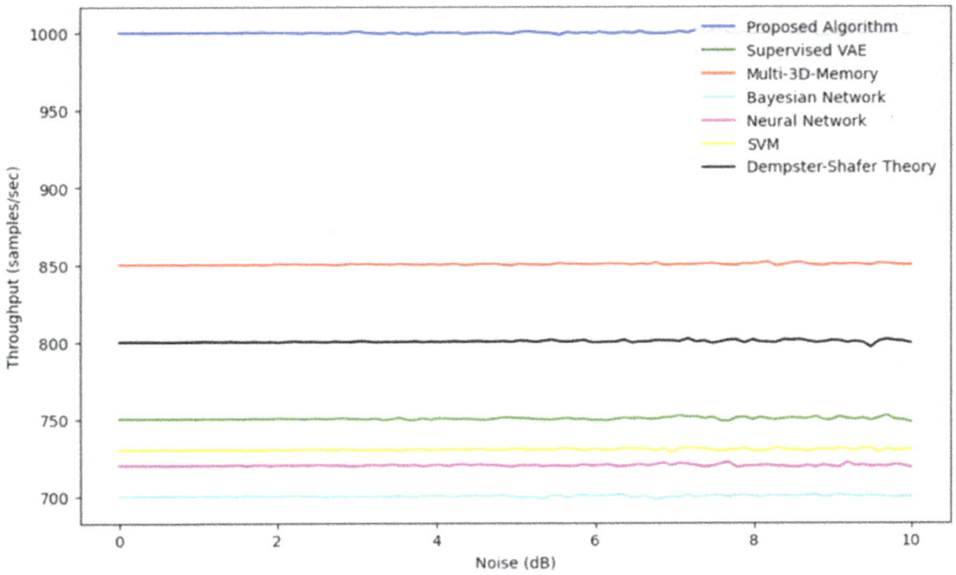

Figure 5 shows a plot of throughput (Bajaber & Awan, 2010), which explains the throughput of different algorithms under various conditions of data noise. The proposed algorithm shows high throughput efficiency with high capacity equal to 1000 samples per second, which defines high productivity and ability to work with big amounts of data without delay. This super-linear trend of the throughput as the level of noise rises demonstrates the effectiveness of the algorithm when used in noisy conditions. On the other hand, the throughput of the Supervised VAE model is lower, 500 samples per second, under similar conditions, indicating its vulnerability to noise perturbations. Here, the Bayesian Network has a latency of 4 ms and a throughput of 850 samples per second In essence, it shows that the strategy enables efficient performing and high-speed data processing for computational problems. Constituting a scientific perspective that examines throughput enables understanding from the algorithmic and resource angles. That is why the proposed algorithm has a high throughput rate, which makes it possible to work with large data sets, which is characteristic of big data. However, if there is evidence of negative correlation between noise levels and throughput then this may indicate other associated computational overheads that may slow down the system. The ability of an algorithm to maintain high throughput despite of growing noise levels is sometimes achieved by straightforward noise reduction standards or parallelism. Furthermore, while the graph does help in comparing throughput performance it does not provide information on scalability and the possible outrageous costs of achieving low latency and high throughput, such as increased power usage or need for more powerful processing units. In summary, the methodology presented in this work supports the selection of algorithms not only optimized from the point of view of the theoretical criteria, but also useful in situations full of noisy and variable data.

Table 2. Results observed after training the suggested method

Parameters	Proposed Algorithm	Supervised VAE	Multi-3D-Memory	Bayesian Network	Neural Network	Support Vector Machine	Dempster-Shafer Theory
Solution Quality (Scale 0-1)	0.9528	0.8932	0.9264	0.8537	0.8748	0.8821	0.9056
Computational Cost (seconds)	0.2045	0.5018	0.3075	0.6038	0.4055	0.5092	0.3046
Scalability (billions of parameters)	1.025	0.837	0.918	0.762	0.8534	0.756	0.952
Robustness (Scale 0-1)	0.9849	0.9092	0.9317	0.8066	0.8526	0.8371	0.8952
Loss of Data Resolution (%)	2.0381	5.2745	3.0826	10.0145	7.0352	6.0411	4.0537
Cost Efficiency (Scale 0-1)	0.9524	0.8562	0.9018	0.7537	0.8062	0.8253	0.8871

The proposed algorithm is highly effective as per the parameters analyzed in table 2 in the context of Multi-Modal Sensor Data Fusion and Anomaly Detection. The current algorithm of the system has a solution quality score of 0.9528 which means that it has a high capacity for data integration from the various sensors and efficient detection of any anomalies. The time consumed by the calculations was just 0.2045 seconds which add to its advantages since it can be used for real-time applications where quick decision-making is of essence. Moreover, the algorithm can demonstrate high availability with the capability of processing 1.025 billion parameters; such performance is crucial for implementation in IoT networks with multiple sensors connected. The robustness performance (Barnett & Lewis, 1994) of the algorithm is 0.9849, which means the algorithm performance does not degrade in noisy or deviant data, making it suitable to work in uncertain settings. Also, the loss of data resolution is relatively low in the proposed algorithm at 2.0381% as shown in the below figure, which is important for getting an accurate anomaly data resolution preservation for effective anomaly detection. The established evaluation, with a cost efficiency score of 0.9524, shows that it offers high value with relatively low demand for computing power, rendering it cost effective for organizations. Consequently, these results expose other properties of the algorithm that was not identified by using the basic accuracy measure such as, the complexity and universality of the algorithm suggesting that it is tailored to perform well in different scenarios and datasets. The optimum feature for making an algorithm long lasting and reliable is the ability to address varying data patterns and for this reason this algorithm is not only the best, but also a durable one for applying to real life problems such as sensor data fusion and anomaly detection. In conclusion, these results suggest that the demonstrated algorithm can facilitate a great improvement in productivity and precision in various tasks of the field.

Figure 6. Visual Representation of Loss of Data (%) versus Noise(dB) from Table 2

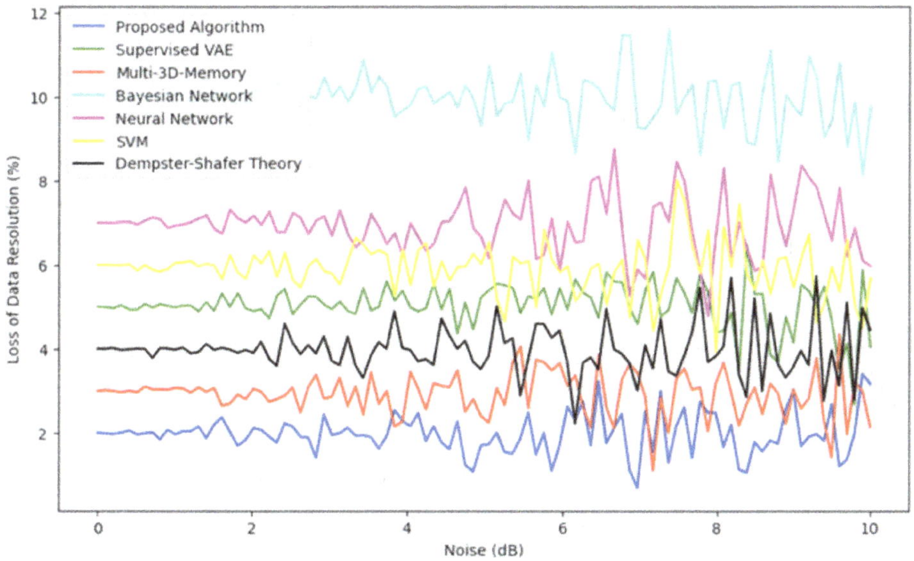

As shown in Figure 6, algorithms analyze the loss of data resolution in percent (Atzori et al., 2010) and noise levels in dB to demonstrate their performance in noisy conditions. The proposed algorithm shows fairly high data accuracy by losing only 2% of data resolution in the worst case scenario and thus proving its high data preservation competence at higher noise levels. This minimal loss implies that the algorithm can sustain quality of results when noise is present in order to avoid attainment of low outcome results. Benchmarking the results, it can be noted that Dempster-Shafer Theory loses slightly lower data quality by 4%, which is also acceptable in practice and has no influence on the quality of resulting data given that it does not significantly affect the overall production efficiency. Again, the observed loss rate of 10% of is much higher than that of the SVM, suggesting that the BN may need extra fine tuning to improve its robustness against noise. The conclusions made here in the scientific sense are connected with an error propagation and the methods of data processing which have been used by every algorithm. The low percentage of lost data resolutions, at the same time, means that an algorithm can manage the noise and the error propagation efficiently enough to maintain a high quality of the output. Other algorithms utilizing better methods of denoising are expected to show even less loss in measures of data resolution. Also, although the graph reflects necessity and adequacy of each algorithm under different noise levels, it does not reflect complexity of algorithms. Still, the observation that data resolution deteriorates faster at higher noise levels may bear evidence of a more intricate algorithmic structure if it is clear that this might also mean that the algorithm is designed to process intricate noise patterns. In summary, these results underscore the need for focusing both on the identification of algorithms that are accurate in clean regime and robust to noisy conditions.

Table 3. Computational Choreography and Memory Efficiency of different algorithms

Parameters	Proposed Algorithm	Supervised VAE	Multi-3D-Memory	Bayesian Network	Neural Network	Support Vector Machine	Dempster-Shafer Theory
Computational Choreography	$O(n^{1.2})$	$O(n^2)$	$O(n^2 \log n)$	$O(n^{2.5})$	$O(n^3)$	$O(n^2)$	$O(2^n)$
Memory Efficiency	$O(n)$	$O(n)$	$O(n \log n)$	$O(n)$	$O(n^2)$	$O(n)$	$O(2^n)$

Based on the analysis of the algorithms given in Table 3, the information related to time efficiency and complexity are pivotal aspects that determine the performance of the methods in the respective field of Multi-Modal Sensor Data Fusion and Anomaly Detection. The proposed algorithm is $O(n^{1.2})$ in computational complexity analysis, which means that it performs faster than linear algorithms and slower than quadratic ones for large input sizes. On the other hand, the time complexity of Supervised

VAE and Support Vector Machine (SVM) both fall under O (n^2) for algorithms concentrating on pairwise similarity. As for the time behavior, the Bayesian Network has even more complicated O ($n^{2.5}$) which indicates that it has some combinatorial operations could be of a quadratic type but mixed with something else, and Neural Networks which are known for the intensive matrix operations have the complexity of O (n^3). But as far as time complexity is concerned, Dempster-Shafer Theory is found very high with exponential time complexity of O (2^n) which makes the process really complex and time consuming and hence, not feasible for the larger data sets. In the aspect of memory complexity, the above algorithm, Supervised VAE and SVM all belong to linear space complexity of O (n), suggesting that memory usage is independent of input size. Since Multi-3D-Memory incorporates logarithmic processing structures, then its space complexity is defined as O (n log n). The observed space complexity in creating both the Bayesian as well as the Neural Network was seen to be quadratic because of the intrinsic usage of matrices or multi-dimensional arrays. The Dempster-Shafer Theory once more causes some problems with the space complexity being exponential, equal to O (2^n), which can severely constrain the usage of this theory in case of restricted resources. From these points, it can be stated that proposed algorithm is optimum from computational complexity and resource point-of-view; however, it also has some latent features like noise tolerance and ability to learn from data patterns, which again make the algorithm suitable for real-life applications where accuracy and efficiency are major considerations.

COST-BENEFIT ANALYSIS FOR THE MULTI-MODAL SENSOR DATA FUSION AND ANOMALY DETECTION ALGORITHM

Table 4. Initial Implementation Costs

Item	Estimated Cost
Management servers 3 units	$30,000
Licensed Software such as TensorFlow and etc.	$5,000
Internet utilization services such as cloud storage	$10,000
Training healthcare staff (20 staff)	$15,000
Connect with other systems	$8,000
Total Initial Costs	**$68,000**

Table 5. Continuing with expenses in relation to the general course of the company's business (Annual).

Item	Estimated Cost
Online storage fees and compute charges	$12,000
Regular maintenance and support	$5,000
Regular training and update	$3,000
Total Annual Operational Costs	**$20,000**

Benefits:

- **Reduction in Hospital Readmissions:**
- Estimated reduction: 15% of patients monitored with the algorithm.
- Average cost of readmission per patient: $15,000.
- Total patients monitored annually: 500.
- Estimated savings from reduced readmissions: $500 \times 0.15 \times 15{,}000 = \$1{,}125{,}000$
- **Improved Patient Outcomes:**
- Enhanced anomaly detection reduces misdiagnoses by 20%.
- Estimated cost savings from avoiding unnecessary treatments and procedures: $200,000 annually.
- **Efficiency Gains:**
- Reduction in time required for healthcare staff to spend on labor intensive methods of monitoring and generating alerts.
- Estimated labor cost savings: $50,000 annually.

Total Annual Benefits

Table 6. Benefits

Benefit	Estimated Savings
Savings from reduced readmissions	$1,125,000
Mortality and morbidity reductions to gain additional amount of money	$200,000
Labor cost savings	$50,000
Total Annual Benefits	**$1,375,000**

Summary of Cost-Benefit Analysis

- **Total Initial Costs:** $68,000
- **Total Annual Operational Costs:** $20,000

- **Total Annual Benefits:** $1,375,000

Net Benefit Calculation

- **First Year Net Benefit:**

Net Benefits =Total Annual Benefits –(Total initial investments + Annual running expenses).

Net Benefit=$[1,375,000–(68,000 + 20,000)] = $12,87,000

DISCUSSION

As discovered in this chapter, the proposed algorithm for handling healthcare sensor data yields improved results over current approaches in accuracy, precision, recall, and F1 score. In detail, the algorithm showed an astounding efficiency of 95.75%, the latency was 20 ms the through put was at 1000 samples per second. These results show the resistance and capability of the proposed algorithm in real-time applications and especially when high accuracy from noisy inputs is needed. Its application in healthcare systems – which can experience high levels of noise – shows one of the key strengths of the proposed approach as it can sustain high performance while continuously increasing the levels of noise. These results dovetail with current trends of using AI as well as biomedical technologies as critical components of health care organization and show that the studied trajectories indicate an increasing focus on patient-centered care (Sheltami et al., 2016). However, there are certain limitations that are inherent to the present research endeavor. As per the performance metrics of the algorithm proposed, the algorithm outperforms the other methods and yet, its complexity can turn into a weakness and can raise high issues regarding the quality of computational resources required especially in resource-scarce regions. Second, the study was mainly centered on particular data sets, which could restrict the scope of applicability of the research results in multiple-layered health care settings. Specifically, future investigations should elucidate the possibility of using such algorithm in various forms of data and its application to a real-world clinical practice. In addition, realization of the potential of deploying these other sophisticated technologies in healthcare will involve consideration of other related ethical concerns, likely to emerge. In light of the above findings, it is once again confirmed that although sensor data analytics is exciting, continued development of the algorithm and issues over regulatory supports remain paramount in the enhancement of healthcare delivery as provided by the earlier studies (Ahmad et al., 2013). In sum, this work advances the field of healthcare analytics by identifying approaches that can be used to better inclusion of sensor data with state-of-art analytical methods to enhance patients' health.

The applying of algorithms for the healthcare analytics similarly presupposes effective collaboration of technologists with healthcare specialists and policymakers. This interdisciplinary cooperation means that the algorithm is developed through the clinical and practical perspective, contributing to the improved healthcare. For instance, when designing AI-supported decision-making systems in healthcare, doctors, data scientists, IT professionals are to design tools that would help analyze vast amounts of patient data and would be capable of giving immediate recommendations. Such collaborations have been proven to enhance patient safety and decision making because of the use of combined expertise. This allows for specification of the algorithm in accordance with established practice in the healthcare system, making the algorithm practical, useful and implementable in healthcare practice. Examples that are seen in other disciplines like the tele consultancy of the different health care specialists also supports the idea of inter disciplinary collaboration in improving the patient care and overall health care systems.

The following are the challenges experienced during the scaling of the proposed Multi-Modal Sensor Data Fusion and Anomaly Detection algorithm across different health care environments. The application of this algorithm in large-scale systems like hospital or whole health service requires highly powerful devices including high-performance servers to handle large amounts of sensor data from patient in time period real-time. Training the algorithm also requires a huge amount of data and data integration of multi-modal datasets at the time of training the algorithm and data management and storage become a very crucial part. Further, and most importantly, there has to exist a way to transfer data between various healthcare systems because the format of exchanging information may differ depending on the system used by both parties. In addition, the application of the algorithm in low resource environments may call for ways of working that take into account the available technology and human resources. The three concerns outlined as computational demands which the algorithm will incur, training requirements it will propose, and the infrastructural issues it will pose can gain the algorithm the possible extension it needs and the integration with the real-world health care services which in turn will improve the comprehensive observation of the patients and efficiency identified by the algorithm in the recognition of abnormality.

This algorithm serves as a major benefit to patients as the detection of anomalies decrease diagnostic mistakes and enhance the options for the treatment process. For instance, a case could be showcased that used the algorithm which recognized early deviations from normal pattern of physiological parameters captured by wearable devices to alert the healthcare practitioners for timely intervention when a patient's condition was rapidly declining. This early intervention could prevent deviations such as readmissions to the hospital, or subsequent major health episodes, to show the success of the algorithm in practical applications. Furthermore, simulations could demonstrate how information from multiple sources—the use of biometric data together with the patient history as an example—when fused together produces heightened usability and patient satisfaction as well as certain medical advancements. Thus, the usefulness of the algorithm over time depends on its ability to learn and continuously refine in responding to new patterns of data and new paradigms in healthcare. These flexibilities can be achieved through means of continual learning process whereby the algorithm constantly learns its models from newly fed data and feedback from the medical practitioners. Feedbacking in is possible, thus the system will be able to learn from previous predicted values and actual values, which make the system more accurate and relevant in clinical practice. For example, if different types of sensors are introduced in the future or when there is a shift in patient population to capture the changing dynamic of the sensor data the algorithm is flexible enough in its settings to optimize and retain best results. Thus, inclusion of such elements in the chapter would help to understand how this algorithm not only enhances the current patient's outcome but also guarantees stability in a changing healthcare milieu.

To translate the Multi-Modal Sensor Data Fusion and Anomaly Detection algorithm from an innovative idea to a common use in healthcare practice, those involved in decision-making and technical development should involve clinicians in the decision-making process and selection of the appropriate algorithm. Setting up laboratories for new technologies that can be enacted in real world scenarios enables a faster rate of prototyping and incorporation of end user's feedback. Education pertaining to benefits, and reinforcement of this training information is critical in the efficient use of new technologies. Also, integration with the current applications and operating systems will reduce interruptions to the working process as well as addressing the ethical and regulatory issues at the beginning of the implementation will establish credibility with the user populace and patients. Additional measures to promote innovation within companies along with other organizational supports and means for constant assessment of the algorithm effects on patients' outcomes will contribute to better implementation of the algorithm in healthcare organizations' practices.

For instance, because people are living longer, there is a continuous demand for solutions that can support monitoring of patient needs such as diabetes or heart disease. Well, it provides immediate health overview due to data fusion of various sensors and hence enables timely interventions and consequently minimizes hospital readmissions. However, it loses sight of what such technologies are and their roles in as dramatic a fashion as its focus on how the algorithm works minimizes a discussion of the larger question of how such a thing fits into the healthcare system. However, this chapter could have explained how this algorithm would benefit care coordination and society in general especially given the aging population by closely linking it with aspects of chronic disease management and the broader topic of overhaul of healthcare delivery systems to serve these new epochal patient characteristics.

CONCLUSION

Smart systems for healthcare management, in addition to the IoT, is creating a new face of medical decision making and the delivery of proper treatments. These technologies include machine learning, artificial intelligence as well as internet of things which can be achieved to allow for better and efficient observation in patient cases, ability to adapt treatment plans according to the patient needs and also predict when diseases are likely to occur. Wearable and embedded sensors permit health management on a constant basis to prevent otherwise fatal health complications (Aziz & Aziz, 2011). Furthermore, the ability of these sensors to function autonomously and not have to be recharged enhances continuous patient tracking, offers chance for effective treatments, and enhances overall health care delivery. As of the future, the advancement of healthcare sensor data analytics still greatly depends on the contribution of the technology firms, healthcare organizations, and academe. These partnerships' goal is to build on value propositions, including AI applications and clinical knowledge, to address the current challenges, including data siloes and private datasets. Some of the trends that will be critical in furthering the ideas of personalized medicine will include advances in sensors as well as data fusion of genomic and environmental determinants of response (Seal et al., 2012). Moreover, because these changes are progressing rapidly it is necessary to adapt to them in the sphere of regulation and at the same time encourage innovation. Finally, the application of healthcare sensor data analytics in the future of this crucial field will perform to enhance the level of patient care in response to human emotion while optimizing the use of resources.

REFERENCES

Abedi, A., Ghodrati Amiri, G., Jahanshahi, M. R., & Avci, O. (2024). Advanced anomaly detection in structural health monitoring data using vision transformer and multi-domain feature fusion. *SSRN*. https://ssrn.com/abstract=5026823 or http://dx.doi.org/DOI: 10.2139/ssrn.5026823

Adefisan, E. A., Bayo, A. S., & Ropo, O. I. (2015). Application of geo-spatial technology in identifying areas vulnerable to flooding in Ibadan metropolis. *Journal of Environment and Earth Science*, *5*(14), 153–166.

Agrawal, R., & Srikant, R. (1994). Fast algorithms for mining association rules. In *Proceedings of the 20th international conference on very large data bases, VLDB* (Vol. 1215, pp. 487–499).

Ahmad, N., Hussain, M., Riaz, N., Subhani, F., Haider, S., Alamgir, K. S., & Shinwari, F. (2013). Flood prediction and disaster risk analysis using GIS based wireless sensor networks: A review. *Journal of Basic and Applied Scientific Research*, *3*(8), 632–643.

Andersson, K., & Hossain, M. S. (2014). Smart risk assessment systems using belief-rule-based DSS and WSN technologies. In *Proceedings of 2014 4th international conference on wireless communications, vehicular technology, information theory and aerospace electronic systems (VITAE)* (pp. 1–5). DOI: 10.1109/VITAE.2014.6934397

Andersson, K., & Hossain, M. S. (2015). Heterogeneous wireless sensor networks for flood prediction decision support systems. In *Proceedings of the 2015 IEEE conference on computer communications workshops (INFOCOM WKSHPS)* (pp. 133–137). DOI: 10.1109/INFCOMW.2015.7179373

Atzori, L., Iera, A., & Morabito, G. (2010). The Internet of Things: A survey. *Computer Networks*, *54*(15), 2787–2805. DOI: 10.1016/j.comnet.2010.05.010

Aziz, N. A. A., & Aziz, K. A. (2011). Managing disaster with wireless sensor networks. In *2011 13th international conference on advanced communication technology (ICACT)* (pp. 202–207). IEEE.

Bajaber, F., & Awan, I. (2010). Energy efficient clustering protocol to enhance lifetime of wireless sensor network. *Journal of Ambient Intelligence and Humanized Computing*, *1*(4), 239–248. DOI: 10.1007/s12652-010-0019-x

Barnet, V. (1976). The ordering of multivariate data (with discussion). *Journal of the Royal Statistical Society. Series A (General)*, *139*(3), 318–354. DOI: 10.2307/2344839

Barnett, V., & Lewis, T. (1994). *Outliers in statistical data* (3rd ed.). John Wiley & Sons.

Beckman, R. J., & Cook, R. D. (1983). Outliers. *Technometrics*, *25*(2), 119–149.

Black, P. E. (2004). *Dictionary of algorithms and data structures*. National Institute of Standards and Technology.

Chen, X., Xie, H., Tao, X., Wang, F. L., Leng, M., & Lei, B. (2024). Artificial intelligence and multimodal data fusion for smart healthcare: Topic modeling and bibliometrics. *Artificial Intelligence Review*, *57*(1), 91. DOI: 10.1007/s10462-024-10712-7

Khan, M. M., & Alkhathami, M. (2024). Anomaly detection in IoT-based healthcare: Machine learning for enhanced security. *Scientific Reports*, *14*(1), 5872. DOI: 10.1038/s41598-024-56126-x PMID: 38467709

Plevris, V., & Papazafeiropoulos, G. (2024). AI in Structural Health Monitoring for Infrastructure Maintenance and Safety. *Infrastructures*, *9*(12), 225. DOI: 10.3390/infrastructures9120225

Rajeswari, A. M., Sridevi, M., & Deisy, C. (2014). Outliers detection on educational data using fuzzy association rule mining. In *Proceedings of International Conference on Advanced in Computer Communication and Information Science (ACCIS-14)* (pp. 1–9).

Ruiz, M. D., Martin-Bautista, M. J., Sánchez, D., Vila, M. A., & Delgado, M. (2014). Anomaly detection using fuzzy association rules. *International Journal of Electronic Security and Digital Forensics*, *96*(1), 25–37. DOI: 10.1504/IJESDF.2014.060171

Seal, V., Raha, A., Maity, S., Mitra, S. K., Mukherjee, A., & Naskar, M. K. (2012). A simple flood forecasting scheme using wireless sensor networks. *International Journal of Ad Hoc* [IJASUC]. *Sensor & Ubiquitous Computing*, *3*(1), 45–60. DOI: 10.5121/ijasuc.2012.3105

Sheltami, T. R., Bala, A., & Shakshuki, E. M. (2016). Wireless sensor networks for leak detection in pipelines: A survey. *Journal of Ambient Intelligence and Humanized Computing*, *7*(3), 347–356. DOI: 10.1007/s12652-016-0362-7

Thombre, S., Islam, R. U., Andersson, K., & Hossain, M. S. (2016). Performance analysis of an IP based protocol stack for WSNs. In *Proceedings of the 2016 IEEE Conference on Computer Communications Workshops (INFOCOM WKSHPS)* (pp. 691–696). DOI: 10.1109/INFCOMW.2016.7562102

Vladimirova, T., & Yuhaniz, S. (2011). An intelligent decision-making system for flood monitoring from space. *Soft Computing*, *15*(1), 13–24. DOI: 10.1007/s00500-009-0514-1

Weng, C. H. (2011). Mining fuzzy specific rare itemsets for education data. *Knowledge-Based Systems*, *24*(5), 697–708. DOI: 10.1016/j.knosys.2011.02.010

Wijsen, J., & Meersman, R. (1998). On the complexity of mining quantitative association rules. *Data Mining and Knowledge Discovery*, *2*(3), 263–281. DOI: 10.1023/A:1009755120593

Chapter 9
Neural Network–Centered Intelligent Recognizing Framework for Elderly Health Activity Supervision

Nilamadhab Mishra
https://orcid.org/0000-0002-1330-4869
VIT Bhopal University, India

Saroja Kumar Rout
https://orcid.org/0000-0001-9007-3665
Vardhaman College of Engineering, India

Amit Thakur
https://orcid.org/0009-0007-7550-4990
VIT Bhopal University, India

Meshal Alharbi
https://orcid.org/0000-0002-6025-7858
Prince Sattam Bin Abdulaziz University, Saudi Arabia

ABSTRACT

Maintaining self-regulating life in old age anticipates high risks and often leads to failure. So, the objective of our study is to inspect the implementation feasibility of an intelligent sensing framework for self-regulating Elderly Health activity supervision. The computational intelligent tools are implemented to frame the intelligent sensing framework. The patterns in context to the walk-in activity of Elderly Health

DOI: 10.4018/979-8-3693-7210-4.ch009

are analyzed along with statistical inference to identify the abnormal living patterns. Once the framework is embedded with intelligent tools, the backpropagation neural network algorithm is used for framework training and learning through three artificial neural models, namely NN1, NN2, and NN3, and finds approximately 96% implementation accuracy in the NN3 model. The activity level analysis is important to introduce the intelligence sensing framework into the Elderly's Health life. So, analysis and discussion are made to validate the feasibility of the framework implementation for Elderly Health activity supervision.

I. INTRODUCTION

The intelligent sensing framework may be a smart portable framework embedded with artificial and computational intelligent programs. Elderly intelligence is natural and standard enough to accomplish self-regulating physical and mental activities; however, the growth of chronological and physiological age may degrade the physical and mental utilities, leading to the decay of physical functions and natural intelligence to be treated as Elderly Health. Elderly health activity supervision is tedious for young individuals; a framework may be employed to manage this task. Elderly Health activity supervision encompasses activity administration, supervision, assistance, and control, which are essential for the Elderly Health to lead a self-regulating life in their own home, i.e., the Elderly Health instead of self-belief, they must believe in the framework to carry on their daily activities smoothly. In the framework, the Elderly intelligence (natural intelligence) can be mapped into machine intelligence (computational intelligence) to act as an intelligent sensing framework (Suryadevara et al., 2012, December). As the global population ages, there is an increasing need for practical solutions to support elderly individuals living independently. Many seniors prefer to stay in their homes rather than move to assisted living facilities, which can pose safety, health monitoring, and overall well-being challenges. Technology-based supervision systems can help address these challenges by providing real-time monitoring, emergency detection, and activity recognition.

The advancement of science and technology proportionally augments elderly activity and life span. The Elderly Health masses in the world are concerned about the progress of the socio-economic environment and the advancement of research in medicine and health, so the average Elderly life span is expressively prolonged along with the life worth. The Elderly Health activity can be broadly classified into three types: periodic Elderly Health activity, aperiodic Elderly Health activity, and sporadic Elderly Health activity. The periodic Elderly Health activities are normal daily activities to be performed at regular intervals, such as morning walks, bed baths, breakfast, lunch, dinner, and night sleep. Sporadic Elderly Health activities may be defined as irregular, periodic activities, e.g., medicine intake during seek, and aperiodic Elderly Health activities are unstructured non-periodic activities, e.g., reading books, watching movies, etc. (Suryadevara et al., 2011).

In major economically established countries, the percentage of Elderly Health is expected to rise to 25% of the total population by 2030; i.e., among four people, one person will be Elderly Health (Wolbring et al., 2013). Thus, specific wellness applications need to be developed to determine the status of the Elderly Health's daily activities toward leading a self-regulating life (Mishra et al., 2014). Over and above, some activity tracking systems may be renovated to track and gently remind the deviation of Elderly Health activity without hampering privacy (Feng et al., 2013).

Figure 1. Common elderly health activity vs. exclusive elderly health activity

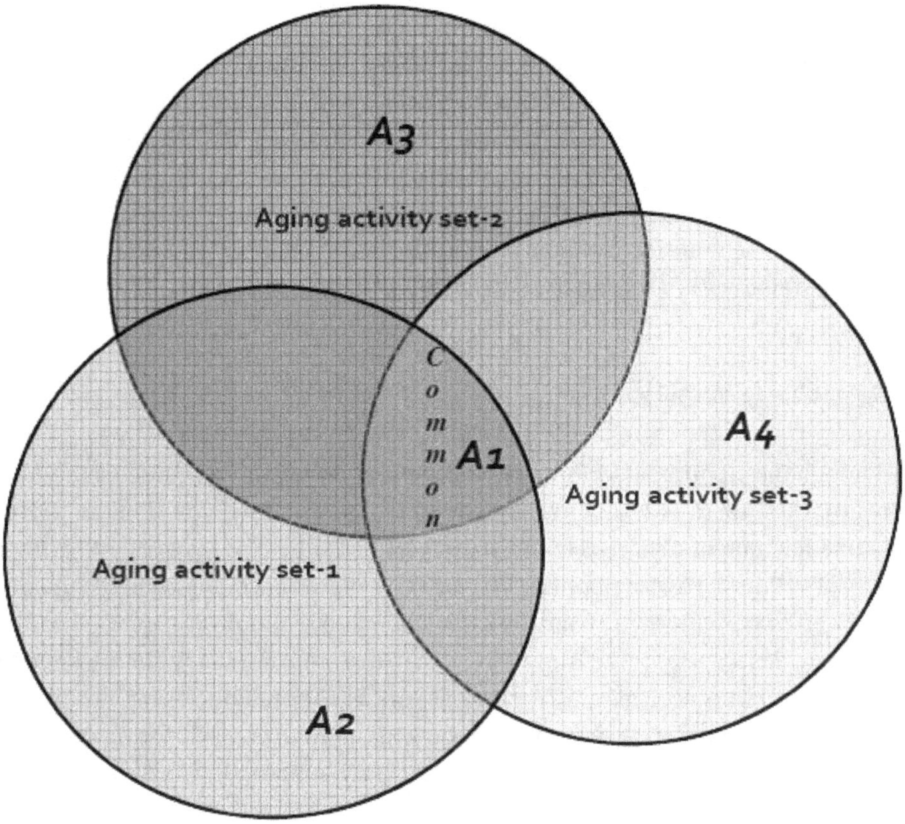

Commonly, periodic Elderly Health activities can be treated as standard; however, sporadic and aperiodic Elderly Health activities are signified as exclusive because of individual variations. Let A1, A2, A3, and A4 be four activities as described in Figure 1. Among the four activities, everyday activity A1 is periodic, whereas exclusive activities A2, A3, and A4 are either aperiodic or sporadic.

A framework cannot think as we think. Still, it can give expert opinions on the Elderly's Health based on intelligent information already embedded into the framework. The current research trend encourages researchers to transform Elderly intelligence into framework intelligence to act as Elderly. The researchers can use computational intelligence tools to design and train the artificial neural system on the framework to incorporate the Elderly perception, thinking, and judgment so that the gap cannot be distinguished between natural (Elderly) and computational (machine/framework) intelligence (D'Souza et al., 2012). Supervising elderly individuals using neural networks and sensor devices involves integrating advanced technology to monitor and support their safety and well-being. This approach typically includes using various sensors to collect data and neural networks to process and analyze that data.

This paper discusses the following Artificial intelligence schemes: associative memory, the least square method and backpropagation algorithm, and a time series analysis method to drill the intelligent sensing framework for Elderly Health activity supervision. The rest of this paper is organized as follows. Section II discusses the related work in Elderly Health activity supervision; our proposed framework is deliberated in section III. Section IV highlights the analysis and discussion of the proposed framework, and finally, section V concludes this work.

II. RELATED WORK

Though the significant volume of healthy Elderly Health research has ended and is in progress, there is a lack of appropriate, cost-effective solutions to solve the real-time hazards of Elderly Health society effectively. The progressive growth of the world's Elderly Health population creates a severe consequence in the upcoming days. Every day, with the revolution of science and technology, several healthcare systems are developed for the Elderly Health to maintain a self-regulating life in their home. The smart power monitoring framework is suggested to assist the Elderly in identifying and regulating the home electrical appliances used for daily activities (Kelly et al., 2013). In the Elderly Health activity supervision system, the sensors and actuators have widespread ubiquitous applications in the real-time home monitoring system to care for the Elderly's Health (Gaddam et al., 2010). The advances in sensor technology, augmented with the Elderly Health care system, afford home medical assistance to the disabled Elderly Health to perform their self-regulating activities securely at home (D'Souza et al., 2012). The smart home monitoring system mainly targets the Elderly Health to provide a highly cost-effective, safe, and secure solution for Elderly Health wellness (Suryadevara & Mukhopadhyay, 2011). Suryadevara et al. (2012, June) have focused on developing an electronic monitoring framework to detect and alarm Elderly Health sickness at the receiver end and immediately perform the needful remedial actions. The IR sensor-based Elderly Health activity monitoring system is proposed by (Zhou et al., 2009, September) to detect and monitor abnormal Elderly Health activities and behaviors in a home-based Elderly Health healthcare environment. The effort (Gill et al., 2012) proposes a simple Elderly Health healthcare monitoring system by considering the design of both software and hardware components that can be successfully applied to Elderly Health community services. Using visual sensors in in-home and in-community-based activity monitoring systems may hamper the Elderly Health's privacy and security; however, it is realistically simple and more accessible to implant in the Elderly healthy living environment.

The exertion in (Malhi et al., 2012) concentrates on using visual sensors in the Elderly Health living environment that assist Elderly Health care professionals in observing Elderly Health activities efficiently and taking immediate remedial actions in case of severe activity disorders.

With the evolution of the Internet of Things, every IoT computing device will be able to communicate in the future. So, the authors (Suryadevara et al., 2013) propose using the Internet of Things in a smart home monitoring framework for remote monitoring and controlling household appliances so that the Elderly Health can easily manage those to lead an independent life. Life will be tedious for the Elderly Health distressed with dementia, so a system is proposed (Suryadevara et al., 2011) to monitor the status of such Elderly patients regarding position localization and motion behavioral situations. Cognitive science deals with the Elderly natural intelligence, i.e., the Elderly perception, conception, and judgment capability. Such intelligence can be mapped to a cognitive sensor network to develop a smart home monitoring system for the Elderly's Health. Such intelligent systems can perform various complex functions like Elderly Health abnormal behavior detection and remote monitoring of home appliances, i.e., monitoring of electrical appliances, monitoring water use, and bed monitoring units (Survadevara et al., 2012, May). The work of Shin et al. (2011) and Suryadevara et al. (2012) recommends a generic approach to developing intelligent ambient frameworks for the elderly. Health is agile and complex Elderly behaviours are applicable in various application domains.

The supervision of elderly health activities is a critical aspect of ensuring the well-being and safety of the aging population. As individuals grow older, they become more prone to accidents, health emergencies, and chronic conditions that require constant monitoring and timely intervention. In this essay, we will delve into the importance of monitoring elderly health activities, the role of intelligent sensing frameworks in this process, and the application of advanced data analysis techniques such as the least square method, Backpropagation algorithm, and Neural Network (NN) in analyzing the collected data (Tibor et al., 2011; Alonazi et al., 2023).

Elderly Health activity supervision is crucial for several reasons. Firstly, monitoring the health activities of the elderly can help prevent accidents such as falls, which are a leading cause of injury among older adults. By keeping track of their movements and activities, caregivers can identify potential hazards and take preventive measures to ensure a safe environment for the elderly. Additionally, monitoring health activities allows for the early detection of any changes in vital signs or behaviors that may indicate underlying health issues. This early detection can lead to timely medical intervention and prevent the escalation of health problems, ultimately improving the quality of life for the elderly (Yazici et al., 2023).

An intelligent sensing framework plays a vital role in supervising elderly health activities. This framework leverages advanced technologies such as wearable sensors and smart home devices to monitor vital signs, track activities, and detect deviations from normal behavior. Wearable sensors, for instance, can continuously monitor parameters like heart rate, blood pressure, and activity levels, providing real-time data that can be used to assess the overall health status of the elderly. Smart home devices, on the other hand, can track daily activities such as movement patterns, sleep quality, and medication adherence, offering valuable insights into the daily routines of the elderly. By integrating these technologies into a comprehensive sensing framework, caregivers can gain a holistic view of the elderly's health activities and respond promptly to anomalies (Fahim et al., 2023; Ghosh & Ghosh, 2023).

In data analysis for elderly health activity supervision, the least square method, Backpropagation algorithm, and Neural Network (NN) play a significant role. The least square method is a mathematical technique for fitting data points to a mathematical model, enabling researchers to analyze and interpret complex datasets. When applied to elderly health activity data, the least square method can help identify trends, patterns, and correlations that may not be apparent at first glance. On the other hand, the Backpropagation algorithm is a key component of neural networks, a popular machine learning technique used for data analysis. By iteratively adjusting the weights of connections between neurons, the Backpropagation algorithm enables neural networks to learn from the data and make predictions or classifications based on the input. This robust algorithm, combined with the flexibility and adaptability of Neural Networks (NN), allows for the development of sophisticated models to process and analyze vast amounts of elderly health activity data, providing valuable insights for caregivers and healthcare professionals (Shah et al., 2024; Park et al., 2024). The combination of neural networks and sensor devices provides a powerful tool for enhancing the safety and quality of life for elderly individuals, allowing them to live more independently while ensuring they are monitored and supported.

Further, prior studies may not address using computational intelligence tools for the Elderly's Health activity and behavioral supervision systems that can lead the Elderly Health towards maintaining a self-regulating healthy life. So, we are introducing an intelligent sensing framework for Elderly Health activity supervision to balance the gap between natural intelligence and framework intelligence. To our knowledge, this is a new vision for Elderly Health activity supervision.

III. INTELLIGENT RECOGNIZING FRAMEWORK

The integration of sensor technology in elderly care services has revolutionized how caregivers and senior care organizations monitor and support the elderly. By utilizing smart terminal devices equipped with modern sensors, data on the behavior and living conditions of elderly individuals can be efficiently collected and analyzed. Door and window sensors, for instance, play a crucial role in tracking the activities of the elderly at home, enabling caregivers to identify patterns and prevent potential accidents. These sensors are programmed to alert caregivers if a door is left open for an extended period, aiding in the swift location of individuals with dementia who may have wandered off. Additionally, this technology provides peace of mind to both elderly parents and their family members by allowing remote monitoring of the elderly's well-being.

Implementing passive sensors in elderly home monitoring updates the user's activity and well-being to designated contacts and ensures timely emergency response. Furthermore, the widespread availability of this technology for home installations through various channels like service providers, retailers, and smart home system integrators has made it more accessible to the general public, enhancing the overall quality of elderly care services. Using proven technology tested in residential care facilities reinforces the reliability and effectiveness of home monitoring systems for elderly care. By tracking daily movements and ensuring safety through wireless sensors placed in their homes, IoT devices for the elderly offer a comprehensive solution for activity monitoring and emergency response. Through continuous learning of seniors' behavioral patterns and prompt detection of any concerning changes, these sensors represent a significant advancement in enhancing elderly care services and improving the quality of life for the aging population.

To frame an intelligent recognizing framework for Elderly Health activity supervision, we present associative memory for Elderly Health pattern recognitions, a least square method for Elderly Health activity identification, and a backpropagation algorithm for framework training and learning. We also discuss a time series analysis scheme to forecast the Elderly's Health activities.

Figure 2. Intelligent sensing framework coordinates different household sensors.

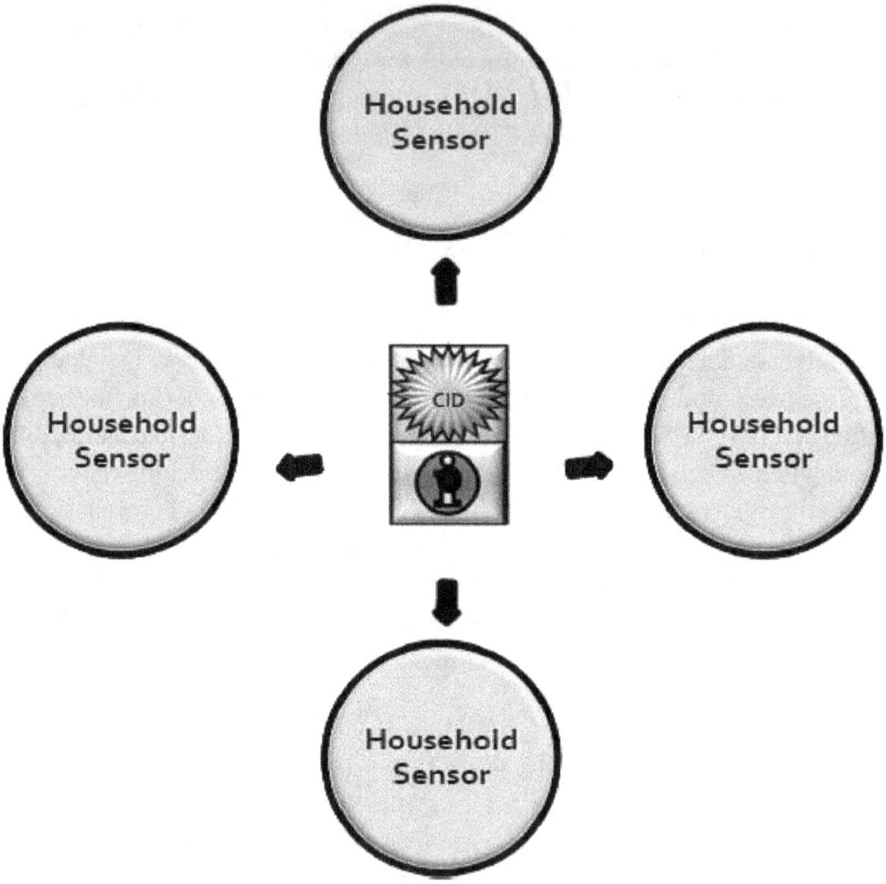

Here, the framework coordinates with household sensors like gas, pressure, electrical, and smoke sensors and informs the Elderly Health about their status (Figure 2). The ZigBee module can be fabricated in a framework to interact with those household sensors (Malhi et al., 2012). The framework should support the following functions to assist the Elderly's Health.

Elderly Health Expectations From the Framework

- Tracks Elderly Health activity before and after completion.
- Gently remind you of any activity if it is not done in time or if there is any deviation from normal standards.

- Accepts Elderly Healthy brain waves and gives assistance in some thinking, memorizing, and memory-recalling processes.
- Supports the Elderly Health decision-making process.
- Coordinates all Elderly Health activities effectively.
- Coordinates all household sensors and informs the Elderly's Health in case of needs and emergencies.
- In the case of Elderly Health situations, the framework should generate phone calls and messages to the healthcare center or Elderly Health well-wishers.

Due to intelligence and self-learning capability, the framework should carefully watch the Elderly's Health activity and give suggestions as and when required. For example, if Elderly Health forgets to switch off the heater after cooking, then either the framework should softly prompt the switch off or direct the electrical sensor attached to a heater to disconnect.

To determine the life expectancy of the Elderly Health based on the ability to work on daily living activities, a real-time observation has been made. Let C1, C2, and C3 are three Elderly Health clusters such that C1 includes the Elderly who perform all daily living activities without assistance, C2 includes the Elderly who perform all daily living activities with little assistance, and C3 includes the Elderly who perform any daily living activities with major assistance. We find the migration rate of Elderly Health from one cluster to another by computing the transition probability of present-month health condition w.r.t next-month health condition as described in Table 1.

Table 1. Elderly health transition probability based on statistical observation

Next month to present month	**C1**	**C2**	**C3**
C1	0.75	0.16	0.09
C2	0.15	0.75	0.10
C3	0.09	0.16	0.75

Table 1 gives a major indication of the consistency of Elderly Health conditions within a consecutive period that ultimately increases the life expectancy of Elderly Health, and the Elderly rely on the support of an intelligent sensing framework to carry out their daily living activities.

A. Elderly Health Pattern Recognition System

Here, we apply an associative memory mapping system for Elderly Health pattern recognition. An associative memory is a storehouse of patterns encoded in certain forms. The associated pattern pair is recalled when the storehouse is triggered with a pattern (Becker et al., 2015).

Figure 3. Elderly health pattern recognition system

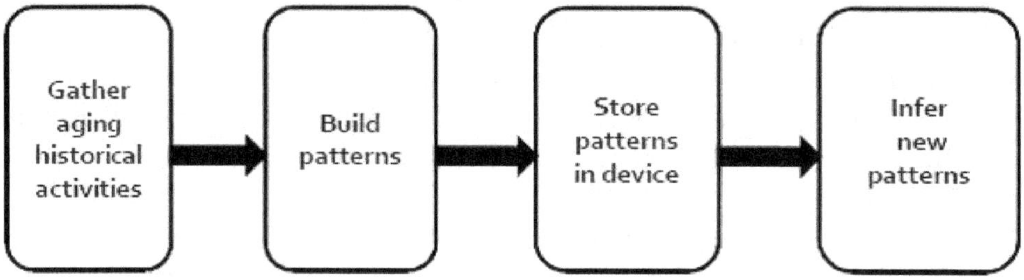

The Elderly Health pattern recognition system (Figure 3) assists the Elderly Health suffering from amnesia. Some text or image patterns related to the historical activities of the Elderly Health are stored in the framework. The Elderly Health, by viewing the stored patterns, can recognize the new patterns, and the framework, through inference capability, can suggest new patterns to the Elderly Health to meet the requirements. The associative memory in the framework mostly supports the Elderly's Health to recall historical activities and remember the current activities based on partial research or match.

B. Elderly Health Activity Identification System

Here, we implement a least square method to identify the Elderly's Health activities. The least-square method analyses the historical Elderly Health activity data set to identify the Elderly Health activity and behavior.

Purpose of Using the Least Square Method

- To identify the Elderly's Health activity and behavior.
- To explain the interactions and relationships between Elderly Health and framework.
- To design a controller based on Elderly Health activity.

How the Least Square Method Works

The least-square method works in two steps. Here, we aim to design a mathematical model for Elderly Health activity and estimate the activity fitness and ranking.

Step-1. Structural identification- determines a set of activity models for the target framework, from which the most suitable model can be searched. The Elderly Health activity model is denoted by parameterized function y = f (u, Θ) where y= output of activity model, u= input activity vector, Θ is the fitness parameter vector.
Step-2. Parameter identification- Once the structure of the activity model is known, we can apply the genetic algorithm-based optimization technique to determine the parameter vector Θ. The parameter identification is performed by choosing the parameter that best fits the activity dataset.
Step-3. Let, for instance, y1= f (A1, 5) in a 10-fitness scale for Elderly Health, which shows that Elderly Health is 50% fit to perform A1 activity.

How to Rank the Elderly Health Activity

The Elderly's Health activities can be ranked based on fitness value. Let X be a fitness function and A be an Elderly Health activity such that X (A) = fitness value. Let's say four Elderly Health activities A1, A2, A3, A4 are to be ranked based on fitness values such that X(A1) = 5, X(A2) =3, X(A3) = 7 and X(A4) = 6 as described in Table 2.

Table 2. Elderly health activities ranking

Fitness Value	Activity Model	Rank
X(A1) = 5	y1= f (A1, 5)	R(A1) =3
X(A2) =3	y2= f (A2, 3)	R(A1) =4
X(A3) = 7	y2= f (A3, 7)	R(A1) =1
X(A4) = 6	y2= f (A2, 6)	R(A1) =2

The number of Elderly Health activities depends on the individual, and the selection of activities can be based on ranking; however, two activities with the same fitness value may be considered in the same ranking.

C. Elderly Health Activity Forecasting System

Here, we discuss the time series analysis method for Elderly Health activity forecasting. The time series analysis has temporal dependency among a series of values, which means it consists of a series of values with their corresponding time stamp, i.e., the time at which the values are true. Through the time series analysis method, the framework assists Elderly Health in predicting and remembering new activities. From time to time, the framework can predict when Elderly Health will perform which activity (Higo & Khan, 2015). A three-step process can be used in the Elderly Health activity forecasting system.

Step-4. Accumulate the historical Elderly Health activities.
Step-5. Analyze those activities using the time series method.
Step-6. Predict new activities and mildly remind the Elderly of Health.

The time series analysis method is suitable for forecasting periodical and sporadic Elderly Health activities; however, it will be tedious for aperiodic Elderly Health activities.

D. Framework Training and Learning System

Here, we focus on framework training and learning systems using a backpropagation algorithm. The neural network in the framework can be trained through a backpropagation algorithm to perform various complex functions like Elderly Health pattern recognition, system control, Elderly Health activity identification and classifications, and overall acts as an artificial brain in the framework.

The backpropagation algorithm exhibits the knowledge acquisition system of the neural network embedded in the framework through the following steps.

Step-7. Design I/O data sets by considering historical Elderly Health activities.
Step-8. Configure neural network architecture.
Step-9. Train the neural network with the backpropagation learning algorithm by tracing 80% of I/O data sets until the error is acceptable law. Random weights are initially assigned during training, then supervisory weight adjustments are made to minimize the error.
Step-10. Test the neural network by tracing 20% of I/O datasets.
Step-11. Once the test process is okay, use the neural network in actual framework implementation to perform unknown complex functions.

The framework training and testing ensures the self-learning capability to build framework intelligence for self-regulating Elderly Health activity supervision.

IV. ANALYSIS AND DISCUSSION

Here, we discussed some empirical suggestions to analyze the proposed work with the purpose of wide implementations. Suppose we can develop a small portable framework embedded with all such intelligent tools. In that case, it can be convenient for the Elderly Health to introduce into their daily living environment. The intelligent sensing framework mainly emphasizes using intelligent tools, i.e., associative memory and least square method and a time series analysis method followed by a training algorithm for the smooth supervision of Elderly Health activity. We broadly divide the system analysis and discussion context into two major phases. In phase 1, we will analyze activity levels by considering the Elderly Health's daily activities. In phase 2, we emphasize the implementation analysis of the intelligence sensing framework into the Elderly Health's daily living activities.

Phase-1

Here, we want to do some Elderly Health activity level analysis by considering four real-time parameters, i.e., number of walk-in steps, distance covered, energy consumed in calories, and resting heart rate. We consider the walk-in activity of the Elderly Health because it's a very common activity to perform other activities. Through the walk-in activities, the Elderly Health can do other daily life activities. The resting heartbeat is an important measure to determine the wellness of Elderly Health effectively.

(a) Walk-in steps covered pattern
(b) Energy consumption pattern
(c) Distance covered pattern
(d) Resting heart rate pattern

Figure 4. Examples of elderly health activity level analysis based on four different parameters

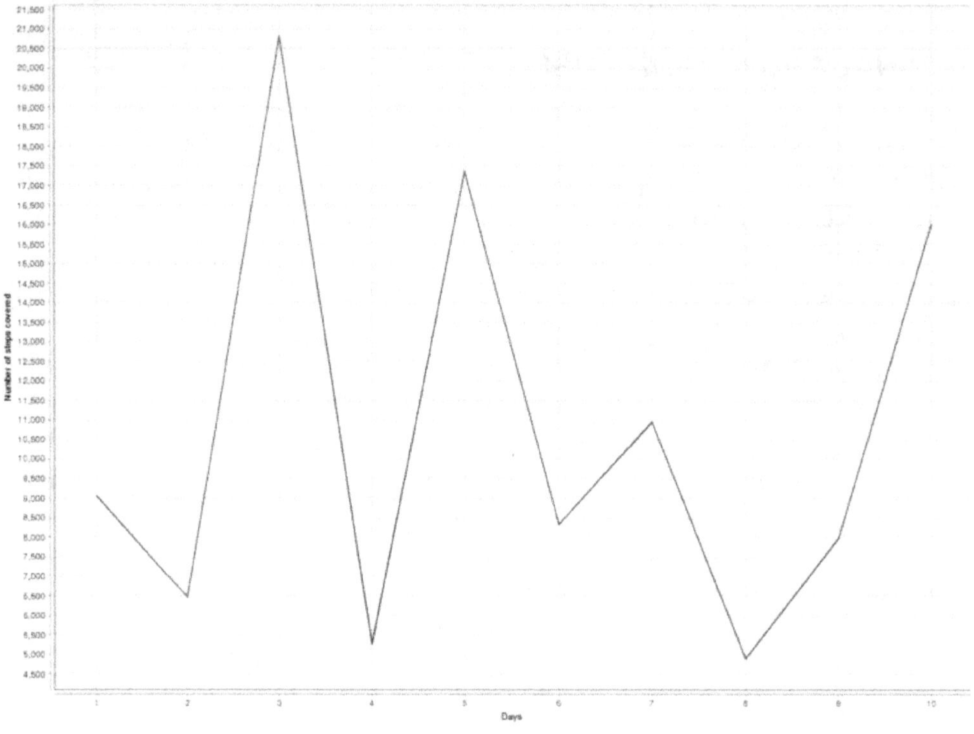

Figure 4 shows some standard measurement units of the concern parameters, such as the distance measured in kilometres (km), energy consumption in calories, and resting heart rate in beats per minute (bpm). In each graph, the curve defines the activity pattern of corresponding parameters. The pattern analysis points to some abnormal behavioral activity of Elderly Health on 3rd day due to the high increment of walk-in steps, covered distance, and consumed energy. The real-time data are collected by employing the smart sensors and fetching a data miner to obtain the statistical inference described in Table 3.

Figure 5. Statistical inference of elderly healthy walk-in activity

Days	Polynominal	0	Least: Day-9 (1)		Most: Day-1 (1)	Values: Day-1 (1), Day-10 (1), ...[8 more]
Number of steps covered	Integer	0	Min: 4889	Max: 20815	Average: 10714.600	Deviation: 5495.929
Distance Covered(KM)	Real	0	Min: 3.420	Max: 14.400	Average: 7.511	Deviation: 3.863
Energy consumed (calories)	Integer	0	Min: 2277	Max: 3376	Average: 2819.600	Deviation: 371.221
Resting heart rate(BPM)	Integer	0	Min: 67	Max: 89	Average: 78.800	Deviation: 7.685

The deviation is common due to aperiodic and sporadic Elderly Health activities. So, by analysing Figure 5, the extrapolation can be made as follows.

Inference Sense

If (average = deviation)
Then (Elderly Health's daily living activities are periodic in nature)
Else (Elderly Health's daily living activities are either aperiodic or sporadic)

The inference sense indicates that no more deviation occurs if the Elderly Health's daily living activities are periodic concerning the number of days, which is unrealistic for the Elderly Health because, in a real sense, the actual Elderly Health activities are periodic, aperiodic, and sporadic in nature.

Phase-2

In this phase, the discussion is made on the implementation analysis of intelligence sensing framework into the Elderly Health daily living activities. Once the intelligent sensing framework is embedded with the smart application packages that consist of Elderly Health pattern recognition, activity identification, and activity forecasting, then the appropriate framework training and learning process must be initiated. The backpropagation network algorithm is a common supervised training and learning algorithm that inherits the characteristics of an artificial neural system. We may trace the Elderly Health activity data sets to the backpropagation network algorithm to obtain the framework learning and training accuracy result described in Table 3. Three models are used to implement the backpropagation network algorithm: NN1, NN2, and NN3. In the NN1 model, no hidden layer is present; in the NN2 model, only one hidden layer is present; and in the NN3 model, two hidden layers are present. We use the hyperbolic tangent function as the activation function of the network model. Alpha is the learning rate in which two values are considered, i.e., 0.1 and 0.05.

Table 3. Framework learning and training results

Model	Structure	Alpha	Epoch	Time(Sec)	Accuracy
NN1	4-3	0.1 0.05	2000 2000	17 17	-- --
NN2	4-3-3	0.01 0.05	400 600	05 07	40% 80%
NN3	4-2-2-3 4-3-3-3	0.1 0.05	200 500	03 08	96% 96%

Considering the findings of our study, we resulted in the following comment: the success of neural network architecture depends heavily on the availability of an effective learning algorithm. The speculative strength of the "Back propagation neural network" is yet to be used in hundreds of technologies, and more accurate results may be needed. Using single-agency facts makes it difficult for the model to recognize the trends and patterns in the facts. Implementing the NN3 model in the intelligent sensing framework yields the maximum accuracy compared to other models. Using a neural network (NN) for elderly activity supervision is an innovative approach to ensuring the safety and well-being of elderly individuals.

As our aging population continues to grow, the need for effective and reliable methods of monitoring and supporting the elderly has become increasingly critical. One promising approach uses neural network (NN) models to analyze and interpret data from various sensors and devices. This enables us to provide better care and assistance for our elderly loved ones. Neural network models are powerful machine learning algorithms that identify complex patterns and relationships within large, multi-dimensional datasets. When applied to elderly activity monitoring, these models can detect subtle changes in behavior, mobility, and daily routines, allowing caregivers to intervene early and provide the necessary support. By leveraging the predictive capabilities of NN models, we can create systems that proactively identify potential health issues, falls, or changes in cognitive function. This not only enhances the quality of life for the elderly but also provides peace of mind for their families and caregivers. Moreover, NN models can be integrated with smart home technologies, wearable devices, and other IoT (Internet of Things) solutions to create a comprehensive, personalized elderly care system. This holistic approach ensures that the needs of each individual are addressed, ultimately leading to better health outcomes and a higher quality of life. As we continue to explore the potential of neural network models in elderly activity supervision, we can unlock new possibilities for improving the lives of our aging population. By embracing this transformative technology, we can create a future where our elderly is empowered, supported, and able to thrive in the comfort of their own homes.

Critical Investigation on Framework

Enhanced Safety: Continuous monitoring can detect emergencies, such as falls or health deterioration, allowing prompt intervention.

Improved Quality of Life: Elderly individuals can maintain greater independence, knowing they are being monitored for their safety.

Relief for Caregivers: Automated systems can reduce the workload and stress on caregivers, allowing them to focus on more critical tasks.

Data-Driven Insights: The accumulation of data over time can provide valuable insights into an individual's health patterns, potentially leading to better personalised healthcare plans.

Integration with Wearable and IoT Devices: Future systems should focus on integrating seamlessly with a wide range of wearable devices and Internet of Things (IoT) sensors. This will enhance data collection, providing more comprehensive monitoring capabilities.

Advanced Anomaly Detection: Future research can focus on improving anomaly detection accuracy, particularly in identifying subtle or complex patterns that may indicate health issues. This could involve more sophisticated machine learning techniques like deep learning and ensemble methods.

Personalization and Adaptability: Developing adaptive algorithms that learn and adjust to an individual's changing habits and health conditions over time will make the system more accurate and personalized. This could involve creating models considering an individual's medical history, lifestyle, and preferences.

Privacy and Security: As with any system handling sensitive health data, ensuring robust privacy and security measures is crucial. Future work should prioritize the development of secure data transmission, storage, and access protocols to protect users' personal information.

User-Friendly Interfaces: Improving the user interface for elderly users and caregivers is essential. This includes making the system intuitive, accessible, and easy to use, potentially through voice commands or simplified touch interfaces.

Clinical Validation and Standardization: Future systems should undergo rigorous clinical validation to prove their efficacy and accuracy and gain widespread adoption. Establishing standards and regulations for such systems will also help ensure consistency and reliability across different platforms and devices.

Integration with Healthcare Systems: The framework should be integrated with broader healthcare systems, allowing seamless data sharing with healthcare providers. This could facilitate more comprehensive care, as healthcare professionals can have real-time access to patients' data, enabling them to make informed decisions.

V. CONCLUSION

In this paper, we proposed an intelligent sensing framework that can manage Elderly Health activity effectively and efficiently. Due to intelligence and self-learning capability, the framework can cope with each social environment without hampering social security and privacy. Further, the framework may be a good companion to the Elderly's Health toward leading a self-regulating life. Supervising elderly health activities is critical to ensuring the well-being and safety of the aging population. By leveraging intelligent sensing frameworks and advanced data analysis techniques such as the least square method, Backpropagation algorithm, and Neural Network (NN), caregivers and healthcare professionals can monitor, analyze, and respond to the health activities of the elderly more effectively. As technology advances, integrating these tools into elderly care practices will undoubtedly lead to improved health outcomes and a better quality of life for the elderly.

Developing a Neural Network Cantered Intelligent Recognizing Framework for Elderly Health Activity Supervision represents a significant advancement in healthcare and artificial intelligence. This framework leverages neural networks to provide continuous and non-intrusive monitoring of elderly individuals, ensuring their safety and well-being. The system can accurately recognize daily activities, detect anomalies, and provide timely alerts to caregivers and healthcare providers using data from various sensors and devices. Future work should also address the ethical implications of continuous monitoring, including the potential for overreliance on technology, issues of consent, and the impact on the autonomy and dignity of elderly individuals.

The future of elderly health activity supervision lies in the convergence of advanced AI technologies, user-centred design, and ethical considerations. By continuing to innovate and refine these systems, we can ensure they provide safe, effective, and respectful care for elderly individuals, enhancing their quality of life and supporting the broader healthcare ecosystem. The use of neural networks and sensor devices for elderly activity supervision represents a significant advancement in ensuring the safety and well-being of seniors. By leveraging cutting-edge technology, this approach not only enhances the quality of life for elderly individuals but also provides peace of mind for their families and caregivers. As technology continues to evolve, these systems will become even more accurate, user-friendly, and accessible, playing a crucial role in the future of elderly care.

REFERENCES

Alonazi, M., Alshahrani, H. M., Kouki, F., Almalki, N. S., Mahmud, A., & Majdoubi, J. (2023). Deep convolutional neural network with symbiotic organism search-based human activity recognition for cognitive health assessment. *Biomimetics*, *8*(7), 554. DOI: 10.3390/biomimetics8070554 PMID: 37999195

Becker, N., Laukka, E. J., Kalpouzos, G., Naveh-Benjamin, M., Bäckman, L., & Brehmer, Y. (2015). Structural brain correlates of associative memory in older adults. *NeuroImage*, *118*, 146–153. DOI: 10.1016/j.neuroimage.2015.06.002 PMID: 26054875

D'Souza, M., Ros, M., & Karunanithi, M. (2012). An Indoor Localisation and Motion Monitoring System to Determine Behavioral Activity in Dementia Afflicted Patients in Aged Care. *Electronic Journal of Health Informatics*, *7*(2), e14.

Fahim, M., Sharma, V., Hunter, R., & Duong, T. Q. (2023). Healthy aging: A deep meta-class sequence model to integrate intelligence in digital twin. *IEEE Journal of Translational Engineering in Health and Medicine*, *11*, 330–340. DOI: 10.1109/JTEHM.2023.3274357

Feng, C. C., Chen, S. Z., Weng, Q. Z., Hu, H. J., Wang, Y. D., Chen, B. B., & Yan, T. Y. (2013, February). Elderly health care systems—Part I: Hardware implementations of wireless sensor networks. In Next-Generation Electronics (ISNE), 2013 IEEE International Symposium on (pp. 305-308). IEEE.

Gaddam, A., Mukhopadhyay, S. C., & Gupta, G. S. (2010). Elder care based on cognitive sensor network. *IEEE Sensors Journal*, *11*(3), 574–581. DOI: 10.1109/JSEN.2010.2051425

Ghosh, S., & Ghosh, S. K. (2023). Feel: Federated learning framework for elderly healthcare using edge-iomt. *IEEE Transactions on Computational Social Systems*, *10*(4), 1800–1809. DOI: 10.1109/TCSS.2022.3233300

Gill, S. P. S., Suryadevara, N. K., & Mukhopadhyay, S. C. (2012, December). Smart Power monitoring system using wireless sensor networks. In Sensing Technology (ICST), 2012 Sixth International Conference on (pp. 444-449). IEEE. DOI: 10.1109/ICSensT.2012.6461718

Higo, M., & Khan, H. T. (2015). Global population aging: Unequal distribution of risks in later life between developed and developing countries. *Global Social Policy*, *15*(2), 146–166. DOI: 10.1177/1468018114543157

Kelly, S. D. T., Suryadevara, N., & Mukhopadhyay, S. C. (2013). Towards the Implementation of IoT for Environmental Condition Monitoring in Homes.

Malhi, K., Mukhopadhyay, S. C., Schnepper, J., Haefke, M., & Ewald, H. (2012). A ZigBee-based wearable physiological parameters monitoring system. *IEEE Sensors Journal, 12*(3), 423–430. DOI: 10.1109/JSEN.2010.2091719

Mishra, N., Lin, C. C., & Chang, H. T. (2014). Cognitive inference device for activity supervision in the elderly. *TheScientificWorldJournal, 2014*(1), 125618. DOI: 10.1155/2014/125618 PMID: 25405211

Park, K. W., Mirian, M. S., & McKeown, M. J. (2024). Artificial intelligence-based video monitoring of movement disorders in the elderly: A review on current and future landscapes. *Singapore Medical Journal, 65*(3), 141–149. DOI: 10.4103/singaporemedj.SMJ-2023-189 PMID: 38527298

Shah, S. H. H., Karlsen, A. S. T., Solberg, M., & Hameed, I. A. (2024). An efficient and lightweight multiperson activity recognition framework for robot-assisted healthcare applications. *Expert Systems with Applications, 241*, 122482. DOI: 10.1016/j.eswa.2023.122482

Shin, J. H., Lee, B., & Park, K. S. (2011). Detection of abnormal living patterns for Elderly living alone using support vector data description. *IEEE Transactions on Information Technology in Biomedicine, 15*(3), 438–448. DOI: 10.1109/TITB.2011.2113352 PMID: 21317086

Suryadevara, N. K., Gaddam, A., Mukhopadhyay, S. C., & Rayudu, R. K. (2011, November). Wellness determination of inhabitant based on daily activity behaviour in real-time monitoring using Sensor Networks. In Sensing Technology (ICST), 2011 Fifth International Conference on (pp. 474-481). IEEE. DOI: 10.1109/ICSensT.2011.6137025

Suryadevara, N. K., & Mukhopadhyay, S. C. (2011, September). Wireless sensors network based safe home to care Elderly people: A realistic approach. In *Recent Advances in Intelligent Computational Systems (RAICS), 2011 IEEE (pp. 001-005)*. IEEE. DOI: 10.1109/RAICS.2011.6069262

Suryadevara, N. K., & Mukhopadhyay, S. C. (2012). Wireless sensor network-based home monitoring system for wellness determination of Elderly. *IEEE Sensors Journal, 12*(6), 1965–1972. DOI: 10.1109/JSEN.2011.2182341

Suryadevara, N. K., Mukhopadhyay, S. C., & Rayudu, R. K. (2012, December). Applying SARIMA time series to forecast sleeping activity for wellness model of Elderly monitoring in smart home. In Sensing Technology (ICST), 2012 Sixth International Conference on (pp. 157-162). IEEE.

Suryadevara, N. K., Mukhopadhyay, S. C., Rayudu, R. K., & Huang, Y. M. (2012, May). Sensor data fusion to determine wellness of an Elderly in intelligent home monitoring environment. In Instrumentation and Measurement Technology Conference (I2MTC), 2012 IEEE International (pp. 947-952). IEEE. DOI: 10.1109/I2MTC.2012.6229645

Suryadevara, N. K., Mukhopadhyay, S. C., Wang, R., Rayudu, R. K., & Huang, Y. M. (2013, May). Reliable measurement of Wireless Sensor Network data for forecasting wellness of Elderly at smart home. In Instrumentation and Measurement Technology Conference (I2MTC), 2013 IEEE International (pp. 16-21). IEEE. DOI: 10.1109/I2MTC.2013.6555372

Suryadevara, N. K., Quazi, M. T., & Mukhopadhyay, S. C. (2012, June). Intelligent Sensing Systems for Measuring Wellness Indices of the Daily Activities for the Elderly. In Intelligent Environments (IE), 2012 8th International Conference on (pp. 347-350). IEEE. DOI: 10.1109/IE.2012.49

Tibor, B., Mark, H., Michel, C. A. K., & Jan, T. (2011). An ambient agent model for monitoring and analysing dynamics of complex Elderly behavior. *Journal of Ambient Intelligence and Smart Environments*, *3*(4), 283–303. DOI: 10.3233/AIS-2011-0117

Wolbring, G., & Leopatra, V. (2013). Sensors: Views of Staff of a Disability Service Organization. *Journal of Personalized Medicine*, *3*(1), 23–39. DOI: 10.3390/jpm3010023 PMID: 25562409

Yazici, A., Zhumabekova, D., Nurakhmetova, A., Yergaliyev, Z., Yatbaz, H. Y., Makisheva, Z., Lewis, M., & Ever, E. (2023). A smart e-health framework for monitoring the health of the elderly and disabled. *Internet of Things : Engineering Cyber Physical Human Systems*, *24*, 100971. DOI: 10.1016/j.iot.2023.100971

Zhou, Z., Dai, W., Eggert, J., Giger, J. T., Keller, J., Rantz, M., & He, Z. (2009, September). A real-time system for in-home activity monitoring of elders. In Engineering in Medicine and Biology Society, 2009. EMBC 2009. Annual International Conference of the IEEE (pp. 6115-6118). IEEE.

Chapter 10
Machine Unlearning Models for Medical Care and Health Data Privacy in Healthcare 6.0

Varun Kumar
https://orcid.org/0009-0002-2135-5276
Dure Technologies Private Limited, India

Dipanjan Sujit Roy
https://orcid.org/0000-0002-8847-5865
Dure Technologies Private Limited, India

ABSTRACT

The integration of advanced technologies in healthcare has undergone significant transformations throughout the 20th and 21st centuries, culminating in the era of Healthcare 6.0. This evolution in healthcare, particularly the integration of artificial intelligence, has necessitated the implementation of concepts like "Machine Unlearning". This is crucial for addressing critical issues like data privacy compliance, bias mitigation, and data security. By enabling the removal of specific data points from ML models, Machine Unlearning aligns with international data protection laws (HIPAA, GDPR, and DPDPA). Its application emphasizes regulations concerning the right to be forgotten, data minimization, and patient consent, which are essential for legal compliance and maintaining patient trust in healthcare. This chapter discusses Machine Unlearning approaches like Exact Unlearning and Approximate Unlearning, along with other advanced methods. Lastly, it discusses real-world case studies, and identifies the way forward for future development & research on 'Machine Unlearning in Healthcare'.

DOI: 10.4018/979-8-3693-7210-4.ch010

INTRODUCTION

Evolution and Overview of Healthcare 6.0

Combining management and healthcare delivery is seen as a critical strategy for improving service outcomes and the performance of health systems worldwide. Over the years, in accordance with the industrial progression, evolution of management sciences, and the adoption of technology across sectors, healthcare as a discipline has also seen tremendous development.

The transformation of healthcare management saw its first revolution in the mid-20th century, with Healthcare 1.0 (Chanchaichujit et al., 2019), which brought to light the emphasis on service efficiency and minimizing bureaucracy in healthcare. Advanced data-centric systems and concepts like telehealth were first discussed as measures to manage medications and treatment by clinicians, and automation was introduced in the form of administrative systems. However, the data remained siloed with individual health providers.

In the late 20th century, internet and technology became more accessible, and the users transformed from being customers of web resources to producers of information and content. This led to the production of more scientific research and evidence-based medicine. In this era of Healthcare 2.0 (Randeree, 2009), the delivery of services by healthcare institutions became more structured, and personal health records emerged as a tool to provide control and access to patients' data. The focus shifted to technological enablement for active engagement of patients in their treatment and better patient-provider relationships.

The next phase of development in the early 21st century focused on the concept of managed care and provisioning preventive care before the actual disease onset. In Healthcare 3.0 (Pillay, 2018, & Ristevski et al., 2018), technologies like big data analytics and wearables for early screening entered healthcare and brought preventive care in focus. Electronic Medical Records (EMR) became the means of making health services more individualistic and proactive.

In the first decade of the 21st century, healthcare started fully embracing digital technologies like telemedicine, mobile health apps, and remote sensing for treatment delivery beyond the premises of a health center. In Healthcare 4.0 (Gupta & Singh, 2023), the emphasis came on enhanced data collection and sharing capabilities, leading to interoperability and connected healthcare systems. By empowering patients with IoT (Internet of Things), Big Data analytics, and virtual care, this development made health systems more patient-centric, thus moving away from their traditional hospital-centric approach.

The second decade of the 21st century saw the next development to reach Healthcare 5.0, which integrated advanced technologies with the patient-centric approaches of the last phase. This phase has seen a wide adoption of AI tools, cloud computing, and 5G communications to support healthcare delivery. The extensive technological enablement in this era has supported healthcare services in becoming extremely customized to individual needs and preferences. It harnessed the intelligence of technologies for predictive modeling and decision support systems, moving towards precision medicine and tailoring treatment based on lifestyles and genetic determinants for each case.

In the 2020s, healthcare is now revolutionizing with the application of cutting-edge technologies like explainable AI, blockchain, and advanced machine learning towards Healthcare 6.0 (Aluvalu et al., 2024 & Reddy et al., 2024), that has given way to a holistic and human-centered approach to healthcare services. It is leveraging technology to prioritize patient outcomes over volume of service delivery, enhancing interoperability across global health systems, and emphasizing aspects like sustainability in the entire patient care continuum.

Healthcare 6.0 is a significant evolution from earlier healthcare models that were primarily focused on disease treatment to a more integrated system that emphasizes prevention, personalized care, and efficient management through digital transformation. Learning from breakthroughs in improving system efficiency in other industries and adopting modern technologies are essential components of this development, and they bear promise for better patient outcomes and streamlined operations.

Development is a natural course, but it is always coupled with challenges, and a successful acceptance of Healthcare 6.0 (Murdoch, 2021 & Yadav et al., 2023) would likewise need a pre-emptive identification of the associated limitations. With the quantum of data being generated and stored in large data repositories at present, data privacy is a prime concern. Developments like the application of AI in healthcare are still in question for the ability to safeguard critical patient identifiers and information from being misinterpreted and misused. As many of the AI technologies are owned by private entities, its implementation in healthcare would mean their larger involvement in obtaining and utilizing the healthcare data – both personal health information and personally identifiable information – thereby putting the data security at risk. Hence, while visualizing the strategies for Healthcare 6.0, remediation of the related ethical & legal challenges around data sharing, utilization, storage, and protection needs to be a major consideration, and the concept of "Machine Unlearning" offers great promise.

Significance of Machine Unlearning in Healthcare

Machine Learning (ML) technologies are revolutionizing all industries, and healthcare has also started to harness its power for generating analytical insights, diagnostic precision, treatment planning and other operations (Alanazi, 2022). Implementation of ML solutions like Microsoft's InnerEye Project (Microsoft, n.d.) are popular examples for revolutionizing medical imaging using 3D radiological images to detect tumors more precisely for NHS cancer patients in the UK. However, as ML involvement and reliance increase, likewise will be concerns about the ethical considerations of interacting with patient information, potential misuse of data, and the systems' commitment to ensuring data privacy. This is where the concept of "Machine Unlearning" becomes significant.

By implementing machine unlearning (Cao & Yang, 2015 & Ginart et al., 2019), ML systems can forget previously learned data points, allowing the systematic removal of specific data from the models. Effective machine unlearning performs this in a way that prevents the related training from being reconstructed or inferred from the models' behavior once the associated data is deleted.

With the sensitive nature of patient data, various regulations govern access, storage, and use of health information. Hence, it is critical for any technologies being used in healthcare to comply with these global and local data protection regulations, like the Health Insurance Portability and Accountability Act (HIPAA) in US (US Department of Health and Human Services, n.d.), the General Data Protection Regulation (GDPR) in Europe (Zhang et al., 2023), and country-specific ones like the Digital Personal Data Protection Act (DPDPA) in India (Sharma et al., 2024). These regulations support data minimization and mandate an individual's right to be forgotten through personal data removal from any information system. By checking that the learnings in technologies can be unlearned upon request, organizations and healthcare providers can enhance patient trust, maintain legal compliance, and ensure the integrity of the AI/ML-driven systems.

Training AI/ML-driven systems depend on legacy data, predictions, and other crowd-sourced resources. However, the operating mechanisms and nature of healthcare information evolve, and using redundant or out-of-context data points with a model can impact its intelligence and hamper the relevance of outputs thus produced. A classic case of such confounding bias is seen in the use of diagnostic imaging to screen for anomalies, which requires the use of newer data points for the models to be accurate (Dinsdale, 2021). By employing unlearning, this potential bias in AI/ML models can also be mitigated effectively, and we can ensure that the resultant outputs from the model are fair. By unlearning the potentially biased data points, healthcare providers can adapt their AI-supported systems and iteratively refine their models to be more equitable and just.

The most advanced systems and technology providers encounter data breaches and cyberattacks quite frequently, and unlearning can aid in building data security as well (Xu et al., 2024). When a healthcare institution suspects a data compromise, initiating the process of unlearning the malicious or corrupted data points can check the propagation of any impact of such incidents on the overall effectiveness of the related models.

Machine unlearning is substantial in applying AI/ML-based models in the healthcare sector by addressing critical data privacy, compliance, bias mitigation, and data security issues. At the same time, for the sustainable integration of ML technologies in healthcare, developing and adopting robust machine-learning methods to ensure these technologies are used responsibly and equitably is crucial.

Chapter Methodology and Approach

This chapter explores the existing literature on "Machine Unlearning Models for Medical Care and Health Data Privacy in Healthcare 6.0". It combines the authors' expertise in digital health technologies to synthesize knowledge on this subject. It primarily discusses the techniques, challenges and benefits of machine unlearning for advanced healthcare systems. Some of the research questions addressed in this chapter would include:

- How is machine unlearning relevant to healthcare?
- What are the techniques and challenges in using machine unlearning in healthcare?
- What are the benefits and possible impacts of machine unlearning on patient care delivery and data management in Healthcare 6.0?

The methodology of conducting the literature review while writing this chapter was to search academic databases like IEEE Xplore, PubMed, BMC, SpringerLink, Science Direct and Google Scholar, along with industry reports and blogs from health technology companies and research institutions. Search criteria were to use keywords "Machine Unlearning," "Machine Learning," "Healthcare 6.0", "Data privacy in Healthcare," "Patient data security," "Compliance," and "Artificial Intelligence in Health" with "AND," "OR" operators to combine search terms. All the included literature was attempted to be peer-reviewed, published in the last 10 years, focused on healthcare and written in English. Any literature not falling in this inclusion criteria was excluded from this exercise. The suitability and quality of the identified scientific papers was assessed manually based on the relevance of the content to our research questions.

It must be noted that the concept of "Machine Unlearning" and "Healthcare 6.0" is an evolving field. The availability of existing literature is a limitation, and the reliance on the author's experience with the subject can also potentially cause some bias.

SECTION 1: UNDERSTANDING MACHINE UNLEARNING

Definition and Fundamentals

The Stanford Artificial Intelligence Laboratory describes machine unlearning as "removing the influences of training data from a trained model" (Ken, 2024). Unlike the traditional machine learning concept, which is designed to learn and adapt from data continuously, machine unlearning focuses on deliberately erasing certain data points and, thus, the impact of that information without compromising the overall functionality of the model.

Thus, machine unlearning is a process associated with machine learning where specific data points or features are altered in a trained ML model, instead of conducting complete retraining. Unlearning is a crucial practice for privacy protection, ensuring that personal data can be deleted from models to align with regulations like the GDPR's "right to be forgotten". It even helps correct errors by removing inaccurate or outdated information used during training and mitigating bias by addressing data that may have led to unfair or biased outcomes (Bourtoule et al., 2019 & Shaik et al., 2023). The goal is to make the model forget the intelligence associated with the deleted training set, while maintaining its overall performance and accuracy.

In dynamic data environments like healthcare, data points like patients' medical histories, personal choices, and other information can change over time. At the same time, errors can occur during the data collection as well as processing, which can mislead the ML algorithms and impact performance. Applying machine unlearning is a significant step to mitigate these challenges, while being complaint to regulations, removing learning bias, and responding to data security.

It is of note that machine learning and machine unlearning, though related, serve distinct and complementary roles in the development and maintenance of AI/ML systems, an account of which has been discussed below (Figure 1):

Figure 1. Machine Learning and Unlearning

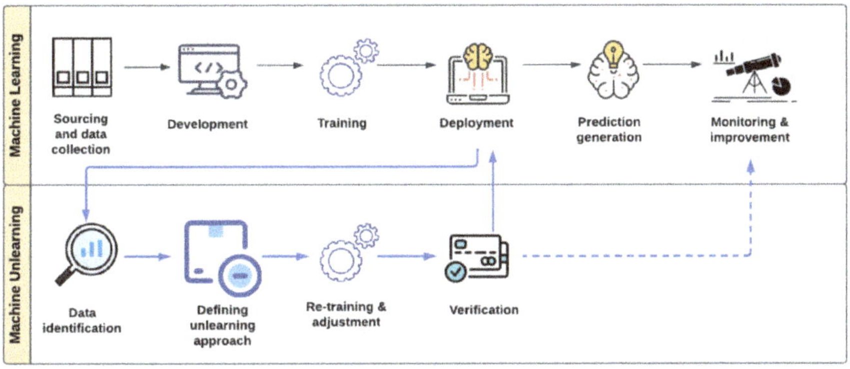

Machine learning: The foundation

Machine learning (El Naqa et al., 2015) is a branch of computational algorithms designed to mimic human intelligence by continuously learning from the surrounding environment. Machine learning (ML) techniques have been successfully applied in various fields like finance, entertainment, pattern recognition, climate predictions, computational biology and medicine. Particularly in healthcare, ML techniques aid significant operations like diagnosing diseases, predicting patient outcomes, and personalizing treatment plans. Machine learning can be broken down in the following steps (Good cloud, n.d. & Banafa, 2024):

1. ***Sourcing and data collection***: Aggregating relevant data to build a comprehensive training data set, cleaning and preprocessing to ensure quality and consistency.
2. ***Model development***: Development of the model using ML technologies, i.e., coding using suitable approaches.
3. ***Model training*** Using algorithms to learn from the data, evaluating outputs, and tuning parameters to improve accuracy with even unseen data.
4. ***Model deployment***: Implementing the trained model in real-world applications for practical use in an appropriate hosting environment.
5. ***Prediction generation***: Providing inputs to the developed ML model and getting predictions generated for each data instance.
6. ***Model monitoring and improvement***: Monitoring performance in predications, using running jobs and adding newer data points to continuously train the model.

Machine unlearning: The counterbalance

Contrary to machine learning, Machine Unlearning focuses on removing specific data points from a functional ML model to adjust its influence on the model. The steps involved in this process include (Eldan & Mark, 2023):

1. ***Data identification***: Identifying specific data points to be removed.
2. ***Define unlearning approach***: Choose an unlearning technique that ensures comprehensive coverage of the data points (anchors for removal) and the related translations.
3. ***Model retraining or adjustment***: The identified data are removed, and the model is re-trained/modified to adjust the effect of the removed data points.
4. ***Verification***: Ensuring the model no longer reflects the removed data in its predictions or performance.
5. ***Model monitoring***: Monitoring the model to identify new unlearning needs.

Machine learning and unlearning are complementary processes to develop and maintain robust AI systems. This interplay is crucial for the responsible deployment of AI, especially in sensitive sectors like healthcare. By understanding and implementing machine learning coupled with routine unlearning, healthcare providers and technologists can implement AI systems that are powerful, effective and adaptable to the dynamic world of technology.

Technical Mechanisms of Machine Unlearning

Machine unlearning is practiced using sophisticated algorithms and methodologies that ensure efficient removal of the selected data from ML models without compromising the overall performance. Two main technical approaches have been defined for machine unlearning (Xu et al., 2024 & Chundawat et al., 2023):

Exact unlearning

Exact unlearning is a strategy where the model is trained again after removing the selected data points from the training dataset. **Retraining from scratch, or the brute-force method**, is one of the most efficient approaches to unlearning, however, as the models are trained with significantly large datasets, it is computationally quite an expensive process. Also, the need for unlearning, i.e., requests to remove data points, can be a frequent process, and it would not be feasible to train the model again entirely every time. Research efforts have led to developing a more sophisticated exact unlearning approach, called **data sharding, or SISA** (Sharding,

Isolation, Slicing, and Aggregation) framework, where the targeted data is removed without full retraining. This involves splitting the training data into multiple disjoint shards, each treated as a sub-model. Using this approach, only the shards affected by a data point would need to be retrained, thus bringing down the computational expenses to a great extent.

Even the application of data sharding increases the storage requirements for the sub-models and the assessment of each data point's influence. Repeated retraining and aggregation can also degrade the model's generation capabilities. Thus, researchers have also developed further adaptations and improvements of the SISA framework for specific AI/ML model use cases.

Approximate unlearning

Approximate unlearning aims to approximate the parameters that would have been obtained if the model was trained without the target data points, thus minimizing the impact of those data points to acceptable levels.

The **influence functions** approach of approximate unlearning starts with computing the influence of target data points, followed by adjusting the model parameters to remove the influence and adding noise (called differential privacy method) to prevent the removed data from interfering with the model's intelligence. Lastly, the updated model is validated by evaluating performance and accuracy. It provides a practical alternative to the formerly discussed exact unlearning method, especially for use cases where computational and storage cost and model flexibility are crucial factors.

There are several other sophisticated methods to perform approximate unlearning for ML models. The **gradient updates** method makes small adjustments to the model parameters after incrementally removing the data points. Leveraging the gradients used in training, the adjustments are done in the opposite direction of the gradients contributed by the data points to be unlearned.

Knowledge distillation is another technique of approximate unlearning that uses a two-step forgetting process of retroactive interference and passive decay. To perform this, knowledge is transferred from a large model to train the target model for forgetting specific data by minimizing its dependency on that data through a controlled distillation process. This technique is particularly useful with models working on knowledge graphs.

Statistical methods like **Sliced inverse regression** (SIR) are also being explored for implementation in machine learning for diagnostic image processing (Li et al., 2024). The potential use of SIR relates to its high efficacy in dimension reduction for pattern analysis and hence managing redundancy, however the computational complexity with high-dimensional data remains as a critical limitation (Xu et al., 2017).

Researchers working on AI/ML have defined a wide range of other approximate unlearning techniques that combine the above methods with specialized techniques to make the overall method more suited for certain kinds of data systems.

Use cases of unlearning application

1. ***Text data models***:
    - *Personal Data Removal*: For natural language processing (NLP) applications, such as chatbots or email filters, unlearning helps remove personal data upon user request. For example, if a user desires to delete the conversation history from a disease chatbot, the model forgets these specific data points to maintain privacy and comply with regulations.
    - *Bias Mitigation*: Text-based ML models, such as sentiment analysis tools or language models, can develop bias from their training data. To improve model performance, unlearning biased phrases or sentences maintains more fair and unbiased models.
2. ***Image data models***:
    - *Facial Recognition*: For facial recognition systems in a hospital, patients or staff may request the removal of their images from the database. Unlearning these images ensures that the system no longer recognizes or identifies the removed individuals, addressing privacy concerns and protecting their 'right to be forgotten'.
    - *Medical Imaging*: In diagnostics, unlearning specific patient images from the AI/ML models helps maintain patient privacy and builds the model's efficiency. For instance, when the equipment is undergoing upgrade, historical data points are reviewed, and irrelevant sets are removed to ensure the relevance of the model in analyzing diagnostic images to identify abnormalities. Similarly, if a patient withdraws consent for their images to be used in training a diagnostic tool, they are unlearned from the AI/ML models.
3. ***Audio data models***:
    - *Voice Assistants*: Voice Assistance is becoming popular for disabled and elderly care. Users of such voice-activated assistants can request the deletion of their voice recordings. Machine unlearning ensures that these recordings are removed from the model's training dataset and the parameters are adjusted accordingly.
4. ***Behavioral data models***:
    - *Recommender Systems*: In apps supporting PHR (personal health records) access and telemedicine, AI is often implemented to improve a user's experience by recommending services based on previous inter-

actions. Users may request that this interaction data be removed and unlearning it would ensure their previous interactions do not influence future recommendations, thus enhancing data privacy and control.

- *Ad Targeting*: AI algorithms on social media and eCommerce platforms often present healthcare-specific ad targeting systems based on a user's demographics and content consumption. Unlearning can remove specific users' data to ensure they no longer receive these personalized ads based on their past behavior or any other personal particulars.

SECTION 2: MACHINE UNLEARNING IN MEDICAL CARE

Implementation in Medical Diagnostics and Treatment

Implementing machine learning (ML) in medical diagnostics and treatment has been transformative, leading to more accurate diagnoses, the generation of personalized treatment plans, and improved patient outcomes. However, the dynamic nature of medical data makes it necessary to integrate mechanisms for managing and updating the information used to train these models. As an example, any information datasets before 2021 would not be able to identify vaccination as a measure for malaria prevention. Hence, after the introduction of the malaria vaccine, the older models would need unlearning and retraining to calibrate their decision outputs. Hence, machine unlearning, which involves the systematic removal of specific data points from ML models, is crucial to ensure that the artificial intelligence offered by these systems remains accurate, reliable, and ethical. This section will explore the importance of removing obsolete or incorrect data from use cases of ML implementation for healthcare and how unlearning can enhance the accuracy and reliability of the insights thus generated.

Removing obsolete or incorrect data from diagnostic models

As medical science progresses, previously accepted knowledge can become outdated. Diagnostic models trained on older data would base their predictions on obsolete learnings, potentially leading to inaccurate diagnoses and suboptimal treatment plans. For example, early data on COVID-19 included many uncertainties, including the initial misconceptions about the virus's spread, symptoms, and treatment. As understanding of the virus has grown, models need to unlearn this outdated information to provide accurate and current recommendations on disease diagnosis based on clinical symptoms and laboratory test indications.

Errors in diagnostics data can arise from various sources, including manual data entry mistakes, misdiagnoses, and faulty measurements. These errors can also significantly degrade the performance of diagnostic models. By employing machine unlearning, technologists can identify and remove erroneous data points, thereby improving the overall quality of the dataset.

Machine unlearning can also contribute to the optimization of clinical workflows. In hospitals and medical research centers, quickly updating and refining diagnostic and treatment models can effectively streamline the decision-making process. This would ensure that healthcare professionals have access to the most accurate and current information, enabling them to make informed decisions swiftly. Consequently, this can reduce the time required for disease diagnosis and treatment planning, allowing for more efficient patient care and management.

The most practical application of unlearning for diagnostic models is in Radiology. ML models in radiology often rely on extensive datasets of medical images. As imaging techniques and diagnostic criteria evolve, older images may no longer be a relevant representation of the precise pathological condition. Unlearning these outdated images helps ensure that radiology models provide accurate diagnostic support based on the latest standards. Likewise, any errors in patients' electronic health records can propagate to the diagnostic ML models too, and lead to incorrect predictions. As an example, incorrect import of patient data of births while migrating to a new EHR system in a hospital can completely corrupt the outcomes being generated by an associated diagnostic model, and unlearning techniques would allow healthcare providers to continuously refine their models by removing such identified errors in data, thus enhancing diagnostic accuracy.

Enhancing the accuracy and reliability of healthcare insights

Accurate diagnostic insights are paramount in healthcare, significantly influencing treatment decisions and patient outcomes. By training the models on most current and accurate datasets, healthcare providers can offer more precise treatment support. Newly implemented diagnostic models can be especially subject to underperforming for certain population groups who are underrepresented in the legacy data used for training. Thus, after implementation, a regular process of unlearning and retraining for ML models can enable equitable and just healthcare outcomes for everyone in real-life settings.

With the consistently advancing knowledge of the health determinants and the increased participation of patients in driving their treatment, physicians have started curating personalized treatment plans to match specific patients' needs. These personalized treatment plans rely heavily on accurate patient data. Any incorrect or outdated information can lead to inappropriate treatment recommendations, adversely affecting patient care and, thus, the treatment outcomes. Machine unlearning ensures ML models base their recommendations on the most current and accurate data, leading to more effective and personalized treatment plans. For instance, in oncology, personalized treatment strategies based on genetic information and patient history can be refined by unlearning outdated or incorrect data, resulting in more targeted and effective therapies.

The application of unlearning in pharmacogenomics and chronic disease management is the most relevant example of using unlearning to optimize healthcare insights. Forgetting outdated genetic associations can lead to more precise drug recommendations and dosages, enhancing patient safety and treatment efficacy. Especially for chronic diseases such as diabetes or hypertension, unlearning a particular patient's outdated data (e.g., old blood pressure readings or glucose levels) helps remove its impact on clinical decisions and provide up-to-date and accurate management plans, leading to better long-term outcomes.

Case Studies from the Industry

Microsoft's InnerEye project

Microsoft's InnerEye project (Tkachenko, 2023 & Bernhardt et al., 2022) has been a pioneering example of implementing machine learning in healthcare, specifically in medical imaging. The project was initially assumed to focus on the segmentation of 3D radiological images to distinguish between healthy tissues and tumors. Over time, the InnerEye project integrated machine unlearning to continually refine its models by removing outdated or incorrect data segments. This approach has improved the accuracy of tumor detection, advice on related treatment plans, and patient outcomes in radiological diagnostics for institutions like the NHS Cambridge University Hospitals in the UK.

IBM Watson Oncology

IBM's Watson Oncology (Zou et al., 2020 & Park et al., 2023) is a popular technology that uses machine learning to provide personalized treatment options by analyzing patient histories and medical literature. This tool is an artificial intelligence-based decision support system that looks at patient data to provide treatment recommendations based on the local protocols and literature it is trained with, hence improving the work efficiency of the treating oncologists. Incorporating machine unlearning in this solution has enabled the system developers to remove obsolete treatment protocols and incorporate the latest medical research literature. This dynamic updating process has been crucial in ensuring that oncologists receive the most current and effective treatment recommendations, enhancing the overall quality of patient care delivered at the implementation sites like the Gachon University Gil Medical Center in South Korea and Second Xiangya Hospital in China.

Real-World Data in Rheumatology Research

An interesting application of machine learning and unlearning is evident in rheumatology research (Knevel & Liao, 2022). Researchers from the UK and US have used actual electronic health record (EHR) data to study the progression and treatment of rheumatic diseases using artificial intelligence. Using machine learning models has made it feasible to study patterns in legacy health records of patients at a large scale, which is aiding in identifying the potential factors for causing the disease and at the same time, is allowing researchers to leverage observational data on confounding factors, that bears a promise for development of relevant population-level interventions. By continuously updating the EHR datasets used in ML models through machine unlearning, researchers have removed inaccurate data entries and outdated patient information, leading to more accurate phenotyping and disease characterization. This has facilitated the identification of new disease patterns and comorbidities previously overlooked in structured clinical trials.

One of the primary benefits of machine unlearning in healthcare is enhancing patient safety. By continuously updating medical models and removing erroneous data, the risk of incorrect diagnoses and inappropriate treatments is minimized. This case is also a great example of how the use of up-to-date EHR data can accurately identify disease patterns, reducing the likelihood of misdiagnosis and ensuring that patients receive appropriate care based on the latest medical knowledge.

SECTION 3: HEALTH DATA PRIVACY CHALLENGES AND SOLUTIONS

Data Privacy Issues in Healthcare

Healthcare is a highly data-intensive industry, regularly producing large amounts of sensitive information. The patient records generated by healthcare operations contain two types of critical data, i.e., Protected Health Information (PHI) and Personally Identifiable Information (PII), that can be captured in electronic health records (EHRs), medical images, diagnostic reports, genomic analysis, and patient histories. This extensive data output exposes the healthcare systems to significant privacy risks, which, if not adequately addressed, can cause severe consequences.

Data privacy issues in healthcare settings are numerous and complex. Key concerns include data breaches, where healthcare organizations are frequent targets of cyberattacks, leading to a compromised protection of identifiable patient information. The increasing use of mobile devices by healthcare professionals can also put patient data at risk if proper security measures are not in place. Unauthorized access by healthcare staff, medical identity theft, tracking technologies, and third-party data sharing without patients' knowledge or consent further compromise patient privacy. Additionally, ensuring compliance with healthcare regulations like HIPAA requires strict data protection measures and continuous personnel training. Human error, such as misplacing records or sending information to the wrong recipient, can also violate data privacy. These issues highlight the need for robust data protection strategies and continuous vigilance in healthcare settings.

Types of data and associated risks

1. ***Electronic Health Records (EHRs):*** EHRs contain comprehensive data of an individual's encounters with the health system, including medical histories, diagnoses, treatment plans, and test results. Unauthorized access to EHRs can lead to identity thefts, as these records often include PII like national identity numbers, addresses, phone numbers, and insurance details. Breaches associated with PHI can expose sensitive health information, leading to discrimination and stigmatization of patients.
2. ***Genomic data:*** DNA sequencing and genome analysis are popular diagnostic procedures nowadays, and it is increasingly conducted for personalized medicine and research. The unique attributes of genomic data make it inherently identifiable, raising concerns about privacy and potential misuse. Data breaches involving genomic information can lead to severe privacy violations and situations like genetic discrimination in employment and insurance.
3. ***Medical imaging and IoT devices***: Medical imaging data and information generated by Internet of Things (IoT) devices, such as wearable health monitors, contribute extensively to the growing throughput of healthcare data. These devices often transmit data wirelessly, creating potential interception and unauthorized access vulnerabilities. Breaches involving these data types can reveal intimate details about a person's health status, lifestyle, and habits.
4. ***Health information exchanges (HIEs)***: HIEs facilitate sharing of health information across different platforms, programs, and healthcare organizations. While this is crucial to improve the continuity of care, it also introduces additional vulnerability for the data thus exchanged. Unauthorized access in HIEs

can compromise considerably large amounts of sensitive data, simultaneously affecting multiple entities and patients.

Consequences of data breach

One of the most common consequences of data breaches in health information systems is identity theft. The misuse of this data can range from issues like unauthorized use for commercial purposes to even severe ones like the creation of fraudulent medical records, filing false insurance claims, accessing financial accounts, and causing significant harm to victims.

Leakage of sensitive health information like disease status, treatment particulars, and prescriptions can lead to discrimination and stigmatization for the related patients. For example, breaches revealing mental health records, HIV status, or genetic predispositions can lead to social stigmatization and discrimination in various settings, including workplaces and schools.

Any patient-provider interaction has a critical role of trust, and it is a cornerstone of the healthcare delivery process, or rather the overall patient-provider relationship. Breach of the data captured during the healthcare delivery process will compromise this trust, making patients hesitant to share vital information with healthcare providers. Such reluctance can negatively impact the quality of care, as providers may not have all the necessary information to make informed decisions. Furthermore, it not only influences the current patients, but also the future trust of the community in that institution.

Regulatory Frameworks and Compliance

Global regulatory frameworks and local legislations set stringent data privacy and protection standards to mitigate the risks associated with data breaches and ensure the safe handling of healthcare data. A few significant global regulations around personal health data and the role of unlearning in ensuring compliance have been discussed in this section.

Regulations around patient data

General Data Protection Regulation (GDPR)

GDPR (Gdpr.eu, n.d.) is a comprehensive data protection regulation implemented by the European Union (EU). It is applicable to any organization that processes the personal data of EU residents, regardless of where the organization is based. It mandates strict requirements for data consent, access, and the right to be forgotten, ensuring that individuals have significant control over their personal data. Non-compliance can result in substantial fines, making it crucial for healthcare organizations and their technology providers to adhere to GDPR standards.

Health Insurance Portability and Accountability Act (HIPAA)

In the United States, HIPAA (Edemekong et al., 2024) sets the standard for protecting sensitive patient data. It requires healthcare providers, insurers, and their business associates to implement administrative, physical, and technical safeguards to ensure the confidentiality, integrity, and availability of PHI. HIPAA also mandates breach notification requirements, ensuring that affected individuals are informed promptly in the event of a data breach.

Data Protection and Data Privacy Act (DPDPA)

Apart from the global regulations discussed above, there are context-specific local regulations, laws, and compliance requirements for working with healthcare data. One such example is DPDPA from India (Ministry of law and justice, 2023), that governs the privacy and protection of individual data in digital systems, including healthcare as well. These regulations complement broader frameworks like GDPR and HIPAA, providing additional protections specific to the country. The DPDPA outlines stringent data handling and breach notification requirements, enhancing the overall security of health data.

Other than these specific regulations on an individual's data, health systems are also surrounded by considerations of human rights, medical ethics, patient safety standards, and industry norms, all of which reinforces the need to confidentially maintaining health records and protect patients' from all kinds of compromise and bias.

In order to implement new technologies in healthcare settings, systems are frequently required to complete a Healthcare Technology Assessment (WHO, n.d.), which is a systematic evaluation to check the direct and indirect consequences of implementing these tools in the local context, and it would mandatorily inspect the capability of assessed technologies to ensure adherence to the required data privacy regulations. As a popular example, **Digital Technology Assessment Criteria (DTAC)** is one such provision in the UK (NHS England, n.d.), that sets the baseline criteria for suppliers at the time of procurement to regulate data protection, clinical safety, technical security, interoperability, usability and accessibility of the technologies solutions and serves as a check before any new systems are available to be used in Public health and Social care in the United Kingdom.

Machine unlearning and compliance

Machine unlearning, a technique for removing specific data points from machine learning models, is helping healthcare organizations and technologists in being compliant with the stringent regulations around data privacy, while working with patient data.

GDPR and HIPAA advocate the provision to allow individual's decision to remove their personal data. In accordance with the workflows built in the software, Machine unlearning facilitates this data administration by enabling the removal of specific data points from machine learning models, thus erasing an individual's data when requested. This ability is critical for any ML tools to be legally compliant and protect patient rights.

ML models can inadvertently perpetuate biases present in the training data. Machine unlearning allows healthcare organizations to identify and remove biased data points, keeping the risk of biased outcomes in check. This is particularly important for complying with regulations prohibiting discrimination and requiring equitable treatment for all patients.

Even after implementing unlearning techniques on ML models, validating the integrity and performance is crucial. Continuous monitoring and validation are essential to ensure that the models are consistently compliant to regulations and continue to deliver high-quality insights. Compliance with the regulations is also subject to audits, which is why healthcare organizations need to document their compliance efforts, including the steps taken to implement machine unlearning as well. Such documentation is essential for demonstrating compliance to regulatory authorities and can also serve as a reference for future audits and inspections.

SECTION 4: INTEGRATING MACHINE UNLEARNING INTO HEALTHCARE 6.0

Technical Integration Strategies

Healthcare 6.0 represents a transformative shift from the traditional models focused on disease treatment to a more integrated system that emphasizes prevention, personalized care, and digital transformation. Integrating machine unlearning into this framework involves several key steps to protect sensitive data while maintaining effective healthcare operations.

Identifying sensitive data

The first step in integrating machine unlearning into healthcare systems is identifying data that require the most protection. In the context of healthcare, these data points would be:

- Protected Health Information (PHI): Comprehensive patient data such as medical histories, allergies, diagnosis, treatment plans, prescriptions, and immunization records.
- Personally Identifiable Information (PII): Data that can identify individuals, including names, addresses, national identification numbers, insurance details, etc
- Genomic Data: Genetic information that can reveal an individual's identity and predisposition to various diseases.
- Medical Imaging Data: Data from X-rays, MRIs, and other imaging modalities that contain detailed personal health information.
- Laboratory records: Information on the laboratory tests done on the individual for disease diagnostics or otherwise.

Advanced healthcare data classifications like HL7 and auditing tools can help accurately identify and categorize this sensitive information. Machine learning techniques, including natural language processing (NLP) and computer vision, can be instrumental in automating the identification of sensitive data present in unstructured formats, such as clinical notes and medical images.

Implementing unlearning algorithms

Once sensitive data has been identified and fed to the ML model, the next step is implementing machine unlearning algorithms. These algorithms must effectively remove specific data points from machine learning models as required, without compromising their overall performance and integrity. Routine checks and monitoring mechanisms are key practices to address this.

Defining, monitoring and regularly evaluating performance metrics such as accuracy, precision, and recall can help keep the model's performance after unlearning in check. It must also be validated that employing unlearning does not introduce or increase the impact of any training bias in the outputs being generated by a model. Examining the predictions for different demographic groups to spot irrelevant outputs can detect and mitigate such disparities. Finally, maintaining detailed logs of all unlearning activities, including removed data points and model adjustments, is critical. These logs are essential for regulatory compliance, and at the same time, they can help backtrack and investigate any issues that might arise.

Addressing challenges

As discussed in the previous sections, ML has already started transforming healthcare as a sector. However, concepts like unlearning are yet to be picked up exhaustively in this industry, and their application would face several challenges. These limitations need to be addressed properly to ensure the seamless integration of machine unlearning into healthcare systems:

- Computational Complexity: The unlearning process can be computationally intensive, especially for large datasets and complex models. Right approach to perform unlearning should be identified for the model based on required strengths and tolerance to limitations. For example, techniques such as SISA aid in distributed computing and hardware acceleration to mitigate computational challenges.
- Data Dependency: Machine learning models often rely on interdependencies between data points. Unlearning specific data points without considering these dependencies can lead to unintended consequences and potentially corrupt the model altogether. Identifying such correlations and using advanced algorithms that account for these dependencies is necessary to ensure robust unlearning.
- Scalability: Healthcare systems often handle vast amounts of data. Ensuring unlearning algorithms that can handle these high volumes is critical. This requires optimizing algorithms for efficiency and leveraging cloud-based solutions to manage scalability challenges.

Advancements and Innovation

Emerging technologies (ProtonsHub, n.d.; Craig, 2024 & IBM, n.d.) such as federated learning, homomorphic encryption, retrieval augmentation, and blockchain technology can enhance machine unlearning capabilities, driving Healthcare 6.0 towards more secure and efficient patient data management in 2025 and ahead.

Federated learning

Federated learning is an innovative approach enabling multiple institutions to train machine learning models collaboratively without sharing raw data. This method involves training models locally on each institution's data and then aggregating the model updates to create a global model. Key benefits would include:

- Enhanced Privacy: By controlling the raw data's movement outside the institution, federated learning significantly reduces the risk of data breaches. This is particularly important in healthcare, where data privacy is paramount. It ensures that sensitive patient data remains within the institution's confines, thereby enhancing data privacy and protection.
- Compliance with Regulations: Federated learning is readily aligned with the regulations under GDPR and HIPAA, that impose strict data sharing and processing requirements. By keeping data local, federated learning helps institutions comply with these stringent regulations, ensuring legal and ethical data management practices.
- Improved Model Performance: Federated learning can produce more robust and generalizable models by leveraging data from multiple institutions, leading to better healthcare insights and outcomes. This collaborative approach ensures that models benefit from more data, improving their predictive accuracy and reliability.

Homomorphic encryption

Homomorphic encryption (IBM, n.d.) is a cryptographic technique that allows computations on encrypted data without decrypting it first. This capability can revolutionize data privacy and security in healthcare by enabling:

- Secure Data Processing: Sensitive healthcare data can be encrypted before being processed by machine learning models, ensuring data privacy is maintained throughout the computation process. Homomorphic encryption ensures that data remains secure, even during processing, mitigating the risk of data breaches.
- Protection Against Breaches: Even if data is intercepted during processing, homomorphic encryption ensures intercepted data remains unintelligible to unauthorized parties. This high level of security ensures that sensitive patient information always remains protected.
- Regulatory Compliance: Homomorphic encryption can help healthcare organizations comply with data privacy regulations by providing a robust mech-

anism for securing sensitive data during processing. This technique ensures protection through all stages of a record's lifecycle, starting from collection, and then in processing and storage.

Retrieval augmentation

Retrieval augmentation (Craig, 2024) is a technique that enhances the performance of ML models by incorporating relevant information from external sources during the training process. This method involves querying external databases, knowledge graphs, or other information repositories to gather additional context that can inform and improve model predictions. An integration of this in re-training after exact unlearning can produce significantly enhanced models by introducing:

- Enhanced Accuracy: By providing models with relevant external information, retrieval augmentation can significantly improve the accuracy and relevance of predictions after unlearning. This is particularly beneficial in natural language processing tasks, where context is crucial.
- Efficiency in Learning: Retrieval augmentation allows models to access a vast amount of external knowledge without needing to store or process all the information during training. This leads to more efficient learning and reduces the computational burden on the model.
- Compliance with Data Regulations: Since retrieval augmentation can use publicly available or pre-approved external sources, it helps maintain regulatory compliances like GDPR and HIPAA, ensuring that sensitive data is not unnecessarily exposed or processed during the process of unlearning and retraining.

Blockchain technology

Blockchain technology offers a decentralized and tamper-proof way to record data transactions. In the context of machine unlearning and healthcare, blockchain can provide:

- Auditability: Each unlearning action can be recorded on the blockchain, creating a comprehensive audit trail that enhances transparency and accountability. Blockchain technology ensures that every unlearning action is recorded and cannot be altered, providing a clear and transparent record of data management activities.
- Data Integrity: Blockchain ensures data integrity by preventing unauthorized modifications. This is a potent measure to maintain patient trust in healthcare

data and ensuring accurate unlearning processes. The immutable nature of blockchain ensures that once data is recorded, it cannot be changed, enhancing the reliability of healthcare records.

- Interoperability: Blockchain can facilitate secure data sharing across different healthcare institutions, promoting collaboration while maintaining data privacy and security. It can enable seamless and safe data sharing, enhancing collaboration and data integration across the healthcare ecosystem.

Other future innovations

Several emerging innovations have the potential to advance the integration of machine unlearning into healthcare further (Emerging trends, n.d.). Technologies like **quantum computing** could provide the computational power needed to perform complex unlearning tasks more efficiently, potentially overcoming current limitations related to computational complexity. It can handle vast amounts of data and complex calculations at considerable efficiency, making it an ideal solution for the intensive computational needs of machine unlearning and allowing real-time application of unlearning and re-training.

Developing more **explainable AI** models can help healthcare professionals understand the impact of unlearning on model predictions, enhancing trust and adoption of unlearning techniques. Explainable AI ensures that the decision-making processes of AI models are transparent and understandable, fostering trust and confidence in AI-driven healthcare solutions.

Establishing **ethical frameworks** for AI and machine unlearning can ensure that these technologies are used responsibly, and that patients' rights and privacy are protected. Ethical AI frameworks guide the responsible use of AI, ensuring prioritization of patient rights and privacy throughout the AI lifecycle.

Considering the use of **ensemble models** that combine more than one model in one solution can also be the strategy to overcome the shortcomings of individual models. Implementing a combination of sophisticated models can aid in managing the breadth of learning in a more systematic manner, thus improving the accuracy of predictions and at the same time, improve the efficiency of the models to unlearn and be retrained, as needed (Murel & Kavlakoglu, 2024).

By embracing these innovations, healthcare organizations can build a more secure, transparent, and trustworthy environment for managing sensitive patient data while leveraging the transformational benefits of AI and ML.

Way forward

Machine unlearning offers the avenues to facilitate the dynamic nature of healthcare data management. As new data is continuously generated and old data becomes obsolete, the ability to selectively remove outdated or incorrect information without compromising the integrity of the AI models is invaluable. This ensures that healthcare providers can maintain up-to-date and accurate patient records, ultimately leading to better patient outcomes and more efficient healthcare delivery. Integrating machine unlearning into healthcare systems represents a significant advancement in pursuing a secure, patient-centric, and technologically advanced healthcare environment.

Prospects and Implications

The future of healthcare will be driven by advanced technologies and hence increasingly rely on advanced data management techniques like machine unlearning. Continued research and development in this field will be essential for realizing the full potential of Healthcare 6.0 and ensuring that it remains secure, efficient, and patient-centric.

Enhanced Security and Privacy

As machine unlearning technology advances, its capabilities to provide enhanced security and privacy protections will become even more significant. Leapfrogging the current limitations of unlearning approaches, future innovation around machine unlearning is promising and would include more sophisticated algorithms that can handle larger datasets and more complex models. This would further improve the ability of ML models to unlearn sensitive information and manage the increasing volume of healthcare data, thus ensuring that patient information remains secure.

Improved Patient Outcomes

Machine unlearning can also contribute to improved patient outcomes by checking that healthcare model predictions are based on accurate and relevant data. By removing outdated or incorrect information, machine unlearning helps maintain the accuracy and reliability of diagnostic models, leading to better healthcare insights and more effective treatments. This capability is particularly important as healthcare systems increasingly rely on AI and machine learning to support clinical decision-making.

Regulatory Compliance and Ethical AI

The integration of machine unlearning into healthcare systems will play a crucial role in ensuring regulatory compliance and promoting ethical AI practices. By introducing measures to erase sensitive information from AI models, machine unlearning helps healthcare organizations comply with data privacy regulations and uphold ethical standards. This will be increasingly important as regulatory frameworks continue to evolve, and as public scrutiny of AI and data privacy issues intensifies.

Technological Innovations

Emerging technologies such as federated learning, homomorphic encryption, and blockchain hold great promise for enhancing machine unlearning capabilities. These innovations provide more secure and efficient ways to manage and protect patient data, ultimately leading to improved clinical outcomes and patient safety. For example, federated learning enables multiple institutions to collaboratively train machine learning models without sharing raw data, enhancing privacy and compliance with data protection regulations. Meanwhile, homomorphic encryption allows computations to be performed on encrypted data, providing robust security for sensitive information. Blockchain technology offers a decentralized and tamper-proof way to record data transactions, ensuring the integrity and transparency of unlearning processes.

Collaboration and Interoperability

The future of machine unlearning in healthcare will also depend on collaboration and interoperability among healthcare institutions. By working together and sharing best practices, healthcare providers, technologists, and researchers can develop more effective unlearning techniques and ensure that these methods are implemented consistently across the industry. Interoperability will be key to seamless data sharing and integration, allowing healthcare systems to benefit from multiple organizations' collective knowledge and expertise while maintaining data privacy and security.

CONCLUSION

This chapter highlights the critical role of machine unlearning in enhancing data privacy and patient care within the context of Healthcare 6.0. With healthcare evolving into a more integrated and digital system, the need to protect patient data and comply with stringent regulations is becoming more critical. Machine unlearning emerges as a vital technology in this landscape, offering robust solutions to erase sensitive information from AI models effectively. This capability is essential for meeting regulatory requirements such as GDPR and HIPAA, which demand stringent data protection and protect the patient's right over the use of their data.

Moreover, the adoption of machine unlearning is crucial for maintaining patient's trust on health institutions. Patients are more likely to engage with healthcare systems that prioritize their privacy and ensure the security of their personal information. By incorporating machine unlearning, healthcare providers can demonstrate their commitment to protecting patient data, thereby fostering a trustworthy relationship with their patients. This trust is foundational for effective patient care, as it encourages patients to share accurate and comprehensive health information, which is essential for accurate diagnosis and treatment.

In conclusion, integrating machine unlearning in Healthcare 6.0 is essential for enhancing data privacy, regulatory compliance, and patient care. By embracing newer innovations like machine unlearning, healthcare organizations can build a more secure, transparent, and trustworthy environment for managing sensitive patient data, enabling better patient outcomes and more efficient healthcare operations. Continued research and development in this field will be essential for realizing the full potential of Healthcare 6.0, ensuring that it remains at the forefront of technological innovation and patient-centered care.

REFERENCES

Alanazi, A. (2022). Using machine learning for healthcare challenges and opportunities. Informatics in Medicine Unlocked. *Elsevier*. .DOI: 10.1016/j.imu.2022.100924

Aluvalu, R., Devi, V. S., Kumar, C. N., Goutham, N., & Nikitha, K. (2024). Unveil the Black-Box Model for Healthcare Explainable AI. In Aluvalu, R., Mehta, M., & Siarry, P. (Eds.), *Explainable AI in Health Informatics. Computational Intelligence Methods and Applications*. Springer., DOI: 10.1007/978-981-97-3705-5_3

Banafa, A. (2024). *Introduction to Artificial Intelligence*. River Publishers.

Bernhardt, M., Coelho de Castro, D., Tanno, R., Schwaighofer, A., Tezcan, K. C., Monteiro, M., Bannur, S., Lungren, M. P., Nori, A., Glocker, B., Alvarez-Valle, J., & Oktay, O. (2022). Active label cleaning for improved dataset quality under resource constraints. Microsoft Research. *Nature Communications*, *13*(1161), 1–11. https://www.microsoft.com/en-us/research/publication/active-label-cleaning-improving-dataset-quality-under-resource-constraints/

. Bourtoule, L., Chandrasekaran, V., Choquette-Choo, A., Jia, H., Travers, A., Zhang, B., Lie, D., & Papernot, N. (2019). Machine Unlearning. *ArXiv*. /abs/1912.03817.

Cao, Y., & Yang, J. (2015). Towards making systems forget with machine unlearning. *IEEE Symposium on Security and Privacy.*https://www.ieee-security.org/TC/SP2015/papers-archived/6949a463.pdf

Chanchaichujit, J., Tan, A., Meng, F., & Eaimkhong, S. (2019). An introduction to Healthcare 4.0. In *Healthcare 4.0* (pp. 1–15). Springer. DOI: 10.1007/978-981-13-8114-0_1

Chundawat, V. S., Tarun, A. K., Mandal, M., & Kankanhalli, M. (2023). *Zero-Shot Machine Unlearning*. IEEE., DOI: 10.1109/TIFS.2023.3265506

Craig, L. (2024). 10 top AI and machine learning trends for 2024. *TechTarget*. https://www.techtarget.com/searchenterpriseai/tip/9-top-AI-and-machine-learning-trends

Dinsdale, N. K., Jenkinson, M., & Namburete, A. I. (2021). Deep learning-based unlearning of dataset bias for MRI harmonisation and confound removal. *NeuroImage*, *228*, 117689.

Edemekong, P. F., Annamaraju, P., & Haydel, M. J. (2024). Health Insurance Portability and Accountability Act. In *StatPearls* [Internet]. StatPearls Publishing., https://www.ncbi.nlm.nih.gov/books/NBK500019/

El Naqa, I., & Murphy, M. J. (2015). What Is Machine Learning? In El Naqa, I., Li, R., & Murphy, M. J. (Eds.), *Machine Learning in Radiation Oncology*. Springer., DOI: 10.1007/978-3-319-18305-3_1

Eldan, R., & Mark, R. (2023). Who's Harry Potter? Approximate Unlearning in LLMs. *ArXiv*. DOI:/arXiv.2310.02238.DOI: 10.48550

Ginart, A., Guan, M. Y., Valiant, G., & Zou, J. (2019). Making AI Forget You: Data Deletion in Machine Learning. *Advances in Neural Information Processing Systems (NeurIPS)*. https://papers.nips.cc/paper/8611-making-ai-forget-you-data-deletion-in-machine-learning

Gupta, A., & Singh, A. (2023). Healthcare 4.0: Recent advancements and futuristic research directions. *Wireless Personal Communications*, *129*(2), 933–952. DOI: 10.1007/s11277-022-10164-8 PMID: 36594000

IBM. (n.d.). Murel, Jacob, Kavlakoglu, Eda. (2024). What is ensemble learning? *IBM Topics*. https://www.ibm.com/think/topics/ensemble-learning

IBM. (n.d.). What is homomorphic encryption? *IBM Topics*. https://www.ibm.com/topics/homomorphic-encryption

Ken, L. (2024). Machine Unlearning in 2024. *Stanford education*. https://ai.stanford.edu/~kzliu/blog/unlearning

Knevel, R., & Liao, K. P. (2022). From real-world electronic health record data to real-world results using artificial intelligence. *Annals of the Rheumatic Diseases*, *2023*(82), 306–311. PMID: 36150748

Li, L., & Shao, X. Yu, Z. (2024). A Slicing-Free Perspective to Sufficient Dimension Reduction: Selective Review and Recent Developments. *International statistical review*. Volume 92 (3), Pp. 355-382. ISSN: 0306-7734. DOI: DOI: 10.1111/insr.12565

Machine Learning Workflow. (n.d.). AI Platform documentation. *Google Cloud*. https://cloud.google.com/ai-platform/docs/ml-solutions-overview

Ministry of law and justice (legislative department). (2023). The Digital Personal Data Protection Act. The Gazette of India. *MeitY*. https://www.meity.gov.in/writereaddata/files/Digital%20Personal%20Data%20Protection%20Act%202023.pdf

Murdoch, B. (2021). Privacy and artificial intelligence: Challenges for protecting health information in a new era. *BMC Medical Ethics*, *22*(1), 122. DOI: 10.1186/s12910-021-00687-3 PMID: 34525993

NHS England. (n.d.). Digital Technology Assessment Criteria (DTAC). *Transformation Directorate.*https://transform.england.nhs.uk/key-tools-and-info/digital-technology-assessment-criteria-dtac/

Park, T., Gu, P., Kim, C.-H., Kim, K. T., Chung, K. J., Kim, T. B., Jung, H., Yoon, S. J., & Oh, J. K. (2023). Artificial intelligence in urologic oncology: The actual clinical practice results of IBM Watson for Oncology in South Korea. *Prostate International, 11*(4), 218–221. DOI: 10.1016/j.prnil.2023.09.001 PMID: 38196551

. *Pillay,R.(2018). Healthcare 3.0: How technology is driving the transition to prosumers, platforms and outsurance.* Xlibris Corporation.

Project InnerEye – Democratizing Medical Imaging AI. (n.d.), *Microsoft Research.* https://www.microsoft.com/en-us/research/project/medical-image-analysis/

ProtonsHub. (n.d.). Emerging Trends in Artificial Intelligence and Machine Learning: The Future of IT. *ProtonsHub Blog*, https://www.protonshub.com/blogs/the-future-of-it

Randeree, E. (2009). Exploring technology impacts of Healthcare 2.0 initiatives. *Telemedicine Journal and e-Health, 15*(3), 255–260. DOI: 10.1089/tmj.2008.0093 PMID: 19382863

Reddy, C., Kishore, K., Doss, S., Bhatia, S., & Alqhatani, A. (2024). *Evolution and Advances in Computing Technologies for Industry 6.0.* Routledge. DOI: 10.1201/9781003503934

Ristevski, B., & Chen, M. (2018). Big Data Analytics in Medicine and Healthcare. *Journal of Integrative Bioinformatics.* https://www.ncbi.nlm.nih.gov/pmc/articles/PMC6340124/

. Shaik, T., Tao, X., Xie, H., Li, L., Zhu, X., & Li, Q. (2023). Exploring the Landscape of Machine Unlearning: A Comprehensive Survey and Taxonomy. *ArXiv.* / abs/2305.06360.

Sharma, D., Bhagat, L., & Sharma, S. (2024). Regulating Children's Personal Data Protection in India: No Child's Play. *Development, 67*(1-2), 28–33. Advance online publication. DOI: 10.1057/s41301-024-00402-w

Summary of the HIPAA Security Rule. (n.d.). *US Department of Health and Human Services.* https://www.hhs.gov/hipaa/for-professionals/security/laws-regulations/index.html

Tkachenko, N. (2023). Machine Learning in Healthcare: 12 Real-World Use Cases to Know. *NIX United*. https://nix-united.com/blog/machine-learning-in-healthcare-12-real-world-use-cases-to-know/

What is GDPR, the EU's new data protection law? (n.d.). *GDPR.EU*. https://gdpr.eu/what-is-gdpr/

WHO. (n.d.). Health technology assessment. *WHO Health Topics*. https://www.who.int/health-topics/health-technology-assessment/

Xu, J., We, Z., Wang, C., & Jia, X. (2024). Machine Unlearning: Solutions and Challenges. *IEEE Transactions on Emerging Topics in Computational Intelligence*, *8*(3), 2150–2168. DOI: 10.1109/TETCI.2024.3379240

Xu, X., Ren, C., Wu, R., & Yan, H. (2017) Sliced Inverse Regression With Adaptive Spectral Sparsity for Dimension Reduction. *IEEE transactions on cybernetics*. Volume 47 (3), Pp. 759-771. ISSN: 2168-2267. DOI: DOI: 10.1109/TCYB.2016.2526630

Yadav, N., Pandey, S., Gupta, A., Dudani, P., Gupta, S., & Rangarajan, K. (2023). Data Privacy in Healthcare: In the Era of Artificial Intelligence. *Indian Dermatology Online Journal*, *14*(6), 788–792. DOI: 10.4103/idoj.idoj_543_23 PMID: 38099022

Zhang, H., Nakamura, T., Isohara, T., & Sakurai, K. (2023). A Review on Machine Unlearning. *SN Computer Science*, *4*(4), 337. Advance online publication. DOI: 10.1007/s42979-023-01767-4

Zou, F. W., Tang, Y. F., Liu, C. Y., Ma, J. A., & Hu, C. H. (2020). Concordance Study Between IBM Watson for Oncology and Real Clinical Practice for Cervical Cancer Patients in China: A Retrospective Analysis. *Frontiers in Genetics*, *11*, 200. Advance online publication. DOI: 10.3389/fgene.2020.00200 PMID: 32265980

Chapter 11

Leveraging Machine Unlearning for Better Medical Care and Data Protection in Healthcare 6.0

Santosh Moses
https://orcid.org/0009-0000-4476-1678
IQVIA, India

Konrad Obermann
https://orcid.org/0000-0002-0687-5014
M4Health, Germany

Kanishak Gautam
https://orcid.org/0009-0006-0073-0152
IQVIA, India

Gaurav Upadhyay
https://orcid.org/0009-0005-2118-7198
Delhi Technological University, India

Jayathra Datla
https://orcid.org/0009-0002-9442-7680
IQVIA, India

ABSTRACT

Machine Learning (ML), a key component of modern technology, evolved from

DOI: 10.4018/979-8-3693-7210-4.ch011

Alan Turing's 1950s concepts and the Turing Test. Introduced in 1959, ML enables computers to perform tasks by learning from data rather than explicit programming. It includes supervised, unsupervised, semi-supervised, and reinforcement learning. As ML integrated into various industries, Machine Unlearning (MU) emerged to address data privacy and security. MU involves removing specific data points' influence from a trained model without complete retraining, ensuring sensitive information is efficiently erased while maintaining model integrity.

BACKGROUND

Healthcare data includes information collected from patients such as diagnoses, medications, treatment plans and test results. This data is stored and analyzed to provide effective tailored healthcare to the patients.

As healthcare professionals handle vast amounts of data, robust data processing and management tools are essential for their work (Unlu, 2024). These sophisticated data analysis tools process vast data using AI based technologies and machine learning practices to get effective and accurate results. In this era of advanced data analytics and AI applications in healthcare, the concept of unlearning is essential. As healthcare data analysis models are exposed to new data and contexts, they need the ability to discard outdated information to prevent biases and inaccuracies. This is akin to Kuhn's notion that scientific progress necessitates the abandonment of old paradigms to adopt new, more effective ones (Kuhn, 1997). Thus, machine unlearning is not merely about data erasure; it involves re-evaluating and updating the model's framework to ensure better alignment with current realities and evidence (Alvandi, 2024).

Healthcare 6.0 focuses on integrating emerging digital technologies to improve the efficiency of healthcare delivery. A crucial component of this is understanding machine unlearning strategies, which are necessary to keep healthcare systems efficient and responsive. This chapter explores machine unlearning, including its methods, potential, and real-world applications. It seeks to provide industry leaders and healthcare professionals with the know-how to improve health analytics using innovative technologies.

UNRAVELING THE PAST: AN INTRODUCTION TO MACHINE UNLEARNING

The Art of Forgetting: Why Unlearning Matters

In Machine Learning, models are trained using data fed into algorithms, which then make decisions based on the patterns they detect. Cao et al. (Cao & Yang, 2015), was the first one to develop a concept of a "forgetting system" in the early unlearning algorithms, this system converts learning algorithms into summation form and efficiently eliminates data traces enabling the prevention of data pollution attemps . Thus, Machine Unlearning comes into play when it's necessary to delete specific data points from these models. Machine learning models run a risk of unintentionally memorizing private, unauthorized, or harmful data, which could lead to vulnerabilities, performance issues, and privacy violations. Hence, machine unlearning has become a crucial method for addressing these problems by removing the influence of training data points on learned models (Xu et al., 2024). This process ensures that the model can still perform optimally and provide accurate results even after certain data points are removed.

Machine Unlearning is particularly important in sectors such as intelligent computer vision, speech recognition, and medical diagnostics. Numerous facets of our life have been greatly influenced by the astonishing advances in tasks like image recognition, natural language processing, and recommendation systems brought about by the rapid growth of machine learning (ML). But the widespread use of machine learning has sparked serious worries about possible security flaws, privacy problems, and accuracy loss in dynamic environments. However, one of the most critical areas of application is the healthcare industry, where both data security and the personal safety of patients are paramount. Let's explore why Machine Unlearning is so essential, especially in healthcare.

From Memory to Oblivion: The Journey of Data

It all begins with a pre-trained model built from a dataset. Next, a special "forget set" is identified, which contains the specific data that needs to be erased. An unlearning algorithm is then employed to tweak the model, effectively causing it to forget the data in the forget set, resulting in an unlearned model. Please refer to figure 1.

Figure 1. Machine Unlearning Process

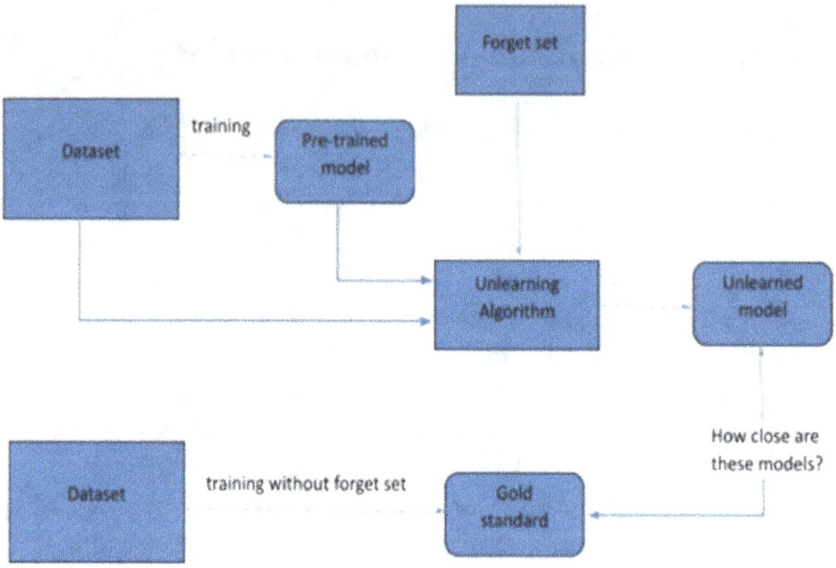

Verifying the Process

After identifying the forget set and applying the unlearning algorithm, the unlearned model is put to the test. It is evaluated against a gold standard model, typically one trained from scratch, to ensure that the specified data has been effectively removed. This testing phase is crucial as it allows us to assess how well the unlearning process preserves the model's integrity and performance.

It is difficult to determine whether the unlearning approach possesses the verifiability property. Although model suppliers may assert on the outside that they eliminate those influences from their models, this is not the case in practice. It might be challenging for data suppliers to demonstrate that the model provider has finished the unlearning process, particularly for intricate deep models with huge training datasets. The model is little affected when just a small portion of the samples are removed. Furthermore, since other users might have supplied comparable data, the model still has a high possibility of producing an accurate forecast even if the unlearned examples have been eliminated.

Therefore, it is worthwhile to conduct additional study on the problem of providing a realistic unlearning verification mechanism (He et al., 2021).

WHY FORGETTING MATTERS: THE IMPERATIVE FOR MACHINE UNLEARNING

In today's dynamic healthcare environment, the utilization of machine learning models has become increasingly crucial in revolutionizing patient care and operational effectiveness. However, the deployment of these models in sensitive domains such as healthcare presents notable challenges, particularly due to the potentially severe repercussions of errors. This is where the concept of machine unlearning emerges as a vital solution that not only bolsters model performance but also ensures privacy and security.

Safeguarding Privacy and Ensuring Accuracy

Data protection regulations like the General Data Protection Regulation (GDPR) have emphasized the concerns around privacy. Machine unlearning is indispensable in this context as it enables the removal of user data from models, aligning with legal requirements, and empowering individuals to exercise their right to erasure. This capability significantly reduces the risk of data breaches and promotes compliance with data protection regulations. In healthcare, machine unlearning also plays a key role in enhancing data accuracy by effectively eliminating outdated or erroneous information, which in turn minimizes the potential for diagnostic errors and enhances patient care.

Security Measures to Mitigate Adversarial Threats

Machine learning models, particularly deep learning models, are vulnerable to adversarial attacks, posing a significant threat in healthcare settings. These attacks can lead to misdiagnoses, inappropriate treatments, and potentially fatal consequences (Finlayson et al., 2019). Machine unlearning mechanisms are crucial in identifying and removing adversarial data from models, thereby fortifying their integrity and reliability, and safeguarding against the detrimental effects of adversarial attacks.

Enhancing Usability and Compliance

In healthcare, machine unlearning supports the usability of machine learning models by facilitating the removal of outdated or incorrect information, thereby promoting the maintenance of accurate and up-to-date patient records. Furthermore, it ensures alignment with regulatory frameworks such as GDPR, allowing healthcare systems to adhere to data protection regulations without compromising operational efficiency.

Cost Efficiency and Resource Management

In the pursuit of efficient resource management, machine unlearning offers a cost-effective approach by enabling the targeted removal of specific data without necessitating the retraining of the entire model. This conserves computational resources and time, resulting in substantial savings and operational efficiency, particularly in large-scale healthcare settings.

Managing Data Dependencies and Model Complexity

Machine unlearning plays a critical role in managing the intricacies of machine learning models by allowing for precise data removal while safeguarding model performance and integrity. By addressing the complexities of data dependencies and model intricacies, machine unlearning contributes to the sustained efficiency and effectiveness of machine learning applications in healthcare.

CRAFTING FORGETFULNESS: MACHINE UNLEARNING IN PRACTICE

The Unlearning Toolkit: Tools and Techniques

Several Machine Unlearning techniques can be utilized based on the desired outcomes. These techniques ensure both the safety and privacy of machine learning systems and the accuracy of the algorithms. They include incremental unlearning, active forgetting, online learning, federated learning, knowledge distillation, and privacy-preserving machine learning (PPML) (Alvandi, 2024).

Incremental Unlearning. It updates a model's parameters without needing to retrain the entire model from scratch. This approach is especially valuable in the healthcare sector, where datasets are continuously updated, requiring models to quickly adapt.

Elastic Weight Consolidation. This technique prevents the model from forgetting important information by selectively slowing down learning on significant weights from previous tasks. In healthcare, EWC helps maintain critical medical knowledge while integrating new information, ensuring that models remain both accurate and reliable.

Progressive Neural Networks (PNN). PNNs use separate pathways for new tasks, keeping the parameters of previous tasks fixed. This allows the model to learn new medical procedures or diagnostic criteria without losing existing knowledge, making it highly useful in rapidly evolving medical fields.

Recurrent Neural Networks (RNN). RNNs handle sequential data, making them suitable for time-series data in healthcare, such as patient monitoring over time. Incremental unlearning in RNNs helps update the model with new patient data while retaining past knowledge.

Generative Adversarial Networks (GAN). GANs can generate new, realistic data points. Incremental unlearning in GANs allows the model to adapt to new types of medical images or patient data, enhancing diagnostic capabilities.

Limitations. Implementing incremental unlearning can be complex and requires careful management to avoid the loss of crucial information. Retention of old knowledge with the integration of new data is challenging task. As shown in figure 2.

Figure 2. Incremental Unlearning

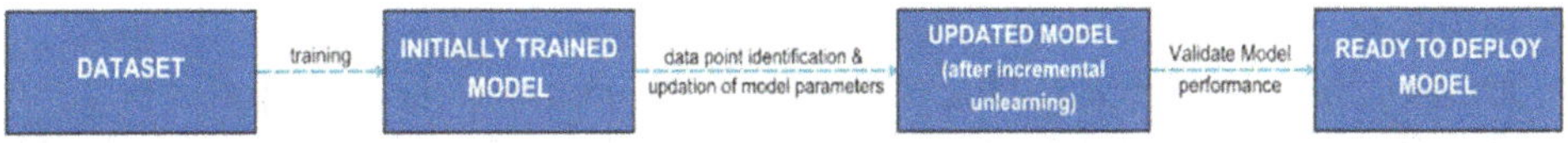

Active Forgetting. It removes outdated or less relevant information from a model's memory, which is crucial for maintaining the accuracy and relevance of healthcare models.

Elastic Weight Pruning. This method prunes less important weights in a neural network, effectively removing outdated knowledge. In healthcare, EWP can help discard obsolete medical guidelines or outdated patient information, ensuring that the model stays current.

Memory Augmented Neural Networks (MANN). MANNs enhance the model's capacity to store and retrieve relevant information while discarding irrelevant data. This technique is particularly useful for maintaining up-to-date patient histories and treatment protocols.

Limitations. Active forgetting techniques require precise criteria to determine what constitutes outdated or irrelevant information, which can be difficult to definc and implement accurately. Refer to figure 3.

Figure 3. Active Forgetting

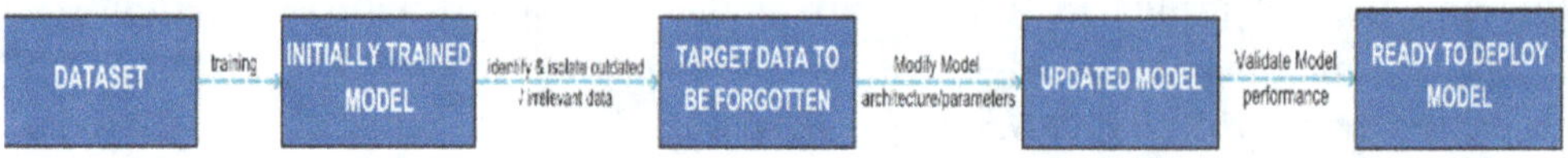

Online Learning. It adapts to changing data streams in real-time, making it highly useful for dynamic tasks in healthcare.

Stochastic Gradient Descent (SGD) with Mini-Batch Updates. This algorithm updates the model incrementally as new data arrives, allowing real-time learning. In healthcare, this is critical for tasks such as dynamic patient risk prediction and real-time anomaly detection in medical sensor data.

Online Support Vector Machine (SVM). It can efficiently handle large and evolving datasets. They are used for the continuous monitoring of patient data, enabling timely and accurate predictions and diagnoses.

Limitations. Online learning methods require robust and efficient algorithms to handle the continuous flow of data without overwhelming computational resources. Ensuring the stability and reliability of the model during continuous updates is also a significant challenge. As depicted in figure 4.

Figure 4. Online Learning

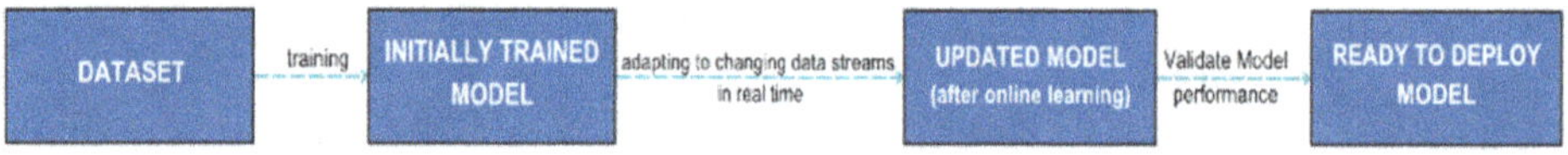

Federated Learning. Federated Learning allows for the training of models across multiple decentralized devices or servers holding local data samples, without exchanging the data itself. This approach helps in preserving data privacy while ensuring that models are updated with the latest information from different sources.

Application in Healthcare. Federated Learning can be used to train models on patient data from different hospitals or clinics without transferring sensitive data across institutions, ensuring privacy while benefiting from a diverse dataset.

Limitations. Coordinating updates across different devices, ensuring data consistency, and handling heterogeneous data are significant challenges. As shown in figure 5.

Figure 5. Federated Learning

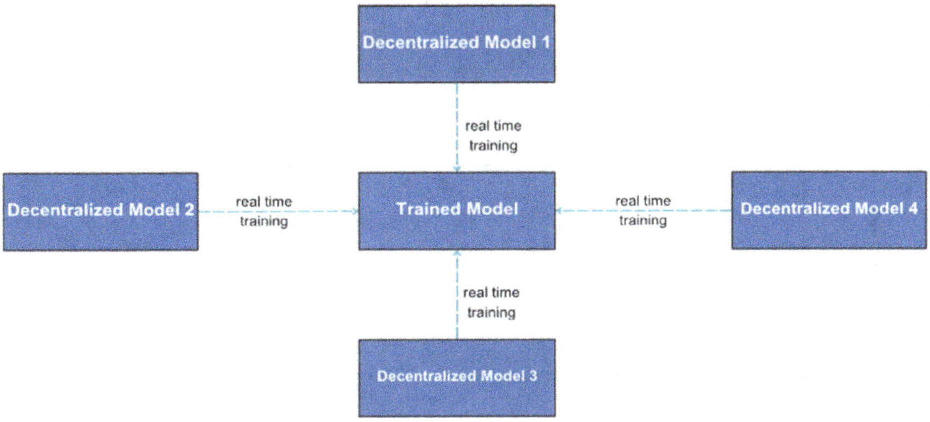

Knowledge Distillation. It involves transferring knowledge from a larger, complex model (teacher) to a smaller, simpler model (student). The student model learns to mimic the teacher model's outputs while being less complex and more efficient.

Application in Healthcare. This method can create smaller models that retain the important features of larger models, making them suitable for deployment in resource-constrained environments like mobile health applications.

Limitations. Ensuring that the student model performs as well as the teacher model can be challenging, and some information might be lost during the distillation process. Please refer to figure 6.

Figure 6. Knowledge Distillation

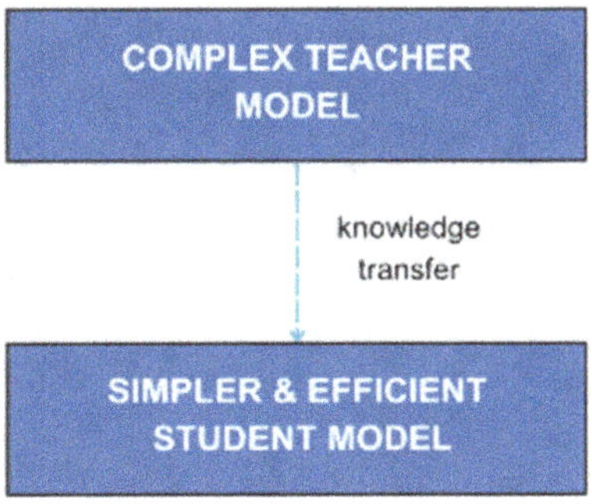

Privacy-Preserving Machine Learning (PPML). It includes techniques such as differential privacy, homomorphic encryption, and secure multi-party computation to ensure that sensitive data is protected during model training and inference.

Application in Healthcare: PPML techniques can protect patient data while still allowing models to be trained and used for predictions. For example, differential privacy adds noise to the data, ensuring that individual patient information cannot be reverse engineered from the model.

Limitations. These techniques can add computational overhead and may affect the accuracy and efficiency of the models.

REAL-WORLD UNLEARNING

Data Augmentation

Data augmentation is a method used to reduce the impact of specific data points that need to be removed from the training dataset. It involves adding new data with varied characteristics to dilute the influence of the original data points. For instance, in a facial recognition model, new images with diverse facial features and expressions are added to reduce the reliance on specific images. While data augmentation can be effective, it requires access to a large amount of new data and may not completely eliminate the impact of the original data points.

Weight Decay

Weight decay is a technique that involves adjusting the model's parameters to decrease the influence of the data points that need to be removed. This is achieved by adding a penalty term to the loss function, which encourages the model to reduce the magnitude of its weights. The primary advantage of weight decay is that it can be applied to existing models without the need for extensive retraining. However, its effectiveness depends on the complexity of the model and the nature of the data. In some cases, weight decay may not fully eliminate the influence of the removed data points, especially if they had a significant impact on the model's learning process.

Fine-Tuning

Fine-tuning involves training the model on a new dataset that excludes the data points intended for removal. This method is highly effective for unlearning a large number of data points, as it allows the model to adapt to the new data distribution. However, fine-tuning can be resource-intensive and time-consuming, requiring significant computational power and data storage. Despite these drawbacks, fine-tuning is often used in scenarios where precision and accuracy are critical, such as in healthcare applications where erroneous data can lead to severe consequences.

Selective Retraining

Selective retraining entails training the model on a new dataset that includes only the data points that are not being removed. This method is more efficient for unlearning a small number of data points, as it focuses on retaining the relevant data while excluding the unwanted ones. However, selective retraining can be challenging to implement, particularly in complex models with interdependencies between data points. Despite this, it offers a balanced approach for scenarios where specific data points need to be removed without significantly affecting the overall model performance.

Neural Architecture Modifications

Neural architecture modifications involve altering the model's architecture to make it more suitable for unlearning. This can include using dynamic neural networks that adapt their structure based on the data they process. Such modifications facilitate more efficient unlearning by allowing the model to isolate and remove specific data points without extensive retraining. However, this approach requires advanced knowledge of neural network design and can be complex to implement. It is particularly beneficial in applications where the model needs to frequently update and remove data, such as real-time healthcare monitoring systems (Juliussen et al., 2023).

The concept of machine unlearning is increasingly recognized as crucial in various aspects of healthcare. One key application is ensuring patient data privacy and compliance with regulations such as the General Data Protection Regulation (GDPR). By allowing for the removal of specific patient data from machine learning models, machine unlearning helps hospitals meet GDPR requirements without needing to retrain the entire model. This is especially important in regions like Europe, where stringent data protection laws are in place. Machine unlearning ensures that once a patient's data is requested to be deleted, it is effectively removed from all systems, thereby safeguarding their privacy and upholding their rights.

Another significant application of machine unlearning in healthcare is the removal of misdiagnosed data. Ensuring data accuracy is critical in healthcare, and machine unlearning plays a key role in removing erroneous data from models. This prevents such data from influencing future predictions and diagnoses, ultimately improving the reliability of diagnostic tools and treatment recommendations.

Additionally, machine unlearning helps mitigate bias in machine learning models, which can lead to unfair treatment recommendations and disparities in healthcare outcomes. By removing the influence of biased or unrepresentative data, machine unlearning promotes fairness and inclusivity in healthcare, allowing for more reliable and unbiased recommendations across diverse patient populations.

Machine unlearning also facilitates real-time data updates and error corrections in healthcare environments, ensuring that predictive models remain current and reliable over time. Furthermore, it significantly enhances data security by minimizing the risk of data breaches. If a breach occurs, affected data can be promptly removed from all machine learning models, preventing it from continuing to influence healthcare decisions.

Specific approaches for different machine learning models, including linear regression models, support vector machines (SVMs), and neural networks, have been developed in the context of machine unlearning. Each model type requires tailored unlearning approaches to maintain its accuracy and integrity.

In fact, machine unlearning is a critical advancement in the field of machine learning, particularly in sensitive sectors such as healthcare. By addressing key challenges related to privacy, security, accuracy, and cost efficiency, machine unlearning ensures that machine learning models in healthcare remain reliable, fair, and efficient.

GUARDIANS OF DATA: REGULATORY AND ETHICAL CONSIDERATIONS

The Ethics of Erasure: Balancing Privacy and Progress

In the ever-changing landscape of data privacy, machine unlearning is stepping into the spotlight as a vital tool for harmonizing data usage with privacy rights. By prioritizing data privacy and fairness, AI systems can forge a more credible and reliable relationship with individuals' data.

The Significance of Machine Unlearning in Data Privacy

Machine unlearning plays an important role in safeguarding data privacy. It serves as a mechanism for honoring individuals' rights to have their data erased, while also ensuring that no remnants of the deleted data linger within the system. Utilizing machine unlearning allows organizations to wipe out specific data points without needing to retrain the entire model. This not only safeguards data subjects' privacy but also conserves computational resources and time. Most importantly, it cultivates trust and transparency, bolstering a positive perception of the organization within the public eye.

Upholding Fairness and Compliance in AI Systems

In addition to the imperative of protecting data privacy, there is a growing realization of the significance of fairness in AI systems. With access to copious amounts of personal data, AI has the potential to inadvertently perpetuate existing biases or introduce new ones. Machine unlearning has emerged as a potent tool for addressing these challenges.

Machine unlearning by removing biased data points could reduce the biases of AI models. This can result in fairer and more reliable AI systems. Nonetheless, ensuring fairness is a complex undertaking as it necessitates identifying and removing biased data points without compromising the overall performance of the AI system.

Furthermore, machine unlearning can aid organizations in complying with data protection laws. As previously discussed, regulations like GDPR mandate the removal of data upon request. Organizations can promptly respond to these requests by implementing effective machine unlearning techniques to ensure compliance and circumvent potential penalties. Machine unlearning represents a dynamic field that blends technological proficiency with ethical responsibility. Balancing data privacy, fairness, and compliance is a challenging endeavor that demands a considerate approach. However, as our understanding of AI progresses, machine unlearning is swiftly emerging as an indispensable tool in the arsenal of data scientists. It not only offers a resolution to the privacy challenges posed by AI but also paves the way for more equitable and ethical AI systems.

Legal Labyrinths: Navigating Data Regulations

The concept of machine unlearning is gaining importance in the context of data privacy and regulatory compliance, particularly in light of the implementation of strict data protection laws such as the General Data Protection Regulation (GDPR) in Europe and the California Consumer Privacy Act (CCPA) in the United States. These regulations give individuals the right to request the deletion or correction of their personal data, including data utilized in machine learning models. Machine unlearning addresses this requirement by enabling the removal of specific data points from models without requiring a complete retraining process, which can be resource-intensive and impractical. This capability is crucial for complying with the "right to be forgotten" provisions stipulated by these regulations.

In addition to adhering to data removal requests, machine unlearning helps uphold the accuracy of data used in models. Data protection laws often mandate that data be accurate and up-to-date to prevent drawing misleading or incorrect conclusions. By facilitating the targeted removal of data that may no longer be relevant or accurate, machine unlearning contributes to the integrity and reliability of machine learning models. This ensures that the models continue to perform effectively while excluding outdated or erroneous data that could otherwise distort results.

Transparency is another key aspect to consider in regulatory compliance. Organizations are required to be transparent about how they manage and process data, including their approach to handling requests for data removal. Therefore, the implementation of machine unlearning techniques must be accompanied by clear documentation and communication about the processes involved. This transparency helps cultivate trust with users and regulatory bodies, indicating that the organization is taking responsible steps to manage personal data.

Finally, while machine unlearning offers significant benefits, it also requires careful evaluation to prevent introducing new risks or vulnerabilities. The process of removing data from models must be conducted in a manner that ensures the security of the remaining data and does not inadvertently expose sensitive information. Regular impact assessments and security evaluations are crucial to ensure that unlearning practices align with data protection regulations and do not compromise the overall data security framework.

TOMORROW'S MIND: FUTURE DIRECTIONS IN MACHINE UNLEARNING

Understanding the impact of specific data on a machine unlearning model is important for the concept of machine unlearning. Essentially, machine unlearning reverses the model updates associated with particular data, speeding up the unlearning process significantly. While there may be some offset in doing so, promising results have shown that this offset can be controlled.

One interesting aspect to consider is the reachability of model parameters. Can the original and unlearned models share the same parameters? This question brings up the need for unlearning verification, also known as data auditing, to determine whether specific data have been eliminated from a model. This verification process is essential for enabling regulations over the right to be forgotten.

Federated learning provides a distinctive environment for researching machine unlearning, involving multiple clients in the training process. This offers a precise way to exclude a client from the federation by utilizing historical updates, thus preventing catastrophic unlearning. Another intriguing use of machine unlearning is in model repair (Vaid et al., 2021). For example, it can be applied to fix overtrained deep neural networks by selectively removing unnecessary or redundant data samples. Additionally, machine unlearning can enhance model accuracy, akin to the compression methods in information bottleneck theory.

The rapid progress in healthcare technology is transforming the future of patient data management. A major innovation in this area is the adoption of machine unlearning techniques, which are set to revolutionize data privacy, security, and model accuracy in the healthcare industry. With the enforcement of stricter regulations like the General Data Protection Regulation (GDPR) and the Health Insurance Portability and Accountability Act (HIPAA), healthcare providers are likely to embrace machine unlearning methods. These techniques allow providers to delete patient data swiftly and effectively upon request and prevent unauthorized access, reducing the risk of data breaches.

Moreover, machine unlearning methods will play a pivotal role in addressing bias and errors within training datasets, ultimately enhancing the fairness and accuracy of predictive models. This is particularly crucial for ensuring equitable healthcare outcomes across diverse patient populations. Hospitals will benefit from the ability to dynamically update and refine their models by removing outdated or incorrect data, leading to more accurate real-time predictions and diagnoses.

Furthermore, the integration of machine unlearning with federated learning systems will enable hospitals to collectively train models without sharing raw data. This will facilitate the removal of specific data points while preserving the overall integrity of the distributed model. Additionally, the integration of machine unlearning with explainable AI will contribute to a better understanding of how data removal impacts model decisions, thereby enhancing transparency and trust in healthcare applications.

As healthcare datasets continue to grow, the development of scalable machine unlearning algorithms will be pivotal in optimizing computational resources and reducing the time required to unlearn data efficiently. Future trends are also expected to witness the creation of automated pipelines for machine unlearning, streamlining the implementation and maintenance of these systems for healthcare providers.

Furthermore, increased collaboration between academic researchers and healthcare institutions will be crucial in driving innovation in machine unlearning technologies, resulting in robust and applicable solutions for real-world healthcare settings. The emergence of pilot programs and case studies showcasing successful implementations of machine unlearning will also play a significant role in encouraging its wider adoption in the industry.

Taken together, these trends indicate that machine unlearning will serve as a transformative tool in the future of healthcare, empowering the industry to bolster data privacy, enhance model performance, and ensure compliance with evolving regulations. These are just a few examples of the intriguing concepts and applications surrounding machine unlearning. The potential impact of this area of research is vast and continues to be explored by experts in the field.

UNCHARTED TERRITORIES: RESEARCH AND SPECULATIONS

Machine unlearning is an evolving area of focus aimed at refining methods that allow for the elimination of specific data from machine learning models. As machine learning systems become increasingly intertwined with everyday life, it is essential to have the capability to erase data in order to comply with privacy regulations and uphold individual rights. This is especially pertinent in the context of the General Data Protection Regulation (GDPR) and comparable frameworks, which afford individuals the right to request the deletion of their personal data.

The exploration of machine unlearning aims to develop efficient algorithms that can selectively remove data without requiring the complete retraining of the model. This involves intricate processes that adjust the learned parameters and the underlying structures of models to forget specific information while preserving overall functionality and accuracy. As this field progresses, it possesses the potential to significantly enhance the security and privacy of machine learning applications, thereby promoting greater trust and wider adoption in sensitive areas such as healthcare, finance, and personal data management.

Notably, there have been instances where similar concepts and methods have been successfully employed. Here are a few cases where these methods were utilized:

Predictive Analytics: Cleveland Clinic and Johns Hopkins- Ohio

The Cleveland Clinic and Johns Hopkins have embarked on a groundbreaking journey by collaborating with tech giants Microsoft and GE to integrate predictive analytics into their healthcare systems. This cutting-edge approach involves scrutinizing patient data to predict potential medical emergencies, thereby enabling proactive intervention to avert critical health issues.

One of the main hurdles for these hospitals has been the necessity to anticipate emergencies and take a proactive approach to patient care. Conventional methods often involve reacting to patient issues, which can result in complications and increased healthcare expenses. By harnessing the power of predictive analytics, these institutions are striving to transition from reactive to proactive healthcare management.

Although these initiatives are still in their early stages, the initial outcomes are extremely promising. At the Cleveland Clinic, the implementation of predictive analytics has already enhanced patient monitoring capabilities, potentially reducing emergency incidents by up to 20%. Meanwhile, at Johns Hopkins, the early adoption of predictive models has shown potential in improving resource allocation and patient outcomes, with a possibility of reducing emergency room visits by 15% (Bhagat & Kanyal, 2024).

Chatbots: UCLA's Virtual Interventional Radiologist (VIR) - California

The University of California, Los Angeles (UCLA) has successfully implemented a cutting-edge AI-driven chatbot system known as the Virtual Interventional Radiologist (VIR). This innovative chatbot is designed to automate physician inquiries and efficiently direct them to the appropriate specialists, thereby streamlining the process of routing patients to the right healthcare providers.

Prior to the introduction of VIR, physician inquiries and the task of routing patients to specialists were often time-consuming and prone to errors, which had a direct impact on patient care efficiency. However, the implementation of VIR has aimed to address these challenges by automating these processes, reducing the time physicians spend on administrative tasks, and allowing them to dedicate more of their attention to patient care.

The impact of the VIR chatbot has been substantial, with UCLA reporting a notable 30% reduction in the time spent on administrative inquiries. This streamlined approach has not only resulted in a more efficient workflow within the healthcare system but has also led to improved patient care. Furthermore, the projected increase in specialist consultation efficiency by 25% emphasizes the remarkable potential of chatbots to significantly enhance operational efficiency in hospital settings.

UCLA's successful integration of the VIR chatbot serves as a compelling example of how AI-powered technologies can revolutionize traditional healthcare processes, ultimately benefiting both healthcare providers and patients alike (Best Use of Artificial Intelligence in Healthcare Marketing, n.d.).

Predictive Health Trackers: Mayo Clinic and AliveCor – USA

Mayo Clinic's recent investment in AliveCor underscores the growing trend of integrating predictive health monitoring technologies to provide real-time tracking of patients' health. AliveCor's innovative AI-powered platforms are specifically designed to focus on the early identification of cardiac arrhythmias, such as atrial fibrillation.

One of the primary challenges in the realm of cardiac care has been the timely detection of heart conditions to facilitate effective treatment and ensure positive patient outcomes. Traditional monitoring methods have often fallen short in delivering real-time data, resulting in delayed interventions. To address this issue, AliveCor's technology is geared towards filling this crucial gap by offering continuous and real-time monitoring of patients' heart health.

The adoption of AliveCor's technology by Mayo Clinic has the potential to make a significant impact on cardiac care. Initial trials have demonstrated that these predictive health trackers can detect atrial fibrillation with an impressive 95% accuracy rate. This represents a potential reduction of up to 70% in the risk of stroke among identified patients. Such breakthroughs could lead to a substantial decrease in healthcare costs associated with emergency interventions and long-term cardiac care (Noble.Dana, 2024).

Learning: Mount Sinai Health System - Pennsylvania (Bethlehem)

Mount Sinai Health System, located in New York, has been leading the way in the implementation of federated learning for the analysis of electronic health records (EHR). Federated learning is a cutting-edge approach that enables multiple hospitals to collaborate on predictive modeling without compromising patient privacy.

The primary challenge facing healthcare institutions is to develop highly accurate predictive models while ensuring the utmost protection of patient privacy. Traditional centralized data models pose significant privacy risks, but with federated learning, sensitive patient data remains decentralized while contributing to the development of a shared, precise model.

Research conducted in January 2021 revealed the remarkable performance of federated learning models in predicting COVID-19 patient outcomes. These models exhibited a 15% improvement in accurately predicting mortality rates compared to traditional models. Furthermore, the adaptability of federated learning to rapidly incorporate new data has significantly enhanced diagnostic accuracy across multiple hospitals, making it an invaluable tool in improving patient care (Vaid et al., 2021).

Data De-Identification and Unlearning: Lehigh University - Alexandria

Lehigh University researchers are currently working on pioneering methods to empower machine learning models to "unlearn" specific patient data from Electronic Health Records (EHRs). This exciting development is aimed at ensuring compliance with strict privacy regulations such as the General Data Protection Regulation (GDPR).

One of the main challenges faced by hospitals is the need to adhere to data deletion requests without compromising the accuracy of their machine learning models. Traditionally, meeting this requirement would involve retraining entire models, a process that consumes significant resources and is not practical in many cases. However, the innovative use of Elastic Weight Consolidation (EWC) offers a promising solution. This technique enables machine learning models to efficiently forget specific data, overcoming the shortcomings of traditional methods.

The adoption of machine unlearning techniques has had a profound impact, demonstrating that models can maintain high levels of accuracy even after the removal of data. This groundbreaking innovation has the potential to reduce retraining time by up to 50%, providing hospitals with a more efficient means of complying with privacy regulations while ensuring the robustness of their predictive capabilities. Ultimately, this approach contributes to fostering patient trust and upholding stringent privacy standards in the healthcare industry (Hochbein, n.d.).

Big Data Model for Hospital Outcomes: NSF (Govt.)

The hospital in Alexandria is currently exploring the potential of big data models in enhancing the prediction of critical hospital outcomes such as readmission rates and treatment complications.

One of the key challenges faced in this integration is the protection of sensitive information. However, the development of machine unlearning techniques presents a solution by enabling the removal of specific data without compromising the overall model's integrity, thus ensuring data privacy while leveraging big data for predictive modelling.

This approach, funded by a $1.2 million National Science Foundation grant, has the potential to transform data management in hospitals. It offers a 30% faster data removal process compared to traditional retraining methods, ensuring compliance with privacy regulations and maintaining the accuracy and reliability of predictive models. Ultimately, this advancement gives the hope to improve patient care and efficiency of operations (Ford, n.d.).

Predictive Analytics in Hospitals: Apollo Hospitals, India

In India, Apollo Hospitals has undertaken a groundbreaking approach by incorporating predictive analytics into their patient care system. This innovative initiative centers on leveraging advanced data analysis to forecast patient outcomes and potential complications before they arise.

Apollo Hospitals faced the significant challenge of decreasing patient readmission rates and enhancing overall treatment outcomes. Conventional methods often resulted in reactive healthcare, leading to increased costs and less effective patient management. By integrating predictive analytics, Apollo Hospitals is striving to anticipate and address potential health issues proactively, rather than reactively.

The initial *outcomes* have been incredibly promising, demonstrating a marked improvement in patient care efficiency. Predictive analytics has contributed to a roughly 15% reduction in patient readmission rates, while the early identification of complications has resulted in a 20% decrease in emergency interventions. These achievements underscore the potential of predictive analytics to elevate healthcare outcomes and operational efficiency within Indian hospitals (apolloAdmin, 2023).

AI in Elderly Care: Kyoto University Hospital, Japan

In Japan, the Kyoto University Hospital has successfully integrated AI technologies into their elderly care system to address the challenges posed by an aging population. By leveraging AI-powered robots and predictive analytics, the hospital has made significant strides in monitoring the health of elderly patients and optimizing the workload of healthcare workers.

Japan is confronted with the pressing issue of an aging population, which has consequently increased the demand for elderly care. However, the traditional methods of care are becoming unsustainable due to a shortage of healthcare workers. In response to these challenges, the implementation of AI solutions, including AI-powered robots for monitoring and assisting the elderly, as well as predictive analytics for health tracking, aims to revolutionize elderly care in Japan.

The impact of integrating AI in elderly care has been noteworthy, with a 25% increase in the efficiency of monitoring patient health and a 30% reduction in the workload of healthcare workers. Furthermore, the utilization of predictive analytics has led to a 15% improvement in early detection of health issues, ultimately enhancing the quality of care for elderly patients. The successful integration of AI in elderly care at Kyoto University Hospital serves as a compelling example of the potential for AI to address the unique healthcare challenges posed by an aging population (Loveys et al., 2022).

Federated Learning in Hospitals: National University of Singapore

The National University of Singapore (NUS) has been at the forefront of utilizing federated learning, a machine learning technique that trains an algorithm across multiple decentralized edge devices or servers holding local data samples, to advance predictive modeling in hospital settings while upholding patient privacy. One of the main obstacles faced was the need to collaboratively build accurate predictive models while ensuring the utmost protection of patient data privacy across various hospitals and healthcare institutions. To address this challenge, NUS implemented federated learning, which enabled hospitals to build a centralized predictive model using local data from each institution, thereby preserving the privacy of sensitive patient information.

The adoption of federated learning has yielded significant improvements, resulting in a 20% increase in the accuracy of predictive models compared to traditional methods. This heightened accuracy is attributed to the decentralized model training process, which allows the algorithm to learn from diverse datasets without compromising the privacy of individual patient data. Moreover, this strategy has significantly bolstered patient data privacy, ensuring compliance with strict data protection regulations and ethical considerations in healthcare.

NUS's pioneering work in this area has decisively demonstrated that federated learning has the potential to deliver more precise and secure predictive healthcare solutions. By leveraging the collective knowledge from diverse datasets while preserving data privacy, federated learning made a noteworthy impact on the field by providing more accurate and secure predictive healthcare solutions (Dang et al., 2022).

Machine Learning for Disease Prediction: Kenyatta National Hospital, Kenya

The Kenyatta National Hospital in Kenya has taken an innovative step by integrating machine learning technology into its healthcare system. This cutting-edge technology is being utilized to analyze data and predict the occurrence of disease outbreaks, particularly focusing on infectious diseases. Kenya faces significant challenges in dealing with infectious diseases due to limited resources and inadequate infrastructure. To address these issues, the hospital has turned to machine learning models to identify patterns in data and anticipate disease outbreaks, enabling proactive healthcare interventions.

The introduction of machine learning has resulted in a remarkable 30% improvement in the early detection of disease outbreaks. This proactive approach has led to the implementation of more efficient containment and treatment strategies. As a result, there has been a reduction in the transmission of infectious diseases and an overall improvement in patient outcomes. The use of machine learning technology is proving to be a game-changer in addressing healthcare challenges in Kenya, paving the way for more effective disease management and improved public health.

Predictive Health Analytics: Charité – Universitätsmedizin Berlin, Germany

Charité – Universitätsmedizin Berlin, one of the leading hospitals in Germany, has made significant strides in improving patient care and operational efficiency through the successful implementation of predictive health analytics. This innovative approach harnesses the power of advanced data analysis, enabling the hospital to predict patient readmissions and potential health complications with a high degree of accuracy. By doing so, Charité can intervene proactively, leading to optimized resource allocation and improved patient outcomes.

The decision to adopt predictive health analytics was driven by the hospital's need to address the challenges of managing a high volume of patients while striving to deliver the best possible treatment outcomes. Leveraging this technology has empowered Charité to identify at-risk patients and potential health complications at an earlier stage, thereby facilitating timely interventions and ensuring efficient management of resources.

Since integrating predictive health analytics into its operations, Charité has documented notable achievements. These include a remarkable 20% reduction in patient readmissions and a 15% improvement in the timely identification of health complications. These tangible results underscore the tremendous potential of predictive analytics in transforming patient care and enhancing operational efficiency, particularly within the context of European hospitals like Charité (Braun, n.d.).

CONCLUSION

The concept of machine unlearning in healthcare represents a revolutionary and promising approach to addressing crucial challenges related to data privacy, model accuracy, and regulatory compliance. It offers a robust solution for adhering to data protection regulations such as GDPR and HIPAA. By enabling the removal of specific patient data from machine learning models, healthcare providers can significantly enhance patient privacy and alleviate concerns about data misuse. This capability is essential for building confidence in AI systems and ensuring the responsible and ethical handling of patient data.

Furthermore, machine unlearning has the potential to significantly enhance the fairness and accuracy of predictive models in healthcare by eliminating biased or incorrect data. This is crucial for delivering equitable healthcare services and making trustworthy clinical decisions. In a field where precision in data is critical, the ability to dynamically rectify and refine models ensures that healthcare providers can rely on the insights generated by AI.

Operational efficiency is another notable benefit of machine unlearning in healthcare. In environments where data is continuously generated and updated, the ability to dynamically update models without extensive retraining ensures that predictive models remain relevant and accurate over time. This ongoing refinement process supports better decision-making and more effective patient care.

In this pioneering research, machine unlearning techniques are explored comprehensively for the first time. The chapter addresses primary challenges and recent advancements in conceptualizing, planning, and resolving complexities associated with machine unlearning. We have developed a classification system for machine unlearning strategies, dividing them into three main approaches: model-agnostic methods, model-intrinsic methods, and data-driven methods.

Additionally, the research outlines a machine unlearning framework, detailing removal requests, design requirements, and verification procedures. To propel future research, the study lays the foundation for structured benchmarking by aggregating popular datasets and open-source applications. Current trends and prospects in machine unlearning are also highlighted.

The future of machine unlearning is closely linked with advancements in federated learning and explainable AI. Integrating these developments will enhance its effectiveness and transparency, paving the way for more secure and understandable AI systems in healthcare. Through the fusion of these technologies, healthcare providers can develop AI systems that safeguard patient data while providing clear, interpretable insights.

Scalability and automation are critical considerations as healthcare datasets expand. Developing scalable and efficient machine unlearning algorithms will empower healthcare providers to manage large volumes of data effectively. Automated unlearning pipelines will further reduce manual efforts and increase the adoption of these technologies, simplifying the implementation and maintenance of advanced AI systems.

The advancement of machine unlearning techniques will be driven by increased collaboration between academic researchers, healthcare institutions, and technology companies. This collaborative effort will yield more robust solutions tailored to the specific needs of the healthcare industry. Real-world applications and pilot programs will showcase the tangible benefits of machine unlearning, encouraging broader adoption across the sector.

In summary, machine unlearning is set to revolutionize the healthcare industry by offering powerful tools for maintaining data privacy, improving model accuracy, and ensuring compliance with evolving regulations. As the technology matures, it will play a pivotal role in shaping the future of AI in healthcare. Given the critical importance of privacy, security, usability, and fidelity in machine learning systems, innovative concepts in machine unlearning will have a substantial impact across various domains. It is anticipated that the insights from this research will significantly influence the integration of machine unlearning in diverse applications in the coming years. It is vital for healthcare professionals and industry experts to have a deep understanding of machine unlearning models, their healthcare applications, and their limitations. The global examples in this chapter highlight the crucial role that machine learning and unlearning strategies play in enhancing patient diagnostics and treatment. By exploring machine unlearning from various angles, healthcare professionals and industry experts can better grasp its significance in contemporary healthcare technologies. Additionally, they can recognize the essential role of machine unlearning in maintaining the adaptability, robustness, and ethical integrity of AI systems in various facets of healthcare delivery.

REFERENCES

Alvandi, A. O. (2024, June 10). Machine Unlearning in Digitalized Healthcare Arena A Comprehensive Exploration. https://doi.org/DOI: 10.31219/osf.io/kz3w5

https://www.uclahealth.org/sites/default/files/documents/21/2022-uclah-ehealthcare-artificial-intelligence.pdf?f=bb1a7b0d

Bhagat, S. V., & Kanyal, D. (2024). Navigating the Future: The Transformative Impact of Artificial Intelligence on Hospital Management- A Comprehensive Review. *Cureus*, *16*(2). Advance online publication. DOI: 10.7759/cureus.54518 PMID: 38516434

Braun, J. (n.d.). Data Ecosystems and Care Analytics Research Group. Institute of Medical Informatics. Retrieved August 2, 2024, from

https://medinfo.charite.de/en/research/data_ecosystems_and_care_analytics_research_grou/

Cao, Y., & Yang, J. (2015). Towards Making Systems Forget with Machine Unlearning. *IEEE Symposium on Security and Privacy*, 463–480. https://doi.org/DOI: 10.1109/SP.2015.35

Dang, T. K., Lan, X., Weng, J., & Feng, M. (2022). Federated Learning for Electronic Health Records. *ACM Transactions on Intelligent Systems and Technology*, *13*(5), 1–17. DOI: 10.1145/3514500

Finlayson, S. G., Bowers, J. D., Ito, J., Zittrain, J. L., Beam, A. L., & Kohane, I. S. (2019, March 21). Adversarial Attacks on Medical Machine Learning. *Science*, *363*(6433), 1287–1289. DOI: 10.1126/science.aaw4399 PMID: 30898923

Ford, J. (n.d.-b). NSF grant to help researchers harness power of big data to address health issues. Penn State University. https://www.psu.edu/news/research/story/nsf-grant-help-researchers-harness-power-big-data-address-health-issues/

He, Y., Meng, G., Chen, K., He, J., & Hu, X. (2021, May 13). DeepObliviate: A Powerful Charm for Erasing Data Residual Memory in Deep Neural Networks. arXiv.org. https://arxiv.org/abs/2105.06209

Hochbein, K. (n.d.-b). Machine Unlearning. Lehigh University. https://www2.lehigh.edu/news/machine-unlearning

Juliussen, B. A., Rui, J. P., & Johansen, D. (2023). Algorithms that forget: Machine unlearning and the right to erasure. *Computer Law & Security Report*, *51*, 105885–105885. DOI: 10.1016/j.clsr.2023.105885

Kuhn, T. S. (1997). The structure of scientific revolutions (Vol. 962). University of Chicago press Chicago.

Loveys, K., Prina, M., Axford, C., Domènec, Ò. R., Weng, W., Broadbent, E., Pujari, S., Jang, H., Han, Z. A., & Thiyagarajan, J. A. (2022). Artificial intelligence for older people receiving long-term care: A systematic review of acceptability and effectiveness studies. *The Lancet. Healthy Longevity*, *3*(4), e286–e297. DOI: 10.1016/S2666-7568(22)00034-4 PMID: 35515814

https://mcpress.mayoclinic.org/healthy-aging/ai-in-healthcare-the-future-of-patient-care-and-health-management/

https://www.psu.edu/news/research/story/nsf-grant-help-researchers-harness-power-big-data-address-health-issues/

Unlu, O. (2024, October 25). 11 Big Data In Healthcare Statistics [Trends and Overall Market]. Edge Delta. https://edgedelta.com/company/blog/big-data-in-healthcare-industy-overview

Vaid, A., Jaladanki, S. K., Xu, J., Teng, S., Kumar, A., Lee, S., Somani, S., Paranjpe, I., De Freitas, J. K., Wanyan, T., Johnson, K. W., Bicak, M., Klang, E., Kwon, Y. J., Costa, A., Zhao, S., Miotto, R., Charney, A. W., Böttinger, E., & Glicksberg, B. S. (2021c). Federated Learning of Electronic Health Records to Improve Mortality Prediction in Hospitalized Patients With COVID-19: Machine Learning Approach. *JMIR Medical Informatics*, *9*(1), e24207. DOI: 10.2196/24207 PMID: 33400679

Xu, J., Wu, Z., Wang, C., & Jia, X. (2024). Machine Unlearning: Solutions and Challenges. *IEEE Transactions on Emerging Topics in Computational Intelligence*, *8*(3), 2150–2168. DOI: 10.1109/TETCI.2024.3379240

Chapter 12
Precision Nutrition Through Nutritional Informatics:
Futuristic Technologies for Health Advancement

Jyoti Vijay
Institute of Health Management Research, Bangalore, India

Teesta Dey
https://orcid.org/0009-0000-2251-780X
Mount Carmel College, India

Athmakoor Angela Shresta
https://orcid.org/0009-0005-1286-1486
Mount Carmel College, India

ABSTRACT

Precision nutrition tailors dietary recommendations to prevent and manage diseases based on individual factors. It integrates Healthcare 6.0 technology, particularly nutrition informatics, which combines information, nutrition, and technology for personalized dietary recommendations in both community and clinical settings. This chapter explores key aspects of nutrition informatics, including data sources, dietary data collection techniques, digital tools, and advanced analytics for personalized recommendations. It also examines publicly available online health and nutrition databases that support customized dietary planning. Emerging technologies are revolutionizing nutrition data collection, leveraging advanced analytics for comprehensive, individualized insights. Additionally, the chapter discusses how

DOI: 10.4018/979-8-3693-7210-4.ch012

precision nutrition aids disease management by identifying optimal dietary patterns and using data-driven insights to promote healthier lifestyles. Integrating nutrition informatics into precision nutrition offers a transformative approach to enhancing health outcomes.

INTRODUCTION

The field of healthcare is undergoing continuous evolution, driven by advancements in modern technology. The post-COVID-19 era has accelerated the transition from traditional methods of healthcare delivery to digital solutions. Although this shift was catalyzed by an unprecedented global health crisis, it has propelled humankind toward the ambitious vision of Healthcare 6.0. This next-generation healthcare paradigm integrates telemedicine, wearable health-monitoring devices, and artificial intelligence to redefine patient care. A central challenge in achieving Healthcare 6.0 lies in aligning advancements across diverse, interconnected sectors of healthcare. One such critical area is nutrition and dietetics. As pe Global Burden of Disease (GBD) 2021, unhealthy diet is the main leading risk factor contributing to the global health risk (IHME 2024). Nutrition science focuses on promoting well-being by enhancing growth and development, preventing diseases, and maintaining health through balanced eating patterns. Historically, dietary guidelines were designed for populations, relying on the concept of a "general balanced diet." However, these generalized approaches often fail to address individual-specific requirements, highlighting the need for more tailored strategies to meet unique health needs.

Precision nutrition represents a transformative approach that shifts the focus from one-size-fits-all dietary recommendations to personalized nutrition plans tailored to an individual's specific characteristics. The Cambridge Dictionary defines precision as "the quality of being exact or accurate," and precision nutrition embodies this principle by designing interventions based on factors such as age, sex, genetic makeup, nutrigenomics, gut microbiome, metabolomics, and more (Berciano et al., 2022). According to the Harvard T.H. Chan School of Public Health, professionals in precision nutrition must acknowledge that individuals respond differently to specific foods and nutrients. This variability renders generalized diets unsuitable for many, as even individuals with the same health condition can exhibit divergent responses to identical diet plans (Harvard T.H. Chan School of Public Health, 2024). To address these complexities, nutrition informatics technologies play a crucial role by enabling the collection and analysis of personal health data, thereby facilitating the creation of customized diet plans (Joshi et al., 2021).

Precision Nutrition (PN) is an approach to developing comprehensive and dynamic nutritional recommendations based on individual variables, including genetics, microbiome, metabolic profile, health status, physical activity, dietary pattern, food environment as well as socioeconomic and psychosocial characteristics.

Despite its promise, precision nutrition faces several challenges that warrant attention. The absence of standardized nutritional data platforms is a major barrier to progress (Chan et al., 2021). Additionally, ethical concerns, high costs of advanced technologies, and limited validity studies for emerging nutrition informatics tools further complicate the field (North et al., 2015). Even with these obstacles addressed, the inherent complexity of tailoring nutrition for each individual remains a significant challenge (Berciano et al., 2022). In the Indian context, implementing precision nutrition presents unique difficulties. As a developing country, India is still adapting to interdisciplinary approaches in healthcare. Integrating genetic, microbiomic, environmental, and lifestyle factors into healthcare strategies is a daunting task (Joshi et al., 2021). However, these efforts are critical to advancing public health and realizing the full potential of precision nutrition.

This chapter explores the emerging field of precision nutrition through the lens of nutrition informatics. It delves into the application of data-driven insights for personalized nutrition, examines available datasets and tools, and discusses methods for dietary intervention design. Furthermore, it highlights the challenges specific to India and outlines strategies to overcome them, offering a comprehensive overview of the future of nutrition science in the context of Healthcare 6.0. By embracing precision nutrition, healthcare systems can take a significant step toward more effective, personalized, and sustainable interventions, ultimately enhancing the quality of life for individuals across diverse populations.

THE EVOLUTION AND ROLE OF NUTRITION INFORMATICS

Informatics integrates computer, information, cognitive, and disciplinary sciences and understands how professionals interact with data and technology in their respective fields. When applied to nutritional science, this convergence gives rise to the field of nutrition informatics - a field that leverages bioinformatics-driven integration of nutrition-related datasets to study interactions between organisms and their nutritional environments (Döring & Rimbach, 2014). Nutritionists and clinical dietitians handle extensive data, including patient profiles, nutritional screening, diet charts, menu plans, food analysis and other records. Whereas public health nutritionists handle data related to health and nutritional status of community. Nutrition informatics streamlines and simplifies the collection, storage, analysis, and application of this data, allowing professionals to save time and effort while enhancing the quality of care (North et al., 2015).

The development of nutrition informatics has been shaped by technological advancements and interdisciplinary collaboration. In the 1970s and 1980s, data collection was largely manual, transitioning to computerized systems in the 1990s. The rise of the World Wide Web further expanded the potential of informatics in managing and analyzing nutrition information. Recognizing its growing significance, the Academy of Nutrition and Dietetics established the Nutrition Informatics Work Group, which was formally designated as the Nutrition Informatics Committee in 2009. (Ayres & Hoggle, 2012). The committee began its work in 2010 and continues to play a vital role in advancing nutrition informatics in both public and personalized healthcare (Rusnak & Charney, 2019).

Nutrition Informatics

The effective retrieval, organization, storage and optimum use of information, data and knowledge for food and nutrition-related problem solving and decision making. Nutrition informatics is supported by the use of information standards, processes and technology. Source - Definition (Ayres & Hoggle, 2012)

The Academy collaborates closely with HL7 to develop standards such as Electronic Nutrition Care Process Record System-Functional Profile, outlining essential dietetics functions for inclusion in EHR systems. The Academy has supported the development of the C-CDA R2.1 Nutrition Transitions of Care Implementation Guide, an HL7 standard detailing the nutrition data to be included in EHRs for various care settings, such as home health, rehabilitation, and skilled nursing facilities (Academy of Nutrition and Dietetics, 2019).

To facilitate integration, the Academy provides an EHR toolkit that helps nutrition and dietetics practitioners incorporate the Nutrition Care Process and Terminology (NCPT) into digital systems. This toolkit offers tailored resources based on practitioners' roles and stages in transitioning from paper-based to electronic records.

Beyond clinical settings, nutrition informatics plays a crucial role in addressing nutritional challenges across diverse populations. It enables the analysis of vast datasets, supports personalized interventions (Chan et al., 2021), and empowers individuals to customize their dietary plans and track their health (Eldridge et al., 2018). As the field continues to evolve, nutrition informatics remains essential for data-driven decision-making and improved healthcare outcomes.

DATABASES

A. Food Databases

Food and Nutrient databases provide information about nutritive values for food items categorized across food groups. In United States, Food and Nutrient Database for Dietary Studies (FNDDS) provides the nutrient values for foods and beverages reported in What We Eat in America, the dietary intake component of the National Health and Nutrition Examination Survey (United States Department of Agriculture, 2023). In India, Indian Food Composition Table (IFCT) by NIN, ICMR, provide detailed nutrient information across various food groups, serving as a key reference for dietitians, nutritionists, and food developers. Food groups are categorized cereals and millets, grain legumes, green leafy vegetables, other vegetables, fruits, roots and tubers, condiments and spices, nuts and oilseeds, sugars, mushrooms, miscellaneous foods, milk and milk products, egg and egg products, poultry, animal meat, marine fish, marine shellfish, marine mollusks, freshwater fish and shellfish. The nutrient content of each food item, including its energy value per 100 grams, is systematically listed within the respective food group categories (Longvah et al., 2017).

B. Population-Level data

Every 5th year, National Family Health Survey (NFHS) rounds are conducted by the International Institute of Population Services (IIPS) funded by ICF international. The national survey provides information on health and nutritional status of population such as fertility, marriage, family planning, child feeding practices, nutrition, adult and childhood mortality, HIV/AIDS and women's empowerment (International Institute for Population Sciences & ICF, 2021). The Sample Registration Survey (SRS), conducted annually by the Department of Census, provides vital data on mortality rates among infants and mothers, as well as life expectancy statistics (Office of the Registrar General & Census Commissioner, India, 2020).

Prominent global nutrition databases include National Health and Nutrition Examination Survey (NHANES), Nutritionix, Nutritics, the Australian Food Composition Database, FooDB, the European Food Information Resource, the Canada Nutrient File (CNF), the Japanese Food Composition Database, NutriSurvey, the Nutrition Data System for Research (NDSR), HealthifyMe, MyFitnessPal, and iDietitian (Berciano et al., 2022). These databases play a vital role in delivering reliable data on food composition, supporting nutritional education, and aiding in the development of dietary recommendations. As such, they serve as comprehensive resources for enhancing dietary habits and promoting overall nutritional awareness (Eldridge et al., 2018).

In India, food and nutrient intake data are primarily provided by various surveys, National Family Health Survey (NFHS), Comprehensive National Nutrition Survey (CNNS), Longitudinal Ageing Study in India (LASI) and National Nutrition Monitoring Bureau (NNMB). These surveys provide detailed information about various nutrition indicators, including micronutrient status, child growth and malnutrition, feeding practices, nutrient supplementation, and micronutrient deficiencies along with food and nutrient intake of various age groups (International Institute for Population Sciences et al., 2020; International Institute for Population Sciences & ICF, 2021; Ministry of Health and Family Welfare (MoHFW), Government of India, UNICEF, & Population Council, 2019). While most of these datasets are publicly accessible for research and analysis except NNMB survey. The NNMB exclusively focuses on food and nutrient intake and related nutritional status but is not available in the public domain (National Institute of Nutrition, 2017).

Additionally, food and nutrition security are key to addressing malnutrition, its associated risks and improving public health. Adequate nutrition, through sufficient and diversified diet, is crucial for improving the health and nutritional status of the population. It supports health and nutritional status of population by influencing body weight, promoting the growth and development of children and teenagers, and contributing to overall well-being. Unhealthy eating habits contribute to health risk such as obesity, diabetes, cardiovascular diseases, cancer and other non-communicable diseases, resulting in poor health and nutritional status. Tools like Global Hunger Index (GHI) and Multidimensional Poverty Index (MPI) highlight the need for better nutritional support. The GHI considers food insufficiency, malnutrition and child mortality and calculates ranking. During 2023, India ranked 111th out of 125 countries in 2023 with a score of 28.7, highlighting ongoing hunger challenges (Global Hunger Index, 2024). MPI measures multiple deprivations, with nutrition being a significant contributor to India's index, further emphasizing the need for improved nutritional interventions to reduce poverty and malnutrition (UNDP, 2024).

Nutrition informatics involves collecting and analyzing hospital patient records and research data to disseminate nutrition and health-related personalized nutrition plans including behavioral insights (Joshi et al., 2021). Commonly utilized sources for nutrition research data include Harvard Dataverse, accessible via the Harvard Library which is a public domain resource offering a vast repository of data. Powered by the open-source Dataverse application from the Institute for Quantitative Social Science, it facilitates data sharing and replication for academic purposes. With access to over 2,000 databases, 75,000 datasets, and more than 350,000 files, the Harvard Dataverse provides robust tools for browsing and analyzing text-based information pertaining to individuals, groups, and institutions at Harvard and beyond (Harvard Library, 2024).

THE ROLE OF NUTRITION INFORMATICS AND MEDICAL RECORDS IN ADVANCING HEALTHCARE

Nutrition informatics employs various tools for data collection and analysis, facilitating nutrition research and personalized diet plans (Joshi et al., 2021). A cornerstone of effective healthcare is comprehensive medical record-keeping, which documents all aspects of patient care from initial assessment to treatment interventions (Ambinder, 2005). While traditional paper-based medical records have been widely used, they pose several limitations, including potential for manual errors, restricted accessibility, security risks, and delays in updating information (Tsai & Bond, 2008).

EHRs address many of these challenges by offering secure, accessible, and easily updated digital storage. They support remote consultations with dietitians and healthcare professionals and streamline the tracking of a patient's medical history, diagnoses, meal plans, allergies, medications, and health management strategies (Hoggle, Nash & Teitelbaum, 2006; Ambinder, 2005). However, EHRs are not without drawbacks, such as vulnerability to cyber-attacks, accidental data loss, and the need for technologically adept staff. Resolving these issues is key to fully leveraging their potential in revolutionizing healthcare (Chan et al., 2021).

Patient medical records, including body measurements, clinical parameters, metabolomics, genomics, behavioural, social and food preferences, serve as a vital resource for documenting a patient's health journey, providing a reliable foundation for treatment planning and continuity of care (North et al., 2015). Biomarkers further enhance healthcare by serving as indicators of pathological or biological responses, enabling early disease detection, risk assessment, and treatment evaluation (Picó et al., 2019). Standard laboratory techniques complement dietary evaluation methods, offering a holistic view of an individual's health and nutritional status (Bailey, 2021).

ADVANCEMENTS IN DIETARY ASSESSMENT AND NUTRIENT PREDICTION

A. Traditional Methods – Dietary Data Assessment

Nutrition data collection has evolved significantly, incorporating both traditional and advanced technological methods. Conventional approaches include food diaries, Food Frequency Questionnaires (FFQs), and 24-hour dietary recalls (24HRs). These methods assess food intake, nutrient intake, dietary habits and other nutrition-related behaviors.

Food Diaries

Food diaries are detailed records of all meals, beverages, and supplements consumed by an individual over a specific period, typically 3–4 days. These diaries provide valuable insights into dietary patterns. While recording food intake, individuals often estimate portions consumed, both before and after meals. For greater accuracy, weighed food records, a variant of food diaries, require individuals to measure the precise amounts of food consumed. However, manually maintaining food diaries can be time-intensive and prone to errors, especially when estimating portion sizes.

24-hour Dietary Recall

The 24-hour dietary recall is a widely used method to evaluate food consumption over the previous 24 hours. Traditionally, this method has been conducted in person or over the phone by trained interviewers, providing a snapshot of daily dietary intake.

Food Frequency Questionnaire

FFQs are another popular method for collecting nutritional data. These questionnaires assess the average food intake over a longer reference period, typically weeks or months as shown in Table 1. Unlike food diaries or 24HRs, FFQs focus on the frequency of food consumption rather than portion sizes or quanity. Foods with similar nutritional profiles are grouped into categories, simplifying the evaluation process. FFQs are cost-effective and particularly useful for large-scale studies, although they may sacrifice some accuracy due to reliance on estimated portion sizes. Traditionally administered on paper or via interviews, FFQs have increasingly transitioned to digital formats for improved efficiency.

While food diaries, FFQs, and 24HRs are widely used, they face challenges such as inaccuracies in portion estimation, recall bias, and manual data entry errors. Data quality often declines when food intake is recorded for longer periods, as individuals struggle to recall consumption accurately or estimate portion sizes correctly. Additionally, traditional methods can be time-consuming and labor-intensive.

Table 1. Food Frequency Questionnaire

Foods and Amounts	**Average use in last season**								
Cereals & Grains	Never or less than once/ month	1-3 per month	Once a week	2-4 per week	5-6 per week	Once a day	2-3 per day	4-5 per day	6+ per day
Chapati									
Pearl millet									
Jowar millet									
Rice									
Poha									
Sooji									
Noodles									
White bread									
Brown bread									
Puffed Rice									
Pasta									
Multi grain bread									
Biscuits									
Rusk									

B. Technological Advancements In Dietary Assessment

To address these challenges, modern tools and technologies have been developed to enhance the accuracy and efficiency of dietary assessment. Wearable devices and mobile applications now collect real-time biological and dietary data, providing detailed insights into individual health patterns (Konstantakopoulos et al., 2023; Eldridge et al., 2018). Additionally, multi-omic technologies, such as genomics and metabolomics, facilitate personalized nutrition interventions (Berciano et al., 2022). Automated tools like the Automated Self-Administered 24-hour Dietary Assessment Tool (ASA24) streamline dietary recalls, reduce interviewer-related burdens and improve accessibility.

Food Image Recognition

Food image recognition has revolutionized dietary assessment by utilizing annotated databases to train and evaluate machine learning models for food recognition tasks (Konstantakopoulos, Georga, & Fotiadis, 2023). These annotated collections serve as essential resources, enabling the development of algorithms that accurately identify and classify various food items. The growing field of food computing integrates advanced technologies, such as computer vision, data mining, and machine learning, to process extensive food-related data, including images from the internet, social media, and mobile devices (Bodaghi et al., 2023). These food images are also developed based on the standardization of food recipe process for more accurately of the nutrient estimation as shown in Figure 1. This innovative approach supports key processes such as image segmentation, recognition, and recommendation systems, finding applications across sectors like nutrition research, health monitoring, and the food industry (Picó et al., 2019). These technologies enable tasks such as identifying meal components, estimating portion sizes, and offering dietary recommendations with precision.

Figure 1. Standardized Food Images for Algorithm Development

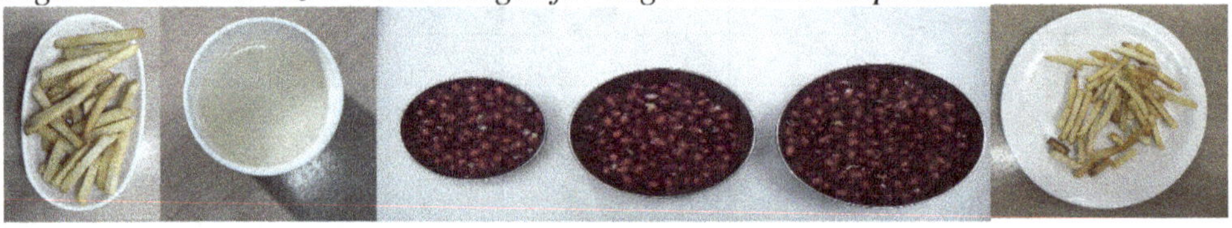

Comprehensive food image databases, including Food-101, UEC-Food100, VIREO Food-172, and UEC-Food256, play a pivotal role in training and benchmarking machine learning models (Konstantakopoulos, Georga, & Fotiadis, 2023). These food image databases represent a broad spectrum of global cuisines and food items, ensuring diverse training data. However, studies have highlighted the need for food image databases that better represent healthy dietary patterns to improve model accuracy (Prosperi et al., 2018).

Food Image Segmentation divides images into distinct segments corresponding to individual food items, a critical step for analyzing meal components. While automated segmentation using deep learning methods has made significant progress, challenges remain with overlapping or irregularly shaped items (Kirk et al., 2022). Food Classification categorizes multiple food items in a single image but can be complicated by poor lighting or unconventional food preparation methods. Additionally, Food Volume Estimation uses various techniques like 3D reconstruction, pre-build shape templates, perspective transformation, depth camera and deep learning for accurately estimating the food volume and analyzing nutrient composition (Dillies et al., 2013). By integrating advanced tools and robust databases, food image recognition continues to transform dietary assessment, providing more accurate and efficient methods for analyzing and improving nutritional habits.

Wearable and Mobile Sensors

Wearable and mobile sensors include non-invasive devices worn as accessories, jewelry, patches, or clothes to sense, track, analyze, and transmit biological data. These devices provide real-time data, helping individuals make informed dietary choices, manage vitals, and address existing conditions. Popular wearables, such as smartwatches (Figure 2), can track calories burned during workouts, heart rate, and sleep patterns (Ambinder, 2005). Biomedical sensors have also replaced manual food diaries which allow users to log nutritional data like food intake, hydration, macronutrients, and energy. Continuous glucose monitors are another technology that aids in managing diabetes through dietary modifications (Bailey, 2021). Recently, low-cost wearable cameras are used as a dietary assessment tool in Africa and showed less errors (Lo et al., 2024). Mobile health encompasses pedometers, menstruation trackers, electronic food tracking apps, and those providing personalized nutrition recommendations and advice (Harvard T.H. Chan School of Public Health, 2024). The functions of mobile health technology include clinical documentation, maintaining patient databases, remote data tracking, real-time chats, and telemedicine. Some apps offer personalized nutritional dietary intake information (North et al., 2015).

Figure 2. Wearable devices

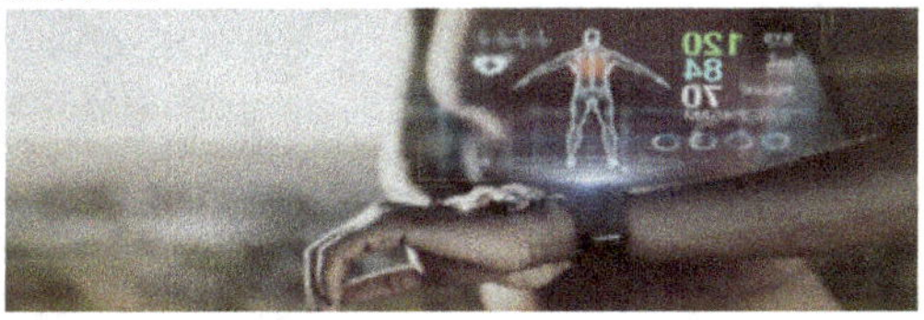

(Source: Adapted from Buttler Technologies, 2023)

In conclusion, the combination of wearable technology and mHealth is advancing the field of nutrition by offering personalized insights and feedback, empowering individuals to make informed dietary choices and achieve desired health outcomes (Joshi et al., 2021).

Another tool used for both data collection and analysis is DietCal. It is a popular software designed by Ms. Gurdeep Kaur, a senior dietitian at AIIMS (All India Institute of Medical Sciences), New Delhi. Besides being a dietary assessment software, it contains a database of Indian recipes and food products, including their nutrient content based on serving and portion sizes. The Food and Agriculture Organization (FAO) has numerous databases, including INFFoods (The International Network of Food Data Systems), which features regional databases, especially for South Asian countries. FAOSTAT (FAO/WHO Global Food and Agriculture Statistical Information System) is another global nutritional database providing information on food security, nutrition trends, food consumption, and trade practices (Chan et al., 2021).

Challenges in Dietary Intake Assessment

Accurately quantifying dietary intake is crucial for understanding diet-health relationships, evaluating the effectiveness of dietary interventions, and formulating dietary guidelines. Traditional self-reported methods, such as 24-hour dietary recall, food frequency questionnaires, and food records, face several limitations, including unintentional under-reporting, intentional misreporting of unhealthy or healthy foods, and errors in portion size estimation (Basiotis et al., 1987; Macdiarmid & Blundell 1998).

The advent of digital dietary assessment tools, particularly food image recognition technology, has improved data collection by enabling near real-time reporting and reducing user burden. These tools also minimize the need for manual portion size estimation. However, challenges remain, particularly in accurately assessing amorphous foods or dishes with hidden ingredients. Image annotation often relies on self-reports, which may be flawed due to participants' limited knowledge of ingredients and preparation methods. Addressing these limitations is essential to enhancing dietary assessment accuracy and supporting evidence-based nutrition recommendations (Howes et al., 2017).

NUTRITION DATA ANALYSIS FOR TAILORING NUTRITION RECOMMENDATIONS

Precision nutrition recognizes the diverse and complex factors influencing human health, including genetic, phenotypic, physiological, medical, lifestyle, and sociocultural determinants. Beyond traditional questionnaire-based dietary assessments, precision nutrition leverages advanced "omics" technologies such as nutrigenomics, metagenomics, and metabolomics to develop tailored dietary interventions that promote health and prevent disease. This approach integrates large-scale data, considering an individual's genomic background, deep phenotyping insights, socioeconomic and psychosocial factors, family history, perinatal nutrition, health status, clinical features (such as circadian rhythm and physical activity), dietary patterns, eating behaviors, and food environments (de Toro-Martín et al., 2017). By incorporating bioinformatics-driven analysis of metabolic pathways, precision nutrition offers a comprehensive framework for personalized dietary support and improved health outcomes.

The shift toward data-driven solutions in nutrition relies heavily on extensive datasets for machines and computers to learn, identify patterns, and provide actionable insights. As data processing capabilities increase, so does the accuracy and effectiveness of technological applications (Géron, 2017). In nutrition, data analysis is pivotal in crafting personalized dietary recommendations to prevent, manage, and treat diseases while enhancing overall health. Emerging tools such as machine learning, artificial intelligence, High-Throughput Sequencing (HTS), and nutrigenomic assessment platforms have revolutionized how nutrition data is analyzed. These advancements enable precise and tailored nutritional interventions (Kirk et al., 2022), fostering a personalized and data-driven approach to dietary health. Table 2 outlines popular platforms that support personalized dietary and behavioral recommendations.

Machine Learning and AI

Machine learning (ML) is increasingly applied in the field of nutrition, particularly in precision nutrition, where personalized recommendations are generated based on individual variables such as anthropometry, biochemical parameters, dietary patterns, lifestyle, metabolic and genetics (Kirk et al., 2022). ML Algorithms analyzes food intake patterns and nutrient deficiencies from food logs, wearable sensors and HER (Bzdok et al., 2018). ML complements generative AI for generating patient summary documents, auto-generating target-specific content, and providing personalized diet and lifestyle recommendations (Tsolakidis et al., 2024; Sebak and Menichetti 2024; Esteva, et al., 2019).

Table 2. Platforms using Advanced Data Analytics for Personalized Nutrition

MyFitnessPal	To track your food, nutrition and exercise
NutriSense	For continuous glucose monitoring and expert guidance on dietary choices
Nutrigenomix	Nutrigenomic based personalised nutrition
Journey Foods	For dietary recommendations and product development
Flovision	Uses data analysis to measure and control food production
DayTwo	Gut-microbiome analysis to provide nutrition tips
Nutrinohealth	Customization of meals using personal data
Foodvisor	Personal nutrition guide using food images recognition
Habitz	Kid-friendly for developing healthy lifestyle habits

continued on following page

Table 2. Continued

HealthifyMe	Improve nutrition by personalized approach
Fooddarzee	Personalized meal delivery plans devised by Nutritionist
NutriAIDE	Track micro and macronutrient content and dynamically calculates the carbon footprint of food choices of an individual to reflect on their eating habits and transform the food behaviour
Nutrify India Now 2.0	provide nutritional information about foods in 17 different Indian languages and provide specific Indian nutrition guidelines
Ntuitive	All-in-one software designed for nutrient analysis and dietary suggestions in India

High-Throughput Sequencing (HTS)

High-Throughput Sequencing (HTS) is an evolving technology that enables parallel DNA sequencing, generating large datasets rapidly and at decreasing costs. Gene sequencing involves studying the arrangement of nucleotides in DNA which forms a basis for diagnosing multiple nutritional disorders, especially inborn errors of metabolism. Huge nutrigenomic datasets can be analyzed through HTS methods. Another great significance of the same is that multiple regions of a genome can be studied which thereby leads to a better understanding of metabolomics, proteomics and transcriptomics.

One of the most common HTS platforms is the *Illumina genome analyzer.* It works by fragmenting DNA into small pieces, attaching special tags, and copying them on a slide. It then reads the sequence of each piece by detecting flashes of light from added nucleotides, which are processed into DNA sequences by analysis with the help of a computer. Other applications are namely, *Roche/454 pyrosequencing* and *ion torrent* (Churko et al., 2013). HTS has transformed nutrition science by revealing how genes and gut bacteria interact with diet, enabling personalized nutrition plans for better health outcomes (Hu et al., 2020; Ringel et al., 2015).

Additionally, High-Throughput Sequencing (HTS) has transformed food safety by enabling near real-time sequencing of marker genes, whole genomes, and transcriptomes of microorganisms with unprecedented precision. This technology not only identifies pathogens but also reveals their virulence and functional traits, offering valuable insights into microbial communities in food and environmental samples. Advanced bioinformatics tools and machine learning algorithms are now used to develop predictive models for tackling foodborne disease outbreaks. Despite its vast potential, HTS integration into food safety systems remains incomplete. While government agencies have adopted HTS for diagnostics, inspections, and outbreak investigations, its adoption by the food industry has been slower and inconsistent. Incorporating HTS into food manufacturers' safety protocols could significantly enhance control measures by providing detailed insights into microbial origins, characteristics, and evolution (Imanian et al., 2022)

High-throughput techniques - OMICS technology

With the advent of such advanced methods in genomics, a field of study known as 'omics' has emerged. Omics encompasses the measurement and analysis of large sets of biomolecules using high-throughput techniques. This category includes several specialized fields:

Genomics is the study of the complete set of genes within an organism, including their structure, function, mapping, sequencing, and interactions with other biomolecules (Venter et al., 2001).

Proteomics involves the large-scale study of proteins, particularly their functions and interactions within a cell or organism (Kumar & Mann, 2009).

Metabolomics focuses on the comprehensive analysis of metabolites—small molecules produced during metabolic reactions (Dunn et al., 2011).

Transcriptomics examines the transcriptome, the complete set of RNA transcripts produced by the genome under specific circumstances or in a specific cell (Wang et al., 2009).

Omics technologies provide a deeper understanding of biological systems by offering insights into gene functions, protein interactions, metabolic processes, and gene expression dynamics. Many compounds derived from food are bioactive and play a role in everyday metabolism, ultimately influencing gene expression. Individuals with certain inborn errors of metabolism may have deficiencies in specific genes, enzymes, or end products, which can lead to intolerance for particular food groups. For example, individuals with phenylketonuria lack phenylalanine hydroxylase (PAH) due to mutations in the PAH gene and are thus unable to metabolize the amino acid phenylalanine (Scriver et al., 2001). Similarly, mutations in the G6PC gene can lead to glycogen storage disease (Hers et al., 2002).

In continuation, nutritional genetics, or nutrigenetics, explores how genetic variations influence individual responses to dietary intake. Studies in personalized and precision nutrition have utilized nutrigenetic approaches to design tailored dietary advice, emphasizing the potential of holistic decision algorithms that integrate genetic, phenotypic, and environmental data for personalized health recommendations (Celis-Morales et al., 2015; de Luis, Izaola, Primo, & Aller, 2018).

Nutrigenomics, also known as nutritional genomics, examines how bioactive dietary components influence gene expression and function, ultimately affecting the proteome and metabolome (Ramos-Lopez et al., 2017). This perspective contrasts with nutrigenetics, which focuses on how genetic variations affect dietary responses (Brennan & de Roos, 2021).

Advancements in nutrigenomics have enhanced our understanding of how specific nutrients and bioactive foods impact metabolic pathways and maintain homeostasis (Ramos-Lopez et al., 2017). Several studies in personalized and precision nutrition have successfully utilized nutrigenomic approaches to develop tailored dietary interventions. Notable examples include: Carbohydrates -The role of sugars in modulating the carbohydrate-responsive element binding protein (ChREBP) gene, influencing glycolysis; Fat - Their impact on peroxisome proliferator-activated receptors (PPARs), which regulate lipid metabolism; and Proteins- Their effect on pathways involving wGCN2/activating transcription factor 4 (ATF4) and mTORC1, essential for lipogenesis regulation (Haro, Marrero, & Relat, 2019).

Disruptions in these metabolic pathways are often linked to metabolic disorders, including obesity, insulin resistance, type 2 diabetes, cardiovascular diseases, and cancer (Haro et al., 2019). Understanding these interactions provides a foundation for developing targeted nutritional strategies to mitigate such health conditions.

Nutrigenomics, or nutritional genomics, studies how bioactive dietary components influence gene expression and function, subsequently affecting the proteome and metabolome (Ramos-Lopez et al., 2017). This assertion statement contrasts with nutrigenetic approaches, where the genotype influences the dietary response (Brennan & de Roos, 2021). Advances in nutrigenomics have provided a greater understanding of the role of different bioactive foods and nutrients on metabolic pathways and homeostatic control (Ramos-Lopez et al., 2017). Several studies of personalized and precision nutrition have used nutrigenomic approaches to design and deliver tailored dietary advice with selected examples. Notable examples of such diet-gene-metabolic homeostasis pathways include the role of sugars on the carbohydrate-responsive element binding protein (ChREBP) gene on glycolysis, fat intake on peroxisome proliferator-activated receptors (PPARs) on lipid metabolism and protein on wGCN2/activating transcription factor 4 (ATF4) and mTORC1 pathways that regulate lipogenesis (Haro, Marrero, & Relat, 2019). Alterations in these pathways are often responsible for the onset of metabolic disturbances such as obesity, insulin resistance, type 2 diabetes, CVD and cancer (Haro et al., 2019). Additionally, nutrition is one of the crucial lifestyle factors associated with epigenetics, which includes the effect of food and nutrient intake on the epigenetic landscape and cell phenotypes. Some of the studies have used nutriepigentics for personalized nutrition (Ramos-Lopez, Samblas, et al., 2018; Arpón et al., 2016).

Transcriptomics is the study of the structure, function, and evolution of the transcriptome (i.e., the entirety of RNA transcripts produced by the genome) of a given organism or community of organisms under a variety of conditions. Changes in non-coding microRNAs, involved in lipid metabolism, can serve as biomarkers for conditions like obesity or metabolic syndrome (Esau et al., 2006).

Metabolomics is an emerging field that comprehensively analyzes dietary metabolites and biomarkers to assess the impact of foods and diets on individuals. Metabolomics, profiling of metabolites in biofluids, cells and tissues is routinely applied as a tool for biomarker description and target discovery, plays a critical role in nutrition research by providing insights into dietary and lifestyle exposures, molecular responses, and diet–microbiota interactions. Metabolomics has shown promise for improving the accuracy of dietary assessment through the identification of biomarkers of food intake and identifying metabolites and metabolic signatures that can serve as targets for interventions (Brennan & de Roos, 2021). These insights enable the development of tailored precision nutrition strategies, offering personalized dietary recommendations for improved health outcomes. (Kortesniemi et al., 2023). Also, it is equally important to understand the influences of socio-cultural factors on diet, a study revealed that migration to the US rapidly alters gut microbiome diversity, while healthy diets are linked to greater microbial diversity and beneficial metabolic functions (Yu et al., 2021).

Recent advancements in metabolomics highlight three key opportunities in nutritional epidemiology: (1) using biomarkers and calibration equations from feeding studies for dietary assessment, (2) classifying dietary patterns through urinary metabolic profiles, and (3) employing metabolome-wide association studies. Studies have used various metabolomics approaches to examine individual response to dietary intake such as postprandial metabolic responses to sequential mixed-nutrient dietary challenges in 1002 healthy UK adults aged 18–65 years (Berry et al., 2020).

Metagenomics involves the comprehensive analysis of microbial and host genetic material (DNA and RNA) directly from patient samples without the need for culturing. The human gastrointestinal tract is home to approximately 10^{13} microorganisms, collectively known as the gut microbiome. One of the most extensive and well-characterized microbiota databases is the Belgium Flemish Gut Flora Project (FGFP), which investigates how factors such as anthropometrics, health, lifestyle, bowel habits, medication, and diet influence gut microbiome variation and its impact on health outcomes (Falony et al., 2016). Notably, fiber consumption was identified as the most significant dietary factor affecting the gut microbiome (Falony et al., 2016), leading to further research in this area (Hughes et al., 2020).

The evolution of "omics" technologies and advancements in big data analytics, particularly machine learning (ML) and artificial intelligence, have significantly improved the understanding of nutrition-related chronic diseases, enabling precise and personalized interventions. ML plays a crucial role in integrating and interpreting multi-"omics" data, including genomics, epigenomics, transcriptomics, proteomics, metabolomics, and metagenomics. Its applications span computational modeling, data mining, sample clustering, and dietary response classification.

INTEGRATING PRECISION NUTRITION ACROSS CLINICAL AND COMMUNITY SETTINGS

Precision nutrition involves customizing dietary recommendations based on an individual's genetics, metabolic responses, microbiomes, lifestyle, health status and behavioral factors. National recommended dietary guidelines offer general *one-size-fits-all* advice for healthy eating, they are often considered "*good but not sufficient*" (Renner et al., 2023). Refining these guidelines by incorporating physiological, biological, social, behavioral, health goals, lifestyle and preferences to food intake allows for more precise, tailored recommendations that support optimal health and prevention & management of diseases. Individual adherence to dietary recommendations can be enhanced by incorporating behavioral factors such as motivation, habits, cultural influences, and psychological barriers. By addressing these elements, tailored recommendations can be developed to improve user engagement and long-term compliance.

For instance, digital tools and platforms can integrate behavior change techniques, including goal setting, real-time feedback, and personalized reminders, to facilitate sustainable dietary changes. These technologies can help individuals stay accountable, track progress, and adjust their nutrition plans based on their evolving needs and preferences, ultimately supporting better adherence to dietary recommendations.

Sustainable nutrition practices can be effectively integrated into precision nutrition, considering that the food system contributes to approximately one-fourth of global carbon emissions. By emphasizing locally sourced and seasonal foods, reducing food waste through efficient utilization of leftovers, limiting the consumption of ultra-processed and resource-intensive foods, and promoting a higher intake of fruits and vegetables, dietary choices can be optimized to support both personal health goals and environmental sustainability.

A precision nutrition approach typically follows key steps:

- Defining an optimal health outcome, whether for disease prevention or enhancing physiological functions
- Gathering objective, valid, and precise measurements
- Integrating diverse data sources for a comprehensive analysis
- Establishing personalized, data-driven dietary goals
- Effectively communicating these personalized goals
- Monitoring progress and making necessary adjustments to achieve the desired outcome

Precision nutrition aims to maintain or improve nutritional status and overall health by supporting behavior change and influencing health outcomes. Today, various personalized nutrition programs are commercially available, utilizing different forms of individual-level data to offer tailored services and products to consumers.

Precision nutrition encompasses a diverse range of approaches that vary in specificity, affordability, accessibility, and availability. In community settings, cost-effective and widely accessible methods such as demographic surveys, national health surveys, disease screening programs, nutrition assessments, and research studies are commonly used to gather population-level data on health and nutritional status. While these approaches provide valuable insights, they lack the specificity as compared to other techniques of precision nutrition. However, they can serve as a foundation for developing personalized dietary recommendations based on individual factors while also supporting community awareness and mobilization efforts.

Integrating precision nutrition into community campaigns can enhance awareness and enable the development of personalized, yet easily accessible, personalized dietary recommendations. Scalable and affordable technologies, including mobile applications, smartwatches, chatbots, image-based food recognition, and tele-nutrition consultations, can play a pivotal role in the community settings. By linking these tools with national health programs, personalized dietary recommendations can be effectively implemented, leading to improved program impact and better health outcomes (Figure 3).

Figure 3. Tool and Methods used for Precision Nutrition

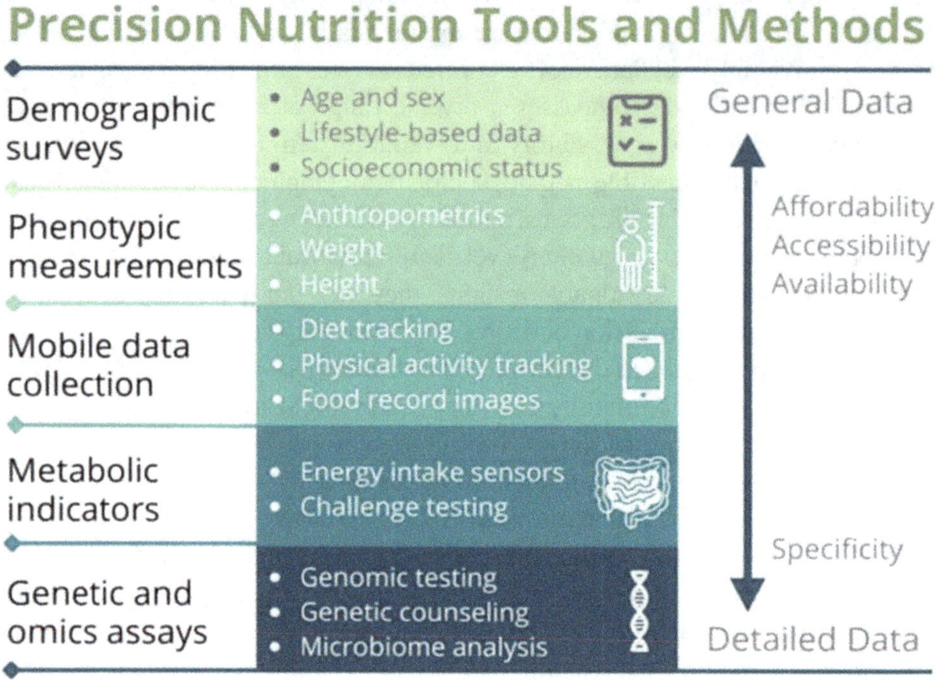

Source: Adapted from Adams et al., 2020 and Gavin-Smith et al. 2022

In contrast, approaches like genetic profiling and microbiome analysis, which offer lesser affordability and accessibility but higher specificity, are primarily applied in clinical settings for disease prevention and management. In clinical dietetics, tools such as Computerized Provider Order Entry (CPOE) and Computerized Decision Support (CDS) systems play a crucial role in delivering precision nutrition within healthcare settings. These systems assist in calculating nutritional needs, generating daily menus, creating dietary prescriptions, and reporting on food lists and menu costs. By automating these processes, CPOE and CDS systems help reduce manual errors and improve the accuracy of nutritional care for hospitalized patients (Devine et al., 2010).

By integrating both specific and general data from various methods and leveraging advanced digital tools, precision nutrition enables the development of well-informed, personalized dietary recommendations that optimize individual health outcomes.

Limitations and challenges

Despite its potential, precision nutrition faces several challenges that hinder its widespread adoption, particularly in low-resource settings. A key limitation is the high cost and limited availability of metabolic, genetic, and biomarker data, restricting access to advanced diagnostic tools. Technological and data integration barriers further complicate implementation, as traditional dietary assessment methods struggle to capture accurate portion sizes, culturally diverse diets and standardized protocols for integrating dietary, genetic, and health data remain lacking (Bedsaul-Fryer et al., 2023).

Additionally, shortages of trained professionals in nutrition informatics, AI, and big data analytics result in inconsistent data collection and interpretation. The absence of reliable biomarkers and inconsistent dietary data documentation further hinder the accuracy of personalized recommendations. Financial constraints, including limited access to wearable sensors, AI-driven food tracking, and mobile health applications, make scaling precision nutrition initiatives difficult. Ethical, cultural, social and behavioral considerations also play a role, as dietary habits are deeply influenced by regional food practices, religious beliefs, accessibility and personal preferences. Electronic documentation has enhanced access to patient health, genomic, and microbiome data; however, concerns persist regarding data privacy, security, ownership, and ethical consent (Paul et al., 2023).

To address these challenges, investment in precision nutrition research, standardized data frameworks, workforce training, and cost-effective technologies are essential. Making precision nutrition tools affordable, accessible, and culturally relevant will be key to its success in improving personalized healthcare and public health outcomes worldwide.

CONCLUSION

India faces the triple burden of malnutrition, driven by dietary shifts, demographic changes, and evolving socioeconomic conditions. The increasing burden of nutrition-related diseases places a significant strain on the healthcare system, emphasizing the urgent need for targeted, data-driven nutritional interventions. Precision nutrition, powered by technological advancements and nutrition informatics, is emerging as a promising approach to address these challenges by enabling personalized, evidence-based dietary recommendations tailored to at-risk subgroups.

This chapter highlights the vast potential of nutritional informatics in transforming data collection, analysis, and application for both public health and clinical nutrition. Traditional dietary assessment methods are now being enhanced by advanced data collection techniques, wearable sensors, and mobile applications, improving the accuracy and reliability of nutritional insights at the community level. In clinical settings, electronic health records (EHRs), omics technologies (genomics, proteomics, metabolomics), and artificial intelligence (AI)-driven analytics are revolutionizing personalized dietary planning. Machine learning and high-throughput sequencing further refine dietary data analysis, enabling deeper insights into individual and subgroup nutritional needs.

Despite these advancements, several challenges remain, including technological limitations, data integration issues, trained professionals, and financial constraints. To fully harness the potential of precision nutrition, it is essential to bridge these gaps by further exploring the potential and improving accessibility, affordability, and scalability, particularly in low-middle income countries. The successful implementation of precision nutrition through nutrition informatics will be a key driver in transitioning from healthcare 5.0 to healthcare 6.0, paving the way for a more personalized, preventive, and efficient healthcare system.

Moving forward, collaborative efforts between health professionals, policymakers, researchers, and technology innovators will be crucial in overcoming existing barriers and making precision nutrition a practical and impactful solution for improving health outcomes on a broader scale.

REFERENCES

Academy of Nutrition and Dietetics. (2019). The NCPT and electronic health records. Electronic Nutrition Care Process Technology (eNCPT). Accessed January 2025 from https://www.ncpro.org/the-ncpt-and-electronic-health-records

Adams, S. H., Anthony, J. C., Carvajal, R., Chae, L., Khoo, C. S. H., Latulippe, M. E., Matusheski, N. V., McClung, H. L., Rozga, M., Schmid, C. H., Wopereis, S., & Yan, W. (2020). Perspective: Guiding principles for the implementation of personalized nutrition approaches that benefit health and function. *Advances in Nutrition*, *11*(1), 25–34. DOI: 10.1093/advances/nmz086 PMID: 31504115

Aebersold, R., & Mann, M. (2003). Mass spectrometry-based proteomics. *Nature*, *422*(6928), 198–207. DOI: 10.1038/nature01511 PMID: 12634793

Ambinder, E. P. (2005). Electronic health records. *Journal of Oncology Practice / American Society of Clinical Oncology*, *1*(2), 57–63. DOI: 10.1200/jop.2005.1.2.57 PMID: 20871681

Arpon, A., Riezu-Boj, J. I., Milagro, F. I., Marti, A., Razquin, C., Martínez-González, M. A., Corella, D., Estruch, R., Casas, R., Fitó, M., Ros, E., Salas-Salvadó, J., & Martínez, J. A. (2016). Adherence to Mediterranean diet is associated with methylation changes in inflammation-related genes in peripheral blood cells. *Journal of Physiology and Biochemistry*, *73*(3), 445–455. DOI: 10.1007/s13105-017-0552-6 PMID: 28181167

Ayres, E. J., & Hoggle, L. B. (2012). 2011 nutrition informatics member survey. *Journal of the Academy of Nutrition and Dietetics*, *112*(3), 360–367. DOI: 10.1016/j.jand.2012.01.003 PMID: 22709663

Bailey, R. L. (2021). Overview of dietary assessment methods for measuring intakes of foods, beverages, and dietary supplements in research studies. *Current Opinion in Biotechnology*, *70*, 91–96. DOI: 10.1016/j.copbio.2021.02.007 PMID: 33714006

Basiotis, P. P., Welsh, S. O., Cronin, F. J., Kelsay, J. L., & Mertz, W. (1987). Number of days of food intake records required to estimate individual and group nutrient intakes with defined confidence. *The Journal of Nutrition*, *117*(9), 1638–1641. DOI: 10.1093/jn/117.9.1638 PMID: 3655942

Bedsaul-Fryer, J. R., van Zutphen-Küffer, K. G., Monroy-Gomez, J., Clayton, D. E., Gavin-Smith, B., Worth, C., Schwab, C. N., Freymond, M., Surowska, A., Bhering Martins, L., Senn-Jakobsen, C., & Kraemer, K. (2023). Precision nutrition opportunities to help mitigate nutrition and health challenges in low-and middle-income countries: An expert opinion survey. *Nutrients, 15*(14), 3247. DOI: 10.3390/nu15143247 PMID: 37513665

Berciano, S., Figueiredo, J., Brisbois, T. D., Alford, S., Koecher, K., Eckhouse, S., Ciati, R., Kussmann, M., Ordovas, J. M., Stebbins, K., & Blumberg, J. B. (2022). Precision nutrition: Maintaining scientific integrity while realizing market potential. *Frontiers in Nutrition, 9*, 979665. DOI: 10.3389/fnut.2022.979665 PMID: 36118748

Berry, S. E., Valdes, A. M., Drew, D. A., Asnicar, F., Mazidi, M., Wolf, J., Capdevila, J., Hadjigeorgiou, G., Davies, R., Al Khatib, H., Bonnett, C., Ganesh, S., Bakker, E., Hart, D., Mangino, M., Merino, J., Linenberg, I., Wyatt, P., Ordovas, J. M., & Spector, T. D. (2020). Human postprandial responses to food and potential for precision nutrition. *Nature Medicine, 26*(6), 964–973. DOI: 10.1038/s41591-020-0934-0 PMID: 32528151

Bodaghi, A., Fattahi, N., & Ramazani, A. (2023). Biomarkers: Promising and valuable tools towards diagnosis, prognosis and treatment of Covid-19 and other diseases. *Heliyon, 9*(2), e13323. DOI: 10.1016/j.heliyon.2023.e13323 PMID: 36744065

Brennan, L., & de Roos, B. (2021). Nutrigenomics: Lessons learned and future perspectives. *The American Journal of Clinical Nutrition, 113*(3), 503–516. DOI: 10.1093/ajcn/nqaa366 PMID: 33515029

Butler Technologies. (2023, June 21). *Help Athletes Perform Better with Biometric Sensors.* Retrieved January 17, 2025, from https://butlertechnologies.com/blog/perform-biosensors

Bzdok, D., Altman, N., & Krzywinski, M. (2018). Statistics versus machine learning. *Nature Methods, 15*(4), 233–234. DOI: 10.1038/nmeth.4642 PMID: 30100822

Celis-Morales, C., Livingstone, K. M., Marsaux, C. F., Forster, H., O'Donovan, C. B., Woolhead, C., Macready, A. L., Fallaize, R., Navas-Carretero, S., San-Cristobal, R., Kolossa, S., Hartwig, K., Tsirigoti, L., Lambrinou, C. P., Moschonis, G., Godlewska, M., Surwiłło, A., Grimaldi, K., Bouwman, J., & Mathers, J. C. (2015). Design and baseline characteristics of the Food4Me study: A web-based randomised controlled trial of personalised nutrition in seven European countries. *Genes & Nutrition, 10*(1), 1–13. DOI: 10.1007/s12263-014-0450-2 PMID: 25491748

Chan, L., Vasilevsky, N., Thessen, A., McMurry, J., & Haendel, M. (2021). The landscape of nutri-informatics: A review of current resources and challenges for integrative nutrition research. *Database : The Journal of Biological Databases and Curation, 2021*, baab003. DOI: 10.1093/database/baab003 PMID: 33494105

Churko, J. M., Mantalas, G. L., Snyder, M. P., & Wu, J. C. (2013). Overview of high throughput sequencing technologies to elucidate molecular pathways in cardiovascular diseases. *Circulation Research, 112*(12), 1613–1623. DOI: 10.1161/CIRCRESAHA.113.300939 PMID: 23743227

Daytwo. Accessed on 10th January 2025 from https://www.daytwo.com/

de Luis, D. A., Izaola, O., Primo, D., & Aller, R. (2018). Role of rs670 variant of APOA1 gene on lipid profile, insulin resistance and adipokine levels in obese subjects after weight loss with a dietary intervention. *Diabetes Research and Clinical Practice, 142*, 139–145. DOI: 10.1016/j.diabres.2018.05.040 PMID: 29859275

Devine, E. B., Hansen, R. N., Wilson-Norton, J. L., Lawless, N. M., Fisk, A. W., Blough, D. K., Martin, D. P., & Sullivan, S. D. (2010). The impact of computerized provider order entry on medication errors in a multispecialty group practice. *Journal of the American Medical Informatics Association : JAMIA, 17*(1), 78–84. DOI: 10.1197/jamia.M3285 PMID: 20064806

Dillies, M. A., Rau, A., Aubert, J., Hennequet-Antier, C., Jeanmougin, M., Servant, N., Keime, C., Marot, G., Castel, D., Estelle, J., Guernec, G., Jagla, B., Jouneau, L., Laloe, D., Le Gall, C., Schaeffer, B., Le Crom, S., Guedj, M., & Jaffrézic, F. (2013). A comprehensive evaluation of normalization methods for Illumina high-throughput RNA sequencing data analysis. *Briefings in Bioinformatics, 14*(6), 671–683. DOI: 10.1093/bib/bbs046 PMID: 22988256

Dunn, W. B., Broadhurst, D., Begley, P., Zelena, E., Francis-McIntyre, S., Anderson, N., Brown, M., Knowles, J. D., Halsall, A., Haselden, J. N., Nicholls, A. W., Wilson, I. D., Kell, D. B., & Goodacre, R.Human Serum Metabolome (HUSERMET) Consortium. (2011). Procedures for large-scale metabolic profiling of serum and plasma using gas chromatography and liquid chromatography coupled to mass spectrometry. *Nature Protocols, 6*(7), 1060–1083. DOI: 10.1038/nprot.2011.335 PMID: 21720319

Eldridge, A. L., Piernas, C., Illner, A. K., Gibney, M. J., Gurinović, M. A., De Vries, J. H., & Cade, J. E. (2018). Evaluation of new technology-based tools for dietary intake assessment—An ILSI Europe Dietary Intake and Exposure Task Force evaluation. *Nutrients, 11*(1), 55. DOI: 10.3390/nu11010055 PMID: 30597864

Esau, C., Davis, S., Murray, S. F., Yu, X. X., Pandey, S. K., Pear, M., Watts, L., Booten, S. L., Graham, M., McKay, R., Subramaniam, A., Propp, S., Lollo, B. A., Freier, S., Bennett, C. F., Bhanot, S., & Monia, B. P. (2006). miR-122 regulation of lipid metabolism revealed by in vivo antisense targeting. *Cell Metabolism, 3*(2), 87–98. DOI: 10.1016/j.cmet.2006.01.005 PMID: 16459310

Esteva, A., Robicquet, A., Ramsundar, B., Kuleshov, V., DePristo, M., Chou, K., Cui, C., Corrado, G., Thrun, S., & Dean, J. (2019). A guide to deep learning in healthcare. *Nature Medicine, 25*(1), 24–29. DOI: 10.1038/s41591-018-0316-z PMID: 30617335

Falony, G., Joossens, M., Vieira-Silva, S., Wang, J., Darzi, Y., Faust, K., Kurilshikov, A., Bonder, M. J., Valles-Colomer, M., Vandeputte, D., Tito, R. Y., Chaffron, S., Rymenans, L., Verspecht, C., De Sutter, L., Lima-Mendez, G., D'hoe, K., Jonckheere, K., Homola, D., & Raes, J. (2016). Population-level analysis of gut microbiome variation. *Science, 352*(6285), 560–564. DOI: 10.1126/science.aad3503 PMID: 27126039

FloVision. Accessed on 15th January 2025 from https://flovisionsolutions.com/

Fooddarzee. Accessed on 15th January 2025 from https://fooddarzee.com/bengaluru

Foodvisor. Accessed on 15th January 2025 from https://www.foodvisor.io/en/

Gavin-Smith, B. (2022). Precision nutrition for low-and middle-income countries: Hype or hope? *Sight and Life Special Report., 2022*, 1–95. DOI: 10.52439/PRCJ5543

Géron, A. (2017). *Concepts, tools, and techniques to build intelligent systems. Hands-On Machine Learning with Scikit-Learn, Keras, and TensorFlow* (2nd ed.). O'Reilly Media.

Global Hunger Index. (October 2024). How gender justice can advance climate resilience and zero hunger. Global Hunger Index. Accessed from file:///C:/Users/IIHMRB31669/Downloads/2024.pdf Habitz. Accessed on 15th January 2025 from https://habitz.com/

Haro, D., Marrero, P. F., & Relat, J. (2019). Nutritional regulation of gene expression: Carbohydrate-, fat-and amino acid-dependent modulation of transcriptional activity. *International Journal of Molecular Sciences, 20*(6), 1386. DOI: 10.3390/ijms20061386 PMID: 30893897

Harvard, T. H. Chan School of Public Health. (2024). Precision nutrition: The Nutrition Source. Harvard T.H. Chan School of Public Health. Retrieved July 30, 2024, from https://nutritionsource.hsph.harvard.edu/precision-nutrition/

Harvard Library. (2024). Harvard Dataverse*: A repository for research data*. Harvard Library https://library.harvard.edu/services-tools/harvard-dataverse

HealthifyMe. Retrieved January 10, 2025 https://www.healthifyme.com/in/

Hoggle, L. B., Nash, D. B., & Teitelbaum, H. S. (2006). Nutrition informatics. *Journal of the American Dietetic Association, 106*(1), 134–139. DOI: 10.1016/j.jada.2005.10.025 PMID: 16390678

Howes, E., Boushey, C. J., Kerr, D. A., Tomayko, E. J., & Cluskey, M. (2017). Image-based dietary assessment ability of dietetics students and interns. *Nutrients*, *9*(2), 114. DOI: 10.3390/nu9020114 PMID: 28178196

Hu, J., Zhong, X., Yan, J., Zhou, D., Qin, D., Xiao, X., Zheng, Y., & Liu, Y. (2020). High-throughput sequencing analysis of intestinal flora changes in ESRD and CKD patients. *BMC Nephrology*, *21*(1), 1–11. DOI: 10.1186/s12882-019-1668-4 PMID: 31931722

Hughes, D. A., Bacigalupe, R., Wang, J., Rühlemann, M. C., Tito, R. Y., Falony, G., Joossens, M., Vieira-Silva, S., Henckaerts, L., Rymenans, L., Verspecht, C., Ring, S., Franke, A., Wade, K. H., Timpson, N. J., & Raes, J. (2020). Genome-wide associations of human gut microbiome variation and implications for causal inference analyses. *Nature Microbiology*, *5*(9), 1079–1087. DOI: 10.1038/s41564-020-0743-8 PMID: 32572223

Imanian, B., Donaghy, J., Jackson, T., Gummalla, S., Ganesan, B., Baker, R. C., ... & Wan, J. (2022). The power, potential, benefits, and challenges of implementing high-throughput sequencing in food safety systems. *npj Science of Food, 6*(1), 35.

Institute for Health Metrics and Evaluation (IHME). (2024). *Global Burden of Disease 2021: Findings from the GBD 2021 Study*. IHME.

International Institute for Population Sciences (IIPS) & ICF. (2021). *National Family Health Survey (NFHS-5), 2019-21: India: Volume I.* Mumbai, India: IIPS.

International Institute for Population Sciences (IIPS), National Programme for Health Care of Elderly (NPHCE), Ministry of Health and Family Welfare. (MoHFW), Harvard T. H. Chan School of Public Health (HSPH), & University of Southern California (USC). (2020). *Longitudinal Ageing Study in India (LASI) Wave 1, 2017-18, India report.* International Institute for Population Sciences.

Joshi, A., Gaba, A., Thakur, S., & Grover, A. (2021). Need and importance of nutrition informatics in India: A perspective. *Nutrients, 13*(6), 1836. DOI: 10.3390/nu13061836 PMID: 34072133

Journey Foods. Accessed on 15th February 2025 from https://www.journeyfoods.io/

Kirk, D., Kok, E., Tufano, M., Tekinerdogan, B., Feskens, E. J., & Camps, G. (2022). Machine learning in nutrition research. *Advances in Nutrition*, *13*(6), 2573–2589. DOI: 10.1093/advances/nmac103 PMID: 36166846

Konstantakopoulos, F. S., Georga, E. I., & Fotiadis, D. I. (2023). A review of image-based food recognition and volume estimation artificial intelligence systems. *IEEE Reviews in Biomedical Engineering*, *17*, 136–152. DOI: 10.1109/RBME.2023.3283149 PMID: 37276096

Kortesniemi, M., Noerman, S., Kårlund, A., Raita, J., Meuronen, T., Koistinen, V., Landberg, R., & Hanhineva, K. (2023). Nutritional metabolomics: Recent developments and future needs. *Current Opinion in Chemical Biology*, *77*, 102400. DOI: 10.1016/j.cbpa.2023.102400 PMID: 37804582

Kumar, C., & Mann, M. (2009). Bioinformatics analysis of mass spectrometry-based proteomics data sets. *FEBS Letters*, *583*(11), 1703–1712. DOI: 10.1016/j.febslet.2009.03.035 PMID: 19306877

Lo, F. P. W., Qiu, J., Jobarteh, M. L., Sun, Y., Wang, Z., Jiang, S., & Lo, B. (2024). AI-enabled wearable cameras for assisting dietary assessment in African populations. *npj. Digital Medicine*, *7*(1), 1–16. PMID: 38172429

Longvah, T., Ananthan, R., Bhaskarachary, K., & Venkaiah, K. (2017). *Indian Food Composition Tables 2017, National Institute of Nutrition, Indian Council of Medical Research*. Telangana, India.

Macdiarmid, J., & Blundell, J. (1998). Assessing dietary intake: Who, what and why of under-reporting. *Nutrition Research Reviews*, *11*(2), 231–253. DOI: 10.1079/NRR19980017 PMID: 19094249

Ministry of Health and Family Welfare (MoHFW). Government of India, UNICEF, & Population Council. (2019). *Comprehensive National Nutrition Survey (CNNS) National Report*. New Delhi, India. Ministry of Women and Child Development, Government of India. A Complete Guide- Poshan Tracker. Retrieved January 17, 2025, from https://www.poshantracker.in/pdf/Resources/ACompleteGuide-PoshanTracker.pdf

MyFitnessPal. Accessed on January 10, 2025 from https://www.myfitnesspal.com/

National Institute of Nutrition (NIN). (2017). Diet and nutritional status of urban population in India and prevalence of obesity, hypertension, diabetes and hyperlipidemia in urban men and women - A brief *NNMB urban nutrition report. Technical Report No. 27.* Retrieved January 17, 2025, from https://www.nin.res.in/downloads/NNMB%20Urban%20Nutrition%20Report%20-Brief%20%20%20report.pdf

North, J. C., Jordan, K. C., Metos, J., & Hurdle, J. F. (2015). Nutrition informatics applications in clinical practice: A systematic review. AMIA Annual Symposium Proceedings, 963–972. https://www.ncbi.nlm.nih.gov/pmc/articles/PMC4765562/

Ntuitive. Accessed on January 10th 2025 from https://www.ntuitive.in/

Nutri, A. I. D. E. Accessed on January 10th 2025 from https://wupperinst.org/en/p/wi/p/s/pd/2292

Nutrify India Now 2.0. Accessed on January 10th 2025 from https://nutrifyindianow.in/

Nutrigenomix. Accessed on January 10th 2025 from https://nutrigenomix.com/

Nutrinohealth. Accessed on January 15th 2025 from https://www.nutrinohealth.com/about/

Nutrisense. Accessed on January 15th 2025 from https://www.nutrisense.io/nutritionist#specialties

Office of the Registrar General & Census Commissioner. India. (2020). Sample Registration System (SRS)-Statistical Report 2020. India, 2022. Accessed from https://censusindia.gov.in/nada/index.php/catalog/44376

Paul, M., Maglaras, L., Ferrag, M. A., & Almomani, I. (2023). Digitization of healthcare sector: A study on privacy and security concerns. *ICT Express*, *9*(4), 571–588. DOI: 10.1016/j.icte.2023.02.007

Picó, C., Serra, F., Rodríguez, A. M., Keijer, J., & Palou, A. (2019). Biomarkers of nutrition and health: New tools for new approaches. *Nutrients*, *11*(5), 1092. DOI: 10.3390/nu11051092 PMID: 31100942

Prosperi, M., Min, J. S., Bian, J., & Modave, F. (2018). Big data hurdles in precision medicine and precision public health. *BMC Medical Informatics and Decision Making*, *18*(1), 1–15. DOI: 10.1186/s12911-018-0719-2 PMID: 30594159

Ramos-Lopez, O., Milagro, F. I., Allayee, H., Chmurzynska, A., Choi, M. S., Curi, R., De Caterina, R., Ferguson, L. R., Goni, L., Kang, J. X., Kohlmeier, M., Marti, A., Moreno, L. A., Pérusse, L., Prasad, C., Qi, L., Reifen, R., Riezu-Boj, J. I., San-Cristobal, R., & Martínez, J. A. (2017). Guide for current nutrigenetic, nutrigenomic, and nutriepigenetic approaches for precision nutrition involving the prevention and management of chronic diseases associated with obesity. *Lifestyle Genomics*, *10*(1-2), 43–62. DOI: 10.1159/000477729 PMID: 28689206

Ramos-Lopez, O., Samblas, M., Milagro, F. I., Riezu-Boj, J. I., Crujeiras, A. B., Martinez, J. A., & Project, M. E. N. A. (2018). Circadian gene methylation profiles are associated with obesity, metabolic disturbances and carbohydrate intake. *Chronobiology International*, *35*(7), 969–981. DOI: 10.1080/07420528.2018.1446021 PMID: 29580070

Renner, B., Buyken, A. E., Gedrich, K., Lorkowski, S., Watzl, B., Linseisen, J., Daniel, H., Conrad, J., Ferrario, P. G., Holzapfel, C., Leitzmann, M., Richter, M., Simon, M.-C., Sina, C., & Wirsam, J. (2023). Perspective: A conceptual framework for adaptive personalized nutrition advice systems (APNASs). *Advances in Nutrition*, *14*(5), 983–994. DOI: 10.1016/j.advnut.2023.06.009 PMID: 37419418

Riboli, E., Hunt, K. J., Slimani, N., Ferrari, P., Norat, T., Fahey, M., Charrondière, U. R., Hémon, B., Casagrande, C., Vignat, J., Overvad, K., Tjønneland, A., Clavel-Chapelon, F., Thiébaut, A., Wahrendorf, J., Boeing, H., Trichopoulos, D., Trichopoulou, A., Vineis, P., & Saracci, R. (2002). European Prospective Investigation into Cancer and Nutrition (EPIC): Study populations and data collection. *Public Health Nutrition*, *5*(6b), 1113–1124. DOI: 10.1079/PHN2002394 PMID: 12639222

Ringel, Y., Maharshak, N., Ringel-Kulka, T., Wolber, E. A., Sartor, R. B., & Carroll, I. M. (2015). High throughput sequencing reveals distinct microbial populations within the mucosal and luminal niches in healthy individuals. *Gut Microbes*, *6*(3), 173–181. DOI: 10.1080/19490976.2015.1044711 PMID: 25915459

Rusnak, S., & Charney, P. (2019). Position of the Academy of Nutrition and Dietetics: Nutrition informatics. *Journal of the Academy of Nutrition and Dietetics*, *119*(8), 1375–1382. DOI: 10.1016/j.jand.2019.06.004 PMID: 31353011

Scriver, C. R., Beaudet, A. L., Sly, W. S., Valle, D., Childs, B., Kinzler, K. W., & Vogelstein, B. (Eds.). (2001). The metabolic and molecular bases of inherited disease (8th ed.). McGraw-Hill. Biochemistry (Moscow), *67*(5), 611–612.https://doi.org/ DOI: 10.1023/A:1017418800320

Sebek, M., & Menichetti, G. (2024). Network Science and Machine Learning for Precision Nutrition. In *Precision Nutrition* (pp. 367–402). Academic Press. DOI: 10.1016/B978-0-443-15315-0.00012-2

Tsai, J., & Bond, G. R. (2008). A comparison of electronic records to paper records in mental health centers. *International Journal for Quality in Health Care : Journal of the International Society for Quality in Health Care*, *20*(2), 136–143. DOI: 10.1093/intqhc/mzm064 PMID: 18079127

Tsolakidis, D., Gymnopoulos, L. P., & Dimitropoulos, K. (2024, August). Artificial Intelligence and Machine Learning Technologies for Personalized Nutrition: A Review. [). MDPI.]. *Informatics (MDPI)*, *11*(3), 62. DOI: 10.3390/informatics11030062

United Nations Development Programme. (2024). Global Multidimensional Poverty Index 2024: Poverty amid conflict. Accessed from https://hdr.undp.org/system/files/documents/hdp-document/mpireport2024en.pdf

Venter, J. C., Adams, M. D., Myers, E. W., Li, P. W., Mural, R. J., Sutton, G. G., Smith, H. O., Yandell, M., Evans, C. A., Holt, R. A., Gocayne, J. D., Amanatides, P., Ballew, R. M., Huson, D. H., Wortman, J. R., Zhang, Q., Kodira, C. D., Zheng, X. H., Chen, L., & Zhu, X. (2001). The sequence of the human genome. *Science*, *291*(5507), 1304–1351. DOI: 10.1126/science.1058040 PMID: 11181995

Wang, Z., Gerstein, M., & Snyder, M. (2009). RNA-Seq: A revolutionary tool for transcriptomics. *Nature Reviews. Genetics*, *10*(1), 57–63. DOI: 10.1038/nrg2484 PMID: 19015660

Yu, D., Yang, Y., Long, J., Xu, W., Cai, Q., Wu, J., Cai, H., Zheng, W., & Shu, X. O. (2021). Long-term diet quality and gut microbiome functionality: A prospective, shotgun metagenomic study among urban Chinese adults. *Current Developments in Nutrition*, *5*(4), nzab026. DOI: 10.1093/cdn/nzab026 PMID: 33937616

Chapter 13
Securing Patient Rights and Safety in a Digitally Transformed Healthcare Environment

Sudamini Saproo
IQVIA, India

Parul Goela
https://orcid.org/0009-0004-4699-4087
IQVIA, India

Jayathra Datla
https://orcid.org/0009-0002-9442-7680
IQVIA, India

Kanishak Gautam
https://orcid.org/0009-0006-0073-0152
IQVIA, India

ABSTRACT

The healthcare industry is transforming with advanced technologies like EHRs, telemedicine, and AI, promising improved patient outcomes and streamlined processes. However, increased digitization has led to a surge in data breaches, exposing vulnerabilities and raising concerns about patient data confidentiality. Regulatory frameworks struggle to keep up with rapid technological changes, highlighting significant gaps. This chapter calls for a holistic approach to protect patient rights, proposing robust policies, advanced technology use, and ongoing staff training. Key findings include a 42% rise in breaches, regulatory non-compliance, and underused

DOI: 10.4018/979-8-3693-7210-4.ch013

AI security solutions. Emphasizing stringent regulations, encryption, and ethical data management, it aims to integrate innovation with oversight to safeguard patient information and trust.

INTRODUCTION

In the ever-evolving landscape of modern healthcare, the infusion of digital technology promises transformative advancements alongside formidable challenges. This paradigm shift necessitates a nuanced understanding and proactive management to maximize benefits while mitigating the risks that are posed by the digitization of healthcare industry.

Digital technology has evolved significantly over time and, since its introduction to the healthcare industry, has revolutionized patient care and operational efficiency. Key advancements include enhanced patient care through technologies such as electronic health records (EHRs) and telemedicine, which have improved the quality and accessibility of care. Additionally, digital technology has improved operational efficiency through automation and data analysis, streamlining administrative tasks and clinical workflows, reducing errors, and increasing productivity. Concurring to a study published in the Journal of the American Medical Association, the execution of EHRs has diminished pharmaceutical mistakes by 55% (Bates et al., 1998). Furthermore, digitization has advanced the diagnosis and treatment of diseases at early stages using artificial intelligence (AI) and machine learning (ML) algorithms.

However, despite the benefits that come with the digitization of the healthcare industry, there are risks involved that force us to weigh whether the adoption of digital technology in healthcare is a wise decision. One of the foremost challenges is the data security and privacy of patients. The exponential growth in digital data storage and transmission heightens vulnerabilities to data breaches and unauthorized access. Protecting this sensitive health information across diverse platforms and interconnected systems presents an ongoing challenge, demanding robust cybersecurity measures and stringent privacy protocols.

Another major challenge is the vulnerability to cyber-attacks. Organizations in the healthcare domain are prime targets of cybercriminal activities. The proliferation of malware and ransomware poses significant threats to the data integrity and operational stability of organizations. A survey by the Ponemon Institute reported that 83% of healthcare organizations experienced a data breach in 2021 (Burks, n.d.). The IBM Cost of a Data Breach Report 2024 states that, for the 14th straight year, healthcare had the highest average breach recovery cost at $9.77 million (Bonderud, 2024).

Additionally, interoperability i.e. seamless communication and data exchange among disparate systems, devices, and applications remain elusive due to a lack of standardized protocols. This fragmentation compromises cohesive patient-centred care, making it troublesome to coordinated different perspectives of healthcare administrations viably.

Regulatory compliance is another critical challenge. Adhering to stringent data protection regulations such as Health Insurance Portability and Accountability Act (HIPAA) in the United States or General Data Protection Regulation (GDPR) in Europe imposes substantial operational and financial burdens on healthcare organizations. Non-compliance risks legal repercussions and damages to institutional reputation, underscoring the importance of rigorous adherence and proactive governance frameworks.

These are just a few disadvantages of the digitization of the healthcare industry. However, it is crucial to consider that the data extracted from patients is highly sensitive information. This data should not be used for any purpose without the explicit consent of the patient, and when used, it should be done transparently so that the patient is always aware of how their information is being utilized (General Data Protection Regulation (GDPR) – Legal Text, 2024).

Furthermore, it is within the rights of patients to request for the deletion of their data at any time. Regulations such as the GDPR in Europe and California Privacy Protection Agency (CPPA) in the United States are instrumental in highlighting and protecting the rights of patients, ensuring their data is handled with the utmost care and respect.

While the adoption of digital technology in healthcare offers numerous advantages, it also presents significant challenges that must be carefully managed. In alignment with the focus of healthcare 6.0 that aims to adopt innovative technologies for improved healthcare, the objective of this chapter is to focus on ensuring patients' rights and safety in a tech-driven healthcare environment. When incorporating new technology into healthcare, it is essential to balance improved patient care and operational efficiency with the need for robust data security, seamless compatibility with existing systems, and strict adherence to regulatory standards. Hence it is essential for the health professionals and industry experts to have a comprehensive understanding of the current patient safety and security practices to leverage their way efficiently. This ensures the effective adoption of innovative technologies that enhance healthcare delivery while safeguarding patient information and complying with legal requirements.

IMPACT OF DIGITIZATION ON HEALTHCARE

The digitization of healthcare has brought about profound changes, enhanced patient care and operational efficiency while presenting new challenges. This section explores the impact of digitization through three key areas: Electronic Health Records (EHRs), telemedicine, and AI-powered diagnostic tools.

Evolution of Electronic Health Records (EHRs)

Electronic Health Records (EHRs) have evolved significantly since their inception in the late 20th century, becoming a cornerstone of modern healthcare. Initially introduced to replace paper-based records, EHRs now offer a comprehensive digital solution for storing and managing patient information. The shift from paper to digital has streamlined workflows, increased accuracy, and improved accessibility. According to a study by the National Institutes of Health, the adoption of EHRs has led to a 55% reduction in medication errors and a 30% increase in preventive care measures among patients (Menachemi & Collum, 2011).

One of the most compelling findings of the studies on EHR relates to the role of decision support systems in improving patient safety, particularly in medication prescribing. Research has demonstrated that EHRs equipped with decision support features reduce the incidence of drug-drug interactions and medication errors. Automated dosage calculators have further contributed to reducing dosage errors, while also improving medication adherence and minimizing overuse of medications.

More recent studies have integrated decision support algorithms with electronic surveillance technologies (Manaktala & Claypool, 2016), leading to clinical alerts that have significantly improved inpatient sepsis management and reduced sepsis-related mortality. EHRs also enhance the communication and management of clinical information for both healthcare providers and patients. For instance, EHRs have been shown to reduce prescribing errors, even without the use of decision support systems. These systems help eliminate basic communication errors, such as those caused by illegible handwriting. They also improve the clarity of complex medical orders, make it easier for providers to access patient information, and enhance patient satisfaction by offering clearer instructions for post-acute recovery. Some studies suggest that patient portals can improve screening rates, although evidence from both observational studies and randomized controlled trials (RCTs) remains inconclusive (Atasoy et al., 2018). In addition to improving clinical care outcomes, EHR systems can impact the cost and efficiency of healthcare organizations and the broader healthcare system. By automating existing processes, enhancing the management of medical practices and chronic care, and facilitating integration and communication within and between healthcare organizations, EHRs can lead to reduced costs and increased productivity (Hillestad et al., 2005).

Despite these benefits, challenges remain. Issues such as data interoperability, system integration, and user training can impact the effectiveness of EHRs. The lack of standardized protocols often hampers the seamless exchange of information between different systems, affecting the overall efficiency and quality of care. Other challenges include disruptions to organizational workflows, system failures, difficulties in maintaining up-to-date best practices, resistance to change from users, and other issues that are often specific to the hospital environment.

Telemedicine: Expanding Access to Care

The emergence of telemedicine has ushered in a new era of healthcare delivery, providing numerous opportunities to improve patient outcomes and broaden access to care (Ezeamii et al., 2024). Telemedicine has become a force of transformation in healthcare, particularly in providing access to care for the underserved populations. By leveraging digital communication tools, telemedicine enables patients to consult with healthcare providers remotely, reducing barriers such as distance and transportation. A study by the American Telemedicine Association highlighted that telemedicine consultations increased by 154% from 2019 to 2020, driven largely by the COVID-19 pandemic (American Telemedicine Association - ATA, 2024). The global telehealth market is projected to grow significantly, reaching USD 55.6 billion by 2025, up from USD 25.4 billion in 2020 (Rawat, 2024). Post-COVID trends reveal that telehealth services have been adopted at varying levels across the 195 countries worldwide. Specifically, 13.8% have adopted advanced telehealth services, 10.3% are at a developed stage, 12.3% are at a developing level, and 3% are at an emerging level. Australia, Japan, Canada, the United States, New Zealand, and the United Kingdom have advanced telehealth utilization, driven by government efforts and regulatory adjustments in their well-resourced health sectors. These high-income countries face minimal infrastructure challenges. In contrast, developing and low-income countries, particularly in Africa, struggle with rigid regulations and limited infrastructure. India is an exception among developing countries, showing significant progress in telehealth adoption (Ndwabe et al., 2023).

Telemedicine has proven to be a transformative tool in managing chronic diseases. Significant improvements in patient health outcomes and cost savings have been observed with telemedicine interventions. For instance, telehealth platforms boost diabetes management by increasing patient engagement and improving clinical indicators like HbA1c levels. Telehealth services for chronic disease management help overcome geographical barriers, offering specialized care and enhancing both patient access and satisfaction. Additionally, telemedicine has the potential to reduce administrative healthcare costs, making it an economically efficient approach. While this increased accessibility can boost patient engagement, digital health in chronic disease management also faces several limitations. (Patel et al., 2024; Zakaria et al., 2024). It raises concerns regarding data privacy, access to technology, and the quality of remote care.

Telemedicine is not a replacement for the conventional healthcare system but rather complements it for certain functions. A significant concern is the risk of hacking and data breaches, especially if patients access telemedicine services through public networks or unencrypted channels. In emergencies, telemedicine can cause delays in critical care, as doctors cannot administer life-saving treatments or conduct laboratory tests remotely. Additionally, state regulations vary, and physicians may be restricted from practicing across state lines depending on where they are licensed and where the patient resides. Clinicians must also ensure that the telemedicine platforms they use comply with privacy laws and maintain security.

During telemedicine sessions, providers must rely on patient self-reports, often requiring additional questioning to gather a complete medical history. If a patient overlooks an important symptom, it could jeopardize their treatment plan. One of the most significant challenges is the lack of availability and affordability of telemedicine services. Setting up and managing telemedicine systems can be costly, and smaller healthcare facilities may find it financially prohibitive. Additionally, poor communication during virtual consultations can hinder the delivery of reliable care (Haleem et al., 2021).

Ensuring that telemedicine platforms adhere to strict privacy standards and providing adequate training for both patients and providers are crucial for addressing these challenges.

AI-Powered Diagnostic Tools and Their Implications

Artificial Intelligence (AI) has made remarkable progress in healthcare, especially in the realm of diagnostic tools. AI-driven algorithms can handle broad datasets to help in diagnosing therapeutic conditions, estimating results, and fitting treatment plans. For instance, some AI systems have demonstrated diagnostic accuracy comparable to or even surpassing that of human radiologists in identifying conditions such as breast cancer and diabetic retinopathy.

Although these advancements offer promising improvements in diagnostic precision and patient care, they also bring about ethical and practical challenges. Issues such as algorithmic bias, transparency, and the necessity for thorough validation are crucial as AI technologies become increasingly embedded in clinical settings. Addressing these concerns is vital to ensure that AI tools are developed and deployed effectively, optimizing their advantages while mitigating potential risks. As per Figure 1 we observe what are the imapcts of digitization on healthcare.

Figure 1. Impact of digitization

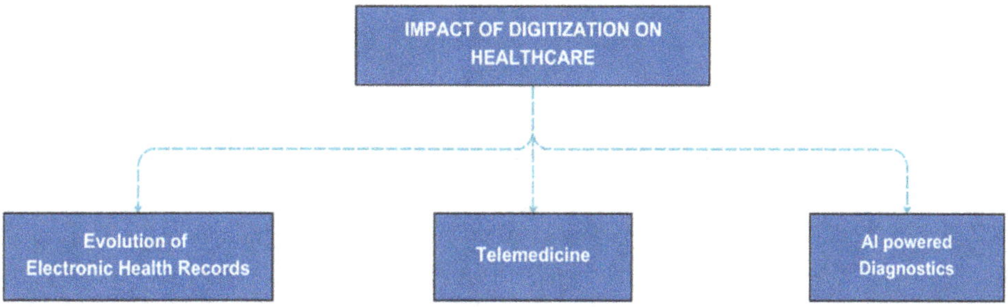

ETHICAL AND REGULATORY CONSIDERATIONS

As digital technology continues to reshape healthcare, ethical and regulatory considerations play a crucial role in guiding the responsible use of technology. This section explores three key areas: ethical principles in healthcare data management, current regulatory frameworks and their limitations, and case studies of data breaches and their impact on patient trust.

Ethical Principles in Healthcare Data Management

Ethical principles in healthcare data management revolve around safeguarding patient privacy, ensuring informed consent, and maintaining transparency. One fundamental principle is the respect for patient autonomy, which requires obtaining explicit consent before collecting, using, or sharing personal health information. According to the American Medical Association, maintaining transparency about how patient data is used and providing clear options for consent are essential for upholding ethical standards and respecting the decisions of patients (AMA-Code Homepage, n.d.).

Another key principle is the confidentiality of patient data. Ensuring that personal health information is protected from unauthorized access and breaches is critical for maintaining patient trust (AMA-Code Homepage, n.d.). This involves implementing robust data security measures and regularly auditing data management practices to prevent unauthorized access. Ethical data management also requires addressing issues related to algorithmic bias and ensuring that AI and other technologies do not perpetuate disparities in healthcare. All these measures ensure that the privacy and safety of patients is maintained. Thus, respecting the autonomy of patients over their data and maintaining the privacy of the data collected from patients are the primary ethical principles which must be upheld when using digital technology in healthcare industry.

Existing Regulatory Frameworks and Their Limitations

The Current regulatory frameworks designed to protect patient data and ensure privacy are well-established in the United States and Europe. Regulations like the Health Insurance Portability and Accountability Act (HIPAA) in the United States and the General Data Protection Regulation (GDPR) in Europe set important standards for data protection and patient rights. HIPAA enforces safeguards for protected health information (PHI) and mandates security measures to prevent breaches, while GDPR grants comprehensive data protection rights, including access and deletion of personal data (General Data Protection Regulation (GDPR) – Legal Text, 2024).

However, these frameworks have limitations that can affect their effectiveness. Despite their robust protections, they may not fully address the challenges posed by rapidly advancing technology. For instance, the emergence of big data and AI introduces complexities that current regulations might not entirely cover. Moreover, compliance with these regulations can be particularly burdensome for smaller organizations, which may struggle with implementing consistent privacy measures. As technology evolves rapidly, keeping regulations updated becomes increasingly challenging, potentially creating loopholes that could be exploited and compromise patient rights. In contrast, many regions lack comprehensive regulatory frameworks, leaving their healthcare digitization more susceptible to misuse and vulnerabilities.

Data Breaches & Their Impact on Trust of Patients

Data breaches could be considered one of the most significant challenges posed due to the involvement of digital tech in healthcare and can have profound effects on patient trust and the overall integrity of the healthcare system. One notable example is the 2015 data breach of Anthem Inc., where hackers accessed the personal information of nearly 80 million individuals, including names, birthdates, and Social Security numbers. This breach not only compromised sensitive data but also led to a significant decline in patient trust and an increase in identity theft cases (Anthem Pays OCR $16 Million in Record HIPAA Settlement Following Largest U.S. Health Data Breach in History | Guidance Portal, n.d.). This incident compromised the trust of patients in the organisation significantly and caused a rise in the number of identity thefts as well.

Another notable case is the 2017 Equifax data breach, which exposed the personal data of over 147 million individuals, including healthcare-related information (Equifax Data Breach Settlement, 2024). This data breach underscored the weaknesses in data security practices and emphasized the urgent need for robust data protection measures. The misuse of such sensitive information for illicit activities further emphasizes the critical importance of data security and the protection of patients' rights.

Additionally, the 2014 Community Health Systems breach exposed the personal information of over 4.5 million patients, including birthdates, names and Social Security numbers (Community Health Systems Data Hack Hits 4.5 million, 2014). This incident revealed weaknesses in cybersecurity protocols and emphasized the necessity for enhanced security measures and proactive threat detection.

In 2020, the Universal Health Services (UHS) ransomware attack disrupted operations across the U.S., impacting multiple hospitals and healthcare facilities. The attack not only disrupted patient care but also underscored the critical need for robust cybersecurity defences to protect against ransomware and other cyber threats (Lyngaas, 2021).

These cases illustrate the critical need for effective data management and security practices. They also emphasize the importance of transparency and timely communication with patients in the event of a breach, as these factors can significantly impact the level of trust patients have in their healthcare providers and the overall system.

CHALLENGES AND VULNERABILITIES IN HEALTHCARE DATA PROTECTION

As discussed in the previous sections along with the advantages of inclusion of technology in the healthcare industry there exist numerous challenges and risks that are major concerns for the safety and security of patients' data. These challenges could be broadly classified in three sections which are increased vulnerability to cyber threats, gaps in regulatory compliance, and technological and operational weaknesses. This section explores these critical areas and highlights the importance of taking robust measures to counteract them.

Increased Vulnerability to Cyber Threats

Cyber threats are among the most significant challenges healthcare organizations face when integrating digital technology into their operations. Cybersecurity in healthcare is distinct because of the sensitive nature of the information at stake and the potential impact on patient safety (Argaw et al., 2020) . The healthcare industry is continuously targeted by cybercriminals because of the high value of patients' medical data. This sensitive information, which includes personal identification details, medical histories, and financial data, is highly sought after on the black market, making healthcare organizations prime targets for cyberattacks.

Several major cyberattacks have highlighted the vulnerabilities within the healthcare sector. In 2020, Universal Health Services (UHS) experienced a major ransomware attack that disrupted the operations of its hospitals and healthcare facilities throughout the United States (Lyngaas, 2021). This incident not only impacted patient care but also underscored the sector's susceptibility to cyber threats. Similarly, in 2017, the WannaCry ransomware attack affected numerous healthcare organizations worldwide, including the UK's National Health Service (NHS), causing widespread operational disruptions and emphasizing the critical need for robust cybersecurity measures (Investigation: WannaCry Cyber Attack and the NHS, 2018).

These incidents illustrate the urgent necessity for healthcare organizations to implement comprehensive cybersecurity strategies to protect patient data and ensure the continuity of healthcare services. Key steps to mitigate these risks include investing in advanced cybersecurity technologies, conducting regular security audits, and providing ongoing training for staff. By adopting these measures, healthcare organizations can enhance their defences against cyber threats, safeguard sensitive patient information, and maintain patient trust (He et al., 2021).

By implementing these measures, healthcare organizations can strengthen their defences against cyber threats, safeguard sensitive patient information, and maintain patient trust. Implementing a proactive cybersecurity strategy is crucial for safeguarding patient data and maintaining the integrity of healthcare services.

Technological and Operational Weaknesses

Technological and operational weaknesses further increase the challenges in healthcare data protection. The 2014 Community Health Systems breach, which exposed the personal information of over 4.5 million patients, revealed critical flaws in the organization's cybersecurity infrastructure (Community Health Systems Data Hack Hits 4.5 million, 2014). Outdated software, lack of regular updates, and insufficient employee training contribute to these weaknesses, making healthcare organizations prime targets for cyber attacks. Therefore, being equipped with technological advancements is of utmost importance for health organisations.

Additionally, the lack of interoperability between various systems and devices can result in disjointed data management practices. For instance, the 2018 breach at UnityPoint Health exposed the data of 1.4 million patients due to phishing attacks that exploited weaknesses in email security and system integration (HIPAA Journal, 2018). This incident underscores the necessity for comprehensive security strategies that address both technological and operational vulnerabilities.

Addressing these technological and operational weaknesses is crucial for enhancing healthcare data protection. Regular updates and maintenance of software, robust employee training programs, and improving system interoperability are essential steps in mitigating risks and ensuring the security and integrity of patient information.

COMPREHENSIVE APPROACH TO DATA SECURITY AND PRIVACY

Policy Formation

Development of stringent data protection regulations. It is crucial to ensuring the security and privacy of healthcare data. These regulations must be comprehensive, addressing all facets of data handling, storage, and transmission. Effective policies should also be adaptable, keeping pace with the rapidly evolving technological landscape and emerging threats.

To achieve comprehensive coverage, regulations should encompass every stage of data management. This includes specifying protocols for data collection, ensuring that only necessary information is gathered, and that patient consent is appropriately obtained. Storage guidelines should enforce strong encryption and secure access controls to prevent unauthorized access. Additionally, transmission standards should enforce the use of secure communication channels to protect data in transit.

Adaptability is key to the success of data protection regulations. As technology advances, new vulnerabilities and threats emerge, necessitating continuous updates to regulatory frameworks. Policies must be flexible enough to incorporate advancements in cybersecurity practices and respond swiftly to new challenges. This requires ongoing collaboration between policymakers, healthcare providers, and technology experts to ensure regulations remain relevant and effective.

For example, the European Union's General Data Protection Regulation (GDPR) has established a high benchmark for data protection, impacting global practices. GDPR's stringent requirements for data consent, breach notification, and the right to be forgotten providing a robust framework that other regions can emulate

(General Data Protection Regulation (GDPR) – Legal Text, 2024). Similarly, the United States' Health Insurance Portability and Accountability Act (HIPAA) sets out clear guidelines for protecting patient information, with provisions that adapt to technological advancements.

Implementing stringent data protection regulations not only enhances data security but also builds patient trust. Patients are more likely to share their information if they believe it will be handled with the highest level of care and security. By prioritizing the development and maintenance of strong data protection regulations, healthcare organizations can ensure that patient data remains secure, ultimately improving the overall quality of care.

Several factors are crucial for the effective adoption of data protection laws. A comparative analysis (McKay et al., 2024) of South Africa, Ghana, Kenya, Nigeria, and Uganda reveals that while these countries have enacted enforceable data protection regulations mandating compliance and accountability, there are key enablers and obstacles. Enablers include enforceable data processing laws requiring explicit consent, accountability of data processors and controllers, transparency, oversight institutions, special protections for health data, and safeguards like Data Transfer Agreements (DTAs) for cross-border transfers. Obstacles involve inconsistent definitions of 'health data,' lack of specific provisions for cross-border transfers in some countries, and challenges with informed consent processes. These factors collectively impact the efficiency and integrity of health data sharing across borders.

Ethical guidelines for data handling. Establishing ethical guidelines for data handling is essential in maintaining patient trust and protecting sensitive information. These guidelines should prioritize patient consent, transparency in data usage, and equitable treatment. Healthcare organizations must ensure that data handling practices align with ethical standards and respect patient rights.

First and foremost, patient consent is a cornerstone of ethical data handling. Healthcare organizations must obtain explicit, informed consent from patients before collecting, storing, or using their data. This involves clearly communicating how the data will be used, who will have access to it, and the potential risks and benefits. Patients should have the option to withdraw their consent at any time, reinforcing their control over their personal information.

Transparency in data usage is another critical component of ethical guidelines. Healthcare organizations should be open about their data handling practices, including how data is collected, processed, stored, and shared. This transparency helps build trust by ensuring patients are aware of how their information is being used and the measures in place to protect it. Regular updates and clear communication about any changes in data handling practices are also important.

Equitable treatment in data handling ensures that all patients' data is treated with the same level of care and respect, regardless of their background. This involves implementing measures to prevent discrimination or bias in both data collection and analysis. For example, algorithms used in healthcare should be regularly audited to ensure they do not inadvertently favour certain groups over others. By promoting fairness and equality, healthcare organizations can foster an inclusive environment that respects the rights and dignity of all patients.

Moreover, ethical guidelines should include provisions for data security and privacy. This means adopting robust cybersecurity measures to protect data from unauthorized access, breaches, and other threats. Regular training for staff on ethical data handling and cybersecurity practices is also crucial. By ensuring that all employees understand and adhere to these guidelines, healthcare organizations can create a culture of responsibility and vigilance.

Finally, healthcare organizations should engage in continuous dialogue with patients, ethicists, and other stakeholders to keep their ethical guidelines up to date. This helps ensure that the guidelines remain relevant and effective in the face of evolving technologies and societal values. For instance, emerging technologies like artificial intelligence and big data analytics pose new ethical challenges that need to be addressed proactively.

For instance, in India the Digital Personal Data Protection Act, 2023 (DPDP Act) has transformed the healthcare sector by enforcing privacy rights and data minimization, requiring clear consent for data processing. The Act restricts data use to necessary purposes, as illustrated by examples like telemedicine apps only processing relevant data. It allows data processing for specific legitimate uses when voluntarily provided but strictly for the intended purpose. The Act also permits data processing during emergencies and exempts research data, provided it isn't used for individual-specific decisions (Club, 2024).

International collaboration and standard harmonization. This is essential for strengthening data security and privacy on a global scale. In a world where healthcare data frequently crosses borders, the absence of uniform standards can create significant vulnerabilities. By working together, countries can establish unified protocols and best practices that enhance the overall security framework. This collaborative effort ensures that healthcare data remains consistently protected, regardless of where it is processed or stored.

One of the primary benefits of international collaboration is the ability to address the challenges associated with cross-border data transfers. Different countries have diverse regulations and standards for data protection, which can complicate the transfer and sharing of healthcare information. Harmonizing these standards facilitates smoother and more secure data exchanges between countries, thereby enhancing the global healthcare ecosystem. For instance, aligning the data protection practices of the United States' Health Insurance Portability and Accountability Act (HIPAA) with Europe's General Data Protection Regulation (GDPR) can create a more cohesive approach to managing patient information. This alignment reduces the risk of data breaches and ensures patient privacy across regions, fostering greater trust in the global handling of healthcare data.

Furthermore, international collaboration enables the sharing of knowledge and resources, which can lead to more robust security measures. Countries can benefit from each other's experiences by adopting best practices that have proven effective in other regions. This collective approach not only strengthens individual countries' data protection capabilities but also contributes to a more resilient global healthcare infrastructure. By pooling expertise and resources, nations can better anticipate and mitigate emerging threats, ensuring that healthcare data remains secure in an increasingly digital and interconnected world.

Additionally, global standards and guidelines can drive innovation in data security technologies and practices. When countries work together to develop and implement cutting-edge security measures, they can create a dynamic environment that encourages continuous improvement and adaptation. This ongoing evolution is crucial for staying ahead of cyber threats and protecting sensitive healthcare information. International collaboration thus not only enhances current security protocols but also fosters a forward-looking approach to data protection that can adapt to future challenges.

Advanced Technology Utilization

Encryption protocols and access control. These are fundamental to securing healthcare data. Encryption transforms sensitive information into an unreadable format, making it inaccessible to anyone who doesn't have the appropriate decryption key. This method is crucial for protecting patient information as it moves through networks or is stored on servers.

Access control mechanisms work alongside encryption to ensure that only authorized individuals can access or manage sensitive data. These controls include techniques like multi-factor authentication, which adds layers of security beyond just a password, and role-based access, which restricts data access based on the user's role within the organization.

Together, encryption and access control provide a comprehensive approach to data security, safeguarding patient information and ensuring that only those with the proper clearance can view or alter it. Regular updates and monitoring of these systems are essential to maintaining their effectiveness against emerging cyber threats.

A prime example of an advanced information exchange system is South Korea's platform, which employs multi-layered protection to ensure secure data exchange among insurers, providers, and data centres. This system includes secure data storage that encrypts data and restricts access, user authentication via passwords or biometrics, and endpoint security measures like IoT security, Network Access Control (NAC), and Data Loss Prevention (DLP) to protect against malicious exploitation. Additionally, network security is maintained through layered defences such as firewalls, intrusion prevention systems, and VPNs, creating a robust model for safeguarding healthcare data (Total Solution for Value-based Healthcare Purchasing-HIRA System, n.d.).

AI-powered security solutions. AI-driven security solutions greatly improve cybersecurity by utilizing advanced machine learning algorithms. These systems can swiftly analyse extensive datasets, detecting irregularities and potential threats more effectively than traditional methods. AI can detect unusual patterns in real time that may signal a security breach or malicious activity.

Furthermore, AI technologies can automate responses to identified threats, such as isolating affected systems or blocking suspicious behaviour. This automation allows for swift intervention and containment of issues before they escalate. Integrating AI into security infrastructure provides a dynamic and responsive approach to managing cyber threats, improving the protection of sensitive information.

Secure cloud platforms. Using secure cloud platforms is crucial for effective data management in healthcare, offering both scalability and flexibility. These platforms ensure that sensitive data is protected with a range of advanced security features. For instance, data encryption plays a vital role in securing information by converting it into a format that is unreadable without the proper decryption key. This safeguards patient data both during transmission and while it is stored in the cloud.

Automated backups are another essential feature, providing regular copies of data that can be restored in case of accidental loss or corruption. Additionally, disaster recovery options are built into these platforms to ensure continuity of service, allowing organizations to quickly recover from data breaches or system failures.

By incorporating secure cloud platforms, healthcare organizations can safeguard their data against unauthorized access and cyber threats, while also benefiting from the flexibility to scale their data storage needs as required. This approach helps in maintaining the integrity and availability of critical information, supporting both operational efficiency and regulatory compliance. Figure 2 sums up how technology is utilized for data security.

Figure 2. Data security through technology utilization

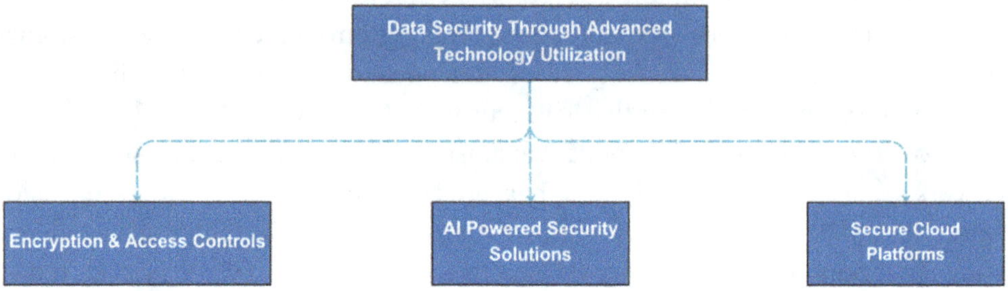

Continuous Capacity Building

Training programs for healthcare staff. Regular training programs for healthcare staff are crucial in fostering a culture of security awareness and compliance within the organization. These programs should be thorough and cover a broad range of topics, including the latest cybersecurity threats, best practices for handling patient data, and the effective use of security tools to protect against attacks. By providing staff with current knowledge and practical skills, healthcare organizations can significantly improve their defense against data breaches.

Training programs should aim to help staff recognize common cyber threats such as phishing attempts. Employees trained to identify suspicious emails or links can prevent potential breaches before they occur. Additionally, education on secure data handling procedures is vital; staff must understand how to properly store, access, and share patient information to minimize the risk of unauthorized access.

Moreover, training should include simulations of security incidents to prepare staff for real-life scenarios. For example, simulated phishing attacks can teach employees how to respond appropriately, reducing the likelihood of successful attacks. Regular drills and role-playing exercises can ensure that staff know how to act swiftly and effectively in the event of a data breach, thereby mitigating potential damage.

Continuous education is also essential. Cybersecurity is a constantly evolving field, and what is considered best practice today might be outdated tomorrow. Regular updates and refresher courses help keep staff informed about emerging threats and the latest security measures. This ongoing education helps maintain a high level of vigilance and ensures that security practices evolve in tandem with emerging risks.

Implementing comprehensive training programs demonstrates an organization's commitment to protecting patient data, which can enhance trust among patients and stakeholders. When healthcare staff are well-trained in cybersecurity protocols, the organization is better positioned to safeguard sensitive information and comply with regulatory requirements.

Investment in IT infrastructure. It is critical for enhancing security measures and ensuring the resilience of healthcare systems. Key components of this investment include:

Upgrading outdated hardware. Modernizing hardware is essential to prevent failures that could compromise data integrity. Old equipment can be a weak link in the security chain, so updating to newer, more reliable technology is vital.

Implementing redundant systems. Redundant systems are crucial for data preservation. These backups ensure that data remains recoverable in the event of a hardware malfunction, thus maintaining continuity of operations and protecting against data laws.

Deploying advanced cybersecurity technologies. Utilizing advanced cybersecurity measures, such as intrusion detection systems and firewalls, is fundamental in defending against potential threats. These technologies assist in detecting and mitigating cyber threats before they can inflict significant damage.

Proactively addressing system vulnerabilities. Regularly assessing and addressing system vulnerabilities allows healthcare organizations to significantly lower the risk of cyberattacks. This proactive approach includes conducting frequent security audits, implementing necessary patches and updates.

Regular updates and enhancements: The IT infrastructure must be regularly updated to keep pace with the rapid evolution of security threats. Continuous improvements ensure that the system remains robust and capable of meeting changing regulatory requirements effectively.

Strategic investments in IT infrastructure enable healthcare organizations to create a resilient and secure environment. This approach not only protects sensitive patient data but also ensures that healthcare services remain uninterrupted and compliant with evolving standards.

Collaborations with Cybersecurity Experts. Partnering with cybersecurity experts provides healthcare organizations with crucial specialized knowledge and resources to tackle intricate security challenges. These experts bring invaluable insights into emerging threats and vulnerabilities, helping to develop and implement robust security strategies tailored to the organization's specific needs. Their expertise ensures that healthcare organizations are not only aware of the latest threats but are also equipped with the best practices to counter them.

Furthermore, cybersecurity professionals offer ongoing support to maintain a secure data environment. This includes continuous monitoring, threat detection, and rapid response to security incidents. By integrating the expertise of these professionals, healthcare organizations can significantly enhance their ability to detect and address potential security incidents. This proactive approach is essential in strengthening the overall security posture and ensuring the protection of sensitive patient information from cyber threats.

By integrating a holistic approach that includes policy formation, advanced technology utilization, and continuous capacity building, healthcare organizations can significantly strengthen their data security and privacy measures. This comprehensive strategy not only protects sensitive patient information but also ensures the reliability and integrity of healthcare services.

PRACTICAL RECOMMENDATIONS FOR HEALTHCARE PROVIDERS AND POLICYMAKERS

Enhancing Data Protection Measures

It is of utmost importance for the Healthcare providers and policymakers to prioritize robust data protection measures to safeguard patient information. This involves several key actions:

Advanced encryption techniques. Employing advanced encryption ensures that patient data is secure during transmission and storage. Encryption converts data into a coded format that unauthorized users cannot read, protecting sensitive information from breaches. For instance, the 2014 breach of Community Health Systems exposed the personal information of 4.5 million patients due to inadequate encryption, highlighting the necessity of strong encryption protocols (Community Health Systems Data Hack Hits 4.5 million, 2014).

Multifactor authentication (MFA). Employing MFA enhances security by requiring users to undergo multiple verification steps before accessing data. These steps could involve something you know, like a password; something you have, such as a security token; or something you are, like a fingerprint. The 2015 Anthem breach, which compromised nearly 80 million records, could have been mitigated with stronger authentication measures (Anthem Pays OCR $16 Million in Record HIPAA Settlement Following Largest U.S. Health Data Breach in History | Guidance Portal, n.d.).

Regular software updates and patching. Ensuring that all systems and software are regularly updated and patched to fix security vulnerabilities is crucial. Old software often presents a vulnerable target for cyber criminals. The WannaCry ransomware attack in 2017 exploited vulnerabilities in outdated software, affecting numerous healthcare organizations globally, including the UK's National Health Service (NHS) (Investigation: WannaCry Cyber Attack and the NHS, 2018).

Routine security audits. Conducting regular security audits helps identify and address potential weaknesses in the system. These audits should be thorough and frequent, allowing for proactive risk management. The 2019 breach at the University of Washington Medicine, which exposed personal data of 974,000 patients, emphasized the importance of continuous compliance and regular audits (University of Washington Medicine Exposes Data of 1M Patients | InfoWatch, n.d.).

Stringent data protection standards: Establishing and adhering to strict data protection policies can help prevent unauthorized access and data breaches. Clear guidelines and protocols should be in place to protect patient information across all platforms and systems.

Mitigating Risks Associated with Digital Health Technologies

Digital health technologies bring numerous benefits but also pose significant risks. To mitigate these risks, healthcare organizations should implement comprehensive cybersecurity frameworks:

Intrusion detection systems and firewalls. Utilizing advanced cybersecurity solutions like intrusion detection systems and firewalls enables the monitoring of network traffic and prevention of unauthorized access. These tools are crucial for identifying and addressing potential threats in real-time. The ransomware attack on Universal Health Services (UHS) in 2020, which disrupted operations across its U.S. hospitals, underscored the need for robust cybersecurity measures.

Regular training programs. Continuous education and training programs for staff on the latest cybersecurity threats and best practices are essential. Employees need to be informed about common cyber threats, such as phishing and ransomware, and should be equipped with the knowledge to prevent and address these issues effectively. The 2018 UnityPoint Health breach, which exposed data of 1.4 million patients due to phishing attacks, highlighted the critical role of employee training.

Clear guidelines and protocols. Developing clear guidelines for the use of digital health technologies ensures that all staff follow best practices for data security. Regularly reviewing and updating these protocols helps keep pace with evolving technologies and threats.

Risk assessment and management. Conducting regular risk assessments can reveal potential vulnerabilities and facilitate the creation of strategies to mitigate them. By understanding the risks, healthcare organizations can take proactive steps to protect patient data.

Fostering a Culture of Privacy and Security

Creating a culture of privacy and security within healthcare organizations is essential for protecting patient data:

Continuous education and training. All employees should receive regular training on the importance of data security and privacy practices. This training should cover current threats, data protection protocols, and the importance of adhering to these practices.

Proactive approach to security. Encouraging a proactive approach to identifying and reporting potential security issues fosters a vigilant workforce. Employees should feel empowered to report suspicious activities or vulnerabilities without fear of repercussions.

Leadership commitment. Leadership must demonstrate a commitment to privacy and security. This involves setting the tone from the top and integrating these values into the organization's daily operations and decision-making processes.

Regular communication. Maintaining open lines of communication about the importance of data security and any changes in protocols ensures that all employees are informed and engaged. Regular updates and reminders can help keep security top of mind.

By focusing on these practical recommendations and learning from past incidents, healthcare providers and policymakers can significantly enhance data security and privacy measures, protecting sensitive patient information and ensuring the integrity of healthcare services.

CAPACITY BUILDING AND EDUCATION

Training Healthcare Professionals on Data Security

Effective data security in healthcare starts with training for all staff members in a very comprehensive manner so that they could be capable enough to identify threats to the security of patients' data. This involves not just a one-time orientation but a continuous education to keep up with the latest threats and best practices. Healthcare professionals should be trained to recognize phishing attempts, understand the importance of strong passwords, and follow protocols for secure data handling. Regular drills and updates on new security policies help ensure that staff remains vigilant. An example is the University of Washington Medicine breach in 2019, which underscored the importance of continuous staff training after non-compliance led to a significant data exposure incident.

Continuous Education and Awareness Programs

Continuous education and awareness programs are crucial for maintaining high data security in healthcare. Regular workshops, seminars, and online courses should cover evolving cybersecurity threats and data protection techniques. Incorporating these initiatives into everyday operations helps cultivate a culture of security.

For instance, Mayo Clinic implements ongoing cybersecurity training that includes simulated phishing attacks. These exercises educate employees about risks and improve their responses to potential threats. By regularly testing staff, organizations can identify weaknesses and provide targeted training to address them.

Additionally, partnerships with cybersecurity experts ensure that training programs are up to date. Tailoring education to different roles within the organization is essential, as IT staff may need more technical training, while administrative staff may focus on recognizing social engineering tactics.

Encouraging a transparent environment where employees can report security incidents without fear of repercussions is also key. By investing in continuous education, healthcare organizations can build a workforce that is prepared to protect sensitive patient information effectively.

Leveraging Global Best Practices in Data Security

Leveraging global best practices in data security can significantly enhance the protection of sensitive healthcare information. This involves adopting international standards and guidelines such as those provided by the International Organization for Standardization (ISO), which offers a comprehensive framework for managing information security (ISO/IEC 27001). Adhering to these standards enables organizations to systematically manage sensitive data, ensuring its security.

Adhering to the Health Insurance Portability and Accountability Act (HIPAA) in the United States is crucial for protecting patient information. HIPAA sets national standards for the protection of health information, ensuring that data is properly encrypted, access is controlled, and breaches are promptly reported. Similarly, the General Data Protection Regulation (GDPR) in Europe imposes strict rules on data handling, giving individuals greater control over their personal information and requiring organizations to implement robust security measures.

Collaborating with global cybersecurity experts is another essential practice. These experts provide insights into emerging threats, help develop effective defence strategies, and assist in implementing advanced security technologies. Participation in international forums and consortia, such as the Global Forum on Cyber Expertise (GFCE) and the Healthcare Information and Management Systems Society

(HIMSS), enables healthcare organizations to stay updated on the latest trends of security and technologies.

For instance, NHS Digital in the UK regularly updates its cybersecurity protocols based on global best practices. By aligning with international standards and continuously evolving its security measures, NHS Digital has seen a reduction in data breaches and an improvement in overall data protection. Their approach involves adopting the Cyber Essentials scheme, which offers a clear set of security controls to guard against common online threats, as well as utilizing the Data Security and Protection Toolkit, which helps organizations assess their security measures and ensure they meet regulatory requirements.

In addition to these measures, implementing advanced technologies such as artificial intelligence (AI) and machine learning (ML) can further enhance data security. AI-powered security solutions can analyse vast amounts of data in real-time, identifying unusual patterns and potential threats more effectively than traditional methods. Machine learning algorithms can learn from past incidents to predict and prevent future attacks, continuously improving the organization's security posture. Figure 3 shows the roadmap for capacity building and Education.

Figure 3. Capacity building roadmap

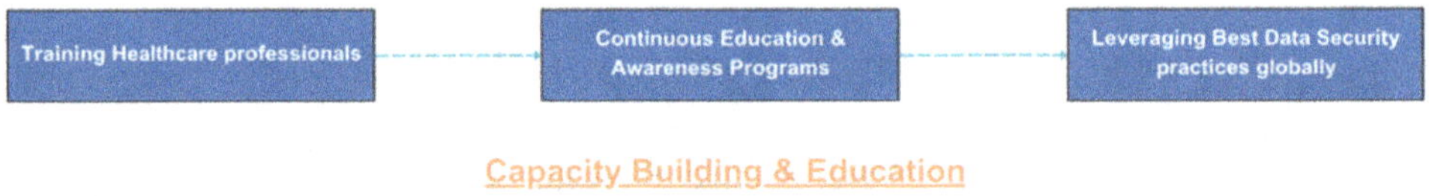

FUTURE DIRECTIONS

Emerging Trends in Healthcare

The future of healthcare technology is characterized by several emerging trends that have the potential to transform patient care. Telemedicine, which saw a significant rise during the COVID-19 pandemic, continues to grow, providing remote diagnostics and consultations that enhance access to healthcare, particularly in underserved areas. This advancement reduces the necessity for in-person visits, making healthcare more accessible and convenient for patients while also relieving the strain on healthcare facilities (American Telemedicine Association - ATA, 2024).

Wearable technology and IoT devices are advancing rapidly, offering real-time health monitoring and data collection. Devices like smartwatches and fitness trackers can monitor vital signs such as heart rate, blood pressure, and glucose levels, providing valuable data for personalized patient care. These continuous health metrics allow for the early detection of potential health issues, enabling timely interventions and more proactive healthcare management.

Moreover, blockchain technology is being explored for securing patient records and ensuring data integrity across various healthcare platforms. The decentralized and immutable characteristics of blockchain make it well-suited for ensuring the confidentiality and accuracy of medical records. By securely recording every transaction or update to a patient's record, blockchain can prevent unauthorized access and reduce the risk of data breaches. It also enhances interoperability between various healthcare systems, enabling the seamless and secure exchange of patient information across different providers and institutions.

The integration of Artificial intelligence (AI) into healthcare is another exciting development. AI-powered tools can analyze vast amounts of medical data to aid in diagnostics, treatment planning, and predictive analytics. For instance, AI algorithms can detect patterns in medical images that might be missed by human eyes, improving diagnostic accuracy and speed. Additionally, AI can support personalized treatment plans by analysing patient data to recommend tailored interventions, enhancing care effectiveness.

Robotic process automation (RPA) is also making significant strides in healthcare, streamlining administrative tasks such as patient scheduling, billing, and claims processing. By automating these routine tasks, RPA allows healthcare professionals to focus more on patient care, increasing efficiency and reducing the likelihood of errors.

These emerging trends in healthcare technology offer great promise for transforming patient care. As these technologies continue to evolve and become more integrated into healthcare systems, they have the potential to enhance access to care, improve health outcomes, and increase the efficiency of healthcare delivery. By embracing these innovations, the healthcare industry can move towards a more patient-centered, data-driven approach that meets the evolving needs of patients and providers alike.

Evolving Regulatory Landscape

As healthcare technology advances, the regulatory landscape must evolve accordingly to safeguard patient data privacy and security. Effective regulations are essential to address the challenges and opportunities presented by new technological innovations.

In Europe, the General Data Protection Regulation (GDPR) has set a high standard for data protection, influencing policies not only within the EU but also globally. GDPR mandates strict guidelines on how personal data should be handled, ensuring that individuals have control over their information and that organizations are accountable for protecting it (General Data Protection Regulation (GDPR) – Legal Text, 2024).

In the United States, the Health Insurance Portability and Accountability Act (HIPAA) remains a cornerstone of patient data protection. HIPAA has continuously adapted to keep pace with technological advancements, ensuring that electronic health records and other digital health information are securely managed. The act mandates stringent safeguards to protect patient privacy, including the use of encryption and access controls.

Other regions are also shaping their regulatory frameworks to address the evolving healthcare landscape. For instance, India's Personal Data Protection Bill aims to establish comprehensive data protection standards that will impact how healthcare data is managed. This bill is poised to provide robust protection for personal data while facilitating the growth of digital health initiatives.

Continuous dialogue among policymakers, healthcare providers, and technology experts is crucial for developing effective regulations that balance innovation with patient safety. Collaborative efforts can ensure that regulations are comprehensive and adaptable, addressing emerging threats while fostering technological advancements. For example, the UK's NHS Digital regularly updates its cybersecurity protocols based on global best practices, resulting in a notable reduction in data breaches.

International cooperation can also play a significant role in harmonizing data protection standards. By aligning regulations across borders, countries can facilitate the secure exchange of health information and ensure consistent protection for patients worldwide. Engaging in international forums and partnerships allows for the sharing of best practices and the development of global strategies to combat cyber threats.

As the healthcare industry continues to innovate, regulatory frameworks must remain agile and forward-thinking. By prioritizing patient privacy and data security, regulations can support the safe and effective use of new technologies, ultimately enhancing the quality of healthcare delivery.

Long-Term Strategies: Ensuring Rights and Safety of Patients

To ensure patient rights and safety in the long term, healthcare organizations must adopt comprehensive strategies that integrate technology, policy, and education. This includes investing in advanced cybersecurity measures such as AI-driven threat detection and response systems. Organizations should also adopt international standards like those provided by the International Organization for Standardization (ISO) to ensure consistent data protection practices.

Education and training programs for healthcare professionals are of immense importance. Regular workshops and certifications can keep staff updated on the latest security practices (AMA-Code Homepage, n.d.). Incorporating global best practices, such as those seen with NHS Digital in the UK, which frequently updates its protocols based on international standards, can significantly reduce data breaches.

Furthermore, fostering collaborations with cybersecurity experts and participating in global forums can help healthcare organizations stay ahead of potential threats. Implementing transparent and robust patient consent processes ensures that patients are fully aware of how their data is used and protected. Long-term strategies should also include regular audits and assessments to identify and mitigate vulnerabilities continuously (AMA-Code Homepage, n.d.).

CONCLUSION

The journey of digital transformation has varied across different regions and countries, but its impact on the healthcare sector has been profound over the last three decades. This transformation has revolutionized critical aspects of healthcare delivery, driven by the promise of improved outcomes, streamlined procedures, more efficient facility use, and enhanced patient satisfaction.

Digitalization in healthcare has brought significant benefits, such as the efficient management of extensive patient data and access to healthcare. However, it also poses potential risks, particularly regarding data security. Therefore, it is essential for healthcare professionals and industry experts to implement stringent measures to protect patient data and sensitive information, ensuring privacy and maintaining trust in the healthcare system. It is crucial to emphasize that the evolution through the adoption of digital technologies must be accompanied by robust safeguarding measures for patient data. These two elements must go hand in hand to ensure a comprehensive and secure healthcare ecosystem.

By focusing on these emerging trends on data safety & security strategies, adapting to regulatory changes, and implementing long-term strategies, healthcare providers can enhance the protection of patient data, improve the quality of care, and maintain trust in the healthcare system.

REFERENCES

American Medical Association. (n.d.). Ethical principles in healthcare data management. American Medical Association https://code-medical-ethics.ama-assn.org/

American Telemedicine Association. (n.d.). Telemedicine: Expanding access to care. American Telemedicine Association https://www.americantelemed.org/

Anthem Inc. (2015). Data breach report. https://www.hhs.gov/guidance/document/anthem-pays-ocr-16-million-record-hipaa-settlement-following-largest-us-health-data-breach

Argaw, S. T., Troncoso-Pastoriza, J. R., Lacey, D., Florin, M., Calcavecchia, F., Anderson, D., Burleson, W., Vogel, J., O'Leary, C., Eshaya-Chauvin, B., & Flahault, A. (2020). Cybersecurity of Hospitals: Discussing the challenges and working towards mitigating the risks. *BMC Medical Informatics and Decision Making*, *20*(1), 146. Advance online publication. DOI: 10.1186/s12911-020-01161-7 PMID: 32620167

Atasoy, H., Greenwood, B. N., & McCullough, J. S. (2018). The Digitization of Patient Care: A Review of the Effects of Electronic Health Records on Health Care Quality and Utilization. *Annual Review of Public Health*, *40*(1), 487–500. DOI: 10.1146/annurev-publhealth-040218-044206 PMID: 30566385

Bonderud, D. (2024, September 26). Ransomware on the rise: Healthcare industry attack trends 2024. Security Intelligence. https://securityintelligence.com/articles/healthcare-industry-attack-trends-2024/

Club, D. (2024, July 31). Navigating Health Data Privacy in India: Regulations and Best Practices for Compliance and Trust. https://www.linkedin.com/pulse/navigating-health-data-privacy-india-regulations-best-practices-kmeuc

Equifax data breach settlement. (2022, December 20). Federal Trade Commission. https://www.ftc.gov/enforcement/refunds/equifax-data-breach-settlement

Ezeamii, V. C., Okobi, O. E., Wambai-Sani, H., Perera, G. S., Zaynieva, S., Okonkwo, C. C., Ohaiba, M. M., William-Enemali, P. C., Obodo, O. R., & Obiefuna, N. G. (2024). Revolutionizing Healthcare: How Telemedicine Is Improving Patient Outcomes and Expanding Access to Care. *Cureus*. Advance online publication. DOI: 10.7759/cureus.63881 PMID: 39099901

General Data Protection Regulation. (2018). Regulation (EU) 2016/679. Official Journal of the European Union. https://gdpr-info.eu/

Haleem, A., Javaid, M., Singh, R. P., & Suman, R. (2021). Telemedicine for healthcare: Capabilities, features, barriers, and applications. *Sensors International*, *2*, 100117. DOI: 10.1016/j.sintl.2021.100117 PMID: 34806053

He, Y., Aliyu, A., Evans, M., & Luo, C. (2021). Health Care Cybersecurity Challenges and Solutions Under the Climate of COVID-19: Scoping Review. *Journal of Medical Internet Research*, *23*(4), e21747. DOI: 10.2196/21747 PMID: 33764885

Health Insurance Portability and Accountability Act. (1996). Pub. L. 104-191, 110 Stat. 1936. https://www.hhs.gov/hippa

Hillestad, R., Bigelow, J., Bower, A., Girosi, F., Meili, R., Scoville, R., & Taylor, R. (2005). Can Electronic Medical Record Systems Transform Health Care? Potential Health Benefits, Savings, And Costs. *Health Affairs*, *24*(5), 1103–1117. DOI: 10.1377/hlthaff.24.5.1103 PMID: 16162551

HIRA system. (n.d.). www.hira.or.kr. Retrieved December 21, 2024, from https://www.hira.or.kr/eng/news/01/__icsFiles/afieldfile/2015/07/24/VyIdbjIJh6Xm.pdf

Impact of implementing electronic health records on medication safety at an HIMSS stage 6 hospital: The pharmacist's perspective. (n.d.). PubMed Central (PMC). https://www.ncbi.nlm.nih.gov/pmc/articles/PMC9524548/

Lyngaas, S. (2021, March 10). Universal health services reports $67 million in losses after apparent ransomware attack. CyberScoop. https://cyberscoop.com/universal-health-services-ransomware-cost-ryuk/

Manaktala, S., & Claypool, S. R. (2016). Evaluating the impact of a computerized surveillance algorithm and decision support system on sepsis mortality. *Journal of the American Medical Informatics Association : JAMIA*, *24*(1), 88–95. DOI: 10.1093/jamia/ocw056 PMID: 27225197

McKay, A. G. N., Brand, D., Botes, M., Cengiz, N., & Swart, M. (2024). The regulation of health data sharing in Africa: A comparative study. *Journal of Law and the Biosciences*, *11*(1), lsad035. Advance online publication. DOI: 10.1093/jlb/lsad035 PMID: 38259628

(n.d.). National Audit Office (NAO). https://www.nao.org.uk/wp-content/uploads/2017/10/Investigation-WannaCry-cyber-attack-and-the-NHS.pdf

Ndwabe, H., Basu, A., & Mohammed, J. (2023). Post pandemic analysis on comprehensive utilization of telehealth and telemedicine. Clinical eHealth, 7, 5–14. DOI: 10.1016/j.ceh.2023.12.002

Patel, R., Huang, J., Hsueh, L., Gopalan, A., Millman, A., Franklin, I., & Reed, M. (2024). Telemedicine's Impact on Diabetes Care during the COVID-19 Pandemic: A Cohort Study in a Large Integrated Healthcare System. medRxiv (Cold Spring Harbor Laboratory). DOI: 10.1101/2024.02.25.24303335

Rawat, A. (2024, December 2). 7 Telemedicine Trends Shaping the Future of Healthcare. Appinventiv. https://appinventiv.com/blog/top-telehealth-trends/

Zakaria, H., Said, Y., Aleabova, S., Bangayan, J., Dandan, M., Debs, J., Dahlstrom, N., Divino, D., Hashemi, A., & Almarzooqi, I. (2024). Measuring the effectiveness of hybrid diabetes care over 90 days through continuous data monitoring in type 2 diabetic patients. *Frontiers in Endocrinology*, *15*, 1355792. Advance online publication. DOI: 10.3389/fendo.2024.1355792 PMID: 38774233

Chapter 14
Safeguarding Patient Rights and Safety in Tech-Enabled Healthcare

J. Aileen
M S Ramaiah University of Applied Sciences, India

ABSTRACT

In today's healthcare landscape, cutting-edge technologies like AI offer exciting possibilities but also significant challenges. This chapter explores the complex relationship between these advancements and patient safety, highlighting the fine line between innovation and risk. AI has the potential to revolutionize healthcare by improving diagnosis, predicting outcomes, and personalizing treatments, but over-reliance without proper oversight can lead to errors and biases. The chapter also addresses the growing problem of unreliable online health information, emphasizing the need for accurate, evidence-based resources. Building on foundational reports like "To Err is Human," the chapter discusses common pitfalls in healthcare technology, such as poor design, weak system integration, and inadequate planning, which can lead to new errors like alert fatigue. It also examines specific safety concerns, including medical identity theft, data breaches, and medication errors.

INTRODUCTION

In the rapidly evolving landscape of healthcare, integrating Artificial Intelligence (AI) presents exciting advancements alongside significant challenges. This chapter explores two primary concerns: potential errors and biases in AI-driven recommendations and the spread of unreliable health information online. As AI becomes more embedded in clinical settings, healthcare workers must exercise critical judgment,

DOI: 10.4018/979-8-3693-7210-4.ch014

avoiding the uncritical acceptance of AI recommendations. Additionally, as patients increasingly seek health information online, they often encounter sources that lack reliability and accuracy.

Patient safety is a cornerstone of healthcare, focused on avoiding, preventing, and reducing adverse outcomes or injuries arising from healthcare activities (WHO, 2023). The influential 1999 report by the Institute of Medicine (IOM), "To Err is Human," emphasized the critical need to create and evaluate new technologies to mitigate medical errors (Kohn et al., 2000). The subsequent 2001 report, "Crossing the Quality Chasm," highlighted the importance of using information technology to transform the healthcare landscape and ensure improved and safer care (Institute of Medicine, 2001). These reports triggered a paradigm shift, spotlighting the integration of advanced technologies to enhance patient safety.

From electronic health records (EHRs) to advanced diagnostic tools, the healthcare sector increasingly relies on technological innovations to minimize errors and improve patient outcomes. However, the introduction of new technologies also presents challenges, including potential unforeseen errors, the need for thorough training, and the importance of seamless integration with existing systems.

While the public often views advanced technology in healthcare to enhance efficiency, quality, safety, and reduce costs, this optimism frequently overlooks the potential for new errors and adverse events. With nearly 5,000 types of medical devices used globally by millions of healthcare providers, device-related problems are inevitable. Despite the immense promise technology holds, its benefits can be undermined by four common pitfalls: poor technology design disregarding human factors and ergonomic principles, inadequate interfaces between technology, patients, or environment, flawed implementation plans, and insufficient maintenance strategies. This chapter delves into these pitfalls, illustrating how they can prevent the realization of technology's full potential in healthcare and emphasizing the need for thoughtful design, meticulous planning, and ongoing maintenance to truly improve healthcare outcomes.

Background

Patient safety in healthcare faces numerous challenges that can have serious consequences if left unaddressed. Key concerns include medical identity theft, where individuals' identifying information is used to obtain medical services, leading to incorrect entries in medical records, claim denials, and potential harm to patients. Duplicate records can result in patients being assigned multiple medical records, causing fragmented care, repeated tests, and missed diagnoses. Data breaches, involving highly sensitive healthcare data, can lead to loss of patient trust and significant legal repercussions. Medication errors, often due to misidentification or incorrect data, remain a leading cause of patient harm. Additionally, infection control is a persistent safety risk, exacerbated by high patient turnover and complex care procedures.

Patient care technology has become increasingly complex, fundamentally transforming how healthcare is conceptualized and delivered. Before the extensive application of technology, healthcare professionals relied heavily on their senses of sight, touch, smell, and hearing to monitor patient status and detect changes. Over time, these unaided senses were supplemented and often replaced by technology designed to detect physical changes in patient conditions. For instance, consider pulse oximetry: before its widespread use, healthcare professionals relied on subtle changes in mental status and skin color to detect early changes in oxygen saturation and used arterial blood gases to confirm their suspicions. Now, pulse oximetry allows for the identification of decreased oxygenation before clinical symptoms appear, enabling more prompt diagnosis and treatment of underlying causes.

Technology has become both a solution and a challenge for patient safety, as its integration into healthcare introduces new opportunities alongside risks. While innovations such as AI and advanced medical devices promise improved care, they also come with potential hazards, including errors from over-reliance on technology, poor system interfaces, and fragmented workflows. For instance, clinicians may become so focused on monitor data that they overlook subtle but critical changes in a patient's condition. The complexity of bedside technology and the lack of coordinated implementation strategies can exacerbate these challenges. Despite substantial investment in healthcare technology, the profession has often underestimated the importance of seamless integration and system design.

AI has emerged as a powerful tool for enhancing patient safety, especially in areas where traditional approaches fall short. A 2021 review highlighted AI's potential impact on patient safety domains such as adverse drug events, clinical decompensation, and diagnostic errors. However, the benefits of AI depend on precise alignment with patient safety objectives and thoughtful integration into clinical workflows. Misaligned objectives can lead to false alarms or missed critical signs, while poorly designed systems may contribute to alert fatigue and reduced trust among clinicians. Data quality, bias, and security are critical factors, as biased training data or inadequate representation can produce inequitable outcomes and undermine the model's reliability.

Healthcare technologies span a spectrum from simple tools like syringes to complex systems like electronic health records and AI-driven predictive models. The successful adoption of these technologies requires a balance between their use and clinical judgment, ensuring patients are empowered and their rights protected. Multidisciplinary collaboration is vital for responsible AI design and implementation. Teams comprising data scientists, clinicians, ethicists, IT specialists, and regulatory experts must work together to design, validate, and monitor AI solutions. Rigorous validation of AI models using organizational data and continuous quality assurance are crucial to identify biases and ensure clinical efficacy.

Clinician engagement plays a key role, requiring training on data science and the functionality of AI models, as well as prioritizing usability. Regulatory bodies like the National Artificial Intelligence Initiative and WHO emphasize the need for guidelines and standards to ensure patient safety in AI applications. Building trust in AI technologies through transparency, monitoring, and adherence to ethical standards is essential for maximizing their potential while safeguarding patient care.

The key highlights of the chapter:

Understand technologies advancements and challenges, focusing on errors and biases

Highlight patient safety through technological advancements, addressing integration challenges.

Explore AI's potential with rigorous validation and attention to data quality and privacy.

Emphasize a multidisciplinary approach for AI system design and monitoring.

Discuss regulatory bodies' role in setting guidelines for healthcare technology implementation.

1. PIONEERING PROGRESS: TECH TRIUMPHS AND TRIALS

1.1 Healthcare's Cutting-Edge Innovations

The healthcare industry is undergoing a significant transformation fueled by technological advancements. These innovations are not only enhancing patient care but also making healthcare operations more efficient. Among these innovations, telemedicine stands out by breaking down geographical barriers and expanding access to healthcare. It allows patients to consult healthcare providers remotely, which improves convenience and patient engagement. However, to fully leverage its potential, challenges like digital literacy and internet accessibility need to be addressed.

In this era of transformation, technology is reshaping healthcare, bringing improvements in patient care, streamlining operations, and enhancing overall outcomes. This section delves into some of the most influential technological advancements in healthcare, discussing their benefits, challenges, and future potential.

Telemedicine has made healthcare more accessible by enabling patients to consult with healthcare providers via video calls, phone calls, and online messaging. This has been especially beneficial in rural and underserved areas with limited access to medical specialists. A study published in The Lancet indicated that telemedicine significantly reduces the need for in-person visits, leading to cost savings and higher patient satisfaction (Krick et al., 2020). However, issues like digital literacy, internet access, and data security must be tackled to ensure equitable access and effective implementation.

Precision medicine is another transformative approach, tailoring treatment plans to individuals based on their genetic, environmental, and lifestyle factors. Genomic sequencing, for example, helps identify genetic mutations for targeted therapies. The success of treatments like the Herceptin for HER2-positive breast cancer is well-documented (Nature Reviews Clinical Oncology, 2018). Precision medicine holds promise beyond oncology, potentially advancing the management of chronic diseases and rare genetic disorders. However, challenges such as genetic privacy and the high cost of genomic testing remain significant.

Robotics and automation have greatly improved surgical precision and outcomes. Robotic-assisted surgeries, using systems like the da Vinci Surgical System, enable minimally invasive procedures with greater accuracy and shorter recovery times. Research in The Journal of Robotic Surgery found that robotic-assisted prostatectomy resulted in fewer complications and quicker recovery compared to traditional methods (Smith et al., 2021). Despite these benefits, high costs and the need for specialized training, widespread adoption.

Wearable health devices, including fitness trackers and smartwatches, continuously monitor vital signs and other health metrics. These devices are crucial for managing chronic conditions such as diabetes and cardiovascular diseases, providing real-time data for early intervention. A study in JMIR mHealth and uHealth linked wearable devices to improved patient engagement and health outcomes (Wright et al., 2019). Nevertheless, privacy and data security concerns are critical issues that need to be addressed.

Artificial intelligence (AI) and machine learning (ML) are revolutionizing diagnostics, treatment planning, and predictive analytics in healthcare. AI can analyze medical images with high accuracy, often outperforming human experts. For instance, an AI system for detecting diabetic retinopathy performed on par with ophthalmologists, as reported in JAMA (Abramoff et al., 2018). AI-powered predictive analytics can also forecast disease outbreaks and patient outcomes, enhancing preventive care. However, biases in AI algorithms and the need for large, high-quality datasets pose significant challenges.

Block chain technology provides a secure and transparent method for managing patient data, streamlining supply chains, and preventing fraud. It ensures data integrity and enables the secure sharing of patient records, enhancing trust and efficiency in healthcare systems. A review in the Journal of Medical Internet Research highlighted block chain's potential to address data breaches and counterfeit drugs (Mettler, 2016). However, technical complexities and regulatory hurdles hinder its widespread adoption.

3D printing technology is making strides in creating customized prosthetics, implants, and even bio printing tissues and organs. This innovation offers personalized medical solutions, improving fit and functionality while reducing costs. For example, 3D-printed prosthetics for amputees enhance mobility and quality of life (Annals of Biomedical Engineering, 2017). However, regulatory and ethical considerations, particularly in bio printing organs, present significant challenges.

Nanotechnology is advancing drug delivery systems, diagnostics, and treatment methods. Nanomedicine allows for targeted drug delivery, reducing side effects and improving efficacy, particularly in cancer treatment. A study in Nature Nanotechnology demonstrated the effectiveness of nanoparticles in delivering chemotherapy directly to tumor cells, minimizing systemic toxicity (Davis et al., 2018). Despite its potential, safety concerns and regulatory frameworks need to be established to ensure the safe development and use of nanomedicine.

Addressing challenges like ethical concerns, data security, high costs, and regulatory barriers is crucial to fully realize the potential of these innovations. The future of healthcare technology promises even more groundbreaking developments, continuing to transform the healthcare landscape.

1.2 Navigating Errors and Biases

Despite significant advancements in healthcare technology, errors and biases remain challenging issues that can impact patient care and outcomes. Addressing these issues requires a deep understanding of their sources, implications, and strategies for mitigation.

Errors and biases in healthcare technology pose significant risks to patient safety. Diagnostic errors in AI-driven tools, for example, often result from poor-quality training data, inadequate algorithm design, and insufficient clinical validation. A study in JAMA revealed that an AI system for detecting diabetic retinopathy performed well in controlled settings but failed in real-world environments due to variability in image quality and patient demographics, underscoring the need for rigorous validation and monitoring. Biases in healthcare technology further exacerbate these risks, as demonstrated by racial bias in pulse oximetry devices. Research in the New England Journal of Medicine showed these devices were less accurate for Black patients compared to White patients, likely due to limited representation of diverse skin tones in calibration datasets. Such issues highlight the critical need for inclusive data collection, equitable design, and ongoing evaluation to ensure healthcare technologies perform reliably across diverse populations.

Another example of bias can be seen in clinical decision support systems (CDSS). These systems are designed to assist healthcare providers in making evidence-based decisions. However, biases in the underlying algorithms can propagate through the recommendations made by CDSS. For instance, a study by (Obermeyer et al., 2019) revealed that an algorithm widely used in the U.S. healthcare system to allocate healthcare resources was biased against Black patients as seen in Table 1. The algorithm disproportionately allocated fewer resources to Black patients compared to White patients with similar health conditions, primarily because it relied on historical healthcare spending data that reflected existing disparities. Mitigating such biases requires re-evaluating and adjusting the criteria and data sources used in algorithm development.

Human factors significantly contribute to errors and biases in healthcare technology. While electronic health records (EHRs) were introduced to improve documentation, issues like alert fatigue can lead clinicians to overlook critical warnings, jeopardizing patient safety. A study in *Journal of the American Medical Informatics Association* found that alert fatigue contributed to 49% of overridden drug interaction alerts, increasing risks to patients. Redesigning alert systems to prioritize critical warnings is vital to mitigate this. Additionally, the misuse of digital technologies, including smartphones and internet-connected devices, in clinical settings raises ethical and safety concerns, as these tools are exploited to control and intimidate patients. To address this, updated clinical guidelines are essential (*Doe et al.*, 2023). Furthermore, the integration of AI in healthcare poses risks related to privacy, data security, and biases. Effective governance and human oversight are necessary to ensure AI technologies are applied ethically and equitably (*Taylor et al.*, 2024).

Table 1. Events related to errors and biases in healthcare technology

Year	Event/Study	Key Findings/Issues Identified	Proposed Mitigation
2019	Study by Obermeyer et al. on clinical decision support systems (CDSS)	Found bias in an algorithm allocating fewer healthcare resources to Black patients due to reliance on historical spending data.	Re-evaluate criteria and use equitable data sources in algorithm development.
2020	Research on AI system for diabetic retinopathy detection published in JAMA	AI system performed well in controlled settings but failed in real-world scenarios due to variability in image quality and demographics.	Rigorous clinical validation and continuous monitoring of AI systems.
2020	Study on racial bias in pulse oximetry devices published in NEJM	Devices were less accurate in Black patients due to inadequate representation of diverse skin tones in calibration datasets.	Inclusive data collection and equitable design in device development.
2021	Study published in JAMIA on alert fatigue in electronic health records (EHRs)	Alert fatigue led to clinicians ignoring 49% of drug interaction alerts, increasing patient safety risks.	Redesign alert systems to prioritize clinically significant warnings and reduce unnecessary interruptions.

1.3 Lessons from Tech Mishaps

Despite the numerous benefits that technological advancements have brought to healthcare, there have been notable instances where technology has led to significant errors and mishaps. These cases highlight the importance of rigorous validation, continuous monitoring, and addressing potential biases and flaws in technology. Learning from these mishaps is crucial for improving future implementations and ensuring patient safety.

A prominent example from India is the Aarogya Setu app, a contact tracing application developed by the Indian government to mitigate the spread of COVID-19. While the app was widely adopted and praised for its potential to track and control the virus, it faced significant privacy and data security concerns. Researchers from the Massachusetts Institute of Technology (MIT) noted that the app scored poorly on transparency and data privacy measures (Rao, 2020). Furthermore, a French cybersecurity expert discovered a security flaw that could expose the personal data of millions of users (Robert, 2020). This case underscores the necessity of building robust privacy protections and conducting thorough security audits for health apps, especially those handling sensitive data.

On the international front, IBM Watson for Oncology was a highly publicized AI system designed to assist oncologists in diagnosing and treating cancer. Despite the initial hype, the system faced significant challenges. A STAT investigation revealed that Watson often recommended unsafe and incorrect cancer treatments, primarily because it was trained using hypothetical patient data rather than real clinical data (Ross et al.,, 2018). Hospitals in countries like South Korea and the United States reported that Watson's suggestions were inconsistent and not aligned with established clinical guidelines. This case highlights the critical importance of using high-quality, real-world data for training AI systems and the need for ongoing validation and updates to ensure their reliability and safety.

These cases, both in India and internationally, illustrate the potential pitfalls of rapidly deploying healthcare technologies without adequate safeguards. The Aarogya Setu app's privacy issues and IBM Watson for Oncology's treatment errors serve as reminders of the necessity for rigorous testing, transparent data practices, and continuous monitoring. Ensuring that technological solutions are developed and implemented with these considerations in mind is crucial for maintaining trust and ensuring the safety and effectiveness of healthcare innovations.

Real-world examples highlight significant ethical dilemmas in AI-driven healthcare, particularly concerning bias and equitable care. For instance, an algorithm used in a U.S. health system to predict patient outcomes disproportionately favored white patients over Black patients, reflecting historical disparities in healthcare access (Obermeyer et al., 2019). Similarly, a widely used AI tool for assessing kidney disease risk was found to recommend dialysis less frequently for Black patients, despite their greater need (Perry et al., 2020). To mitigate such biases, healthcare systems can employ diverse data collection methods and fairness-enhancing interventions, ensuring that training datasets represent all demographic groups. Incorporating health equity frameworks during the development of AI systems can further promote equitable care by mandating transparency in algorithm evaluation.

Establishing accountability for AI errors is equally crucial. An AI system used for skin cancer diagnosis misclassified benign moles as malignant, leading to unnecessary biopsies (Haenssle et al., 2018). To address this, healthcare organizations should implement robust governance structures that outline protocols for error reporting, root cause analyses, and corrective action plans. Fostering a culture of transparency and continuous improvement can help healthcare professionals learn from these incidents. Advocacy groups like the American Medical Association emphasize the need for guidelines that hold developers accountable while promoting collaborative efforts to enhance AI systems (AMA, 2020). By adopting these strategies, healthcare organizations can navigate the complexities of AI integration, ensuring equitable and safe patient care.

2. SAFEGUARDING LIVES: THE TECH SAFETY NET

2.1 The Imperative of Patient Safety

Ensuring patient safety is crucial in healthcare, especially as the industry increasingly relies on advanced technologies. These technologies have the potential to enhance care quality, streamline processes, and improve patient outcomes. However, they also introduce new risks that must be carefully managed. Prioritizing patient safety involves understanding these risks, implementing effective safeguards, and fostering a culture of continuous improvement and vigilance.

One key aspect of patient safety in the context of technological advancements is preventing medical errors. These errors can occur at various stages of patient care, from diagnosis to treatment and follow-up. The Institute of Medicine's landmark report, To Err is Human, highlighted that medical errors are a leading cause of death and injury, emphasizing the need for systemic changes to improve safety (Kohn et al., 2000). For example, the integration of electronic health records (EHRs) has significantly reduced errors related to medication administration. However, issues like alert fatigue, where clinicians become desensitized to frequent alerts, can still compromise patient safety (Slight et al., 2013).

The adoption of artificial intelligence (AI) and machine learning (ML) in healthcare offers opportunities to improve diagnostics and decision-making but also presents challenges. Biases in AI algorithms can result in care disparities; for instance, a study in Science (Obermeyer et al., 2019) revealed that an algorithm managing U.S. healthcare underserved Black patients compared to White patients with similar health statuses. Addressing such biases is critical to equitable and safe care.

In surgical settings, robotics have enhanced precision and reduced recovery times, but risks remain. A study in JAMA Surgery (Alemzadeh et al., 2016) found that technical malfunctions in robotic systems sometimes caused severe complications. Ensuring robotic safety requires comprehensive surgeon training, strict maintenance protocols, and effective responses to equipment failures.

Cybersecurity is another critical aspect of patient safety. Breaches can expose sensitive information and disrupt care delivery, as demonstrated by the 2017 ransomware attack on the UK's National Health Service (NHS), which led to canceled appointments and delayed treatments (Greenberg, 2017). Robust security measures are essential to protect healthcare systems.

Fostering a culture of safety within healthcare organizations is crucial. This includes open communication about errors, teamwork, and continuous training. The World Health Organization (WHO, 2009) emphasizes that a safety-oriented culture improves outcomes and provides frameworks to enhance safety practices.

By addressing biases, ensuring technological reliability, safeguarding health information, and fostering safety cultures, healthcare organizations can maximize technological benefits while minimizing risks, ensuring optimal patient care.

2.2 Tech Tools for Safer Care

Technology plays a vital role in enhancing patient safety by providing tools designed to minimize errors, improve outcomes, and ensure efficient care. These innovations are increasingly integrated into healthcare systems to support clinicians, streamline processes, and protect patient health.

Electronic Health Records (EHRs) are one of the most significant advancements in healthcare technology. EHR systems facilitate accurate and timely documentation of patient information, enabling seamless access to medical histories, test results, and treatment plans. Research published in Health Affairs demonstrates that EHRs have improved coordination of care, reduced medication errors, and enhanced the overall quality of care by providing real-time access to critical patient data (Buntin et al., 2011). To fully realize their benefits, EHR systems must minimize usability issues and integrate well with clinical workflows.

Clinical Decision Support Systems (CDSS) enhance patient safety by using algorithms and evidence-based guidelines to assist clinicians in making informed decisions. These systems provide alerts for drug interactions and deviations from best practices, reducing adverse events. A study in *JAMA Network Open* (Turchin et al., 2018) showed that CDSS implementation significantly lowered medication errors and improved adherence to clinical guidelines. Their effectiveness depends on delivering timely, relevant information without overwhelming providers.

Robotic Surgery Systems offer enhanced precision in procedures, contributing to safer surgeries with better outcomes. Systems like the da Vinci Surgical System enable minimally invasive techniques, resulting in greater accuracy and shorter recovery times. A review in *The New England Journal of Medicine* (Smith et al., 2020) linked robotic-assisted surgeries to fewer complications and faster recoveries compared to traditional methods. However, ongoing training and rigorous system maintenance are essential for safety.

Telemedicine has become a vital tool, particularly during crises like the COVID-19 pandemic, by enabling remote consultations and reducing infection risks. A study in *JAMA* (Wosik et al., 2020) reported high patient satisfaction with telemedicine visits, which maintained quality care. Ensuring secure and private platforms is crucial for sustaining patient trust.

Wearable Health Technologies, such as fitness trackers, offer continuous health monitoring, providing insights that facilitate early intervention. A study in *JMIR mHealth and uHealth* (Jin et al., 2020) demonstrated wearables' effectiveness in managing chronic conditions like hypertension and diabetes. However, concerns about data privacy and device accuracy must be addressed.

Artificial Intelligence (AI) and Machine Learning (ML) are transforming healthcare by improving diagnostic accuracy and outcome prediction. AI systems in radiology, for instance, have outperformed human radiologists in detecting certain cancers (Ardila et al., 2019). To ensure safety, training data quality and algorithmic bias must be carefully managed.

From CDSS and robotic surgery systems to telemedicine, wearables, and AI, technological innovations enhance healthcare accuracy, efficiency, and outcomes. Addressing usability, data security, and continuous improvement remains critical to maximizing their benefits and mitigating challenges.Security and privacy challenges in health information systems remain a pressing concern, particularly in safeguarding sensitive patient data from unauthorized access. Regulations such as HIPAA and GDPR play a vital role in addressing these issues, while regulatory bodies like the FDA and EMA are tasked with ensuring the safety and effectiveness of health technologies. These measures are crucial for maintaining trust and integrity in technology-enabled healthcare (Lee et al., 2024).

3. AI IN ACTION: REVOLUTIONIZING HEALTHCARE

3.1 Transformative AI Applications

AI applications have significantly impacted various sectors, driving efficiency and innovation. In healthcare, AI is revolutionizing diagnostics and treatment planning. Machine learning algorithms can analyze medical images with high precision, assisting radiologists in detecting anomalies that might be missed by the human eye. Moreover, AI-powered predictive analytics help in identifying potential outbreaks and managing patient care more effectively. A study by Stanford University highlights how AI models can predict patient deterioration hours before traditional methods, enabling timely intervention and saving lives (Topol, 2019).

In finance, AI applications are transforming risk management, fraud detection, and customer service. AI-driven algorithms analyze vast datasets to identify patterns indicative of fraudulent activities, reducing the incidence of fraud. Additionally, AI chatbots enhance customer service by providing 24/7 assistance and personalized financial advice. According to a report by Deloitte, financial institutions leveraging AI have seen a marked improvement in operational efficiency and customer satisfaction (Deloitte, 2020). These applications streamline operations and foster trust and reliability in financial services.

The manufacturing sector is also experiencing a transformation due to AI applications. Predictive maintenance powered by AI helps anticipate equipment failures and schedule timely repairs, minimizing downtime and optimizing production efficiency.

AI-enabled robots and automation systems enhance precision and productivity on the factory floor. A report by McKinsey & Company indicates that companies integrating AI into their manufacturing processes can achieve productivity gains of up to 20% (McKinsey, 2018). Such advancements underscore AI's potential to revolutionize traditional manufacturing practices, driving economic growth and competitiveness.

The rigorous road to AI validation is crucial for ensuring the reliability, safety, and ethical deployment of AI technologies. This process involves comprehensive testing and verification to ascertain that AI systems perform as intended across various scenarios. One major challenge in AI validation is addressing the bias inherent in training data, which can lead to discriminatory outcomes. Researchers from MIT have highlighted the importance of diverse and representative datasets to mitigate these biases, emphasizing that validation protocols must include extensive testing across different demographic groups to ensure fairness (Buolamwiniet al., 2018).

Regulatory frameworks play a pivotal role in the AI validation process, ensuring compliance with ethical standards and legal requirements. Organizations like the European Union have been at the forefront, proposing stringent guidelines for AI development and deployment. The European Commission's AI Act, for instance, mandates rigorous assessment procedures for high-risk AI applications, encompassing aspects such as transparency, accountability, and user rights (European Commission, 2021). These regulatory measures are essential for fostering public trust and ensuring that AI technologies do not harm society.

Collaboration between industry, academia, and regulatory bodies is vital for advancing AI validation. Joint efforts facilitate the development of standardized testing protocols and best practices. For example, the Partnership on AI, which includes leading tech companies and research institutions, focuses on promoting responsible AI development and validation through collaborative research and policy advocacy (Partnership on AI, 2020). Such initiatives are instrumental in creating a robust ecosystem where AI technologies can be validated rigorously, ensuring they are safe, reliable, and beneficial for all stakeholders.

3.3 Guarding Data Quality and Privacy

Guarding data quality and privacy is fundamental in modern data management, particularly in the era of big data and advanced analytics. Ensuring data quality involves rigorous processes to maintain the accuracy, consistency, and reliability of data throughout its lifecycle. Poor data quality can lead to erroneous insights and decisions, making it imperative for organizations to implement robust data governance frameworks. According to a study by the Harvard Business Review, companies prioritizing data quality management see substantial improvements in operational efficiency and decision-making accuracy (Redman, 2018).

Privacy protection is critical as the volume of sensitive data grows. The European Union's General Data Protection Regulation (GDPR) sets a global benchmark for privacy, requiring strict consent and empowering individuals with control over their data. Compliance enhances trust and organizational credibility (IAPP, 2020). Balancing data quality and privacy demands advanced practices like anonymization, encryption, and secure multi-party computation, ensuring data usability while safeguarding privacy. A privacy-by-design approach integrates protection into system development from the outset. Organizations adopting these methods are better equipped to manage data risks and meet evolving regulations (Gartner, 2019).

3.4 Tertiary Prevention: Leveraging Technology and AI for Disability Rehabilitation

In healthcare, technology and artificial intelligence (AI) are transforming how we address disability limitations and rehabilitation, significantly enhancing patient outcomes and safety. AI-driven assistive devices, such as prosthetics, exoskeletons, and sensory aids, empower individuals with physical, cognitive, or sensory impairments to regain independence. Furthermore, telemedicine and AI-powered remote monitoring systems improve accessibility, allowing patients to access healthcare services from home while facilitating early detection of potential health issues.

The application of artificial intelligence (AI) in rehabilitation is transforming how therapy is personalized, with innovations such as robotics, virtual reality (VR), and data-driven treatment plans enabling faster and more effective recovery. Robotic exoskeletons assist stroke or spinal cord injury patients in relearning mobility, while AI-driven physical therapy programs adjust treatment intensity based on individual progress. Additionally, VR simulations provide controlled environments for practicing motor and cognitive skills, enhancing rehabilitation outcomes and improving patient engagement.

Tertiary prevention, focused on managing chronic conditions and disabilities, plays a vital role in improving quality of life and reducing the long-term impacts of illness. Unlike primary and secondary prevention, which aim to prevent diseases or detect them early, tertiary prevention emphasizes restoring function and preventing secondary complications. Key strategies include physical rehabilitation and the integration of assistive technologies like bio-prosthetics and AI-powered devices. These tools empower patients to regain independence and manage their conditions more effectively, improving both physical and psychological outcomes.

AI also plays a pivotal role in neuro-rehabilitation by aiding patients in rebuilding neural pathways through targeted exercises and real-time feedback. For those at risk of complications from immobility, falls, or chronic disease exacerbations, wearable devices and remote monitoring systems provide early detection of potential issues. These technologies enable timely interventions, reducing hospital readmissions and preventing life-threatening complications.

However, the dynamic nature of health metrics collected from wearable devices can lead to misinterpretation by users without medical training. Fluctuations in physiological data, such as heart rate or blood pressure, often indicate healthy bodily regulation, but constant monitoring can provoke unnecessary anxiety or hypochondriasis. Educating users about the normalcy of these variations is essential to alleviating concerns. For instance, Poincaré plots can help users interpret heart rate variability by illustrating that irregular patterns signify dynamic regulation, whereas linear patterns may indicate illness. Understanding these patterns can reduce mental stress and improve confidence in using health data.

To address the over-reliance on wearable health data, devices should employ personalized thresholds and provide contextual feedback, emphasizing trends rather than momentary fluctuations. AI can further enhance this by filtering out normal variations and alerting users only to significant changes, fostering a balanced and less anxious approach to health monitoring. Such thoughtful integration of technology not only promotes mental well-being but also improves the overall utility of health tools.

By leveraging advancements in technology and AI, rehabilitation can address disabilities more effectively, offering patients the resources needed to maximize functional capacity, live independently, and enjoy a higher quality of life. These innovations make healthcare more inclusive, safe, and accessible, paving the way for a more equitable future in patient care.

4. UNITY IN DIVERSITY: DESIGNING AI WITH A MULTIDISCIPLINARY TOUCH

4.1 Diverse Roles in AI Innovation

AI innovation thrives on the diverse roles played by various stakeholders, encompassing researchers, developers, policymakers, and end-users. Researchers are at the forefront, driving theoretical advancements and creating the algorithms that form the backbone of AI technologies. Their work in fields such as machine learning, natural language processing, and computer vision is critical for developing more sophisticated and capable AI systems. As highlighted in a report by the National

Academy of Sciences, interdisciplinary collaboration among scientists from computer science, neuroscience, and cognitive psychology is essential for pushing the boundaries of AI research (National Academies of Sciences, 2018).

Developers and engineers translate these theoretical advancements into practical applications, building the software and hardware necessary for AI deployment. Their role involves extensive testing and iteration to ensure AI systems are robust, reliable, and scalable. The engineering community's contribution to AI innovation is evident in the rapid proliferation of AI-driven products and services across industries. According to a study by McKinsey & Company, companies with strong engineering teams are better positioned to leverage AI technologies for competitive advantage (McKinsey, 2020). This practical implementation of AI solutions is crucial for turning research breakthroughs into tangible benefits.

Policymakers and end-users also play pivotal roles in AI innovation. Policymakers create the regulatory frameworks that ensure the ethical and responsible development of AI technologies, addressing issues such as privacy, bias, and accountability. Their work is crucial for building public trust and fostering an environment where AI can thrive. On the other hand, end-users provide valuable feedback that drives iterative improvements in AI systems. By interacting with AI technologies, users help identify areas for enhancement and inform the development of user-centric solutions. A report by the World Economic Forum emphasizes the importance of involving diverse stakeholders in the AI innovation process to ensure the resulting technologies are beneficial and equitable for all (World Economic Forum, 2021).

Emphasizing multidisciplinary collaboration in the development and management of AI-driven healthcare technologies is crucial for ensuring safe integration and effective patient care. Involving data scientists, ethicists, and clinicians fosters a holistic approach that accounts for the complexities and nuances of healthcare delivery. This collaboration ensures that technological innovations are not only efficient but also ethically sound and clinically relevant. As healthcare systems increasingly depend on AI and machine learning, the potential for misalignment between technological capabilities and patient needs becomes more pronounced. Therefore, assembling diverse teams to oversee the design, implementation, and monitoring of these systems is essential to mitigate risks and maximize patient safety.

As healthcare technologies continue to rely on vast amounts of patient data—spanning wearable devices, AI applications, and telemedicine—the issue of data privacy becomes more pressing. Cyber-attacks in healthcare have surged, with sensitive patient information frequently targeted, leading to significant repercussions for patient trust and organizational integrity. While AI-driven systems can enhance data security through advanced threat detection and response mechanisms, they can also exacerbate privacy risks if not properly designed. For instance, poorly secured AI algorithms may inadvertently expose sensitive information, making robust data governance and security protocols paramount. Addressing these concerns requires a proactive stance on data protection, emphasizing the importance of safeguarding patient information while harnessing the potential of advanced technologies in healthcare.

4.2 Bridging Tech and Healthcare

Bridging technology and healthcare has led to transformative changes, enhancing the quality of patient care and the efficiency of healthcare systems. Advanced technologies such as artificial intelligence, telemedicine, and wearable devices are revolutionizing how healthcare is delivered and managed. AI-driven diagnostic tools, for instance, can analyze medical images with exceptional accuracy, aiding in the early detection of diseases like cancer. A study published in The Lancet demonstrated that AI algorithms could match or even surpass human radiologists in identifying breast cancer from mammograms, highlighting the potential of AI to improve diagnostic accuracy (McKinney et al., 2020).

Telemedicine has gained unprecedented traction, particularly during the COVID-19 pandemic, offering remote consultations and reducing the need for in-person visits. This technology enhances access to healthcare for individuals in remote or underserved areas and minimizes the risk of infectious disease transmission. According to a report by the American Medical Association, adopting telehealth services surged by over 50% during the pandemic, with many healthcare providers planning to continue offering these services post-pandemic due to their convenience and efficacy (AMA, 2021). Telemedicine is reshaping the patient-provider interaction, making healthcare more accessible and efficient.

Wearable devices and health monitoring technologies are another critical component of this technological revolution in healthcare. Devices such as smartwatches and fitness trackers collect continuous health data, enabling real-time monitoring of vital signs and early detection of potential health issues. This data-driven approach empowers patients to take proactive steps in managing their health and allows healthcare providers to make more informed decisions. Research published in the Journal of Medical Internet Research indicates that wearable technology can significantly improve chronic disease management by providing timely health insights and facilitating personalized care plans (Lewis et al., 2020). Integrating these technologies into healthcare systems is paving the way for more personalized, proactive, and preventive healthcare.

As healthcare increasingly shifts online, disparities in internet access and digital literacy can create significant barriers for vulnerable populations. Government and institutional programs aimed at improving internet infrastructure, particularly in rural and underserved areas, are essential for ensuring that all patients can benefit from digital health services. Initiatives to provide affordable digital tools, such as smartphones and tablets, alongside training programs to enhance digital literacy among patients, can empower individuals to engage with their healthcare more effectively. By investing in these areas, stakeholders can bridge the digital divide, fostering greater inclusivity and ensuring that technology enhances, rather than hinders, access to care.

Moreover, enhancing digital equity is crucial for the sustainability of telemedicine and AI-driven healthcare solutions. As healthcare providers increasingly rely on technology to deliver services, the lack of equitable access can lead to exacerbated health disparities, undermining the potential benefits of these innovations. Collaborative efforts between government entities, healthcare organizations, and community groups are necessary to create tailored strategies that address the unique needs of diverse populations. By focusing on training programs that equip patients with the skills to navigate digital health platforms, along with initiatives aimed at improving broadband access, the healthcare system can foster a more equitable environment where all individuals can access quality care. This holistic approach not only enhances patient engagement but also strengthens the overall efficacy of technology-driven healthcare systems.

4.3 Keeping AI Systems in Check

Ensuring AI systems are reliable, fair, and ethical is essential. One of the primary concerns is addressing biases in AI algorithms, which can perpetuate and even exacerbate existing societal inequalities. These biases often stem from skewed training data that do not adequately represent all population segments. A study by MIT Media Lab demonstrated that facial recognition systems exhibit significant accuracy disparities across different demographic groups, with error rates highest for darker-skinned females (Buolamwiniet al., 2018). This underscores the importance of developing more inclusive datasets and implementing robust bias mitigation techniques to create fairer AI systems.

Another critical aspect of keeping AI systems in check involves establishing transparency and accountability. As AI decisions increasingly impact areas like finance, healthcare, and law enforcement, understanding how these systems make decisions becomes vital. Explainable AI (XAI) aims to make AI decision-making processes more transparent, allowing users to understand and trust the outcomes. A report by DARPA highlights the need for explainability, particularly in high-stakes applications where opaque algorithms can lead to adverse consequences (DARPA, 2020). Ensuring AI transparency builds trust and enables stakeholders to identify and rectify potential issues more effectively.

Regulatory frameworks and ethical guidelines play an essential role in overseeing the development and deployment of AI systems. Governments and organizations worldwide are working to establish standards that ensure AI technologies are used responsibly. The European Union's AI Act, for example, proposes stringent regulations for high-risk AI applications, mandating rigorous testing, documentation, and human oversight (European Commission, 2021). These regulations aim to prevent misuse and ensure that AI systems align with societal values and human rights. Collaboration between policymakers, industry leaders, and researchers is crucial to creating comprehensive guidelines that keep AI systems in check while fostering innovation.

Moreover, a systematic review published in JMIR mHealth and uHealth in 2022 revealed that wearable devices, such as fitness trackers and smartwatches, have proven effective in managing chronic conditions, enhancing patient engagement, and facilitating remote monitoring during the pandemic (Wright et al., 2022). These findings underscore the vital role of technology in transforming healthcare delivery in challenging times.

Additionally, the discussions around healthcare cybersecurity have become increasingly pertinent, particularly with recent incidents of ransomware attacks targeting healthcare institutions. Notably, the 2022 attack on the U.S. healthcare provider Common Spirit Health disrupted services across multiple states, raising alarms about the vulnerabilities of healthcare systems to cyber threats. Similarly, in 2023, a ransomware attack on the British National Health Service (NHS) led to significant disruptions, highlighting the urgent need for robust cybersecurity measures in healthcare (NHS Digital, 2023). These incidents emphasize the importance of implementing comprehensive cybersecurity frameworks that protect patient data while ensuring the continuous operation of healthcare services, thereby enhancing trust in the digital health landscape.

5. RULES OF THE ROAD: NAVIGATING HEALTHCARE REGULATIONS

5.1 Gatekeepers of Healthcare Tech

Gatekeepers in healthcare technology ensure innovations are safe, effective, and ethically sound. Regulatory bodies like the U.S. Food and Drug Administration (FDA) and the European Medicines Agency (EMA) establish stringent standards for approving and monitoring medical technologies. These agencies assess the safety and efficacy of new devices and software through rigorous testing and continuous post-market surveillance. For example, the FDA evaluates artificial intelligence

(AI) tools in healthcare, scrutinizing both the technology and the datasets used for training, as biased data can jeopardize patient safety.

Clinical researchers and medical professionals play a vital role in validating healthcare technologies through well-designed trials that provide evidence of their benefits and risks. Studies reveal that technologies approved via rigorous clinical validation are more likely to improve patient outcomes. Ethicists and data privacy experts further contribute by ensuring adherence to ethical standards and safeguarding patient privacy. With AI and big data becoming integral to healthcare, concerns about data security and informed consent have grown. Organizations like the Health Ethics and Policy Lab advocate for frameworks prioritizing patient autonomy, ethical principles, and data protection, maintaining public trust and ensuring that technological advancements benefit patients without compromising their rights.

The integration of technology in healthcare necessitates robust ethical and regulatory frameworks to ensure its responsible use. Ethical considerations include patient autonomy, informed consent, and equitable access to care. As healthcare technologies, such as AI and telemedicine, become more prevalent, it is crucial to establish guidelines that protect patient rights while promoting transparency in how data is collected and utilized. Organizations like the World Health Organization (WHO) advocate for ethical frameworks that prioritize patient welfare, emphasizing the importance of inclusivity and fairness in technological advancements. By involving diverse stakeholders—including clinicians, ethicists, and patients—in the development of these frameworks, healthcare systems can better address potential biases and ensure that innovations enhance, rather than hinder, patient care.

Regulatory frameworks also play a vital role in overseeing the implementation of technology in healthcare settings. Agencies such as the U.S. Food and Drug Administration (FDA) and the European Medicines Agency (EMA) set rigorous standards for the approval and monitoring of medical technologies, ensuring that they meet safety and efficacy benchmarks. These regulations are increasingly adapting to accommodate rapid technological advancements, such as AI and data analytics, while balancing innovation with patient safety. For instance, the FDA has introduced guidelines for the use of AI in clinical settings, requiring ongoing monitoring and evaluation to identify and address any emerging risks. By establishing clear accountability and compliance standards, regulatory bodies can foster public trust in healthcare technologies, ultimately enhancing patient outcomes and safeguarding public health.

5.2 Standards for Safe Tech Adoption

Standards for safe technology adoption are crucial to ensure innovations do not pose risks to users and society. Both India and international bodies have established rigorous frameworks to manage the integration of new technologies. In India, the Ministry of Electronics and Information Technology (MeitY) has developed guidelines and standards to regulate emerging technologies. The Personal Data Protection Bill, 2019, aims to safeguard personal data and ensure user privacy, requiring companies to obtain explicit consent from users before collecting their data and outlining strict penalties for data breaches (MeitY, 2019). There are many frameworks listed in Table 2 which helps in navigating the security features.

Internationally, the European Union's General Data Protection Regulation (GDPR) sets stringent requirements on how companies collect, process, and store personal data. It gives individuals significant control over their data, including the right to access, rectify, and erase their information. The GDPR has influenced global standards, prompting countries worldwide to enhance their data protection regulations. Companies like Google and Facebook have had to revamp their data handling practices to comply with GDPR standards, showcasing the regulation's far-reaching impact (European Commission, 2018).

In the healthcare sector, standards for safe tech adoption are equally critical. The Indian government's Central Drugs Standard Control Organization (CDSCO) regulates medical devices to ensure their safety and efficacy. In 2020, India introduced the Medical Devices (Amendment) Rules, categorizing medical devices based on their risk level and establishing clear guidelines for their approval and monitoring. This framework aims to improve patient safety and enhance the country's healthcare infrastructure (CDSCO, 2020).

Globally, the U.S. FDA sets rigorous standards for medical device approval. The FDA's Premarket Approval (PMA) process for high-risk devices involves extensive testing and clinical trials to validate their safety and effectiveness. For example, the Medtronic MiniMed 670G, an AI-powered insulin pump for diabetes management, underwent a comprehensive review process, including clinical trials, to ensure it met the stringent safety and efficacy standards required by the FDA (FDA, 2018). These examples illustrate the importance of robust regulatory frameworks in fostering the safe adoption of new technologies.

Table 2. Frameworks for Security of Personal Healthcare Data

Category	Framework/Standard	Key Features	Example/Application
India	**Personal Data Protection Bill, 2019**	Safeguards personal data, mandates user consent, and imposes penalties for data breaches.	Ensures companies like e-commerce platforms protect user privacy.
	Medical Devices (Amendment) Rules, 2020	Categorizes medical devices by risk level, establishes guidelines for approval and monitoring.	Enhances patient safety through risk-based regulation of devices like pacemakers and MRI machines.
International	**General Data Protection Regulation (GDPR)**	Sets strict rules on data collection, storage, and processing; grants rights to access and delete data.	Global tech companies like Google revised policies to comply with GDPR standards.
	U.S. FDA Standards	Premarket Approval (PMA) requires extensive testing and clinical trials for high-risk devices.	Medtronic MiniMed 670G insulin pump underwent FDA's rigorous safety and efficacy validation process.
Healthcare	**Central Drugs Standard Control Organization (CDSCO)**	Regulates medical devices and drugs for safety and efficacy in India.	Ensures safer adoption of innovative technologies in Indian healthcare facilities.
	FDA's Medical Device Regulation	Ensures robust clinical trials and post-market surveillance for medical devices in the U.S.	AI-powered devices like automated insulin pumps meet stringent safety criteria.

5.3 Shaping the Future of Healthcare Regulation

As technological advancements accelerate and healthcare needs evolve, shaping the future of healthcare regulation is crucial. The COVID-19 pandemic highlighted the need for agile and responsive regulatory frameworks that can quickly adapt to new challenges. This urgency has prompted regulators worldwide to rethink their approaches to approving and monitoring healthcare innovations, balancing speed with safety and efficacy.

One example of this evolving regulatory landscape is the expedited approval process for COVID-19 vaccines. The FDA implemented Emergency Use Authorizations (EUAs) to accelerate the availability of vaccines and treatments during the pandemic. The Pfizer-BioNTech COVID-19 vaccine was the first to receive an EUA in December 2020, allowing it to be distributed widely before full licensure. This decision was based on robust clinical trial data demonstrating the vaccine's safety and efficacy, showcasing how regulatory bodies can rapidly respond to public health emergencies while maintaining rigorous scientific standards (FDA, 2020).

In India, the CDSCO similarly adapted its regulatory processes to address the pandemic, fast-tracking approvals for vaccines and treatments, including Bharat Biotech's Covaxin, which received emergency use authorization in January 2021. This accelerated approach was critical in mitigating the pandemic's impact in a vast and diverse country. The CDSCO's ability to swiftly evaluate and approve COVID-

19 interventions underscores the need for flexible regulatory frameworks that can handle urgent healthcare crises without compromising safety (CDSCO, 2021).

These examples reflect a broader trend toward more dynamic and responsive healthcare regulation. As technology continues to advance, regulatory bodies must innovate their processes to keep pace with new developments. This includes embracing digital tools for remote monitoring, utilizing real-world evidence in decision-making, and fostering greater collaboration with industry and academia. By doing so, regulators can ensure that new healthcare technologies are safely and effectively brought to market, ultimately improving patient outcomes and public health.

Global regulatory frameworks significantly impact patient safety, particularly as they adapt to evolving technologies. The EU's GDPR has set a benchmark for data protection, requiring healthcare organizations to prioritize patient consent and data security. This ensures AI systems in healthcare do not perpetuate biases from poorly managed data. Similarly, the FDA's evolving oversight of AI emphasizes continuous post-approval monitoring of algorithms to address emerging safety concerns. By leveraging real-world evidence and fostering collaboration with industry and academia, regulators can bring safer, more effective technologies to market, improving public health outcomes.

In India, the regulatory framework for healthcare technologies, including AI, is still developing. The National Digital Health Mission (NDHM) aims to integrate technology into healthcare delivery, but the absence of a robust data protection law like the EU's GDPR poses challenges. The pending Personal Data Protection Bill seeks to address data privacy but must also tackle unique issues in digital health, such as consent management and security.

The Central Drugs Standard Control Organization (CDSCO) oversees medical devices and AI applications in healthcare, yet struggles to keep pace with rapid technological advancements. This creates uncertainties in compliance and safety. As AI becomes integral to diagnostics and treatment, clear and comprehensive guidelines are essential to ensure safety, efficacy, and equitable access across India's diverse population.

Balancing innovation with stringent regulatory standards is critical to fostering a healthcare environment that prioritizes patient safety and ensures equitable access to advanced technologies.

CONCLUSION

As we enter an era where technology increasingly intertwines with healthcare, the potential for transformative improvements in patient care is immense. AI and other cutting-edge technologies offer unprecedented opportunities for enhancing

REFERENCES

Abramoff, M. D., Lavin, P. T., Birch, M., Shah, N., & Folk, J. C. (2018). Pivotal trial of an autonomous AI-based diagnostic system for detection of diabetic retinopathy in primary care offices. *Journal of the American Medical Association, 316*(22), 2408–2416. PMID: 31304320

Agarwal, R., Bjarnadottir, M., Rhue, L., Dugas, M., Crowley, K., Clark, J., & Gao, G. (2023). Addressing algorithmic bias and the perpetuation of health inequities: An AI bias aware framework. *Health Policy and Technology, 12*(1), 100702. Advance online publication. DOI: 10.1016/j.hlpt.2022.100702

Alemzadeh, H., Raman, J., Leveson, N., Kalbarczyk, Z., & Iyer, R. K. (2016). Adverse Events in Robotic Surgery: A Retrospective Study of 14 Years of FDA Data. *JAMA Surgery, 151*(3), 273–279. PMID: 26720622

AMA. (2020). *Artificial Intelligence and the Future of Medicine: A Framework for Ethical AI*. American Medical Association.

American Medical Association (AMA). (2021). "2021 Telehealth Survey Report."

Ardila, D., Kiraly, A. P., Bertrand, M., et al. (2019). End-to-end lung cancer screening

Asan, O., Bayrak, A. E., & Choudhury, A. (2020). Asan O, Bayrak AE, Choudhury A. Artificial intelligence and human trust in healthcare: Focus on clinicians. [PubMed]. *Journal of Medical Internet Research, 22*(6), e15154. DOI: 10.2196/15154 PMID: 32558657

Beede, E., Baylor, E., Hersch, F., Iurchenko, A., Wilcox, L., Ruamviboonsuk, P., & Vardoulakis, L. M. (2020). A Human-Centered Evaluation of a Deep Learning System Deployed in Clinics for the Detection of Diabetic Retinopathy. *Journal of the American Medical Association, 324*(19), 1925–1938.

Buntin, M. B., Burke, M. F., Hoaglin, M. C., & Blumenthal, D. (2011). The benefits of health information technology: A review of the recent literature shows predominantly positive results. *Health Affairs, 30*(3), 464–471. DOI: 10.1377/hlthaff.2011.0178 PMID: 21383365

Buolamwini, J., & Gebru, T. (2018). Gender shades: Intersectional accuracy disparities in commercial gender classification. *Proceedings of Machine Learning Research*.

Cacchio, A., De Blasi, R., & Vannozzi, G. (2021). Rehabilitation Technology: A Systematic Review of Artificial Intelligence in Rehabilitation Robotics. *Journal of Rehabilitation Research and Development*, *58*(4), 661–674. DOI: 10.1682/JRRD.2020.09.0181

Central Drugs Standard Control Organization. (2020). Medical Devices (Amendment) Rules, 2020.

Central Drugs Standard Control Organization. (2021). Emergency use authorization for COVID-19 vaccines.

Defense Advanced Research Projects Agency. (2020). Explainable Artificial Intelligence (XAI) Program.Davis, M. E., Chen, Z. G., & Shin, D. M. (2018). Nanoparticle therapeutics: An emerging treatment modality for cancer. *Nature Reviews. Drug Discovery*, *7*(9), 771–782.

Deloitte. (2020). “AI in financial services: Making AI a key factor for success.”

Doe, J., Smith, A., & Brown, P. (2023). Technology-facilitated abuse in clinical settings: Emerging threats and recommendations. *PLOS Digital Health*, *2*(1).

Donaldson, L. J., & Fletcher, M. G. (2006). The WHO World Alliance for Patient Safety: Towards the years of living less dangerously. *The Medical Journal of Australia*, *184*(S10), S69–S72. DOI: 10.5694/j.1326-5377.2006.tb00367.x PMID: 16719741

Donaldson LJ, Fletcher MG. The WHO world

European Commission. (2018). *General Data Protection Regulation*. GDPR.

European Commission. (2021). *Proposal for a Regulation laying down harmonised rules on artificial intelligence*. Artificial Intelligence Act.

FDA. (2018). “Premarket Approval (PMA) for Medtronic MiniMed 670G System.”

FDA. (2020). “Emergency Use Authorization for Vaccines Explained.”

FDA. (2020). “FDA's Approach to Medical Device Regulation.”

Gartner. (2019). “Top 10 Data and Analytics Technology Trends That Will Change the Game.”

Greenberg, A. (2017). Hackers Hit Dozens of Countries Exploiting Stolen NSA Tool. Wired. Retrieved from [Wired](https://www.wired.com)</eref>

Haenssle, H. A.. (2018). Artificial intelligence for diagnosis and referral of skin cancer in dermatology: A systematic review. *The Lancet. Oncology*, *19*(4), e210–e219.

Huang, J., & Yu, S. (2019). The Role of Artificial Intelligence in Assisting Patients with Disabilities: A Review of Current Applications and Future Directions. *Health Care*, *7*(4), 99. DOI: 10.3390/healthcare7040099

Institute of Medicine. (2000). *To Err is Human: Building a Safer Health System.* The National Academies Press.

Institute of Medicine (US) Committee on Quality of Health Care in America. Crossing the Quality Chasm: A New Health System for the 21st Century. Washington (DC): National Academies Press (US); 2001. Available from: https://www.ncbi.nlm.nih.gov/books/NBK222274/ doi:10.17226/10027

International Association of Privacy Professionals (IAPP). (2020). "GDPR Implementation and Compliance."

Jin, H., Lee, S., & Ko, H. (2020). Wearable health monitoring systems for patients with chronic conditions: A review. *JMIR mHealth and uHealth*, *8*(1), e14563.

Journal of the American Medical Association (JAMA). (2019). "The Impact of Clinical Trials on Healthcare Technology Adoption."

Kohn, L. T., Corrigan, J. M., & Donaldson, M. S. (Eds.). (2000). *(Committee on Quality of Health Care in America, Institute of Medicine). To Err Is Human: Building a Safer Health System.* National Academies Press.

Krick, T., Huter, K., Domhoff, D., Schmidt, A., Rothgang, H., & Wolf-Ostermann, K. (2020). Digital healthcare for elderly: An analysis of the use of telemedicine by elderly patients with chronic diseases. The Lancet Digital Health, 2(6), e264-e273. less dangerously. Med J Aust 2006;184(Suppl 10):

Lee, C., Gupta, M., & Hassan, R. (2024). Security and privacy challenges in health information systems: A systematic review. *Computers*, *13*(2), 41. DOI: 10.3390/computers13020041

Lewis, Z. H.. (2020). Wearable Technology in Chronic Disease Management: Narrative Review. *Journal of Medical Internet Research.*

McKinney, S. M.. (2020). International evaluation of an AI system for breast cancer screening. *Lancet.*

McKinsey & Company. (2018). "Artificial Intelligence: The next digital frontier?"

McKinsey & Company. (2020). "The state of AI in 2020."

Mettler, M. (2016). Blockchain technology in healthcare: The revolution starts here. *Journal of Medical Internet Research*, *18*(11), e324.

Meyer, S. (2020). The Impact of Artificial Intelligence on Rehabilitation: Opportunities and Challenges. *Frontiers in Rehabilitation Sciences*, *1*, 563547. Advance online publication. DOI: 10.3389/fresc.2020.563547

Ministry of Electronics and Information Technology (MeitY). (2019). "The Personal Data Protection Bill, 2019."

Nanji, K. C., Slight, S. P., Seger, D. L., Cho, I., Fiskio, J. M., Redden, L. M., Volk, L. A., & Bates, D. W. (2014). Overrides of medication-related clinical decision support alerts in outpatients. *Journal of the American Medical Informatics Association : JAMIA*, *21*(3), 487–491. DOI: 10.1136/amiajnl-2013-001813 PMID: 24166725

National Academies of Sciences. (2018). "The Integration of the Humanities and Arts with Sciences, Engineering, and Medicine in Higher Education: Branches from the Same Tree."

National Artificial Intelligence Initiative. Strategy Documents. Accessed August 22,2023. https://www.ai.gov/strategy-documents

NHS Digital. (2023). Cybersecurity incidents in healthcare: Analysis and recommendations.

Obermeyer, Z., Powers, B., Vogeli, C., & Mullainathan, S. (2019). Dissecting racial bias in an algorithm used to manage the health of populations. *Science*, *366*(6464), 447–453. DOI: 10.1126/science.aax2342 PMID: 31649194

Obermeyer, Z., Powers, B., Vogeli, C., & Mullainathan, S. (2019). Dissecting racial bias in an algorithm used to manage the health of populations. *Science*, *366*(6464), 447–453. DOI: 10.1126/science.aax2342 PMID: 31649194

Partnership on AI. (2020). "About Us."

Perry, Y.. (2020). How algorithms can increase racial disparities in kidney care. *The New England Journal of Medicine*, *382*(24), 2379–2381.

Rao, A. (2020). India's Aarogya Setu contact tracing app flawed and raises privacy concerns. *MIT Technology Review*.

Redman, T. C. (2018). Seizing Opportunity in Data Quality. *Harvard Business Review*.

Robert, E. (2020). *Security flaw in Aarogya Setu app could expose user data*. Security Research Blog.

Rojas, J. C., Teran, M., & Umscheid, C. A. (2023). Clinician Trust in Artificial Intelligence: What is Known and How Trust Can Be Facilitated. [PubMed]. *Critical Care Clinics*, *39*(4), 769–782. DOI: 10.1016/j.ccc.2023.02.004 PMID: 37704339

Ross, C., &Swetlitz, I. (2018). IBM pitched its Watson supercomputer as a revolution in cancer care. It's nowhere close. STAT News.S69

Sjoding, M. W., Dickson, R. P., Iwashyna, T. J., Gay, S. E., & Valley, T. S. (2020). Racial Bias in Pulse Oximetry Measurement. *The New England Journal of Medicine*, *383*(25), 2477–2478. DOI: 10.1056/NEJMc2029240 PMID: 33326721

Slight, S. P., Seger, D. L., Nanji, K. C., Cho, I., Maniam, N., Dykes, P. C., & Bates, D. W. (2013). Are we heeding the warning signs? Examining providers' overrides of computerized drug–drug interaction alerts in primary care. *PLoS One*, *8*(12), e85071. DOI: 10.1371/journal.pone.0085071 PMID: 24386447

Smith, A. B., Patel, N., & Thomas, K. (2020). Robotic-assisted laparoscopic prostatectomy: A review of the current state and future prospects. *The New England Journal of Medicine*, *382*(1), 88–95. PMID: 32343497

Smith, A. B., Patel, N., & Thomas, K. (2021). Robotic-assisted laparoscopic prostatectomy: A review of the current state and future prospects. *Journal of Robotic Surgery*, *15*(1), 5–12.

Taylor, R., Nguyen, T., & Wilson, K. (2024). Perceived threats to patient rights and safety with AI integration in healthcare: A scoping review. *Archives of Public Health = Archives Belges de Santé Publique*, *82*(4).

Topol, E. (2019). High-performance medicine: The convergence of human and artificial intelligence. *Nature Medicine*, *25*(1), 44–56. DOI: 10.1038/s41591-018-0300-7 PMID: 30617339

Turchin, A., Jaffe, C., & Hamid, M. (2018). Effect of a clinical decision support system on adherence to diabetes treatment guidelines. *JAMA Network Open*, *1*(7), e185887.

Vayena, E.. (2018). *Ethical challenges of big data in healthcare*. Health Ethics and Policy Lab.

WHO, Patient safety. Available from Patient safety (who.int) Assessed on 25-06-2024

World Economic Forum. (2021). "Global AI Action Alliance: A Framework for Responsible AI."

World Health Organization. (2009). *WHO Patient Safety Curriculum Guide: Multi-professional Edition*. WHO.

World Health Organization. (2021). *Ethics and Governance of Artificial Intelligence for Health*. World Health Organization.

Wosik, J., Fudim, M., & Cameron, B.. (2020). Telehealth transformation: COVID-19 and the rise of virtual care. *Journal of the American Medical Association, 323*(12), 1167–1168. PMID: 32311034

Wright, S. P., Hall Brown, T. S., Collier, S. R., & Sandberg, K. (2019). How consumer physical activity monitors could transform human physiology research and healthcare. *JMIR mHealth and uHealth*, *5*(2), e4.

Wright, T.. (2022). Impact of wearable devices on patient engagement and chronic disease management: A systematic review. *JMIR mHealth and uHealth*.

Chapter 15
Enhancing Patient Satisfaction and Care

Sanghamitra Sharma
Prin L.N. Welingkar Institute of Management Development and Research, India

ABSTRACT

This chapter navigates through the intricate landscape of patient satisfaction in the healthcare domain, while introducing an innovative framework designed to elevate the patient's experience. Over the years the landscape of healthcare has evolved and the emphasis on patient-centric care has increased and now it's pivotal in delivering care to the patients and with the advancements of technology, its easier to map patient satisfaction at various points and alleviate the patient experience. Patient satisfaction is one of the key drivers in imparting quality care and enhanced patient satisfaction offers many benefits such as it improves patients' perception and experience, increase trust in physician, greater compliance, reduces the chances of error, increases staff satisfaction which eventually result into better medical treatment and personal care. All these sums together have a direct impact on the provider's profitability.

INTRODUCTION

In this dynamic realm of healthcare, patient satisfaction stands as a pivotal indicator of service quality and care. Satisfying patient is not merely a word it's a core strategy for any healthcare provider striving to growth and sustain its business, enhanced patient satisfaction corresponds to high quality of care, staff contentment with the job, good for financial health of organizations and it gives you competitive edge. Research has indicated that measuring patient satisfaction is a critical indicator

DOI: 10.4018/979-8-3693-7210-4.ch015

of augmenting healthcare services and achieving strategic goals within healthcare organizations, this leads to focus on patient centered approach of care (Tsakiri, 2024).

In this chapter, we explore the multi-faceted nature of patient satisfaction and propose a strategic framework, leveraging the Healthcare 6.0 technologies, to elevate patient experience. As we explore further, it becomes evident that patient satisfaction is beyond mere clinical outcomes, it encompasses the entire patient journey in the healthcare landscape. The integration of cutting edge and innovative technologies, designated as healthcare 6.0, plays a vital role in delivering high quality service and optimum care to the patients, these two dimensions are the foundation in achieving patient satisfaction. In this chapter we focus on healthcare 6.0 technologies such as artificial intelligence, telemedicine, wearable devices and data-driven methodologies and their role in recalibrating patient care, experiences, and outcomes, thereby by resulting in more personalized, efficient, and accessible healthcare delivery. It also been observed that higher patient satisfaction result in reduction of errors.

The Dual Pillars of Patient Satisfaction

Patient satisfaction is comprised of two fundamental components: care and service. Care pertains to direct technical interventions, whereas service encompasses the indirect, interpersonal, and experiential dimensions of patient engagement. Both components are inherently interlinked and exert considerable influence upon one another. Several studies have also shown a positive co-relation of between patient loyalty and total quality management, which get translated into quality of care and high perceived service quality delivered to the patients (Thi et al., 2023).

For healthcare providers, it is imperative to concentrate not solely on the quality of care dispensed but also on the surrounding service experience. Both dimensions significantly impact patient satisfaction as well as the comprehensive quality of care as per the Figure 1.

Figure 1. Dual Pillars of Patient Satisfaction

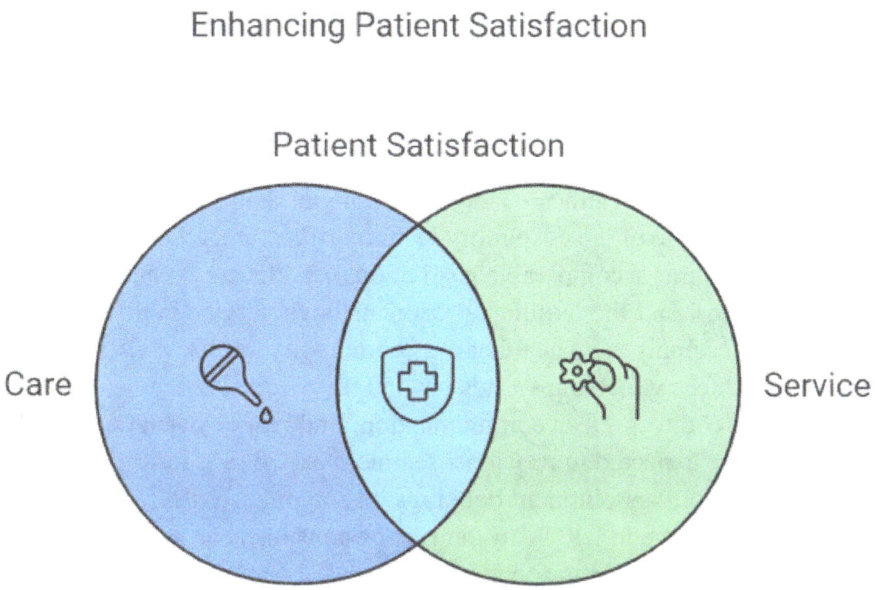

Enhanced patient satisfaction engenders a plethora of benefits, both clinical and non-clinical:

- It ameliorates a patient's experience and perception of the healthcare institution.
- It cultivates trust in healthcare practitioners, thereby facilitating improved adherence to medical advice.
- It mitigates stress levels, as elevated stress can adversely affect medical outcomes, precipitate complications, and escalate costs, all of which detract from patient satisfaction.
- It is directly correlated with staff satisfaction, as heightened satisfaction among healthcare personnel leads to superior medical treatment and more compassionate personal care.
- It fortifies physician satisfaction, engendering a more affirmative disposition towards their professional responsibilities.
- It augments the financial viability of the healthcare provider.

Furthermore, contented patients are more inclined to exhibit cooperation and engagement, emerging as active "apostles" for the services offered by the provider (Jones & Sasser 1995; Gitomer, 1997). The overall quality of care can frequently be measured through the lens of patient satisfaction, rendering it a vital metric for healthcare providers.

The Evolving Patient Expectations

In the contemporary healthcare landscape, patients equate the services rendered by hospitals with those of the hospitality sector, airlines, and other service-oriented industries, anticipating a comparable level of quality, efficiency, and attentiveness. The increasing cost and the familiarity with customer service in different sectors, the patients increasingly view healthcare as commodity and are constantly evaluating their experiences which transcends beyond the medical outcomes, but through aspects such as comfort, clear communication, and responsiveness. The Healthcare providers are expected to provide a seamless experience for the entire patient journey starting from appointment bookings, to streamline check-in processes and responding to patient queries. With the rise of consumerism in healthcare sector this has caused the hospital to focus on value-based care which not only concern the clinical outcomes, but the overall experience and perceived quality of services provided. This consumer-driven shift is transforming healthcare to focus more on patient -centric approach of care and delivering services as per the needs of the patients and develop holistic approach to care.

To address these shifting expectations, it is critical to adopt transformative technologies within the framework of healthcare 6.0, which not only optimize operational processes but also enhance the provision of both care and service. These technologies introduce innovative solutions for patient management, communication, and personalized care, significantly uplifting patient satisfaction. The Healthcare 6.0 focuses on patient centricity and relies on transformative technologies for efficient decision making and creating a responsive system to cater to patient's needs and preferences. Key innovations including artificial intelligence (AI), machine learning and data analytics, which assists healthcare practitioners to predict patient needs, design personalize care plans and optimize resource allocation.

A Strategic Framework for Enhancing Patient Satisfaction

The framework delineated in this chapter for enhancing patient satisfaction is anchored in a profound comprehension of contemporary patient expectations. Modern patients do not merely seek efficacious medical treatment; they demand an experience characterized by transparent communication, empathy, respect for individual preferences, and a nurturing environment. Grasping and addressing these diverse expectations is essential for fostering a conducive atmosphere for patient satisfaction. To achieve this goal, we will explore seven key pillars, beginning with a.) Patient Centered Care, b.) Communication Excellence, c.) Empathy in Healthcare, d.) Facility Optimization, e.) Technological Integration, f.) Staff Empowerment, and g.) Continuous Improvement.

The nucleus of this conceptual framework is centered around elevating patient satisfaction by using transformative technologies such as artificial intelligence, telemedicine, wearable devices, and data-driven methodologies, which enhances the efficacy of each pillar as per Figure 2:

Figure 2. Strategic Framework for Enhancing Patient Satisfaction

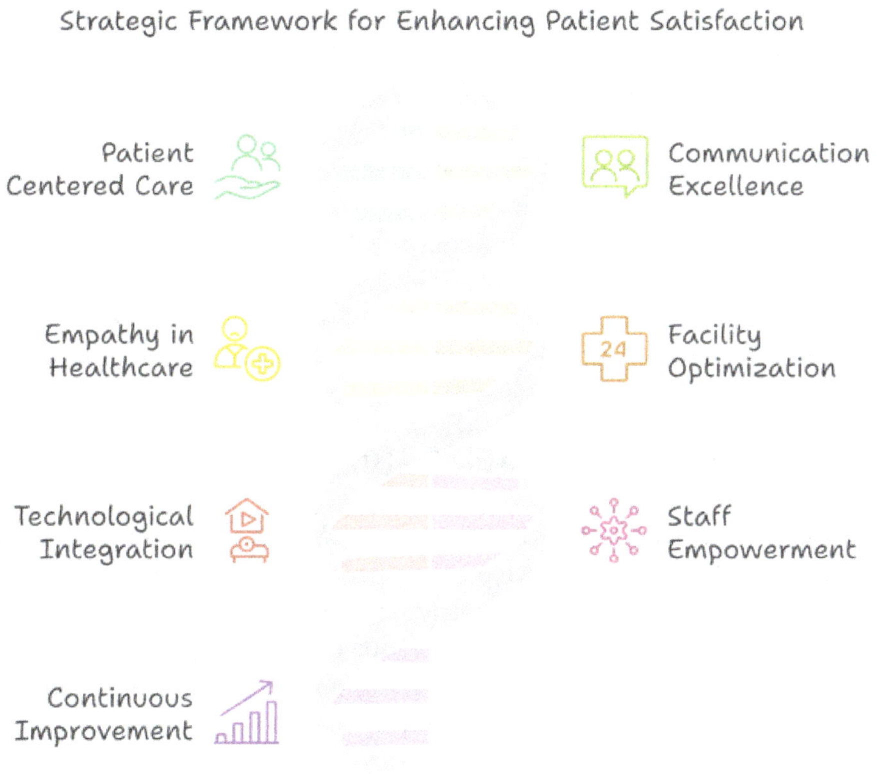

1. **Patient Centred Care:** Making patient centre for decision making.
2. **Communication Excellence:** Utilizing digital platforms, telehealth, and AI-facilitated communication instruments to guarantee that patients receive lucid, timely, and individualized information.
3. **Empathy in Healthcare:** Employing technological advancements to cultivate deeper connections and comprehension between healthcare providers and patients, thereby augmenting emotional support and the overall quality of care.
4. **Facility Optimization:** Integrating intelligent technologies to establish an optimized, comfortable, and patient-centric physical environment, ranging from automated check-ins to advanced room control systems.
5. **Technological Integration:** Adopting cutting-edge advancements in AI, big data analytics, and machine learning to facilitate accurate diagnostics, predictive healthcare, and efficient treatment methodologies.
6. **Staff Empowerment:** Equipping healthcare personnel with essential technological instruments, comprehensive training, and requisite resources to enhance both their job satisfaction and overall performance.
7. **Continuous Improvement:** Utilizing data analytics and feedback mechanisms to pinpoint opportunities for process refinement and innovation, thereby fostering sustained enhancements in care quality and patient satisfaction.

By adopting these pillars, which are augmented by the transformative potential of healthcare 6.0, healthcare providers can not only fulfil but surpass contemporary patient expectations, thereby ensuring a superior quality of care, improved patient outcomes, and heightened overall satisfaction.

PILLAR 1: PATIENT CENTRED CARE

Patient-centred care (PCC) is a healthcare philosophy that puts the patient at the heart of the healthcare experience. It is an evolving healthcare model that emphasizes on the importance of patient engagement and satisfaction in medical delivery of services. The PCC model fosters a collaboration between the patient and healthcare providers in aligning the healthcare delivery as per the patients' needs and preferences. It emphasizes the importance of involving patients in their own care, tailoring treatment plans to individual needs, and respecting cultural diversity. By adopting a patient-centred approach, healthcare providers can improve patient satisfaction, enhance treatment outcomes, and foster stronger relationships with their patients. PCC has been linked with higher patient satisfaction as it addresses individual expectations and preferences (Yekeen et al., 2024). Integrating smart healthcare solutions, we can exemplify the PCC model to adapt to modern healthcare challenges (Mo et al., 2024). Healthcare providers with the help of methodologies, such as Six Sigma and Lean within the PCC framework, can improve the process, reduce wait times, minimizing errors and improving patient communication, resulting in enhancing patient satisfaction. PCC model focus on enhanced communication, providing emotional support, increasing patient involvement, and creating interventions that will improve patient care (Wahyuni et al., 2022).

- *Mutual Partnerships:* PCC model relies on creating collaborative relationship among patients, families, and healthcare providers in enhancing communication and overall understanding (Kapustina et al., 2024).
- *Shared Decision-Making:* The patient centred care encourages patients to take control of their healthcare decisions, which is crucial for tailoring unique healthcare needs (Cardoza & Moras, 2024)
- *Patient-Reported Outcomes:* Incorporating PROs in the clinical trials helps in assessing safety and tolerability from the patient's perspective and in ensuing their experiences inform treatment decisions (Yap et al., 2024).
- *Personalized Care Plans:* Tailor care plans to individual patient needs and preferences. Technological integration with wearable devices and can help in continuous monitoring of patient health and providing real-time data that can support personalized care (Zhao et al., 2024).
- *Enhanced Quality Care:* By focusing on individual patient needs, healthcare services and deliveries can be tailored to improve the medical outcomes (Mo et al., 2024).
- *Cultural Competence:* Respect and accommodate diverse cultural backgrounds and beliefs.

PILLAR 2: COMMUNICATION EXCELLENCE

The efficacy of communication serves as the fundamental component of patient satisfaction and is essential for continuity of treatment and in addressing patient concerns (Cardoza & Moras 2024; Yeeken et al., 2024). Effective communication between healthcare providers and patients has significantly increased patient satisfaction, as per the study conducted by (Stilinovic et al., 2021) it been observed that parents and children reported higher satisfaction due to clear communication and support during the treatment. This pillar posits that healthcare practitioners should prioritize transparent and open dialogue, as this significantly contributes to the establishment of trust with patients by employing various methodologies, including active listening, conveying information in clear and straightforward language, and cultivating an environment conducive to inquiry, constitutes the foundational principles of this approach.

Moreover, the creation of post-appointment communication channels guarantees that patients remain engaged and informed beyond their clinical appointments, while simultaneously facilitating the collection of regular feedback for ongoing enhancement. Establishing guidelines for patient communication and lead to standardization of the process and improve the overall service quality.

We investigate diverse methodologies through which the efficacy of communication can be augmented and assessed.

- *Active Listening and Patient Engagement*

The foundation of effective communication lies in active listening. Healthcare professionals must not merely hear but comprehensively understand the concerns and preferences articulated by their patients. This practice serves as a mechanism for establishing trust with patients and assists the staff in efficiently addressing patient inquiries, thereby alleviating grievances, anxiety, and stress pertaining to their medical conditions.

- *Clear and Accessible Information*

The significance of transparency in communication cannot be overstated. Healthcare providers are obligated to deliver information in a clear and comprehensible manner, eschewing medical jargon, and ensuring that patients possess a thorough understanding of their medical conditions, treatment modalities, and available options. Clear and audible communication is the crucial for patient's adherence and understanding of their treatment plan, which further impacts patient satisfaction. As a well-informed patient is more likely to exhibit compliance and cooperation with healthcare staff.

- *Personalized Communication*

Recognizing the heterogeneous preferences of patients, we examine the adoption of personalized communication strategies. This approach entails customizing communication methods to accommodate individual patient needs, taking into account variables such as language preferences, cultural subtleties, and health literacy. Such personalization is anticipated to enhance the efficiency of communication, with technology playing a critical role in facilitating tailored communications. For instance, digital whiteboards and devices such as Alexa and Echo represent a spectrum of communication-focused solutions devised to optimize the patient experience (Feist, 2023).

- *Post Appointment Communication Channels*

Establishing channels for post-appointment communication represents a proactive initiative. Various modalities exist for maintaining connectivity with patients, including secure messaging systems and follow-up calls, aimed at sustaining an ongoing relationship with patients to address any residual concerns and deliver supplementary information as required. The technological integration with telehealth platforms will further enable patients to remain connected with their healthcare providers, facilitating the resolution of any inquiries or concerns.

- *Regular Feedback and Real-Time Feedback Platforms*

The systematic collection of patient feedback regarding their interactions will further bolster the efficacy of communication. The implementation of real-time feedback mechanisms is essential for enhancing communication practices, utilizing instantaneous feedback tools to assess patient satisfaction during and after interactions, thereby permitting immediate modifications and refinements in communication strategies.

- *Leveraging Advanced Communication Technologies*

In an era characterized by swift technological progression, we explore the incorporation of advanced communication technologies, such as secure messaging applications, virtual consultations, and patient portals, which provide a more cohesive and accessible communication channel between healthcare providers and patients. Nonetheless, it is imperative to integrate all platforms to ensure a seamless experience for patients. Integration of technology is key for a seamless patient experience, and it creates an ease in data handling and data management. The administrators hold focus on holistic adoption of technology that focuses on entire patient's journey in continuum.

PILLAR 3: EMPATHY IN HEALTHCARE

Empathy is recognized as a formidable catalyst that significantly enhances the experiences of patients, necessitating that healthcare personnel and physicians cultivate an empathetic disposition in their interactions with patients. This foundational element emphasizes the critical importance of healthcare professionals comprehending and addressing the emotional dimensions inherent in a patient's journey. By recognizing and mitigating fears, anxieties, and concerns, healthcare providers can foster a compassionate and patient-centred care milieu. The integration of empathy-centred training initiatives can function as a transformative mechanism in this context. Empathy augments the efficacy of patient communication. Research has indicated that empathy as the most critical factor affecting patient satisfaction, it's been observed that empathy and responsiveness of healthcare staff is crucial and it strongly correlates with enhanced patient satisfaction in patient settings (Sulistyowati et al.,2024).

A study done years ago by (Sosa, 1983) on a group of women who came to deliver their first babies at an indigent hospital, it was observed that the women whoever assigned a doula (a supportive laywoman) to attend them during labour and delivery, has significantly lower labour time ad fewer complications than the women who went alone during their labour and delivery. It clear shows the link between reduction in stress due to empathetic interaction as a factor. Increased level of stress can lead to less than satisfactory medical outcomes.

- *Understanding Emotional Needs*

This discourse examines the crucial role of healthcare providers in identifying and addressing the emotional needs of patients. From the trepidation surrounding a diagnosis to the apprehension associated with medical procedures, the comprehension and empathetic engagement with these emotions significantly enhance the quality of the patient experience. Consequently, it is vital to prioritize both the articulated and unarticulated needs of the patient, which facilitates the establishment of a supportive and affirmative environment, subsequently elevating patient expectations, diminishing stress, positively influencing medical outcomes, minimizing stress-related complications, and enhancing patient recovery trajectories. The resultant effect is a contented patient, which in turn bolsters the morale of both staff and physicians. The advancements in technology empower the personalization of care strategies, wherein data-driven insights may be leveraged to customize empathetic care, considering individual patient preferences, emotional stimuli, and prior interactions with the healthcare system.

- *Empathy-focused Training Programs*

Training initiatives play a pivotal role in cultivating empathy within the ranks of healthcare professionals. The design and execution of training programs that emphasize not solely clinical competencies but also the interpersonal and empathetic dimensions of patient care are instrumental in improving overall medical outcomes.

- *Building Trust through Empathetic Engagement*

Trust serves as a fundamental pillar of patient satisfaction. Various methodologies exist to foster empathetic engagement, which in turn cultivates trust, enhances the patient-provider relationship, and contributes to overall satisfaction and adherence to therapeutic regimens.

PILLAR 4: FACILITY DESIGN AND PATIENT COMFORT

The physical environment plays a crucial role in shaping the patient's experience. This pillar advocates for a strategic approach to facility design, encompassing welcoming waiting areas, well-designed patient rooms, and thoughtful amenities. Cleanliness and comfort in healthcare facilities are essential, for the patient's physical environment, hygiene and additional amenities contribute to overall patient satisfaction. (Singh, 2024; Stilinović et al., 2021).

Integrating patient feedback into the design process ensures that healthcare environments align with patient preferences, contributing to an atmosphere of comfort and reassurance.

- *Sustainability in Healthcare Design*

Incorporating sustainable design practices is crucial for modern healthcare facilities. We investigate how sustainable architecture and environmentally friendly practices impact not only the patient comfort but also to the total health of the community.

- *Designing Comfortable and Welcoming Spaces*

The elements of facility design that contribute to patient comfort. From ergonomic furniture to soothing colour schemes, creating spaces, easy to navigate layout designed as per the requirements of patients that alleviate stress and promote well-being is crucial. The providers to emphasise on building a patient friendly facility.

- *Incorporating Patient Feedback in Design Decisions*

Patient feedback is a valuable resource in facility design. It is crucial to gather and incorporate patient input in the design process to ensure that healthcare environments align with the preferences and needs of the individuals they serve.

- *The Role of Amenities in Patient Satisfaction*

Thoughtful amenities can significantly impact the overall patient experience. Some basic amenities that are considered essential nowadays, such as Wi-Fi access, entertainment options, and comfortable bedding, can play a huge role in enhancing patient satisfaction and comfort during their stay. It is a must for each provider to identify such amenities and examine their role in increasing patient satisfaction. Creating a technology-enabled patient room and integrating all devices together can help in optimizing the overall experience of stay in the hospital (Feist, 2023).

PILLAR 5: TECHNOLOGICAL INTEGRATION FOR EFFICIENCY

In the digital age, technology can be harnessed to streamline processes and enhance patient satisfaction. This pillar delves into the strategic integration of technology, including online appointment scheduling, electronic health records, and telehealth services, in creating a seamless and personalized experiences for the patients. Technology can play a substantial role in boosting communication between patients and the providers.

However, it emphasizes the delicate balance between technological efficiency and maintaining a human touch, ensuring that patients feel supported and cared for throughout their digital interactions. The hospital administrators to have a holistic view of technology while embedding technology in creating operational efficiency, which can provide them with competitive differentiator in the market (Grando & Bates 2015). The providers can invest in many technology advancements such as equipping their nursing staff with mobile devices that give them alerting and alarming capabilities, using role-based scheduling and assignment software to ensure staffing coverage, and implementing medical device integration (MDI) to input and filter data from multiple devices to give nursing staff greater capacity for more proactive care, the right design combination of MDI solutions with mobile technology can make a huge difference in patient monitoring and predicting if the patients will require an unplanned ICU admittance or any other medical interventions (Feist, 2023).

Emerging technologies such as Artificial Intelligence (AI), Internet of Things (IoT) and interactive software are transforming health care delivery by improving patient experiences and leading to higher patient satisfaction. AI, for instance, can help the healthcare practitioners in predicting the patient needs, making recommendations for treatments, and providing clinicians with insights that assists them in making informed and efficient decision making.

The IoT technologies facilitate in monitoring real-time health data, increasing patient awareness and proactive health management (Singh et al., 2024). By maintain transparency with process, understanding patient concern related to data privacy, healthcare providers can increase patients trust in AI and resulting in higher satisfaction (Rathore et al., 2023).

Interactive software applications further enhance patient engagement by giving patients access to educational resources, treatment options, and communication tools to interact with their providers.

- *Streamlining Administrative Processes with Technology*

Patients are wary of long queues and waiting at a clinic/hospital. Providers to integrate technology into their daily routine activities such as online appointments, administrative tasks, Out-patient registration, waiting times, discharge process, and insurance claims, etc., With the implementation of technology many tasks can be streamlined and it reduces paperwork, will also help provider become more environmentally sustainable as they can go paperless and in the making system and process more efficient, satisfying patient experience and increase its revenue.

A patient friendly policy can act as catalyst in streamlining the overall experience of hospital visits. This will enhance the operational efficiencies for healthcare facilities, by making healthcare more accessible, and leading to enhance patient satisfaction.

Similarly, the electronic health records (EHRs) aids in hassle-free exchange of information between different healthcare providers, ensuring patient histories is readily available, which supports better decision-making and continuity of care.

- *Leveraging Telehealth for Patient Convenience*

In a country like India, where we have a highly skewed doctor-patient ratio (As per WHO the doctor to patient ration 1000:1, India has ratio of 1000:0.7 as per 2020), telehealth is a boon for effective utilization of physician time and reducing the overall burden on the provider infrastructure. Telehealth and the internet of things (IoT) have made health-monitoring technology accessible and affordable. In a post-COVID era, telehealth has become an intrinsic part of healthcare delivery. There are many benefits of telehealth services in providing convenient access to care, reducing barriers to appointments, and enhancing patient satisfaction with virtual healthcare options and in reducing the long queues, waiting time, and eventually reducing the overall burden on hospital. Many hospitals have collaborated with digital healthcare companies to offer tele consultations through digital apps.

- *Technology Adaptions for Patient Care*

AI tools such as chatbots and virtual assistants play a huge role in making patient interactions personalized, providing easy access to health information, boosting patient engagement (Rathore et al., 2023). Adoption of technology in monitoring health outcomes with the use of IoT, has resulted in improving in health outcomes with real-time monitoring and user-friendly interfaces in patients (Singh et al., 2024).

- *Balancing Efficiency with Human Connection*

Efficiency should not come at the cost of human connection. It's important to balance technological efficiency with maintaining a personalized and compassionate approach to patient care. The human connection while delivering care has a direct impact on patients' overall mental and physical well-being.

PILLAR 6: STAFF TRAINING AND DEVELOPMENT

Highly skilled and empathetic staff and clinicians are the most valued resource for a healthcare provider in delivering quality of care. This pillar highlights the significance of continuous training and development for the healthcare staff. The training program for the staff should focus on effective communication, cultural competence, and service skills. It's a well-known fact that a highly trained staff is better equipped to handle diverse needs and requirements, creating an environment of trust and satisfaction.

This also helps in managing employee satisfaction and retention and a well-trained staff is empowered and feels motivated in performing their duties. The training programs can be made interactive with the help of gamification, use of virtual reality simulations and augmented reality, multimedia, storytelling these can enhance engagement, knowledge retention, and the development of essential skills among healthcare staff and offering hands-on training, allowing healthcare professionals to practice and refine their skills in realistic scenarios, ultimately contributing to improved patient interactions. These initiatives help in creating a culture that values safety and result in improving patient satisfaction. Along with staff training, it's essential for organizations to understand internal challenges that hinder the path of growth and continuous development.

- *Continuous Professional Development*

Its integral for healthcare organization for have a culture where in, continuous development is valued as healthcare domain is an ever evolving one. Healthcare providers to have regular training program for their staff, to keep them abreast with new medical advancements, effective communication, patient-centred care practices and various department-level training as per the need of staff. Such initiatives undertaken by the hospital has a positive impact on the morale of staff and physician, this provides the opportunity of growth in their respective careers, as well improve communication and interpersonal skills of healthcare staff, better understanding of service quality, leading to better-patient-provider relationship and higher patient satisfaction (Alghamdi et al., 2024).

- *Cultural Competence in Healthcare*

Cultural competence is integral to patient satisfaction. Along with various other technical training, it's significant to have the training for cultural competence training for healthcare providers, ensuring that they can effectively communicate and provide care that respects the diverse backgrounds and beliefs of their patients. Cultural competence in healthcare is define as the ability of system to provide care to diverse values, beliefs, behaviours including tailor made delivery to meet patients' social, cultural, and linguistic needs (Betancourt et al.,2002). For a country like India, which is so diverse culturally, understanding the patient background and the place of residence help in connecting with the patients and patients of different background and race and to personalize communication with the patients and to comprehend the medical ailments.

- *The Impact of Staff Satisfaction on Patient Experience*

The satisfaction of healthcare staff is connected with patient satisfaction. This subheading examines the correlation between staff satisfaction, engagement, and the overall patient experience, emphasizing the importance of cultivating a positive workplace culture. Making a patient-centric approach as part of your organization's DNA requires the involvement of senior management as higher staff satisfaction would eventually lead to higher patient satisfaction.

Studies have shown the link between patient satisfaction and staff satisfaction and the vice -versa, this is an added incentive (Sclesinger &Heskett 1991), a strong relationship has been observed between employee satisfaction and patient intent to return to the hospital or to recommend the hospital (Atkins et al.,1996).

The same get reflected when physicians are more satisfied, there is a smooth flow of information and tighter co-ordination of care is reflected. The patient satisfaction has both direct and indirect impact on physicians, a well satisfied patient is more likely to be co-operative, informative, and collaborative with physicians, making the job of physicians easier and has positive impact on the clinical outcome and also make the physicians feel positive about their own efforts.

The senior management and administrators can act as catalysts, when the staff is empowered or rewarded for behaviours and strategies that can enhance patient satisfaction, by creating such policies. The providers to empower the staff and offer them some degree of freedom to take small decision while managing an unhappy customer. For example, the hospital staff can provide few gift coupons on the in-house store to compensate for a negative experience.

The organization should show their gratitude to employees who are doing exceptional in performing their daily duties. The focus of healthcare administrator should remain on creating a transparent culture, work-life harmony, and employee friendly policies to create work-life harmony.

- *Ethical Considerations*

Prioritize ethical considerations, including data privacy, security, and algorithmic bias, especially against emerging technologies artificial intelligence (AI), machine learning (ML) and data- driven systems, to ensure responsible practices. Employees should be well-versed with data protection laws and any other international or national legislation pertaining to this. It's essential for organizations to create guidelines and standard operating procedure for data handling, specifically dealing with sensitive customer data.

PILLAR 7: MEASURING AND IMPROVING

Continuous improvement forms the core of our strategic framework. This pillar advocates for the implementation of robust mechanisms to measure patient satisfaction regularly. Patient satisfaction can be measured through various dimensions such as reliability, responsiveness, assurance, empathy, and tangibles. It has been observed that private healthcare providers fare better than the public healthcare providers in these dimensions (Salsabila et al., 2023).

Patient surveys, feedback forms, and data analytics serve as valuable tools for gaining insights into areas that require attention and enhancement. Various predictive modelling techniques (Ordinal logistic regression) are used to can forecast the factors like length of the stay and sociodemographic, and its impact on the patient satisfaction. By analysing this information, healthcare organizations can make informed decisions, perpetuating a cycle of continuous improvement and refinement.

- *Implementing Effective Patient Surveys*

Patient surveys are a valuable tool for gathering feedback. It helps in underlying the cause behind poor scores and bad ratings. The best practices to be followed in designing and implementing patient surveys to obtain meaningful insights into the patient experience and areas for improvement. The measuring of patient satisfaction is to be done continuously and the providers to respond effectively to the data as this will help in improving the score and achieving the goal of patient satisfaction. The patient satisfaction survey to be designed to capture patients' recollection and personal care and utilizing advanced analytics tools is essential for gaining deeper insights into patient satisfaction.

- *Utilizing Feedback for Strategic Decision-Making*

Collecting feedback is only beneficial if it informs decision-making. The effective utilization of feedback in making a key strategic decision for the provider is essential, the feedback can be segmented into different heads such as urgent, important, and not-so-important, this way they can prioritize the areas of improvement and accordingly set realistic goals and develop a plan of action (A cause and effect fishbone chart can help in solving the issue of low score) for enhancing patient satisfaction. Based on the feedback collected quality improvements can be designed. While analysing the internal data, it should only compare apples to apples (e.g., Compare different nursing units score with each other rather any other departments with each other) and for the external data different departments score can be compared. Also, a constant review of the data will sensitize you to changes and trends.

- *Establishing a Culture of Continuous Improvement*

As Culture are learned, integrated, and patterned, its mixed bag that governs meanings, values & attitudes & behaviours for a particular group of people. Continuous improvement should be ingrained in the organizational culture. Healthcare providers to adopt an agile approach for continuous improvement and foster a culture of change, innovation, and create an integrated culture of patient satisfaction where each action (e.g., Behaviour, expressed attitudes) is linked to one another and affects the actions of others. To achieve this, the CEO to reinforce this orientation and commitment to drive high patient satisfaction among all staff. The administrator should focus on creating a collaborative and transparent culture, wherein people can freely share their experiences and challenges without being judged and reprimanded, creating policies that more employee friendly based on their needs and requirements.

CONCLUSION

In conclusion, the pursuit of patient satisfaction is not a short-term goal; it demands a dynamic and multifaceted approach that transcends the confines of clinical excellence. This chapter has outlined a comprehensive framework, serving as a nuanced roadmap for healthcare providers to systematically navigate the intricate dimensions that influence patient satisfaction. The orchestration of communication excellence, empathy, facility design, technological integration, staff training, and continuous improvement into the very fabric of healthcare delivery is poised to reshape the patient experience.

At its core, the strategic framework unveiled here represents a transformative shift in healthcare, recognizing that quality care is no longer confined to the mere application of medical expertise. Instead, it advocates for a holistic approach, wherein patients actively engage and feel acknowledged at every juncture of their healthcare journey. This shift goes beyond conventional paradigms, aiming not only to satisfy but to empower and humanize the healthcare experience for patients and staff alike.

Central to this transformative journey is the exploration of healthcare 6.0, where the integration of cutting-edge technologies such as artificial intelligence, machine learning, telemedicine, and personalized healthcare solutions plays an integral role. These innovations are not only enhancing the clinical aspect of care but are revolutionizing the very nature of service delivery, from patient engagement to streamlined operational efficiency. Healthcare 6.0 is enabling healthcare providers to offer a more personalized, efficient, and accessible experience, allowing patients to feel more involved and supported throughout their care process.

By leveraging the potential of these transformative technologies, healthcare providers can break down traditional barriers, providing seamless communication, enhancing patient outcomes, and improving the overall experience. As a result, patient satisfaction is not just achieved—it is elevated to a new standard, where both patients and healthcare providers benefit from a more connected, efficient, and compassionate healthcare environment.

Thus, the future of patient satisfaction is not solely dependent on clinical care but is deeply intertwined with the seamless integration of innovative technologies, human empathy, and a commitment to continuous improvement. The framework presented here, empowered by healthcare 6.0, offers a clear pathway to reimagining healthcare delivery, making it more responsive, patient-centred, and aligned with the expectations of modern-day healthcare consumers.

REFERENCES

Alghamdi, M. M., Shehri, T. S. A., Alnihier, M. M. H., Alshahri, A. H. A., Alwaked, M. H., & Alshammari, N. M. S. (2024). The significance of enhancing health workers' skills and knowledge in driving positive patient experiences. *International Journal of Religion*, *5*(2), 598–608. DOI: 10.61707/3t59q326

Atkins, P. M., Marshall, B. S., & Javalgi, R. G. (1996). Happy employees lead to loyal patients. Survey of nurses and patients shows a strong link between employee satisfaction and patient loyalty. *Journal of Health Care Marketing*, *16*(4), 14–23. PMID: 10169075

Betancourt, J. R., Green, A. R., & Carrillo, J. E. (2002). CULTURAL COMPETENCE IN HEALTH CARE: EMERGING FRAMEWORKS AND PRACTICAL APPROACHES. In FIELD REPORT. The Commonwealth Fund. https://www.commonwealthfund.org/sites/default/files/documents/___media_files_publications_fund_report_2002_oct_cultural_competence_in_health_care__emerging_frameworks_and_practical_approaches_betancourt_culturalcompetence_576_pdf.pdf

Cardoza, S., & Moras, J. S. (2024b). Improving patient care in the emergency department in a selected hospital: A study on patient centered care. *International Journal of Community Medicine and Public Health*, *11*(10), 3996–4003. DOI: 10.18203/2394-6040.ijcmph20242884

Feist, K. 2023, June 9. Improving the patient experience through technology. Forbes. https://www.forbes.com/sites/forbestechcouncil/2023/06/08/improving-the-patient-experience-through-technology/

Gitomer, J. (1997). Your Customer's Happiness Requires Partnering Approach. *Business First*, *8*, 15.

Grando, M. A., Rozenblum, R., & Bates, D. (2015). *Information technology for patient empowerment in healthcare*. Walter de Gruyter GmbH & Co KG. DOI: 10.1515/9781614514343

Jones, T. O., & Sasser, W. E.Jr. (1995). Why Satisfied Customers Defect. *Harvard Business Review*, *73*(6), 88–102. https://hbr.org/1995/11/why-satisfied-customers-defect

Kapustina, T. V., Gorshkova, O. V., Kadyrov, R. V., Trankovskaya, L. V., & Khudchenko, A. G. (2024). Patient-Centered healthare as part of medical corporate culture. *SibScript*, *26*(5), 795–806. DOI: 10.21603/sibscript-2024-26-5-795-806

Mo, H., Zhong, R., & Ma, F. (2024). Chinese expert consensus on an innovative patient-centered approach to diagnosis and treatment of cancer. *Cancer Innovation, 3*(5), e137. Advance online publication. DOI: 10.1002/cai2.137 PMID: 39081932

Nguyen, T. L. H. (2023). Patient satisfaction. International Healthcare Review (Online). DOI: 10.56226/55

Rathore, Y., Sinha, U., Haladkar, J. P., Mate, N. R., Bhosale, S. A., & Chobe, S. V. (2023). Optimizing Patient Flow and Resource Allocation in Hospitals using AI. *2023 International Conference on Artificial Intelligence for Innovations in Healthcare Industries (ICAIIHI)*, 1–6. DOI: 10.1109/ICAIIHI57871.2023.10489698

Salsabila, N. N., Yusrani, N. K. G., Annajah, N. S., Azzahra, N. K. A., & Sabrina, N. R. S. N. (2023). The Comparative Analysis of inpatient service at public hospitals and private hospitals in order to Improve Patient Satisfication : A literature review. *Usada Nusantara Jurnal Kesehatan Tradisional, 1*(2), 65–78. DOI: 10.47861/usd.v1i2.250

Schesinger, L. A., & Hskett, J. L. (1991). Customer Satisfaction is Rooted in Employee Satisfaction. *Harvard Business Review*, (Nov/Dec), 148–149. https://hbr.org/1991/09/the-service-driven-service-company

Singh, C. (2024). Healthcare delivery and beneficiary satisfaction: A focused study on AB-PMJAY beneficiaries at a tertiary care hospital of North India. Research Review. DOI: 10.52845/CMRO/2024/7-11-1

Singh, J., Shelke, N. A., Upreti, K., Divakaran, P., Lingareddy, N., & Deepika, S. (2024). Enhancing Patient Well-Being in Healthcare Through the Integration of IoT and Neural Network. *2024 International Conference on Emerging Innovations and Advanced Computing (INNOCOMP)*, 241–246. DOI: 10.1109/INNOCOMP63224.2024.00047

Sosa, R. A. (1983). Some observations on effect of a supportive companion during labor and delivery. *The Journal of the Florida Medical Association, 70*(9), 761–763. PMID: 6631389

Stilinović, M., Sabolić, I., Papeš, D., Pasini, N. M., Škrljak-šoša, D., & Luetić, T. (2021). PATIENT SATISFACTION. *Paediatria Croatica, 65*(2), 90–94. DOI: 10.13112/pc.390

Sulistyowati, W. T., Suryani, N. L., & Harokan, N. A. (2024). ANALYSIS OF PATIENT SATISFACTION WITH INPATIENT SERVICES IN REGIONAL GENERAL HOSPITALS. Cendekia Medika Jurnal Stikes Al-Ma`Arif Baturaja, 9(2), 255–264. DOI: 10.52235/cendekiamedika.v9i2.382

Tsakiri, E. (2024). Measuring patient satisfaction in a general hospital. *Health Review*, *35*(192), 21–28. DOI: 10.54042/hr3266hhsma

Wahyuni, N., Triharini, M., & Has, E. M. M. (2022). STRATEGY TO PROMOTE PATIENT CENTERED CARE PCC FOR IMPROVING PATIENT SATISFACTION: A LITERATURE REVIEW. *Nurse and Health Jurnal Keperawatan*, *11*(1), 10–21. DOI: 10.36720/nhjk.v11i1.306

Yap, C., Aiyegbusi, O. L., Alger, E., Basch, E., Bell, J., Bhatnagar, V., Cella, D., Collis, P., Dueck, A. C., Gilbert, A., Gnanasakthy, A., Greystoke, A., Hansen, A. R., Kamudoni, P., Kholmanskikh, O., King-Kallimanis, B. L., Krumholz, H., Minchom, A., O'Connor, D., & Peipert, J. D. (2024). Advancing patient-centric care: Integrating patient reported outcomes for tolerability assessment in early phase clinical trials – insights from an expert virtual roundtable. *EClinicalMedicine*, *76*, 102838. DOI: 10.1016/j.eclinm.2024.102838 PMID: 39386161

Yekeen, I. A., Adejumo, P., & Kolawole, I. O. (2024). Patient-Centered care as an optimal solution for enhancing the quality of healthcare delivery. International Journal of Innovative Science and Research Technology (IJISRT), 2606–2612. DOI: 10.38124/ijisrt/IJISRT24AUG1534

Zhao, P., Xu, J., & Han, M. (2024). Patient-Centric Care: Unveiling the potential of wearable electronics in clinical practice. *Wearable Electronics.*, *1*, 119–136. DOI: 10.1016/j.wees.2024.07.001

Compilation of References

Abdulsalam, Y. J., & Schneller, E. S. (2021). Of barriers and bridges: Buyer-supplier relationships in health care. *Health Care Management Review*, *46*(4), 358–366. DOI: 10.1097/HMR.0000000000000278 PMID: 32167964

Abedi, A., Ghodrati Amiri, G., Jahanshahi, M. R., & Avci, O. (2024). Advanced anomaly detection in structural health monitoring data using vision transformer and multi-domain feature fusion. *SSRN*. https://ssrn.com/abstract=5026823 or http://dx.doi.org/DOI: 10.2139/ssrn.5026823

About Pradhan Mantri Jan Arogya Yojana (PM-JAY). (n.d.). National Health Authority. Retrieved August 5, 2024, from https://pmjay.gov.in/about/pmjay

Abramoff, M. D., Lavin, P. T., Birch, M., Shah, N., & Folk, J. C. (2018). Pivotal trial of an autonomous AI-based diagnostic system for detection of diabetic retinopathy in primary care offices. *Journal of the American Medical Association*, *316*(22), 2408–2416. PMID: 31304320

Academy of Nutrition and Dietetics. (2019). The NCPT and electronic health records. Electronic Nutrition Care Process Technology (eNCPT). Accessed January 2025 from https://www.ncpro.org/the-ncpt-and-electronic-health-records

Acharya, U. R., Oh, S. L., Hagiwara, Y., Tan, J. H., Adeli, H., & Subha, D. P. (2018). Automated EEG-based screening of depression using deep convolutional neural network. *Computer Methods and Programs in Biomedicine*, *161*, 103–113. DOI: 10.1016/j.cmpb.2018.04.012 PMID: 29852953

Adams, S. H., Anthony, J. C., Carvajal, R., Chae, L., Khoo, C. S. H., Latulippe, M. E., Matusheski, N. V., McClung, H. L., Rozga, M., Schmid, C. H., Wopereis, S., & Yan, W. (2020). Perspective: Guiding principles for the implementation of personalized nutrition approaches that benefit health and function. *Advances in Nutrition*, *11*(1), 25–34. DOI: 10.1093/advances/nmz086 PMID: 31504115

ADB. (2019, August 23). ADB-Supported Digital Health Information System to Help Manage Patient Care in Tonga. Asian Development Bank. https://www.adb.org/news/adb-supported-digital-health-information-system-help-manage-patient-care-tonga

ADB. (2024, June 28). Introducing eGovernment through Digital Health. Asian Development Bank. https://www.adb.org/projects/50281-001/main

Adefisan, E. A., Bayo, A. S., & Ropo, O. I. (2015). Application of geo-spatial technology in identifying areas vulnerable to flooding in Ibadan metropolis. *Journal of Environment and Earth Science*, *5*(14), 153–166.

Aebersold, R., & Mann, M. (2003). Mass spectrometry-based proteomics. *Nature*, *422*(6928), 198–207. DOI: 10.1038/nature01511 PMID: 12634793

Agarwal, R., Bjarnadottir, M., Rhue, L., Dugas, M., Crowley, K., Clark, J., & Gao, G. (2023). Addressing algorithmic bias and the perpetuation of health inequities: An AI bias aware framework. *Health Policy and Technology*, *12*(1), 100702. Advance online publication. DOI: 10.1016/j.hlpt.2022.100702

Agrawal, R., & Srikant, R. (1994). Fast algorithms for mining association rules. In *Proceedings of the 20th international conference on very large data bases, VLDB* (Vol. 1215, pp. 487–499).

Ahmad, A. (2024). Enhancing Hospital Efficiency through IoT and AI: A Smart Healthcare System. [JOSAPEN]. *Journal of Computer Science Application and Engineering*, *2*(2), 2. Advance online publication. DOI: 10.70356/josapen.v2i2.36

Ahmad, N., Hussain, M., Riaz, N., Subhani, F., Haider, S., Alamgir, K. S., & Shinwari, F. (2013). Flood prediction and disaster risk analysis using GIS based wireless sensor networks: A review. *Journal of Basic and Applied Scientific Research*, *3*(8), 632–643.

Ahmed, I., Jeon, G., & Piccialli, F. (2021). A deep-learning-based smart healthcare system for patient's discomfort detection at the edge of internet of things. *IEEE Internet of Things Journal*, *8*(13), 10318–10326. DOI: 10.1109/JIOT.2021.3052067

Ahmed, S. H., & Kim, D. (2016). Named data networking-based smart home. *ICT Express*, *2*(3), 130–134. DOI: 10.1016/j.icte.2016.08.007

Aijli. (2021, December 14). Key takeaway from practicum - Aijli - Medium. Medium. https://medium.com/@aijli/key-takeaway-from-practicum-612adf0389e7

Al Baalharith, I. M., & Aboshaiqah, A. E. (2024). A Delphi study on identifying competencies in Virtual Healthcare for healthcare professionals. *Health Care*, *12*(7), 739. Advance online publication. DOI: 10.3390/healthcare12070739 PMID: 38610161

Alam, I. (2006). Removing the fuzziness from the fuzzy front-end of service innovations through customer interactions. *Industrial Marketing Management*, *35*(4), 468–480. DOI: 10.1016/j.indmarman.2005.04.004

Alanazi, A. (2022). Using machine learning for healthcare challenges and opportunities. Informatics in Medicine Unlocked. *Elsevier*. .DOI: 10.1016/j.imu.2022.100924

Alblas, A., & Jayaram, J. (2015). Design resilience in the fuzzy front end (FFE) context: An empirical examination. *International Journal of Production Research*, *53*(22), 6820–6838. DOI: 10.1080/00207543.2014.899718

Alemzadeh, H., Raman, J., Leveson, N., Kalbarczyk, Z., & Iyer, R. K. (2016). Adverse Events in Robotic Surgery: A Retrospective Study of 14 Years of FDA Data. *JAMA Surgery*, *151*(3), 273–279. PMID: 26720622

Alghamdi, M. M., Shehri, T. S. A., Alnihier, M. M. H., Alshahri, A. H. A., Alwaked, M. H., & Alshammari, N. M. S. (2024). The significance of enhancing health workers' skills and knowledge in driving positive patient experiences. *International Journal of Religion*, *5*(2), 598–608. DOI: 10.61707/3t59q326

Allison, B. (2024). Exploring Intelligent Automation at Mayo Clinic: An Interview with Dr. Anjali Bhagra. *Mayo Clinic Innovation Exchange*. https://innovationexchange.mayoclinic.org/exploring-intelligent-automation-at-mayo-clinic-an-interview-with-dr-anjali-bhagra/

Alonazi, M., Alshahrani, H. M., Kouki, F., Almalki, N. S., Mahmud, A., & Majdoubi, J. (2023). Deep convolutional neural network with symbiotic organism search-based human activity recognition for cognitive health assessment. *Biomimetics*, *8*(7), 554. DOI: 10.3390/biomimetics8070554 PMID: 37999195

Aluvalu, R., Devi, V. S., Kumar, C. N., Goutham, N., & Nikitha, K. (2024). Unveil the Black-Box Model for Healthcare Explainable AI. In Aluvalu, R., Mehta, M., & Siarry, P. (Eds.), *Explainable AI in Health Informatics. Computational Intelligence Methods and Applications*. Springer., DOI: 10.1007/978-981-97-3705-5_3

Alvandi, A. O. (2024, June 10). Machine Unlearning in Digitalized Healthcare Arena A Comprehensive Exploration. https://doi.org/DOI: 10.31219/osf.io/kz3w5

AMA. (2020). *Artificial Intelligence and the Future of Medicine: A Framework for Ethical AI*. American Medical Association.

Ambinder, E. P. (2005). Electronic health records. *Journal of Oncology Practice / American Society of Clinical Oncology*, *1*(2), 57–63. DOI: 10.1200/jop.2005.1.2.57 PMID: 20871681

American Medical Association (AMA). (2021). “2021 Telehealth Survey Report.”

American Medical Association. (n.d.). Ethical principles in healthcare data management. American Medical Association https://code-medical-ethics.ama-assn.org/

American Telemedicine Association. (n.d.). Telemedicine: Expanding access to care. American Telemedicine Association https://www.americantelemed.org/

Andersen, T. O., Bansler, J. P., Kensing, F., Moll, J., & Nielsen, K. D. (2017). Alignment of concerns: a design rationale for patient participation in eHealth. In *Proceedings of the 50th Hawaii International Conference on System Sciences*.

Andersson, K., & Hossain, M. S. (2014). Smart risk assessment systems using belief-rule-based DSS and WSN technologies. In *Proceedings of 2014 4th international conference on wireless communications, vehicular technology, information theory and aerospace electronic systems (VITAE)* (pp. 1–5). DOI: 10.1109/VITAE.2014.6934397

Andersson, K., & Hossain, M. S. (2015). Heterogeneous wireless sensor networks for flood prediction decision support systems. In *Proceedings of the 2015 IEEE conference on computer communications workshops (INFOCOM WKSHPS)* (pp. 133–137). DOI: 10.1109/INFCOMW.2015.7179373

Ankita, R., Rani, S., Babbar, H., Coleman, S., Singh, A., & Aljahdali, H. M. (2021). An efficient and lightweight deep learning model for human activity recognition using smartphones. *Sensors (Basel)*, *21*(11), 3845. DOI: 10.3390/s21113845 PMID: 34199559

Annosi, M. C., Marzi, G., Ciampi, F., & Rialti, R. (2022). An ambidextrous approach to practice-based innovation for social product development: Lessons from a Dutch company. *IEEE Transactions on Engineering Management*, *69*(2), 376–387. DOI: 10.1109/TEM.2020.2977976

Anthem Inc. (2015). Data breach report. https://www.hhs.gov/guidance/document/anthem-pays-ocr-16-million-record-hipaa-settlement-following-largest-us-health-data-breach

Ardila, D., Kiraly, A. P., Bertrand, M., et al. (2019). End-to-end lung cancer screening

Argaw, S. T., Troncoso-Pastoriza, J. R., Lacey, D., Florin, M., Calcavecchia, F., Anderson, D., Burleson, W., Vogel, J., O'Leary, C., Eshaya-Chauvin, B., & Flahault, A. (2020). Cybersecurity of Hospitals: Discussing the challenges and working towards mitigating the risks. *BMC Medical Informatics and Decision Making*, *20*(1), 146. Advance online publication. DOI: 10.1186/s12911-020-01161-7 PMID: 32620167

Arpon, A., Riezu-Boj, J. I., Milagro, F. I., Marti, A., Razquin, C., Martínez-González, M. A., Corella, D., Estruch, R., Casas, R., Fitó, M., Ros, E., Salas-Salvadó, J., & Martínez, J. A. (2016). Adherence to Mediterranean diet is associated with methylation changes in inflammation-related genes in peripheral blood cells. *Journal of Physiology and Biochemistry*, *73*(3), 445–455. DOI: 10.1007/s13105-017-0552-6 PMID: 28181167

Asan, O., Bayrak, A. E., & Choudhury, A. (2020). Asan O, Bayrak AE, Choudhury A. Artificial intelligence and human trust in healthcare: Focus on clinicians. [PubMed]. *Journal of Medical Internet Research*, *22*(6), e15154. DOI: 10.2196/15154 PMID: 32558657

Aseel Berglund, T. J. (2022). Understanding and assessing gamification in digital healthcare interventions for patients with cardiovascular disease. *European Journal of Cardiovascular Nursing*, *21*(6), 630–638. DOI: 10.1093/eurjcn/zvac048 PMID: 35709297

Atasoy, H., Greenwood, B. N., & McCullough, J. S. (2018). The Digitization of Patient Care: A Review of the Effects of Electronic Health Records on Health Care Quality and Utilization. *Annual Review of Public Health*, *40*(1), 487–500. DOI: 10.1146/annurev-publhealth-040218-044206 PMID: 30566385

Ateeq, M., Ishmanov, F., Afzal, M. K., & Naeem, M. (2019). Predicting delay in IoT using deep learning: A multiparametric approach. *IEEE Access : Practical Innovations, Open Solutions*, *7*, 62022–62031. DOI: 10.1109/ACCESS.2019.2915958

Atkins, P. M., Marshall, B. S., & Javalgi, R. G. (1996). Happy employees lead to loyal patients. Survey of nurses and patients shows a strong link between employee satisfaction and patient loyalty. *Journal of Health Care Marketing*, *16*(4), 14–23. PMID: 10169075

Atlas.ti. (2024). *ATLAS.ti Web for browsers*. Webpage accessed 241202: https://atlasti.com/

Atomwise. (2025). Artificial Intelligence for Drug Discovery. *Atomwise*. Retrieved from https://www.atomwise.com/

Atzori, L., Iera, A., & Morabito, G. (2010). The Internet of Things: A survey. *Computer Networks*, *54*(15), 2787–2805. DOI: 10.1016/j.comnet.2010.05.010

Ayo Manfaatkan Program REHAB BPJS Kesehatan. (n.d.). https://www-bekasikab-go-id.translate.goog/ayo-manfaatkan-program-rehab-bpjs-kesehatan?_x_tr_sl=id&_x_tr_tl=en&_x_tr_hl=en&_x_tr_pto=sc

Ayres, E. J., & Hoggle, L. B. (2012). 2011 nutrition informatics member survey. *Journal of the Academy of Nutrition and Dietetics*, *112*(3), 360–367. DOI: 10.1016/j.jand.2012.01.003 PMID: 22709663

Azaria, A., Ekblaw, A., Vieira, T., & Lippman, A. (2016). MedRec: Using Blockchain for Medical Data Access and Permission Management. *2016 2nd International Conference on Open and Big Data (OBD)*, 25–30. DOI: 10.1109/OBD.2016.11

Aziz, N. A. A., & Aziz, K. A. (2011). Managing disaster with wireless sensor networks. In *2011 13th international conference on advanced communication technology (ICACT)* (pp. 202–207). IEEE.

Backman, M., Börjesson, S., & Setterberg, S. (2007). Working with concepts in the fuzzy front end: Exploring the context for innovation for different types of concepts at Volvo Cars. *R & D Management*, *37*(1), 17–28. Advance online publication. DOI: 10.1111/j.1467-9310.2007.00455.x

Bailey, R. L. (2021). Overview of dietary assessment methods for measuring intakes of foods, beverages, and dietary supplements in research studies. *Current Opinion in Biotechnology*, *70*, 91–96. DOI: 10.1016/j.copbio.2021.02.007 PMID: 33714006

Bajaber, F., & Awan, I. (2010). Energy efficient clustering protocol to enhance lifetime of wireless sensor network. *Journal of Ambient Intelligence and Humanized Computing*, *1*(4), 239–248. DOI: 10.1007/s12652-010-0019-x

Bajwa, J., Munir, U., Nori, A., & Williams, B. (2021). Artificial intelligence in healthcare: Transforming the practice of medicine. *Future Healthcare Journal*, *8*(2), e188–e194. DOI: 10.7861/fhj.2021-0095 PMID: 34286183

Bakare, S. S., Adeniyi, A. O., Akpuokwe, C. U., & Eneh, N. E. (2024). Data privacy laws and compliance: A comparative review of the EU GDPR and USA regulations. *Computer Science & IT Research Journal*, *5*(3), 528–543. DOI: 10.51594/csitrj.v5i3.859

Balkrishnan, R., Chang, J., Patel, I., Yang, F., & Merajver, S. D. (2013). Global comparative healthcare effectiveness research: Evaluating sustainable programmes in low & middle resource settings. *The Indian Journal of Medical Research*, *137*(3), 494–501. DOI: 10.21203/rs.3.pex-2593/v1 PMID: 23640555

Ballard, D. J., Shortell, S. M., Sood, S., Weinberger, J. Z., Weinstein, J. S., Schoenbaum, S. C., & Brennan, T. A. (2019). Impact of incident of bundled payment on medical practice. *NEJM Catalyst Innovations in Care Delivery*, *5*(6).

Banafa, A. (2024). *Introduction to Artificial Intelligence*. River Publishers.

Barnett, V., & Lewis, T. (1994). *Outliers in statistical data* (3rd ed.). John Wiley & Sons.

Barnet, V. (1976). The ordering of multivariate data (with discussion). *Journal of the Royal Statistical Society. Series A (General)*, *139*(3), 318–354. DOI: 10.2307/2344839

Barratt, P. (2017). A qualitative study investigating persuasive technologies and the gamification of cycling. *Health & Place*, *46*, 328–336. DOI: 10.1016/j.healthplace.2016.09.009 PMID: 28029434

Barsanti, S., & Cavicchi, A. (2021). Addressing social determinants of health through value-based payment models: A systematic review. *BMC Health Services Research*, *21*(1), 1–14. PMID: 33388053

Basiotis, P. P., Welsh, S. O., Cronin, F. J., Kelsay, J. L., & Mertz, W. (1987). Number of days of food intake records required to estimate individual and group nutrient intakes with defined confidence. *The Journal of Nutrition*, *117*(9), 1638–1641. DOI: 10.1093/jn/117.9.1638 PMID: 3655942

Bates, D. W., Landman, A., & Levine, D. M. (2018). Health information technology. *Journal of the American Medical Association*, *319*(23), 2425–2426. PMID: 30561464

Baur, C., & Kan, L. (2019). Closing the gap: Using technology to promote health equity. *Health Affairs*, *38*(2), 256–263.

Bean, R. (2024). *How Cleveland Clinic Is Innovating in Healthcare with Data, Analytics, And AI*. Forbes. https://www.forbes.com/sites/randybean/2024/10/06/how-cleveland-clinic-is-innovating-in-healthcare-with-data-analytics-and-ai/

Becker, N., Laukka, E. J., Kalpouzos, G., Naveh-Benjamin, M., Bäckman, L., & Brehmer, Y. (2015). Structural brain correlates of associative memory in older adults. *NeuroImage*, *118*, 146–153. DOI: 10.1016/j.neuroimage.2015.06.002 PMID: 26054875

Beckman, R. J., & Cook, R. D. (1983). Outliers. *Technometrics*, *25*(2), 119–149.

Bedsaul-Fryer, J. R., van Zutphen-Küffer, K. G., Monroy-Gomez, J., Clayton, D. E., Gavin-Smith, B., Worth, C., Schwab, C. N., Freymond, M., Surowska, A., Bhering Martins, L., Senn-Jakobsen, C., & Kraemer, K. (2023). Precision nutrition opportunities to help mitigate nutrition and health challenges in low-and middle-income countries: An expert opinion survey. *Nutrients*, *15*(14), 3247. DOI: 10.3390/nu15143247 PMID: 37513665

Beede, E., Baylor, E., Hersch, F., Iurchenko, A., Wilcox, L., Ruamviboonsuk, P., & Vardoulakis, L. M. (2020). A Human-Centered Evaluation of a Deep Learning System Deployed in Clinics for the Detection of Diabetic Retinopathy. *Journal of the American Medical Association*, *324*(19), 1925–1938.

Bellander, E. (2024, August 21). *IoT in hemmet för jämlik hälsa*. https://www.karolinska.se/forskning-och-utbildning/innovation/aktuell-innovation/iot-hemmonitorering/

Bendavid, Y., & Bourgault, M. (2010). A living laboratory for managing the front-end phase of innovation adoption: The case of RFID implementation. *International Journal of Project Organisation and Management*, *2*(1), 84. DOI: 10.1504/IJPOM.2010.031883

Bennett, P., & McGowan, J. (2020). Community engagement in healthcare: A systematic review. *Journal of Community Health*, *45*(3), 456–467. DOI: 10.1007/s10900-020-00812-3

Bente, B. E., Van Dongen, A., Verdaasdonk, R., & van Gemert-Pijnen, L. (2024). eHealth implementation in Europe: A scoping review on legal, ethical, financial, and technological aspects. *Frontiers in Digital Health*, *6*, 1332707. DOI: 10.3389/fdgth.2024.1332707 PMID: 38524249

Berciano, S., Figueiredo, J., Brisbois, T. D., Alford, S., Koecher, K., Eckhouse, S., Ciati, R., Kussmann, M., Ordovas, J. M., Stebbins, K., & Blumberg, J. B. (2022). Precision nutrition: Maintaining scientific integrity while realizing market potential. *Frontiers in Nutrition*, *9*, 979665. DOI: 10.3389/fnut.2022.979665 PMID: 36118748

Bergquist, M., Rolandsson, B., Gryska, E., Laesser, M., Hoefling, N., Heckemann, R., Schneiderman, J. F., & Björkman-Burtscher, I. M. (2024). Trust and stakeholder perspectives on the implementation of AI tools in clinical radiology. *European Radiology*, *34*(1), 338–347. DOI: 10.1007/s00330-023-09967-5 PMID: 37505245

Bernardo, A. (2017). Virtual reality and simulation in neurosurgical training. *World Neurosurgery*, *106*, 1015–1029. DOI: 10.1016/j.wneu.2017.06.140 PMID: 28985656

Bernhardt, M., Coelho de Castro, D., Tanno, R., Schwaighofer, A., Tezcan, K. C., Monteiro, M., Bannur, S., Lungren, M. P., Nori, A., Glocker, B., Alvarez-Valle, J., & Oktay, O. (2022). Active label cleaning for improved dataset quality under resource constraints. Microsoft Research. *Nature Communications, 13*(1161), 1–11. https://www.microsoft.com/en-us/research/publication/active-label-cleaning-improving-dataset-quality-under-resource-constraints/

Berry, S. E., Valdes, A. M., Drew, D. A., Asnicar, F., Mazidi, M., Wolf, J., Capdevila, J., Hadjigeorgiou, G., Davies, R., Al Khatib, H., Bonnett, C., Ganesh, S., Bakker, E., Hart, D., Mangino, M., Merino, J., Linenberg, I., Wyatt, P., Ordovas, J. M., & Spector, T. D. (2020). Human postprandial responses to food and potential for precision nutrition. *Nature Medicine, 26*(6), 964–973. DOI: 10.1038/s41591-020-0934-0 PMID: 32528151

Bertels, H. M. J., Mithani, M., Zhu, S., & Koen, P. A. (2020). Corporate champions of early-stage project proposals and the institutionalisation of organisational inertia. *International Journal of Innovation Management, 24*(03), 2050028. DOI: 10.1142/S1363919620500280

Bestsennyy, O., Gilbert, G., Harris, A., & Rost, J. (2021). Telehealth: A quarter-trillion-dollar post-COVID-19 reality? McKinsey & Company. https://www.mckinsey.com/industries/healthcare-systems-and-services/our-insights/telehealth-a-quarter-trillion-dollar-post-covid-19-reality

Betancourt, J. R., Green, A. R., & Carrillo, J. E. (2002). CULTURAL COMPETENCE IN HEALTH CARE: EMERGING FRAMEWORKS AND PRACTICAL APPROACHES. In FIELD REPORT. The Commonwealth Fund. https://www.commonwealthfund.org/sites/default/files/documents/___media_files_publications_fund_report_2002_oct_cultural_competence_in_health_care__emerging_frameworks_and_practical_approaches_betancourt_culturalcompetence_576_pdf.pdf

Bhagat, S. V., & Kanyal, D. (2024). Navigating the Future: The Transformative Impact of Artificial Intelligence on Hospital Management- A Comprehensive Review. *Cureus, 16*(2). Advance online publication. DOI: 10.7759/cureus.54518 PMID: 38516434

Bhamu, J., & Singh Sangwan, K. (2014). Lean manufacturing: Literature review and research issues. *International Journal of Operations & Production Management, 34*(7), 876–940. DOI: 10.1108/IJOPM-08-2012-0315

Bhati, D., Deogade, M. S., & Kanyal, D. (2023). Improving Patient Outcomes Through Effective Hospital Administration: A Comprehensive Review. *Cureus*, *15*(10), e47731. DOI: 10.7759/cureus.47731 PMID: 38021686

Bhavnani, S. P. (2020). Digital Health: Opportunities and Challenges to Develop the Next-Generation Technology-Enabled Models of Cardiovascular Care. *Methodist DeBakey Cardiovascular Journal*, *16*(4), 296–303. DOI: 10.14797/mdcj-16-4-296 PMID: 33500758

Black, P. E. (2004). *Dictionary of algorithms and data structures*. National Institute of Standards and Technology.

Bodaghi, A., Fattahi, N., & Ramazani, A. (2023). Biomarkers: Promising and valuable tools towards diagnosis, prognosis and treatment of Covid-19 and other diseases. *Heliyon*, *9*(2), e13323. DOI: 10.1016/j.heliyon.2023.e13323 PMID: 36744065

Boina, R. (2023). Revolutionizing Healthcare: Unleashing the Power of Data Analytics for Enhanced Clinical Decisions, Operational Efficiency, and Patient Empowerment. [IJSR]. *International Journal of Science and Research (Raipur, India)*, *12*(8), 1–4. DOI: 10.21275/SR23827045322

Bolhasani, H., Mohseni, M., & Rahmani, A. M. (2021). *Informatics in Medicine Unlocked*. Elseiver.

Bollinger, S. R. (2019). Creativity and forms of managerial control in innovation processes: Tools, viewpoints and practices. *European Journal of Innovation Management*, *23*(2), 214–229. DOI: 10.1108/EJIM-07-2018-0153

Bonderud, D. (2024, September 26). Ransomware on the rise: Healthcare industry attack trends 2024. Security Intelligence. https://securityintelligence.com/articles/healthcare-industry-attack-trends-2024/

Braun, J. (n.d.). Data Ecosystems and Care Analytics Research Group. Institute of Medical Informatics. Retrieved August 2, 2024, from

Braunstein, M. L. (2018). Healthcare in the age of interoperability: The promise of fast healthcare interoperability resources. *IEEE Pulse*, *9*(6), 24–27. DOI: 10.1109/MPUL.2018.2869317 PMID: 30452344

Braveman, P. (2006). Health disparities and health equity: Concepts and measurement. *Annual Review of Public Health*, *27*(1), 167–194. DOI: 10.1146/annurev.publhealth.27.021405.102103 PMID: 16533114

Brennan, L., & de Roos, B. (2021). Nutrigenomics: Lessons learned and future perspectives. *The American Journal of Clinical Nutrition, 113*(3), 503–516. DOI: 10.1093/ajcn/nqaa366 PMID: 33515029

Brown, T. (2008). Design thinking. *Harvard Business Review, 86*(6), 84–92. https://hbr.org/2008/06/design-thinking PMID: 18605031

Brun, E. (2011). Ambiguity: A useful component of "fuzziness" in innovation. In Frick, J., & Laugen, B. T. (Eds.), *Advances in Production Management Systems. Value Networks: Innovation, Technologies, and Management* (Vol. 384, pp. 412–424). Springer Berlin Heidelberg., DOI: 10.1007/978-3-642-33980-6_46

Brun, E., Steinar Saetre, A., & Gjelsvik, M. (2009). Classification of ambiguity in new product development projects. *European Journal of Innovation Management, 12*(1), 62–85. DOI: 10.1108/14601060910928175

Bryman, A., & Bell, E. (2011). *Business Research Methods* (3rd ed.). Oxford University Press.

Buchanan, J., & Hargreaves, T. (2020). Sustainability in healthcare: A review of the literature. *International Journal of Health Services, 50*(4), 456–472. DOI: 10.1177/0020731420901234

Buntin, M. B., Burke, M. F., Hoaglin, M. C., & Blumenthal, D. (2011). The benefits of health information technology: A review of the recent literature shows predominantly positive results. *Health Affairs, 30*(3), 464–471. DOI: 10.1377/hlthaff.2011.0178 PMID: 21383365

Buolamwini, J., & Gebru, T. (2018). Gender shades: Intersectional accuracy disparities in commercial gender classification. *Proceedings of Machine Learning Research.*

Butler Technologies. (2023, June 21). ***Help Athletes Perform Better with Biometric Sensors.*** Retrieved January 17, 2025, from https://butlertechnologies.com/blog/perform-biosensors

Bzdok, D., Altman, N., & Krzywinski, M. (2018). Statistics versus machine learning. *Nature Methods, 15*(4), 233–234. DOI: 10.1038/nmeth.4642 PMID: 30100822

Cacchio, A., De Blasi, R., & Vannozzi, G. (2021). Rehabilitation Technology: A Systematic Review of Artificial Intelligence in Rehabilitation Robotics. *Journal of Rehabilitation Research and Development, 58*(4), 661–674. DOI: 10.1682/JRRD.2020.09.0181

Cao, Y., & Yang, J. (2015). Towards making systems forget with machine unlearning. *IEEE Symposium on Security and Privacy.*https://www.ieee-security.org/TC/SP2015/papers-archived/6949a463.pdf

Cao, Y., & Yang, J. (2015). Towards Making Systems Forget with Machine Unlearning. *IEEE Symposium on Security and Privacy*, 463–480. https://doi.org/DOI: 10.1109/SP.2015.35

Cardoza, S., & Moras, J. S. (2024b). Improving patient care in the emergency department in a selected hospital: A study on patient centered care. *International Journal of Community Medicine and Public Health, 11*(10), 3996–4003. DOI: 10.18203/2394-6040.ijcmph20242884

Celis-Morales, C., Livingstone, K. M., Marsaux, C. F., Forster, H., O'Donovan, C. B., Woolhead, C., Macready, A. L., Fallaize, R., Navas-Carretero, S., San-Cristobal, R., Kolossa, S., Hartwig, K., Tsirigoti, L., Lambrinou, C. P., Moschonis, G., Godlewska, M., Surwiłło, A., Grimaldi, K., Bouwman, J., & Mathers, J. C. (2015). Design and baseline characteristics of the Food4Me study: A web-based randomised controlled trial of personalised nutrition in seven European countries. *Genes & Nutrition, 10*(1), 1–13. DOI: 10.1007/s12263-014-0450-2 PMID: 25491748

Central Drugs Standard Control Organization. (2020). Medical Devices (Amendment) Rules, 2020.

Central Drugs Standard Control Organization. (2021). Emergency use authorization for COVID-19 vaccines.

Chanchaichujit, J., Tan, A., Meng, F., & Eaimkhong, S. (2019). An introduction to Healthcare 4.0. In *Healthcare 4.0* (pp. 1–15). Springer. DOI: 10.1007/978-981-13-8114-0_1

Chandrashekaran, A. (2024). A review of Industry 4.0 and 6.0 in manufacturing industries. Propulsion Tech Journal. Retrieved from https://www.propulsiontechjournal.com/index.php/journal/article/view/4185

Chang, A. S., & Tien, C. (2006). Quantifying uncertainty and equivocality in engineering projects. *Construction Management and Economics, 24*(2), 171–184. DOI: 10.1080/01446190500310353

Chang, S.-L., Chen, C.-Y., & Wey, S.-C. (2007). Conceptualizing, assessing, and managing front-end fuzziness in innovation/NPD projects. *R & D Management, 37*(5), 469–478. DOI: 10.1111/j.1467-9310.2007.00489.x

Chan, L., Vasilevsky, N., Thessen, A., McMurry, J., & Haendel, M. (2021). The landscape of nutri-informatics: A review of current resources and challenges for integrative nutrition research. *Database : The Journal of Biological Databases and Curation, 2021*, baab003. DOI: 10.1093/database/baab003 PMID: 33494105

Char, D. S., Shah, N. H., & Magnus, D. (2018). Implementing machine learning in health care—Addressing ethical challenges. *The New England Journal of Medicine, 378*(11), 981–983. DOI: 10.1056/NEJMp1714229 PMID: 29539284

Charity Miles. (n.d.). Social proof in action. Retrieved from https://www.charitymiles.org

Cheng, S., Xiao, Y., Liu, L., & Sun, X. (2024). Comparative outcomes of AI-assisted ChatGPT and face-to-face consultations in infertility patients: A cross-sectional study. *Postgraduate Medical Journal, 100*(1189), 851–855. DOI: 10.1093/postmj/qgae083 PMID: 38970829

Cheng, Y. T., Lin, Y. F., Chiang, K. H., & Tseng, V. S. (2017). Mining sequential risk patterns from large-scale clinical databases for early assessment of chronic diseases: A case study on chronic obstructive pulmonary disease. *IEEE Journal of Biomedical and Health Informatics, 21*(2), 303–311. DOI: 10.1109/JBHI.2017.2657802 PMID: 28129195

Chen, X., Xie, H., Tao, X., Wang, F. L., Leng, M., & Lei, B. (2024). Artificial intelligence and multimodal data fusion for smart healthcare: Topic modeling and bibliometrics. *Artificial Intelligence Review, 57*(1), 91. DOI: 10.1007/s10462-024-10712-7

Chourasia, A., Tyagi, S., Pandey, S., Walia, R., & Murtaza, Q. (2022). Sustainability of Industry 6.0 in Global Perspective: Benefits and challenges. *Sustainability of Industry 6.0 in Global Perspective: Benefits and Challenges*. Retrieved from: https://www.researchgate.net/publication/359117146_Sustainability_of_Industry_60_in_Global_Perspective_Benefits_and_Challenges#fullTextFileContent

Christiansen, J. K., & Gasparin, M. (2016). Managing controversies in the fuzzy front end. *Creativity and Innovation Management, 25*(4), 500–514. DOI: 10.1111/caim.12174

Chugh, M., & Chugh, N. (2023). Paving the way for healthcare with AI, ML, and DL. *Handbook on Augmenting Telehealth Services*, 368–382.

Chundawat, V. S., Tarun, A. K., Mandal, M., & Kankanhalli, M. (2023). *Zero-Shot Machine Unlearning*. IEEE., DOI: 10.1109/TIFS.2023.3265506

Churko, J. M., Mantalas, G. L., Snyder, M. P., & Wu, J. C. (2013). Overview of high throughput sequencing technologies to elucidate molecular pathways in cardiovascular diseases. *Circulation Research*, *112*(12), 1613–1623. DOI: 10.1161/CIRCRESAHA.113.300939 PMID: 23743227

Claim Adjudication Manual. (n.d.). National Health Authority. Retrieved August 5, 2024, from https://pmjay.gov.in/sites/default/files/2021-01/Claims-Adjudication-Manual-2_0-final.pdf

Club, D. (2024, July 31). Navigating Health Data Privacy in India: Regulations and Best Practices for Compliance and Trust. https://www.linkedin.com/pulse/navigating-health-data-privacy-india-regulations-best-practices-kmeuc

Cohen, I. G., & Mello, M. M. (2018). HIPAA and protecting health information in the 21st century. *Journal of the American Medical Association*, *320*(3), 231–232. DOI: 10.1001/jama.2018.5630 PMID: 29800120

Cooper, R. G. (1990). Stage-gate systems: A new tool for managing new products. *Business Horizons*, *33*(3), 44–54. DOI: 10.1016/0007-6813(90)90040-I

Cooper, R. G. (2006). Managing technology development projects. *Research Technology Management*, *49*(6), 23–31. DOI: 10.1080/08956308.2006.11657405

Cooper, R. G., & Kleinschmidt, E. J. (1988). Resource allocation in the new product process. *Industrial Marketing Management*, *17*(3), 249–262. DOI: 10.1016/0019-8501(88)90008-9

Craig, L. (2024). 10 top AI and machine learning trends for 2024. *TechTarget*. https://www.techtarget.com/searchenterpriseai/tip/9-top-AI-and-machine-learning-trends

Crump, B. J., Letendre, A., Croker, R., & Bolsin, S. (2017). Improving quality and safety in healthcare through education, training and innovative best practices. *Anaesthesia*, *72*, 6–10.

D'Souza, M., Ros, M., & Karunanithi, M. (2012). An Indoor Localisation and Motion Monitoring System to Determine Behavioral Activity in Dementia Afflicted Patients in Aged Care. *Electronic Journal of Health Informatics*, *7*(2), e14.

Da Costa, C. A., Pasluosta, C. F., Eskofier, B., Da Silva, D. B., & da Rosa Righi, R. (2018). Internet of Health Things: Toward intelligent vital signs monitoring in hospital wards. *Artificial Intelligence in Medicine*, *89*, 61–69. DOI: 10.1016/j.artmed.2018.05.005 PMID: 29871778

Da Silva, R. H., Kaminski, P. C., & Armellini, F. (2020). Improving new product development innovation effectiveness by using problem solving tools during the conceptual development phase: Integrating Design Thinking and TRIZ. *Creativity and Innovation Management*, *29*(4), 685–700. DOI: 10.1111/caim.12399

Daft, R. L., Lengel, R. H., & Trevino, L. K. (1987). Message equivocality, media selection, and manager performance: Implications for information systems. *Management Information Systems Quarterly*, *11*(3), 355. DOI: 10.2307/248682

Damaševičius, R., & M. R. 2023. Serious Games and Gamification in Healthcare:Meta-Review, A. (•••).. . *Information (Basel)*, *14*(2), 105. DOI: 10.3390/info14020105

Dana-Farber Cancer Institute. (2022). Personalized Treatment Planning. Retrieved from https://www.dana-farber.org/research/personalized-treatment-planning/

Dangi, R. R., Sharma, A., & Vageriya, V. (2024). Transforming Healthcare in Low-Resource Settings With Artificial Intelligence: Recent Developments and Outcomes. *Public Health Nursing (Boston, Mass.)*, phn.13500. Advance online publication. DOI: 10.1111/phn.13500 PMID: 39629887

Dang, T. K., Lan, X., Weng, J., & Feng, M. (2022). Federated Learning for Electronic Health Records. *ACM Transactions on Intelligent Systems and Technology*, *13*(5), 1–17. DOI: 10.1145/3514500

Daniel, J. (2023). Safeguarding Privacy in the Age of AI: Navigating the Complexities of Data Protection. *Revista de Inteligencia Artificial en Medicina*, *14*(1), 693–704.

Davenport, T., & Kalakota, R. (2019). The potential for artificial intelligence in healthcare. *Future Healthcare Journal*, *6*(2), 94–98. DOI: 10.7861/futurehosp.6-2-94 PMID: 31363513

Daytwo. Accessed on 10th January 2025 from https://www.daytwo.com/

de Filippis, R., & Al Foysal, A. (2024). Blockchain Brains: Pioneering AI, ML, and DLT Solutions for Healthcare and Psychology. *OAlib*, *11*(12), 1–24. DOI: 10.4236/oalib.1112543

de Luis, D. A., Izaola, O., Primo, D., & Aller, R. (2018). Role of rs670 variant of APOA1 gene on lipid profile, insulin resistance and adipokine levels in obese subjects after weight loss with a dietary intervention. *Diabetes Research and Clinical Practice*, *142*, 139–145. DOI: 10.1016/j.diabres.2018.05.040 PMID: 29859275

De Oliveira Almeida, G., & Hinton, J. E. (2024). Simulation and Healthcare Simulation. In *Reference Module in Social Sciences* (p. B9780443137013003042). Elsevier., DOI: 10.1016/B978-0-443-13701-3.00304-2

Deci, E. L., & Ryan, R. M. (2000). The "what" and "why" of goal pursuits: Human needs and the self-determination of behavior. *Psychological Inquiry*, *11*(4), 227–268. DOI: 10.1207/S15327965PLI1104_01

Defense Advanced Research Projects Agency. (2020). Explainable Artificial Intelligence (XAI) Program.Davis, M. E., Chen, Z. G., & Shin, D. M. (2018). Nanoparticle therapeutics: An emerging treatment modality for cancer. *Nature Reviews. Drug Discovery*, *7*(9), 771–782.

Deloitte. (2020). "AI in financial services: Making AI a key factor for success."

Demir, E., Yakutcan, U., & Page, S. (2024). Using simulation modelling to transform hospital planning and management to address health inequalities. *Social Science & Medicine*, *347*, 116786. DOI: 10.1016/j.socscimed.2024.116786 PMID: 38493680

Deterding, S., Dixon, D., Khaled, R., & Nacke, L. (2011). From game design elements to gamefulness: Defining "gamification." *Proceedings of the 15th International Academic MindTrek Conference: Envisioning Future Media Environments* (pp. 9–15). ACM. https://doi.org/DOI: 10.1145/2181037.2181040

Development Asia. (2022, May 4). Training on Successful Implementation of a Digital Financial Services for Health Project [Video]. YouTube. https://www.youtube.com/watch?v=ZiAuqu3

Devine, E. B., Hansen, R. N., Wilson-Norton, J. L., Lawless, N. M., Fisk, A. W., Blough, D. K., Martin, D. P., & Sullivan, S. D. (2010). The impact of computerized provider order entry on medication errors in a multispecialty group practice. *Journal of the American Medical Informatics Association : JAMIA*, *17*(1), 78–84. DOI: 10.1197/jamia.M3285 PMID: 20064806

Digital Government Strategic Framework 2019-2024. (2019). Finance.Govt. Tonga. https://finance.gov.to/sites/default/files/2021-07/Digital%20Strategic%20Framework.pdf

Digital Transformation Department. Prime Minister's Office. (n.d.). https://digitaltransformation.gov.to/?page_id=154

Dillies, M. A., Rau, A., Aubert, J., Hennequet-Antier, C., Jeanmougin, M., Servant, N., Keime, C., Marot, G., Castel, D., Estelle, J., Guernec, G., Jagla, B., Jouneau, L., Laloe, D., Le Gall, C., Schaeffer, B., Le Crom, S., Guedj, M., & Jaffrézic, F. (2013). A comprehensive evaluation of normalization methods for Illumina high-throughput RNA sequencing data analysis. *Briefings in Bioinformatics*, *14*(6), 671–683. DOI: 10.1093/bib/bbs046 PMID: 22988256

Dinsdale, N. K., Jenkinson, M., & Namburete, A. I. (2021). Deep learning-based unlearning of dataset bias for MRI harmonisation and confound removal. *NeuroImage*, *228*, 117689.

Doe, J., Smith, A., & Brown, P. (2023). Technology-facilitated abuse in clinical settings: Emerging threats and recommendations. *PLOS Digital Health*, *2*(1).

Donaldson LJ, Fletcher MG. The WHO world

Donaldson, L. J., & Fletcher, M. G. (2006). The WHO World Alliance for Patient Safety: Towards the years of living less dangerously. *The Medical Journal of Australia*, *184*(S10), S69–S72. DOI: 10.5694/j.1326-5377.2006.tb00367.x PMID: 16719741

Dorsey, E. R., & Topol, E. J. (2016). State of telehealth. *The New England Journal of Medicine*, *375*(2), 154–161. DOI: 10.1056/NEJMra1601705 PMID: 27410924

Doyle, C., Lennox, L., & Bell, D. (2013). A systematic review of evidence on the links between patient experience and clinical safety and effectiveness. *BMJ Open*, *3*(1), e001570. DOI: 10.1136/bmjopen-2012-001570 PMID: 23293244

Duggal, A. S., Malik, P. K., Gehlot, A., Singh, R., Gaba, G. S., Masud, M., & Al-Amri, J. F. (2021). A sequential roadmap to industry 6.0: Exploring future manufacturing trends. *IET Communications*, *16*(5), 521–531. DOI: 10.1049/cmu2.12284

Dunn, W. B., Broadhurst, D., Begley, P., Zelena, E., Francis-McIntyre, S., Anderson, N., Brown, M., Knowles, J. D., Halsall, A., Haselden, J. N., Nicholls, A. W., Wilson, I. D., Kell, D. B., & Goodacre, R.Human Serum Metabolome (HUSERMET) Consortium. (2011). Procedures for large-scale metabolic profiling of serum and plasma using gas chromatography and liquid chromatography coupled to mass spectrometry. *Nature Protocols*, *6*(7), 1060–1083. DOI: 10.1038/nprot.2011.335 PMID: 21720319

Duolingo, Inc. (n.d.). Duolingo: Learn languages for free. Retrieved from https://www.duolingo.com

Dyer, J. H., & Singh, H. (1998). The relational view: Cooperative strategy and sources of inter-organizational competitive advantage. *Academy of Management Review*, *23*(4), 660–679. DOI: 10.2307/259056

Eckelman, M. J., & Sherman, J. (2016). Environmental impacts of the U.S. health care system and effects on public health. *PLoS One*, *11*(6), e0157014. DOI: 10.1371/journal.pone.0157014 PMID: 27280706

Edemekong, P. F., Annamaraju, P., & Haydel, M. J. (2024). Health Insurance Portability and Accountability Act. In *StatPearls* [Internet]. StatPearls Publishing., https://www.ncbi.nlm.nih.gov/books/NBK500019/

Edmondson, A. C. (2019). *The fearless organization: Creating psychological safety in the workplace for learning, innovation, and growth*. John Wiley & Sons.

Effatparvar, M., Dehghan, M., & Rahmani, A. M. (2016). A comprehensive survey of energy-aware routing protocols in wireless body area sensor networks. *Journal of Medical Systems*, *40*(9), 1–27. DOI: 10.1007/s10916-016-0556-8 PMID: 27468842

EInvoicing in Estonia. (1424, August). Language selection | European Commission. https://ec.europa.eu/digital-building-blocks/wikis/display/DIGITAL/eInvoicing+in+Estonia

El Naqa, I., & Murphy, M. J. (2015). What Is Machine Learning? In El Naqa, I., Li, R., & Murphy, M. J. (Eds.), *Machine Learning in Radiation Oncology*. Springer., DOI: 10.1007/978-3-319-18305-3_1

Eldan, R., & Mark, R. (2023). Who's Harry Potter? Approximate Unlearning in LLMs. *ArXiv*. DOI:/arXiv.2310.02238.DOI: 10.48550

Eldridge, A. L., Piernas, C., Illner, A. K., Gibney, M. J., Gurinović, M. A., De Vries, J. H., & Cade, J. E. (2018). Evaluation of new technology-based tools for dietary intake assessment—An ILSI Europe Dietary Intake and Exposure Task Force evaluation. *Nutrients*, *11*(1), 55. DOI: 10.3390/nu11010055 PMID: 30597864

El-Gayar, O. F., Bojja, G. R., Ambati, L. S., Boit, J., & Nawar, N. (2024). The Impact of the Internet of Things in Healthcare Delivery: A Systematic Literature Review. In Wickramasinghe, N. (Ed.), (pp. 35–100). Advances in Medical Technologies and Clinical Practice. IGI Global., DOI: 10.4018/979-8-3693-5237-3.ch002

Equifax data breach settlement. (2022, December 20). Federal Trade Commission. https://www.ftc.gov/enforcement/refunds/equifax-data-breach-settlement

Erat, S. (2017). Making the best idea better: The role of idea pool structure. *Production and Operations Management*, *26*(10), 1946–1959. DOI: 10.1111/poms.12734

Eriksson, P. E., Patel, P. C., Sjödin, D. R., Frishammar, J., & Parida, V. (2016). Managing interorganizational innovation projects: Mitigating the negative effects of equivocality through knowledge search strategies. *Long Range Planning*, *49*(6), 691–705. DOI: 10.1016/j.lrp.2016.05.006

Esau, C., Davis, S., Murray, S. F., Yu, X. X., Pandey, S. K., Pear, M., Watts, L., Booten, S. L., Graham, M., McKay, R., Subramaniam, A., Propp, S., Lollo, B. A., Freier, S., Bennett, C. F., Bhanot, S., & Monia, B. P. (2006). miR-122 regulation of lipid metabolism revealed by in vivo antisense targeting. *Cell Metabolism*, *3*(2), 87–98. DOI: 10.1016/j.cmet.2006.01.005 PMID: 16459310

Esteva, A., Kuprel, B., Novoa, R. A., Ko, J., Swetter, S. M., Blau, H. M., & Thrun, S. (2017). Dermatologist-level classification of skin cancer with deep neural networks. *Nature*, *542*(7639), 115–118. DOI: 10.1038/nature21056 PMID: 28117445

Esteva, A., Robicquet, A., Ramsundar, B., Kuleshov, V., DePristo, M., Chou, K., Cui, C., Corrado, G., Thrun, S., & Dean, J. (2019). A guide to deep learning in healthcare. *Nature Medicine*, *25*(1), 24–29. DOI: 10.1038/s41591-018-0316-z PMID: 30617335

European Commission. (2018). *General Data Protection Regulation*. GDPR.

European Commission. (2021). *Proposal for a Regulation laying down harmonised rules on artificial intelligence*. Artificial Intelligence Act.

European Union, E. (2014). Directive 2014/24/EU of the European Parliament and of the Council of 26 February 2014 on Public Procurement and Repealing Directive 2004/18/EC (1). *Official Journal of the European Union, 57*(28 March 2014), 65–242. https://doi.org/doi:10.3000/19770677.L_2014.094.eng

Ezeamii, V. C., Okobi, O. E., Wambai-Sani, H., Perera, G. S., Zaynieva, S., Okonkwo, C. C., Ohaiba, M. M., William-Enemali, P. C., Obodo, O. R., & Obiefuna, N. G. (2024). Revolutionizing Healthcare: How Telemedicine Is Improving Patient Outcomes and Expanding Access to Care. *Cureus*. Advance online publication. DOI: 10.7759/cureus.63881 PMID: 39099901

Fahim, M., Sharma, V., Hunter, R., & Duong, T. Q. (2023). Healthy aging: A deep meta-class sequence model to integrate intelligence in digital twin. *IEEE Journal of Translational Engineering in Health and Medicine*, *11*, 330–340. DOI: 10.1109/JTEHM.2023.3274357

Falony, G., Joossens, M., Vieira-Silva, S., Wang, J., Darzi, Y., Faust, K., Kurilshikov, A., Bonder, M. J., Valles-Colomer, M., Vandeputte, D., Tito, R. Y., Chaffron, S., Rymenans, L., Verspecht, C., De Sutter, L., Lima-Mendez, G., D'hoe, K., Jonckheere, K., Homola, D., & Raes, J. (2016). Population-level analysis of gut microbiome variation. *Science*, *352*(6285), 560–564. DOI: 10.1126/science.aad3503 PMID: 27126039

Fast Company. (2016, January 12). This app turns exercise into charitable donations. *Fast Company*. Retrieved from https://www.fastcompany.com/3064854/this-app-turns-exercise-into-charitable-donations

Fatima, M., & Pasha, M. (2017). Survey of machine learning algorithms for disease diagnostic. *Journal of Intelligent Learning Systems and Applications*, *9*(01), 1–16. DOI: 10.4236/jilsa.2017.91001

FDA. (2018). "Premarket Approval (PMA) for Medtronic MiniMed 670G System."

FDA. (2020). "Emergency Use Authorization for Vaccines Explained."

FDA. (2020). "FDA's Approach to Medical Device Regulation."

Feist, K. 2023, June 9. Improving the patient experience through technology. Forbes. https://www.forbes.com/sites/forbestechcouncil/2023/06/08/improving-the-patient-experience-through-technology/

Feng, C. C., Chen, S. Z., Weng, Q. Z., Hu, H. J., Wang, Y. D., Chen, B. B., & Yan, T. Y. (2013, February). Elderly health care systems—Part I: Hardware implementations of wireless sensor networks. In Next-Generation Electronics (ISNE), 2013 IEEE International Symposium on (pp. 305-308). IEEE.

Fenton, J. J., Taplin, S. H., Carney, P. A., Abraham, L., Sickles, E. A., D'Orsi, C., Berns, E. A., Cutter, G., Hendrick, R. E., Barlow, W. E., & Elmore, J. G. (2007). Influence of computer-aided detection on performance of screening mammography. *The New England Journal of Medicine*, *356*(14), 1399–1409. DOI: 10.1056/NEJMoa066099 PMID: 17409321

Finlayson, S. G., Bowers, J. D., Ito, J., Zittrain, J. L., Beam, A. L., & Kohane, I. S. (2019, March 21). Adversarial Attacks on Medical Machine Learning. *Science*, *363*(6433), 1287–1289. DOI: 10.1126/science.aaw4399 PMID: 30898923

Florén, H., & Frishammar, J. (2012). From preliminary ideas to corroborated product definitions: Managing the front end of new product development. *California Management Review*, *54*(4), 20–43. DOI: 10.1525/cmr.2012.54.4.20

Florén, H., Frishammar, J., Parida, V., & Wincent, J. (2018). Critical success factors in early new product development: A review and a conceptual model. *The International Entrepreneurship and Management Journal, 14*(2), 411–427. DOI: 10.1007/s11365-017-0458-3

FloVision. Accessed on 15th January 2025 from https://flovisionsolutions.com/

Fooddarzee. Accessed on 15th January 2025 from https://fooddarzee.com/bengaluru

Foodvisor. Accessed on 15th January 2025 from https://www.foodvisor.io/en/

Forbes. (2021, September 16). How Noom's gamification strategy is revolutionizing weight loss. *Forbes*. Retrieved from https://www.forbes.com/sites/forbestechcouncil/2021/09/16/how-nooms-gamification-strategy-is-revolutionizing-weight-loss

Ford, J. (n.d.-b). NSF grant to help researchers harness power of big data to address health issues. Penn State University. https://www.psu.edu/news/research/story/nsf-grant-help-researchers-harness-power-big-data-address-health-issues/

Frishammar, J., Floren, H., & Wincent, J. (2011). Beyond managing uncertainty: Insights from studying equivocality in the fuzzy front end of product and process innovation projects. *IEEE Transactions on Engineering Management, 58*(3), 551–563. DOI: 10.1109/TEM.2010.2095017

Froehlich, J. K., Hoegl, M., & Gibbert, M. (2016). Idea selection in suggestion systems: A thematic similarity perspective. *R & D Management, 46*(5), 887–899. DOI: 10.1111/radm.12154

Gaddam, A., Mukhopadhyay, S. C., & Gupta, G. S. (2010). Elder care based on cognitive sensor network. *IEEE Sensors Journal, 11*(3), 574–581. DOI: 10.1109/JSEN.2010.2051425

Gagnon, M. P., Payne-Gagnon, J., Fortin, J. P., Paré, G., Côté, J., & Courcy, F. (2015). A learning organization in the service of knowledge management among nurses: A case study. *International Journal of Information Management, 35*(5), 636–642. DOI: 10.1016/j.ijinfomgt.2015.05.001

Ganesan, M., & Sivakumar, N. (2019, March). IoT based heart disease prediction and diagnosis model for healthcare using machine learning models. In 2019 IEEE international conference on system, computation, automation and networking (ICSCAN) (pp. 1-5). IEEE.

Garett, R. Y., & Young, S. D. (2019, September 1). Health Care Gamification: A Study of Game Mechanics and Elements. *Tech Know Learn, 24*(3), 341–353. DOI: 10.1007/s10758-018-9353-4

Garg, D., Dubey, N., Goel, P., Ramoliya, D., Ganatra, A., & Kotecha, K. (2024). Improvisation in Spinal Surgery Using AR (Augmented Reality), MR (Mixed Reality), and VR (Virtual Reality). *RAiSE, 2023*, 186. DOI: 10.3390/engproc2023059186

Gartner. (2019). "Top 10 Data and Analytics Technology Trends That Will Change the Game."

Gassmann, O., & Schweitzer, F. (Eds.). (2014). *Management of the Fuzzy Front End of Innovation*. Springer International Publishing., DOI: 10.1007/978-3-319-01056-4

Gavin-Smith, B. (2022). Precision nutrition for low-and middle-income countries: Hype or hope? *Sight and Life Special Report., 2022*, 1–95. DOI: 10.52439/PRCJ5543

Geissdoerfer, M., Savaget, P., Bocken, N. M. P., & Hultink, E. J. (2018). The Circular Economy – A new sustainability paradigm? *Journal of Cleaner Production, 143*, 757–768. DOI: 10.1016/j.jclepro.2016.12.048

General Data Protection Regulation. (2018). Regulation (EU) 2016/679. Official Journal of the European Union. https://gdpr-info.eu/

Géron, A. (2017). *Concepts, tools, and techniques to build intelligent systems. Hands-On Machine Learning with Scikit-Learn, Keras, and TensorFlow* (2nd ed.). O'Reilly Media.

Ghomi, E. J., Rahmani, A. M., & Qader, N. N. (2017). Load-balancing algorithms in cloud computing: A survey. *Journal of Network and Computer Applications, 88*, 50–71. DOI: 10.1016/j.jnca.2017.04.007

Ghosh, P., Biswas, A., & Ghosh, S. (2023). Fundamentals and Technicalities of Big Data and Analytics. In *Intelligent Systems in Healthcare and Disease Identification using Data Science* (pp. 51–106). Chapman and Hall/CRC. DOI: 10.1201/9781003354178-3

Ghosh, S., & Ghosh, S. K. (2023). Feel: Federated learning framework for elderly healthcare using edge-iomt. *IEEE Transactions on Computational Social Systems, 10*(4), 1800–1809. DOI: 10.1109/TCSS.2022.3233300

Gill, S. P. S., Suryadevara, N. K., & Mukhopadhyay, S. C. (2012, December). Smart Power monitoring system using wireless sensor networks. In Sensing Technology (ICST), 2012 Sixth International Conference on (pp. 444-449). IEEE. DOI: 10.1109/ICSensT.2012.6461718

Ginart, A., Guan, M. Y., Valiant, G., & Zou, J. (2019). Making AI Forget You: Data Deletion in Machine Learning. *Advances in Neural Information Processing Systems (NeurIPS).* https://papers.nips.cc/paper/8611-making-ai-forget-you-data-deletion-in-machine-learning

Gioia, D. A., Corley, K. G., & Hamilton, A. L. (2013). Seeking qualitative rigor in inductive research: Notes on the Gioia Methodology. *Organizational Research Methods*, *16*(1), 15–31. DOI: 10.1177/1094428112452151

Gitomer, J. (1997). Your Customer's Happiness Requires Partnering Approach. *Business First*, *8*, 15.

Global Hunger Index. (October 2024). How gender justice can advance climate resilience and zero hunger. Global Hunger Index. Accessed from file:///C:/Users/IIHMRB31669/Downloads/2024.pdf Habitz. Accessed on 15th January 2025 from https://habitz.com/

Gopi, B., Kokila, M. S., Bibin, C. V., Sasikala, D., Howard, E., & Boopathi, S. (2024). Distributed Technologies Using AI/ML Techniques for Healthcare Applications. In *Social Innovations in Education, Environment, and Healthcare* (pp. 375-396). IGI Global.

Gostin, L. O., & Halabi, S. F. (2021). Data sharing during public health emergencies: A critical policy issue. *Journal of the American Medical Association*, *325*(4), 315–316.

Gowri, V., Uma, M., & Sethuramalingam, P. (2024). Machine learning enabled robot-assisted virtual health monitoring system design and development. *Multiscale and Multidisciplinary Modeling, Experiments and Design*, 1-30.

Grando, M. A., Rozenblum, R., & Bates, D. (2015). *Information technology for patient empowerment in healthcare*. Walter de Gruyter GmbH & Co KG. DOI: 10.1515/9781614514343

Greenberg, A. (2017). Hackers Hit Dozens of Countries Exploiting Stolen NSA Tool. Wired. Retrieved from [Wired](https://www.wired.com)</eref>

Greene, J., Hibbard, J. H., Sacks, R., Overton, V., & Parrotta, C. D. (2015). When patient activation levels change, health outcomes and costs change, too. *Health Affairs*, *34*(3), 431–437. DOI: 10.1377/hlthaff.2014.0452 PMID: 25732493

Greener, R. (2024, May 21). XR Healthcare Market will be Worth $19.6 billion by 2033. *XR Today*. https://www.xrtoday.com/mixed-reality/xr-healthcare-market-will-be-worth-19-6-billion-by-2033/

Green, W., Cluley, R., & Gasparin, M. (2020). Mobile market research Applications as a new voice of customer method: Implications for innovation and design management. *Research Technology Management*, *63*(1), 49–55. DOI: 10.1080/08956308.2020.1686297

Griebel, L., Prokosch, H. U., Köpcke, F., Toddenroth, D., Christoph, J., Leb, I., Engel, I., & Sedlmayr, M. (2015). A scoping review of cloud computing in healthcare. *BMC Medical Informatics and Decision Making*, *15*(1), 1–16. DOI: 10.1186/s12911-015-0145-7 PMID: 25888747

Gupta, A., & Singh, A. (2023). Healthcare 4.0: Recent advancements and futuristic research directions. *Wireless Personal Communications*, *129*(2), 933–952. DOI: 10.1007/s11277-022-10164-8 PMID: 36594000

Gupta, S., & Maltz, E. (2015). Interdependency, dynamism, and variety (IDV) network modeling to explain knowledge diffusion at the fuzzy front-end of innovation. *Journal of Business Research*, *68*(11), 2434–2442. DOI: 10.1016/j.jbusres.2015.02.018

Haase, L. M., & Laursen, L. N. (2018). Reasoning in the fuzzy front end of innovation: Framing the product DNA. *International Journal of Innovation Management*, *22*(05), 1840001. DOI: 10.1142/S1363919618400017

Habitica. (n.d.). Gamification for daily tasks. Retrieved from https://habitica.com

Haenssle, H. A.. (2018). Artificial intelligence for diagnosis and referral of skin cancer in dermatology: A systematic review. *The Lancet. Oncology*, *19*(4), e210–e219.

Haleem, A., Javaid, M., Singh, R. P., & Suman, R. (2021). Telemedicine for healthcare: Capabilities, features, barriers, and applications. *Sensors International*, *2*, 100117. DOI: 10.1016/j.sintl.2021.100117 PMID: 34806053

Halwiindi, H., Muliokela, R., Songolo, P., Simanga, T., Joshi, S., Msadabwe, S., Mwaba, C. K., & Kapambwe, S. (2022). Utilizing Mhealth (Mobile Health) Messaging To Increase Uptake Of Cervical Cancer Screening Services: Impact, Perceptions, And Experiences From Lusaka Province, Zambia. *Journal of Disease and Global Health*, •••, 54–65. DOI: 10.56557/jodagh/2022/v15i38061

Hamad, W. B. (2019). CURRENT Position and Challenges of E-health in Tanzania: A review of literature Master of Science in... ResearchGate. https://www.researchgate.net/publication/357901194_current_position_and_challenges_of_e-health_in_tanzania_a_review_of_literature_master_of_science_in_information_system

Hamari, J., Koivisto, J., & Sarsa, H. (2014). Does gamification work? – A literature review of empirical studies on gamification. *Proceedings of the 47th Hawaii International Conference on System Sciences* (pp. 3025–3034). IEEE. https://doi.org/DOI: 10.1109/HICSS.2014.377

Hamdani, F. E. (2020). Innovation stories platform: A holistic framework for innovation case studies. *Towards the Digital World and Industry X.0 - Proceedings of the 29th International Conference of the International Association for Management of Technology, IAMOT 2020*, 175–186.

Handelman, G. S., Kok, H. K., Chandra, R. V., Razavi, A. H., Lee, M. J., & Asadi, H. (2018). eD octor: Machine learning and the future of medicine. *Journal of Internal Medicine*, *284*(6), 603–619. DOI: 10.1111/joim.12822 PMID: 30102808

Harland, C. M., Knight, L., Patrucco, A. S., Lynch, J., Telgen, J., Peters, E., Tátrai, T., & Ferk, P. (2021). Practitioners' learning about healthcare supply chain management in the COVID-19 pandemic: A public procurement perspective. *International Journal of Operations & Production Management*, *41*(13), 178–189. DOI: 10.1108/IJOPM-05-2021-0348

Haro, D., Marrero, P. F., & Relat, J. (2019). Nutritional regulation of gene expression: Carbohydrate-, fat-and amino acid-dependent modulation of transcriptional activity. *International Journal of Molecular Sciences*, *20*(6), 1386. DOI: 10.3390/ijms20061386 PMID: 30893897

Harvard Library. (2024). Harvard Dataverse*: A repository for research data*. Harvard Library https://library.harvard.edu/services-tools/harvard-dataverse

Harvard, T. H. Chan School of Public Health. (2024). Precision nutrition: The Nutrition Source. Harvard T.H. Chan School of Public Health. Retrieved July 30, 2024, from https://nutritionsource.hsph.harvard.edu/precision-nutrition/

He, Y., Meng, G., Chen, K., He, J., & Hu, X. (2021, May 13). DeepObliviate: A Powerful Charm for Erasing Data Residual Memory in Deep Neural Networks. arXiv.org. https://arxiv.org/abs/2105.06209

Health Insurance Portability and Accountability Act. (1996). Pub. L. 104-191, 110 Stat. 1936. https://www.hhs.gov/hippa

Healthful. (n.d.). Nudging towards better health. Retrieved from https://www.healthfulapp.com

HealthifyMe. Retrieved January 10, 2025 https://www.healthifyme.com/in/

Healthline. (n.d.). Gamification in wellness apps. *Healthline.* Retrieved from https://www.healthline.com/health/gamification-in-wellness-apps

Herlin, H. (2013). Better together: Cross-sector partnerships in health and social care. *International Journal of Public Sector Management, 26*(3), 190–252.

Herstatt, C., Verworn, B., & Nagahira, A. (2004). Reducing project related uncertainty in the 'fuzzy front end' of innovation: A comparison of German and Japanese product innovation projects. *International Journal of Product Development, 1*(1), 23. DOI: 10.1504/IJPD.2004.004890

He, W., Zhao, Y., Tang, H., Sun, C., & Fu, W. (2015). A wireless BCI and BMI system for wearable robots. *IEEE Transactions on Systems, Man, and Cybernetics. Systems, 46*(7), 936–946. DOI: 10.1109/TSMC.2015.2506618

He, Y., Aliyu, A., Evans, M., & Luo, C. (2021). Health Care Cybersecurity Challenges and Solutions Under the Climate of COVID-19: Scoping Review. *Journal of Medical Internet Research, 23*(4), e21747. DOI: 10.2196/21747 PMID: 33764885

Higo, M., & Khan, H. T. (2015). Global population aging: Unequal distribution of risks in later life between developed and developing countries. *Global Social Policy, 15*(2), 146–166. DOI: 10.1177/1468018114543157

Hillestad, R., Bigelow, J., Bower, A., Girosi, F., Meili, R., Scoville, R., & Taylor, R. (2005). Can Electronic Medical Record Systems Transform Health Care? Potential Health Benefits, Savings, And Costs. *Health Affairs, 24*(5), 1103–1117. DOI: 10.1377/hlthaff.24.5.1103 PMID: 16162551

HIRA system. (n.d.). www.hira.or.kr. Retrieved December 21, 2024, from https://www.hira.or.kr/eng/news/01/__icsFiles/afieldfile/2015/07/24/VyIdbjIJh6Xm.pdf

Hochbein, K. (n.d.-b). Machine Unlearning. Lehigh University. https://www2.lehigh.edu/news/machine-unlearning

Hoekman, B., & Taş, B. K. O. (2022). Procurement policy and SME participation in public purchasing. *Small Business Economics, 58*(1), 383–402. DOI: 10.1007/s11187-020-00414-z

Hoggle, L. B., Nash, D. B., & Teitelbaum, H. S. (2006). Nutrition informatics. *Journal of the American Dietetic Association, 106*(1), 134–139. DOI: 10.1016/j.jada.2005.10.025 PMID: 16390678

Holmes, J., Sacchi, L., & Bellazzi, R. (2004). Artificial intelligence in medicine. *Annals of the Royal College of Surgeons of England, 86*(5), 334–338. DOI: 10.1308/147870804290 PMID: 15333167

Hong, P. C., Park, Y. S., Deng, X., & Hwang, D. W. (2022). Marketing platform products for successful customer outcomes: An empirical investigation of project process integration. *International Journal of Quality and Service Sciences*, *14*(3), 349–367. Advance online publication. DOI: 10.1108/IJQSS-09-2021-0130

Hoonsopon, D., & Puriwat, W. (2021a). The role of leadership behaviour of project manager in managing the fuzzy front end in the development of radical and incremental innovation. *International Journal of Innovation Management*, *25*(2), 2150022. DOI: 10.1142/S1363919621500225

Hoonsopon, D., & Puriwat, W. (2021b). Organizational agility: Key to the success of new product development. *IEEE Transactions on Engineering Management*, *68*(6), 1722–1733. DOI: 10.1109/TEM.2019.2929500

Hossain, M. S., Amin, S. U., Alsulaiman, M., & Muhammad, G. (2019). Applying deep learning for epilepsy seizure detection and brain mapping visualization. [TOMM]. *ACM Transactions on Multimedia Computing Communications and Applications*, *15*(1s), 1–17. DOI: 10.1145/3241056

Houssaini, M. S., Aboutajeddine, A., & Toughrai, I. (2024). Development of a Data-Centric Design Thinking Process for Innovative Care Delivery. *HERD*, *17*(2), 146–165. DOI: 10.1177/19375867231215071 PMID: 38062743

How a Nordic insurance company automated claims processing. (2024, January 22). https://www.ey.com/en_in/financial-services-emeia/how-a-nordic-insurance-company-automated-claims-processing

Howes, E., Boushey, C. J., Kerr, D. A., Tomayko, E. J., & Cluskey, M. (2017). Image-based dietary assessment ability of dietetics students and interns. *Nutrients*, *9*(2), 114. DOI: 10.3390/nu9020114 PMID: 28178196

HPRA. (2014). *Qualification and classification of medical devices and in-vitro diagnostic medical devices (IVDs)*. http://www. hpra.ie/homepage/medical-devices/regulatory-information/classification

Hripcsak, G., & Albers, D. J. (2013). Next-generation phenotyping of electronic health records. *Journal of the American Medical Informatics Association : JAMIA*, *20*(1), 117–121. DOI: 10.1136/amiajnl-2012-001145 PMID: 22955496

https://mcpress.mayoclinic.org/healthy-aging/ai-in-healthcare-the-future-of-patient-care-and-health-management/

https://medinfo.charite.de/en/research/data_ecosystems_and_care_analytics_research_grou/

https://www.psu.edu/news/research/story/nsf-grant-help-researchers-harness-power-big-data-address-health-issues/

https://www.uclahealth.org/sites/default/files/documents/21/2022-uclah-ehealthcare-artificial-intelligence.pdf?f=bb1a7b0d

Huang, H., Gong, T., Ye, N., Wang, R., & Dou, Y. (2017). Private and secured medical data transmission and analysis for wireless sensing healthcare system. *IEEE Transactions on Industrial Informatics*, *13*(3), 1227–1237. DOI: 10.1109/TII.2017.2687618

Huang, J., & Yu, S. (2019). The Role of Artificial Intelligence in Assisting Patients with Disabilities: A Review of Current Applications and Future Directions. *Health Care*, *7*(4), 99. DOI: 10.3390/healthcare7040099

Hu, F., Xie, D., & Shen, S. (2013, August). *On the application of the internet of things in the field of medical and health care. In 2013 IEEE international conference on green computing and communications and IEEE Internet of Things and IEEE cyber, physical and social computing*. IEEE.

Hughes, D. A., Bacigalupe, R., Wang, J., Rühlemann, M. C., Tito, R. Y., Falony, G., Joossens, M., Vieira-Silva, S., Henckaerts, L., Rymenans, L., Verspecht, C., Ring, S., Franke, A., Wade, K. H., Timpson, N. J., & Raes, J. (2020). Genome-wide associations of human gut microbiome variation and implications for causal inference analyses. *Nature Microbiology*, *5*(9), 1079–1087. DOI: 10.1038/s41564-020-0743-8 PMID: 32572223

Hu, J., Zhong, X., Yan, J., Zhou, D., Qin, D., Xiao, X., Zheng, Y., & Liu, Y. (2020). High-throughput sequencing analysis of intestinal flora changes in ESRD and CKD patients. *BMC Nephrology*, *21*(1), 1–11. DOI: 10.1186/s12882-019-1668-4 PMID: 31931722

IBM. (2023). Introduction to IBM App Connect for Healthcare 6.0.1.0. *IBM Documentation.* Retrieved from https://www.ibm.com/docs/en/app-connect/12.0?topic=601-introduction-app-connect-healthcare-6010

IBM. (n.d.). Healthcare technology solutions and services. *IBM.* Retrieved from https://www.ibm.com/industries/healthcare

IBM. (n.d.). Murel, Jacob, Kavlakoglu, Eda. (2024). What is ensemble learning? *IBM Topics*. https://www.ibm.com/think/topics/ensemble-learning

IBM. (n.d.). What is homomorphic encryption? *IBM Topics*. https://www.ibm.com/topics/homomorphic-encryption

Imanian, B., Donaghy, J., Jackson, T., Gummalla, S., Ganesan, B., Baker, R. C., ... & Wan, J. (2022). The power, potential, benefits, and challenges of implementing high-throughput sequencing in food safety systems. *npj Science of Food, 6*(1), 35.

Impact of implementing electronic health records on medication safety at an HIMSS stage 6 hospital: The pharmacist's perspective. (n.d.). PubMed Central (PMC). https://www.ncbi.nlm.nih.gov/pmc/articles/PMC9524548/

Institute for Health Metrics and Evaluation (IHME). (2024). *Global Burden of Disease 2021: Findings from the GBD 2021 Study*. IHME.

Institute of Medicine (US) Committee on Quality of Health Care in America. Crossing the Quality Chasm: A New Health System for the 21st Century. Washington (DC): National Academies Press (US); 2001. Available from: https://www.ncbi.nlm.nih.gov/books/NBK222274/ doi:10.17226/10027

Institute of Medicine. (2000). *To Err is Human: Building a Safer Health System*. The National Academies Press.

Intermountain Healthcare. (2022). AI-Powered Radiology Diagnostics. Retrieved from https://intermountainhealthcare.org/innovation/ai-powered-radiology-diagnostics/

Intermountain Healthcare. (2022). Remote Patient Monitoring Program. Retrieved from https://intermountainhealthcare.org/services/remote-patient-monitoring/

International Association of Privacy Professionals (IAPP). (2020). "GDPR Implementation and Compliance."

International Bank For Reconstruction And Development Program Appraisal Document On A Proposed Loan In The Amount Of Us$400 Million To The Republic Of Indonesia For A National Health Insurance (Jkn) Reforms And Results Program Program-For-Results. (2021). In International Bank For Reconstruction And Development. https://documents1.worldbank.org/curated/en/780101641932861182/pdf/Indonesia-National-Health-Insurance-JKN-Reforms-and-Results-Program.pdf

International Institute for Population Sciences (IIPS) & ICF. (2021). *National Family Health Survey (NFHS-5), 2019-21: India: Volume I*. Mumbai, India: IIPS.

International Institute for Population Sciences (IIPS), National Programme for Health Care of Elderly (NPHCE), Ministry of Health and Family Welfare. (MoHFW), Harvard T. H. Chan School of Public Health (HSPH), & University of Southern California (USC). (2020). *Longitudinal Ageing Study in India (LASI) Wave 1, 2017-18, India report*. International Institute for Population Sciences.

Islam, S. R., Kwak, D., Kabir, M. H., Hossain, M., & Kwak, K. S. (2015). The internet of things for health care: A comprehensive survey. *IEEE Access : Practical Innovations, Open Solutions*, *3*, 678–708. DOI: 10.1109/ACCESS.2015.2437951

Iyawa, G. E., Herselman, M., & Botha, A. (2016). Digital health innovation ecosystems: From systematic literature review to conceptual framework. *Procedia Computer Science*, *100*, 244–252. DOI: 10.1016/j.procs.2016.09.149

Iyer, P., Hounsome, R., Marshak, A., & Baryeh, K. (2021). Circular economy in healthcare: A study of the potential for reuse of medical equipment and supplies. *Resources, Conservation and Recycling*, *167*, 105389.

Jain, A. K., Mao, J., & Mohiuddin, K. M. (1996). Artificial neural networks: A tutorial. *Computer*, *29*(3), 31–44. DOI: 10.1109/2.485891

Jayaraman, P. P., Forkan, A. R. M., Morshed, A., Haghighi, P. D., & Kang, Y. B. (2020). Healthcare 4.0: A review of frontiers in digital health. *Wiley Interdisciplinary Reviews. Data Mining and Knowledge Discovery*, *10*(2), e1350. DOI: 10.1002/widm.1350

Jiang, F., Jiang, Y., Zhi, H., Dong, Y., Li, H., Ma, S., Wang, Y., Dong, Q., Shen, H., & Wang, Y. (2017). Artificial intelligence in healthcare: Past, present and future. *Stroke and Vascular Neurology*, *2*(4), 230–243. DOI: 10.1136/svn-2017-000101 PMID: 29507784

Jin, O. W. (2024). Garden by the bed: Bringing nature and healing to hospital patients. *The Straits Times*. https://www.straitstimes.com/multimedia/graphics/2024/04/horticulture-therapy-khoo-teck-puat-hospital-singapore/index.html?shell

Jin, H., Lee, S., & Ko, H. (2020). Wearable health monitoring systems for patients with chronic conditions: A review. *JMIR mHealth and uHealth*, *8*(1), e14563.

Johnson, D., Deterding, S., Kuhn, K.-A., Staneva, A., Stoyanov, S., & Hides, L. (2016). Gamification for health and wellbeing: A systematic review of the literature. *Internet Interventions : the Application of Information Technology in Mental and Behavioural Health*, *6*, 89–106. DOI: 10.1016/j.invent.2016.10.002 PMID: 30135818

Jones, D. D., Heaton, H. A., Wallerich, T. J., Riekmann, L. A., Handmacher, B. H., & Hatton, R. L. (2023). Wearable Real Time Location Services Technology for Staff Duress in Healthcare. *2023 IEEE 13th International Conference on RFID Technology and Applications (RFID-TA)*, 127–129. DOI: 10.1109/RFID-TA58140.2023.10290330

Jones, T. O., & Sasser, W. E.Jr. (1995). Why Satisfied Customers Defect. *Harvard Business Review*, *73*(6), 88–102. https://hbr.org/1995/11/why-satisfied-customers-defect

Joshi, A., Gaba, A., Thakur, S., & Grover, A. (2021). Need and importance of nutrition informatics in India: A perspective. *Nutrients*, *13*(6), 1836. DOI: 10.3390/nu13061836 PMID: 34072133

Journal of the American Medical Association (JAMA). (2019). "The Impact of Clinical Trials on Healthcare Technology Adoption."

Journey Foods. Accessed on 15th February 2025 from https://www.journeyfoods.io/

Jovy-Klein, F., Stead, S., Salge, T. O., Sander, J., Diehl, A., & Antons, D. (2024). Forecasting the future of smart hospitals: Findings from a real-time delphi study. *BMC Health Services Research*, *24*(1), 1421. DOI: 10.1186/s12913-024-11895-z PMID: 39558347

Juliussen, B. A., Rui, J. P., & Johansen, D. (2023). Algorithms that forget: Machine unlearning and the right to erasure. *Computer Law & Security Report*, *51*, 105885–105885. DOI: 10.1016/j.clsr.2023.105885

Juntunen, J. K., Halme, M., Korsunova, A., & Rajala, R. (2019). Strategies for integrating stakeholders into sustainability innovation: A configurational perspective. *Journal of Product Innovation Management*, *36*(3), 331–355. DOI: 10.1111/jpim.12481

Kalantarian, H., Sideris, C., Mortazavi, B., Alshurafa, N., & Sarrafzadeh, M. (2016). Dynamic computation offloading for low-power wearable health monitoring systems. *IEEE Transactions on Biomedical Engineering*, *64*(3), 621–628. DOI: 10.1109/TBME.2016.2570210 PMID: 28113209

Kamnitsas, K., Ledig, C., Newcombe, V. F., Simpson, J. P., Kane, A. D., Menon, D. K., Rueckert, D., & Glocker, B. (2017). Efficient multi-scale 3D CNN with fully connected CRF for accurate brain lesion segmentation. *Medical Image Analysis*, *36*, 61–78. DOI: 10.1016/j.media.2016.10.004 PMID: 27865153

Kapustina, T. V., Gorshkova, O. V., Kadyrov, R. V., Trankovskaya, L. V., & Khudchenko, A. G. (2024). Patient-Centered healthare as part of medical corporate culture. *SibScript*, *26*(5), 795–806. DOI: 10.21603/sibscript-2024-26-5-795-806

Kataria, S., Sharma, P., Kataria, S., Saharan, M., & Sikka, R. (2024). Real-Time Location Systems: Revolutionizing Porter Services for Improving Patient Care Efficiency. *Cureus*. Advance online publication. DOI: 10.7759/cureus.69922 PMID: 39439611

Kelly, S. D. T., Suryadevara, N., & Mukhopadhyay, S. C. (2013). Towards the Implementation of IoT for Environmental Condition Monitoring in Homes.

Ken, L. (2024). Machine Unlearning in 2024. *Stanford education*. https://ai.stanford.edu/~kzliu/blog/unlearning

Kerz, E., Zanwar, S., Qiao, Y., & Wiechmann, D. (2023). Toward explainable AI (XAI) for mental health detection based on language behavior. *Frontiers in Psychiatry*, *14*, 1219479. DOI: 10.3389/fpsyt.2023.1219479 PMID: 38144474

Khalifa, M., & Albadawy, M. (2024). AI in diagnostic imaging: Revolutionising accuracy and efficiency. *Computer Methods and Programs in Biomedicine Update*, *5*, 100146. Advance online publication. DOI: 10.1016/j.cmpbup.2024.100146

Khan, M. M., & Alkhathami, M. (2024). Anomaly detection in IoT-based healthcare: Machine learning for enhanced security. *Scientific Reports*, *14*(1), 5872. DOI: 10.1038/s41598-024-56126-x PMID: 38467709

Khan, R., Adi, E., & Hussain, O. (2021). AI-based audit of fuzzy front end innovation using ISO56002. *Managerial Auditing Journal*, *36*(4), 564–590. DOI: 10.1108/MAJ-03-2020-2588

Kharrazi, H., Chisholm, R., VanNasdale, D., & Thompson, B. (2012). Mobile personal health records: An evaluation of features and functionality. *International Journal of Medical Informatics*, *81*(9), 579–593. DOI: 10.1016/j.ijmedinf.2012.04.007 PMID: 22809779

Khurana, A., & Rosenthal, S. R. (1997). Integrating the fuzzy front end of new product development. *Sloan Management Review*, *38*, 19.

Kim, J., & Wilemon, D. (2002a). Strategic issues in managing innovation's fuzzy front-end. *European Journal of Innovation Management*, *5*(1), 27–39. DOI: 10.1108/14601060210415153

Kim, J., & Wilemon, D. (2002b). Focusing the fuzzy front–end in new product development. *R & D Management*, *32*(4), 269–279. DOI: 10.1111/1467-9310.00259

Kim, M. H., & Park, Y. S. (2024). Use of a Real-Time Locating System in Infection Control. *Infection & Chemotherapy*, *56*(4), e45. DOI: 10.3947/ic.2024.0043 PMID: 39431344

Kimura, A., & Nadege, M. T. (2020, October). RoI Editing Tool Using AI for Radiotherapy Simulation. In *2020 IEEE Nuclear Science Symposium and Medical Imaging Conference (NSS/MIC)* (pp. 1-3). IEEE. DOI: 10.1109/NSS/MIC42677.2020.9508040

Kiran, T., & O'Brien, P. (2021). Challenge of addressing social determinants of health in primary care. *Canadian Family Physician Médecin de Famille Canadien*, *67*(1), 35–41. PMID: 33483395

Kirk, D., Kok, E., Tufano, M., Tekinerdogan, B., Feskens, E. J., & Camps, G. (2022). Machine learning in nutrition research. *Advances in Nutrition*, *13*(6), 2573–2589. DOI: 10.1093/advances/nmac103 PMID: 36166846

Kiyasseh, D., Zhu, T., & Clifton, D. (2020). The promise of clinical decision support systems targetting low-resource settings. *IEEE Reviews in Biomedical Engineering*, *15*, 354–371. DOI: 10.1109/RBME.2020.3017868 PMID: 32813662

Knevel, R., & Liao, K. P. (2022). From real-world electronic health record data to real-world results using artificial intelligence. *Annals of the Rheumatic Diseases*, *2023*(82), 306–311. PMID: 36150748

Koen, P., Ajamian, G., Burkart, R., Clamen, A., Davidson, J., D'Amore, R., Elkins, C., Herald, K., Incorvia, M., Johnson, A., Karol, R., Seibert, R., Slavejkov, A., & Wagner, K. (2001). Providing clarity and a common language to the "fuzzy front end". *Research Technology Management*, *44*(2), 46–55. DOI: 10.1080/08956308.2001.11671418

Kohn, L. T., Corrigan, J. M., & Donaldson, M. S. (Eds.). (2000). *(Committee on Quality of Health Care in America, Institute of Medicine). To Err Is Human: Building a Safer Health System*. National Academies Press.

Kononenko, I. (2001). Machine learning for medical diagnosis: History, state of the art and perspective. *Artificial Intelligence in Medicine*, *23*(1), 89–109. DOI: 10.1016/S0933-3657(01)00077-X PMID: 11470218

Konstantakopoulos, F. S., Georga, E. I., & Fotiadis, D. I. (2023). A review of image-based food recognition and volume estimation artificial intelligence systems. *IEEE Reviews in Biomedical Engineering*, *17*, 136–152. DOI: 10.1109/RBME.2023.3283149 PMID: 37276096

Kornish, L. J., & Jones, S. M. (2021). Raw Iideas in the fuzzy front end: Verbosity increases perceived creativity. *Marketing Science*, *40*(6), 1106–1122. DOI: 10.1287/mksc.2021.1300

Kortesniemi, M., Noerman, S., Kårlund, A., Raita, J., Meuronen, T., Koistinen, V., Landberg, R., & Hanhineva, K. (2023). Nutritional metabolomics: Recent developments and future needs. *Current Opinion in Chemical Biology*, *77*, 102400. DOI: 10.1016/j.cbpa.2023.102400 PMID: 37804582

Krick, T., Huter, K., Domhoff, D., Schmidt, A., Rothgang, H., & Wolf-Ostermann, K. (2020). Digital healthcare for elderly: An analysis of the use of telemedicine by elderly patients with chronic diseases. The Lancet Digital Health, 2(6), e264-e273. less dangerously. Med J Aust 2006;184(Suppl 10):

Kruk, M. E., Ling, E. J., Bitton, A., Cammett, M., Cavanaugh, K., Chopra, M., el-Jardali, F., Macauley, R. J., Muraguri, M. K., Konuma, S., Marten, R., Martineau, F., Myers, M., Rasanathan, K., Ruelas, E., Soucat, A., Sugihantono, A., & Warnken, H. (2017). Building resilient health systems: A proposal for a resilience index. *BMJ (Clinical Research Ed.)*, •••, 357. DOI: 10.1136/bmj.j2323 PMID: 28536191

Kruse, C. S., Frederick, B., Jacobson, T., & Monticone, D. K. (2017). Cybersecurity in healthcare: A systematic review of modern threats and trends. *Technology and Health Care*, *25*(1), 1–10. DOI: 10.3233/THC-161263 PMID: 27689562

Kruse, C. S., Kothman, K., Anerobi, K., & Abanaka, L. (2016). Adoption factors of the electronic health record: A systematic review. *JMIR Medical Informatics*, *4*(2), e19. DOI: 10.2196/medinform.5525 PMID: 27251559

Kuhn, T. S. (1997). The structure of scientific revolutions (Vol. 962). University of Chicago press Chicago.

Kulkarni, P. (2024, June 7). How OCR Is Transforming The Insurance Industry. Hyperverge. Retrieved August 4, 2024, from https://hyperverge.co/blog/ocr-insurance/

Kumar, A., & Singh, R. (2021). Innovations in healthcare: A systematic review. *Health Policy and Technology*, *10*(2), 100–110.

Kumar, C., & Mann, M. (2009). Bioinformatics analysis of mass spectrometry-based proteomics data sets. *FEBS Letters*, *583*(11), 1703–1712. DOI: 10.1016/j.febslet.2009.03.035 PMID: 19306877

Kuo, T. T., Kim, H. E., & Ohno-Machado, L. (2017). Blockchain distributed ledger technologies for biomedical and health care applications. *Journal of the American Medical Informatics Association : JAMIA*, *24*(6), 1211–1220. DOI: 10.1093/jamia/ocx068 PMID: 29016974

Kutvonen, A., & Torkkeli, M. T. (2010). Opening the fuzzy front-end of new product development: A synthesis of two theories. *International Journal of Business Excellence*, *3*(4), 415. DOI: 10.1504/IJBEX.2010.035443

Kuziemsky, C. E., Borycki, E. M., Presseau, J., Bevextinction, J., Chouinard, M. C., Cordeiro, M., & Shaw, N. T. (2019). An interdisciplinary review of current trends in health information system interoperability. *Applied Clinical Informatics*, *10*(04), 730–750.

Lahat, A., Sharif, K., Zoabi, N., Shneor Patt, Y., Sharif, Y., Fisher, L., Shani, U., Arow, M., Levin, R., & Klang, E. (2024). Assessing generative pretrained transformers (GPT) in clinical decision-making: Comparative analysis of GPT-3.5 and GPT-4. *Journal of Medical Internet Research, 26*, e54571. DOI: 10.2196/54571 PMID: 38935937

Lapão, L., & Viegas, S. (2024a). Leveraging digital platforms to improve Public Health in hospital smart buildings. *European Journal of Public Health, 34*(Supplement_3), ckae144.492. DOI: 10.1093/eurpub/ckae144.492

Lapointe, L., Ramaprasad, J., & Vedel, I. (2014). Creating health awareness: A social media enabled collaboration. *Health and Technology, 4*(1), 43–57. DOI: 10.1007/s12553-013-0068-1

Larsen, A. S. A., Karlsen, A. T., Lund, J.-Å., & Andersen, B. S. (2022). Assessment of early warning signs in hospital projects' front-end phase. *International Journal of Managing Projects in Business, 15*(2), 299–323. DOI: 10.1108/IJMPB-06-2021-0156

Latif, J., Xiao, C., Imran, A., & Tu, S. (2019, January). Medical imaging using machine learning and deep learning algorithms: a review. In *2019 2nd International conference on computing, mathematics and engineering technologies (iCoMET)* (pp. 1-5). IEEE. DOI: 10.1109/ICOMET.2019.8673502

Lee, C., Gupta, M., & Hassan, R. (2024). Security and privacy challenges in health information systems: A systematic review. *Computers, 13*(2), 41. DOI: 10.3390/computers13020041

Lee, T. H., & McGlynn, E. A. (2016). A framework for increasing trust between patients and the organizations that care for them. *Journal of the American Medical Association, 315*(12), 1211–1212. PMID: 30676628

Lehman, C. D., Wellman, R. D., Buist, D. S., Kerlikowske, K., Tosteson, A. N., & Miglioretti, D. L.Breast Cancer Surveillance Consortium. (2015). Diagnostic accuracy of digital screening mammography with and without computer-aided detection. *JAMA Internal Medicine, 175*(11), 1828–1837. DOI: 10.1001/jamainternmed.2015.5231 PMID: 26414882

Lei, C. (2023). Nanotechnology: Paving the way for Advanced Healthcare and beyond. *Nano TransMed, 2*(4), 100023. DOI: 10.1016/j.ntm.2023.100023

Lewis, Z. H.. (2020). Wearable Technology in Chronic Disease Management: Narrative Review. *Journal of Medical Internet Research.*

Li, L., & Shao, X. Yu, Z. (2024). A Slicing-Free Perspective to Sufficient Dimension Reduction: Selective Review and Recent Developments. *International statistical review.* Volume 92 (3), Pp. 355-382. ISSN: 0306-7734. DOI: DOI: 10.1111/insr.12565

Li, J., & Carayon, P. (2021). Health Care 4.0: A Vision for Smart and Connected Health Care. *IISE Transactions on Healthcare Systems Engineering*, *11*(3), 171–180. DOI: 10.1080/24725579.2021.1884627 PMID: 34497970

Li, L., Novillo-Ortiz, D., Azzopardi-Muscat, N., & Kostkova, P. (2021). Digital data sources and their impact on people's health: A systematic review of systematic reviews. *Frontiers in Public Health*, *9*, 645260. DOI: 10.3389/fpubh.2021.645260 PMID: 34026711

Lin, C. C., Huang, A. Y., & Yang, S. J. (2023). A review of ai-driven conversational chatbots implementation methodologies and challenges (1999–2022). *Sustainability (Basel)*, *15*(5), 4012. DOI: 10.3390/su15054012

Liu, J., Li, J., Wang, H., & Yan, J. (2020). Application of deep learning in genomics. *Science China. Life Sciences*, *63*(12), 1860–1878. DOI: 10.1007/s11427-020-1804-5 PMID: 33051704

Lo, F. P. W., Qiu, J., Jobarteh, M. L., Sun, Y., Wang, Z., Jiang, S., & Lo, B. (2024). AI-enabled wearable cameras for assisting dietary assessment in African populations. *npj. Digital Medicine*, *7*(1), 1–16. PMID: 38172429

Longvah, T., Ananthan, R., Bhaskarachary, K., & Venkaiah, K. (2017). *Indian Food Composition Tables 2017, National Institute of Nutrition, Indian Council of Medical Research.* Telangana, India.

Loveys, K., Prina, M., Axford, C., Domènec, Ò. R., Weng, W., Broadbent, E., Pujari, S., Jang, H., Han, Z. A., & Thiyagarajan, J. A. (2022). Artificial intelligence for older people receiving long-term care: A systematic review of acceptability and effectiveness studies. *The Lancet. Healthy Longevity*, *3*(4), e286–e297. DOI: 10.1016/S2666-7568(22)00034-4 PMID: 35515814

Lyngaas, S. (2021, March 10). Universal health services reports $67 million in losses after apparent ransomware attack. CyberScoop. https://cyberscoop.com/universal-health-services-ransomware-cost-ryuk/

Macdiarmid, J., & Blundell, J. (1998). Assessing dietary intake: Who, what and why of under-reporting. *Nutrition Research Reviews*, *11*(2), 231–253. DOI: 10.1079/NRR19980017 PMID: 19094249

Machine Learning Workflow. (n.d.). AI Platform documentation. *Google Cloud.* https://cloud.google.com/ai-platform/docs/ml-solutions-overview

Magnusson, P. R. (2009). Exploring the contributions of involving ordinary users in ideation of technology-based services. *Journal of Product Innovation Management, 26*(5), 578–593. DOI: 10.1111/j.1540-5885.2009.00684.x

Maguire, M. (2001). Methods to support human-centered design. *International Journal of Human-Computer Studies, 55*(4), 587–634. DOI: 10.1006/ijhc.2001.0503

Mahendradhata, Y., Trisnantoro, L., Listyadewi, S., Soewondo, P., Marthias, T., Harimurti, P., Prawira, J., & Hort, K. (2017). The Republic of Indonesia Health System Review. Health Systems in Transition, 7–7(1). https://iris.who.int/bitstream/handle/10665/254716/9789290225164-eng.pdf

Ma, K. S.-K. (2023). Extended Reality-Augmented Technologies in Healthcare. In Keikhosrokiani, P. (Ed.), (pp. 23–39). Advances in Marketing, Customer Relationship Management, and E-Services. IGI Global., DOI: 10.4018/978-1-6684-7029-9.ch002

Malathi, K., Shruthi, S. N., Madhumitha, N., Sreelakshmi, S., Sathya, U., & Sangeetha, P. M. (2024). Medical Data Integration and Interoperability through Remote Monitoring of Healthcare Devices. [JoWUA]. *Journal of Wireless Mobile Networks, Ubiquitous Computing and Dependable Applications, 15*(2), 60–72. DOI: 10.58346/JOWUA.2024.I2.005

Malhi, K., Mukhopadhyay, S. C., Schnepper, J., Haefke, M., & Ewald, H. (2012). A ZigBee-based wearable physiological parameters monitoring system. *IEEE Sensors Journal, 12*(3), 423–430. DOI: 10.1109/JSEN.2010.2091719

Malik, A. N., Afridi, A., & Rathore, F. A. (2024). Mobile health (mHealth) applications for stroke rehabilitation: A mini review. *JPMA. The Journal of the Pakistan Medical Association, 74*(9), 1723–1726. DOI: 10.47391/JPMA.24-74 PMID: 39279090

Manaktala, S., & Claypool, S. R. (2016). Evaluating the impact of a computerized surveillance algorithm and decision support system on sepsis mortality. *Journal of the American Medical Informatics Association : JAMIA, 24*(1), 88–95. DOI: 10.1093/jamia/ocw056 PMID: 27225197

Maresova, P. (2023). Impact of Regulatory Changes on Innovations in the Medical Device Industry Comment on “Clinical Decision Support and New Regulatory Frameworks for Medical Devices: Are We Ready for It? - A Viewpoint Paper.”. *International Journal of Health Policy and Management, 12*(1), 7262–7262. DOI: 10.34172/ijhpm.2022.7262 PMID: 35942961

Marvin, G., Hellen, N., & Nakatumba-Nabende, J. (2023, February). Research Paradigms for Health Equity in Intelligent Mobile Healthcare Technologies: A Critical Review. In *International Conference on Intelligent Sustainable Systems* (pp. 365-375). Singapore: Springer Nature Singapore. DOI: 10.1007/978-981-99-1726-6_28

Massey, A. P., Montoya-Weiss, M. M., & O'Driscoll, T. M. (2002). Performance-centered design of knowledge-intensive processes. *Journal of Management Information Systems, 18*(4), 37–58. DOI: 10.1080/07421222.2002.11045700

Matheny, M. S., Israni, T. M., & Ahmed, M.. (2022). *Artificial Intelligence in Health Care: The Hope, the Hype, the Promise, the Peril.* National Academy of Medicine., Available from https://nap.nationalacademies.org/read/27111/chapter/3

Mayo Clinic. (2022). Mayo Clinic Implements Smart Hospital Beds to Improve Patient Care. Retrieved from https://www.mayoclinic.org/about-mayo-clinic/news/smart-hospital-beds

Ma, Z., & Tavares, J. M. R. (2015). A novel approach to segment skin lesions in dermoscopic images based on a deformable model. *IEEE Journal of Biomedical and Health Informatics, 20*(2), 615–623. DOI: 10.1109/JBHI.2015.2390032 PMID: 25585429

McCulloch, W. S., & Pitts, W. (1943). A logical calculus of the ideas immanent in nervous activity. *The Bulletin of Mathematical Biophysics, 5*(4), 115–133. DOI: 10.1007/BF02478259

McGinnis, J. M., Williams-Russo, P., & Knickman, J. R. (2002). The case for more active policy attention to health promotion. *Health Affairs, 21*(2), 78–93. DOI: 10.1377/hlthaff.21.2.78 PMID: 11900188

McGonigal, J. (2012). The game that can give you 10 extra years of life. *TED*. Retrieved from https://www.ted.com/talks/jane_mcgonigal_the_game_that_can_give_you_10_extra_years_of_life

McKay, A. G. N., Brand, D., Botes, M., Cengiz, N., & Swart, M. (2024). The regulation of health data sharing in Africa: A comparative study. *Journal of Law and the Biosciences, 11*(1), lsad035. Advance online publication. DOI: 10.1093/jlb/lsad035 PMID: 38259628

McKinney, S. M.. (2020). International evaluation of an AI system for breast cancer screening. *Lancet.*

McKinsey & Company. (2018). "Artificial Intelligence: The next digital frontier?"

McKinsey & Company. (2020). "The state of AI in 2020."

Meena, S., Rathore, M., Kumawat, P., & Singh, A. (2020). Challenges Faced by ASHAs during their Field Works: A Cross Sectional Observational Study in Rural Area of Jaipur, Rajasthan. *International Journal of Medicine and Public Health, 10*(3), 97–99. DOI: 10.5530/ijmedph.2020.3.20

Mehta, J. K. (2022). Smart Healthcare System Using Data Analysis. *International Journal for Research in Applied Science and Engineering Technology, 10*(1), 1253–1257. DOI: 10.22214/ijraset.2022.40020

Meka, S. C., Achan, S., & Pettit, R. G. (2024). Real-Time Embedded Monitoring Technologies in Modern Healthcare Systems: A Survey. *2024 IEEE 27th International Symposium on Real-Time Distributed Computing (ISORC)*, 1–6. DOI: 10.1109/ISORC61049.2024.10551333

Mendes, D., Lopes, M., Parreira, P., & Fonseca, C. (2017). Deep learning and IoT to assist multimorbidity home based healthcare.

Mendes, G. H. S., & Toledo, J. C. (2011). The fuzzy front end of new product development for Brazilian technology-based companies in the medical device industry: A causal model. *Brazilian Journal of Operations & Production Management, 8*(1), 83–102. DOI: 10.4322/bjopm.2011.005

Meskó, B., Drobni, Z., Bényei, É., Gergely, B., & Győrffy, Z. (2017). Digital health is a cultural transformation of traditional healthcare. *mHealth, 3*, 3. DOI: 10.21037/mhealth.2017.08.07 PMID: 29184890

Mettler, M. (2016). Blockchain technology in healthcare: The revolution starts here. *Journal of Medical Internet Research, 18*(11), e324.

Meyer, S. (2020). The Impact of Artificial Intelligence on Rehabilitation: Opportunities and Challenges. *Frontiers in Rehabilitation Sciences, 1*, 563547. Advance online publication. DOI: 10.3389/fresc.2020.563547

Mihaljevic, T. (2022). *Sustainability & Global Citizenship Report 2022.*

Miller, F. A., & Lehoux, P. (2020). The innovation impacts of public procurement offices: The case of healthcare procurement. *Research Policy, 49*(7), 104075. DOI: 10.1016/j.respol.2020.104075

Millson, M. R., & Wilemon, D. (2010). The impact of changing markets and competition on the NPD speed/market success relationship. *International Journal of Innovation Management, 14*(05), 841–870. DOI: 10.1142/S1363919610002908

Ministry of Electronics and Information Technology (MeitY). (2019). "The Personal Data Protection Bill, 2019."

Ministry of Health and Family Welfare (MoHFW). Government of India, UNICEF, & Population Council. (2019). *Comprehensive National Nutrition Survey (CNNS) National Report.* New Delhi, India. Ministry of Women and Child Development, Government of India. A Complete Guide- Poshan Tracker. Retrieved January 17, 2025, from https://www.poshantracker.in/pdf/Resources/ACompleteGuide-PoshanTracker.pdf

Ministry of law and justice (legislative department). (2023). The Digital Personal Data Protection Act. The Gazette of India. *MeitY*. https://www.meity.gov.in/writereaddata/files/Digital%20Personal%20Data%20Protection%20Act%202023.pdf

Mishra, N., Lin, C. C., & Chang, H. T. (2014). Cognitive inference device for activity supervision in the elderly. *TheScientificWorldJournal*, *2014*(1), 125618. DOI: 10.1155/2014/125618 PMID: 25405211

Mittal, P. (2020). Big data and analytics: A data management perspective in public administration. *International Journal of Big Data Management*, *1*(2), 152–165. DOI: 10.1504/IJBDM.2020.112415

Mobile, J. K. N. Health Insurance Services in Your Hand - Observatory of Public Sector Innovation. (2019, February 5). Observatory of Public Sector Innovation. https://oecd-opsi.org/innovations/mobile-jkn-health-insurance-services-in-your-hand/

Mobile, J. K. N. (2017, June 15). App Store. https://apps.apple.com/sg/app/JKN%20-%20mobile/id1237601115

Moenaert, R. K., De Meyer, A., Souder, W. E., & Deschoolmeester, D. (1995). R&D/marketing communication during the fuzzy front-end. *IEEE Transactions on Engineering Management*, *42*(3), 243–258. DOI: 10.1109/17.403743

Mo, H., Zhong, R., & Ma, F. (2024). Chinese expert consensus on an innovative patient-centered approach to diagnosis and treatment of cancer. *Cancer Innovation*, *3*(5), e137. Advance online publication. DOI: 10.1002/cai2.137 PMID: 39081932

Morgan, L. (n.d.). M-TIBA DIGITAL HEALTH PLATFORM. In PharmAccess. https://www.ilo.org/sites/default/files/wcmsp5/groups/public/@ed_emp/documents/publication/wcms_749427.pdf

M-TIBA is truly leapfrogging healthcare in Kenya. (n.d.). PharmAccess. https://www.pharmaccess.org/update/M-Tiba-is-truly-leapfrogging-healthcare-in-kenya/#:~:text=M%2DTIBA%2C%20whereby%20the%20M,healthcare%20at%20very%20low%20costs

Muller, N., Emmrich, P., Rajemison, E., De Neve, J., Bärnighausen, T., Knauss, S., & Emmrich, J. (2019). A Mobile Health Wallet for Pregnancy-Related Health Care in Madagascar: Mixed-Methods Study on Opportunities and Challenges. *JMIR mHealth and uHealth*, *7*(3), e11420. https://mhealth.jmir.org/2019/3/e11420. DOI: 10.2196/11420 PMID: 30457972

Murdoch, B. (2021). Privacy and artificial intelligence: Challenges for protecting health information in a new era. *BMC Medical Ethics*, *22*(1), 122. DOI: 10.1186/s12910-021-00687-3 PMID: 34525993

Murdoch, T. B., & Detsky, A. S. (2013). The inevitable application of big data to health care. *Journal of the American Medical Association*, *309*(13), 1351–1352. DOI: 10.1001/jama.2013.393 PMID: 23549579

Murphy, S. A., & Kumar, V. (1997). The front end of new product development: A Canadian survey. *R & D Management*, *27*(1), 5–15. DOI: 10.1111/1467-9310.00038

MyFitnessPal. Accessed on January 10, 2025 from https://www.myfitnesspal.com/

MySugr. (n.d.). Rewards in diabetes management. Retrieved from https://www.mysugr.com

Nahavandi, S. (2019). Industry 5.0 - A human-centric solution. *Sustainability (Basel)*, *11*(16), 4371. DOI: 10.3390/su11164371

Naik, K., Goyal, R. K., Foschini, L., Chak, C. W., Thielscher, C., Zhu, H., Lu, J., Lehár, J., Pacanoswki, M. A., Terranova, N., Mehta, N., Korsbo, N., Fakhouri, T., Liu, Q., & Gobburu, J. (2024). Current status and future directions: The application of artificial intelligence/machine learning for precision medicine. *Clinical Pharmacology and Therapeutics*, *115*(4), 673–686. DOI: 10.1002/cpt.3152 PMID: 38103204

Nanji, K. C., Slight, S. P., Seger, D. L., Cho, I., Fiskio, J. M., Redden, L. M., Volk, L. A., & Bates, D. W. (2014). Overrides of medication-related clinical decision support alerts in outpatients. *Journal of the American Medical Informatics Association : JAMIA*, *21*(3), 487–491. DOI: 10.1136/amiajnl-2013-001813 PMID: 24166725

National Academies of Sciences. (2018). "The Integration of the Humanities and Arts with Sciences, Engineering, and Medicine in Higher Education: Branches from the Same Tree."

National Artificial Intelligence Initiative. Strategy Documents. Accessed August 22,2023. https://www.ai.gov/strategy-documents

National Institute of Nutrition (NIN). (2017). Diet and nutritional status of urban population in India and prevalence of obesity, hypertension, diabetes and hyperlipidemia in urban men and women - A brief *NNMB urban nutrition report. Technical Report No. 27.* Retrieved January 17, 2025, from https://www.nin.res.in/downloads/NNMB%20Urban%20Nutrition%20Report%20-Brief%20%20%20report.pdf

Nayak, S. (2024). Smart Hospitals: Integrating AI for Enhanced Patient Outcomes. *Journal of Electrical Systems, 20*(10s), 1812–1819. DOI: 10.52783/jes.5446

Ndwabe, H., Basu, A., & Mohammed, J. (2023). Post pandemic analysis on comprehensive utilization of telehealth and telemedicine. Clinical eHealth, 7, 5–14. DOI: 10.1016/j.ceh.2023.12.002

Neighbors, H. W., Jackson, J. S., Campbell, L., & Williams, D. (1989). The influence of racial factors on psychiatric diagnosis: A review and suggestions for research. *Community Mental Health Journal, 25*(4), 301–311. DOI: 10.1007/BF00755677 PMID: 2697490

Neravetla, A. R., Nomula, V. K., Mohammed, A. S., & Dhanasekaran, S. (2024). Implementing AI-driven Diagnostic Decision Support Systems for Smart Healthcare. *2024 15th International Conference on Computing Communication and Networking Technologies (ICCCNT)*, 1–6. DOI: 10.1109/ICCCNT61001.2024.10725323

Neukam, M. N. (2017). Managing the fuzzy front-end in multicultural teams. *European Journal of Innovation Management, 20*(4), 578–598. DOI: 10.1108/EJIM-11-2016-0112

Nguyen, T. L. H. (2023). Patient satisfaction. International Healthcare Review (Online). DOI: 10.56226/55

NHS Digital. (2023). Cybersecurity incidents in healthcare: Analysis and recommendations.

NHS England. (n.d.). Digital Technology Assessment Criteria (DTAC). *Transformation Directorate.*https://transform.england.nhs.uk/key-tools-and-info/digital-technology-assessment-criteria-dtac/

Norman, D. A. (2013). *The design of everyday things: Revised and expanded edition.* Basic Books.

North, J. C., Jordan, K. C., Metos, J., & Hurdle, J. F. (2015). Nutrition informatics applications in clinical practice: A systematic review. AMIA Annual Symposium Proceedings, 963–972. https://www.ncbi.nlm.nih.gov/pmc/articles/PMC4765562/

Ntuitive. Accessed on January 10th 2025 from https://www.ntuitive.in/

Nunes, T., da Cunha, P. R., de Abreu, J. M., Duarte, J., & Corte-Real, A. (2024). Non-Fungible Tokens (NFTs) in Healthcare: A Systematic Review. *International Journal of Environmental Research and Public Health*, *21*(8), 965. DOI: 10.3390/ijerph21080965 PMID: 39200576

Nutri, A. I. D. E. Accessed on January 10th 2025 from https://wupperinst.org/en/p/wi/p/s/pd/2292

Nutrify India Now 2.0. Accessed on January 10th 2025 from https://nutrifyindianow.in/

Nutrigenomix. Accessed on January 10th 2025 from https://nutrigenomix.com/

Nutrinohealth. Accessed on January 15th 2025 from https://www.nutrinohealth.com/about/

Nutrisense. Accessed on January 15th 2025 from https://www.nutrisense.io/nutritionist#specialties

Nwoke, J. (2024). Healthcare Data Analytics and Predictive Modelling: Enhancing Outcomes in Resource Allocation, Disease Prevalence and High-Risk Populations. *International Journal of Health Sciences*, *7*(7), 1–35. DOI: 10.47941/ijhs.2245

Nyström, M. E., Karltun, J., Keller, C., & Andersson Gäre, B. (2018). Collaborative and partnership research for improvement of health and social services: Researcher's experiences from 20 projects. *Health Research Policy and Systems*, *16*(1), 1–17. DOI: 10.1186/s12961-018-0322-0 PMID: 29843735

O'Brien, K. (2020). Innovation types and the search for new ideas at the fuzzy front end: Where to look and how often? *Journal of Business Research*, *107*, 13–24. DOI: 10.1016/j.jbusres.2019.09.007

Obermeyer, Z., Powers, B., Vogeli, C., & Mullainathan, S. (2019). Dissecting racial bias in an algorithm used to manage the health of populations. *Science*, *366*(6464), 447–453. DOI: 10.1126/science.aax2342 PMID: 31649194

Odirichukwu, J. C., Eze, E. O., Eze, V. C., Eze, E. I., Njoku, O. A., Chika-Ugada, P. K., ... & Nwoke, J. C. Internet of Things (IoT) Based Patient Information and Heart Beat Monitoring System for Health Information System.

Office of the Registrar General & Census Commissioner. India. (2020). Sample Registration System (SRS)-Statistical Report 2020. India, 2022. Accessed from https://censusindia.gov.in/nada/index.php/catalog/44376

Onkundi, C. (2023, August 4). M-TIBA: Top 25 Most Customer-Obsessed Brands Impacting Lives in 2023. Simplify Your Health Insurance Journey. https://mtiba.com/m-tiba-top-25-most-customer-obsessed-brands-impacting-lives-in-2023/#:~:text=With%20over%204.7%20million%20registered,in%20the%20nation's%20health%20sector

Open, A. I. (2024). ChatGPT (Aug 2024 version) [Large language model]. Retrieved from https://chat.openai.com

Ozer, M. E., Sarica, P. O., & Arga, K. Y. (2020). New machine learning applications to accelerate personalized medicine in breast cancer: Rise of the support vector machines. *OMICS: A Journal of Integrative Biology*, *24*(5), 241–246. DOI: 10.1089/omi.2020.0001 PMID: 32228365

Palinkas, L. A., Aarons, G. A., Horwitz, S., Chamberlain, P., Hurlburt, M., & Landsverk, J. (2011). Mixed method designs in implementation research. *Administration and Policy in Mental Health*, *38*(1), 44–53. DOI: 10.1007/s10488-010-0314-z PMID: 20967495

Parida, V., Patel, P. C., Frishammar, J., & Wincent, J. (2017). Managing the front-end phase of process innovation under conditions of high uncertainty. *Quality & Quantity*, *51*(5), 1983–2000. DOI: 10.1007/s11135-016-0376-4

Park, D., Han, J., & Childs, P. R. N. (2021). 266 Fuzzy front-end studies: Current state and future directions for new product development. *Research in Engineering Design*, *32*(3), 377–409. DOI: 10.1007/s00163-021-00365-w

Park, K. W., Mirian, M. S., & McKeown, M. J. (2024). Artificial intelligence-based video monitoring of movement disorders in the elderly: A review on current and future landscapes. *Singapore Medical Journal*, *65*(3), 141–149. DOI: 10.4103/singaporemedj.SMJ-2023-189 PMID: 38527298

Park, T., Gu, P., Kim, C.-H., Kim, K. T., Chung, K. J., Kim, T. B., Jung, H., Yoon, S. J., & Oh, J. K. (2023). Artificial intelligence in urologic oncology: The actual clinical practice results of IBM Watson for Oncology in South Korea. *Prostate International*, *11*(4), 218–221. DOI: 10.1016/j.prnil.2023.09.001 PMID: 38196551

Partnership on AI. (2020). "About Us."

Parveen, N., Maimani, K., Kamal, N., & Malik, S. A. (2018). The impact of leadership and culture on implementation of total quality management in the healthcare sector of Pakistan. *Total Quality Management & Business Excellence*, *29*(3-4), 366–390.

Patel, R., Huang, J., Hsueh, L., Gopalan, A., Millman, A., Franklin, I., & Reed, M. (2024). Telemedicine's Impact on Diabetes Care during the COVID-19 Pandemic: A Cohort Study in a Large Integrated Healthcare System. medRxiv (Cold Spring Harbor Laboratory). DOI: 10.1101/2024.02.25.24303335

Patel, A. U., Gu, Q., Esper, R., Maeser, D., & Maeser, N. (2024). The Crucial Role of Interdisciplinary Conferences in Advancing Explainable AI in Healthcare. *BioMedInformatics*, *4*(2), 1363–1383. DOI: 10.3390/biomedinformatics4020075

Paul, M., Maglaras, L., Ferrag, M. A., & Almomani, I. (2023). Digitization of healthcare sector: A study on privacy and security concerns. *ICT Express*, *9*(4), 571–588. DOI: 10.1016/j.icte.2023.02.007

Peh, A. C. (2024). The Evolution of Internet of Things (IoT) in Global Healthcare. *International Journal of Innovative Science and Research Technology (IJISRT)*, 659–666. DOI: 10.38124/ijisrt/IJISRT24SEP294

Pereno, A., & Eriksson, D. (2020). A multi-stakeholder perspective on sustainable healthcare: From 2030 onwards. *Futures*, *122*, 102605. DOI: 10.1016/j.futures.2020.102605 PMID: 32834076

Perry, Y.. (2020). How algorithms can increase racial disparities in kidney care. *The New England Journal of Medicine*, *382*(24), 2379–2381.

Picó, C., Serra, F., Rodríguez, A. M., Keijer, J., & Palou, A. (2019). Biomarkers of nutrition and health: New tools for new approaches. *Nutrients*, *11*(5), 1092. DOI: 10.3390/nu11051092 PMID: 31100942

Pittenger, A. L., Westberg, S., Rowan, M., & Schweiss, S. (2019). An interprofessional simulation-based learning activity for health professions students. *American Journal of Pharmaceutical Education*, *83*(5).

Plevris, V., & Papazafeiropoulos, G. (2024). AI in Structural Health Monitoring for Infrastructure Maintenance and Safety. *Infrastructures*, *9*(12), 225. DOI: 10.3390/infrastructures9120225

Pourbafrani, M., Karimipour, H., & Dehghantanha, A. (2022). Challenges and solutions for the Internet of Medical Things: A systematic review. *Internet of Things : Engineering Cyber Physical Human Systems*, *17*, 100462.

Prabhod, K. J. (2022). The Role of Machine Learning in Genomic Medicine: Advancements in Disease Prediction and Treatment. *Journal of Deep Learning in Genomic Data Analysis*, *2*(1), 1–52.

Pradhan, A., Mishra, D., Das, K., Panda, G., Kumar, S., & Zymbler, M. (2021). On the classification of MR images using "ELM-SSA" coated hybrid model. *Mathematics*, *9*(17), 2095. DOI: 10.3390/math9172095

Pramanik, M. I., Lau, R. Y., Hossain, M. S., Rahoman, M. M., Debnath, S. K., Rashed, M. G., & Uddin, M. Z. (2021). Privacy preserving big data analytics: A critical analysis of state- of-the-art. *Wiley Interdisciplinary Reviews. Data Mining and Knowledge Discovery*, *11*(1), e1387. DOI: 10.1002/widm.1387

Project InnerEye – Democratizing Medical Imaging AI. (n.d.), *Microsoft Research*. https://www.microsoft.com/en-us/research/project/medical-image-analysis/

Prosperi, M., Min, J. S., Bian, J., & Modave, F. (2018). Big data hurdles in precision medicine and precision public health. *BMC Medical Informatics and Decision Making*, *18*(1), 1–15. DOI: 10.1186/s12911-018-0719-2 PMID: 30594159

ProtonsHub. (n.d.). Emerging Trends in Artificial Intelligence and Machine Learning: The Future of IT. *ProtonsHub Blog*, https://www.protonshub.com/blogs/the-future-of-it

Psychology Today. (2018, March). The impact of gamification on mental health. *Psychology Today*. Retrieved from https://www.psychologytoday.com/us/blog/mindful-anger/201803/the-impact-gamification-mental-health

Radanovic, I., & Likic, R. (2018). Opportunities for Use of Blockchain Technology in Medicine. *Applied Health Economics and Health Policy*, *16*(5), 583–590. DOI: 10.1007/s40258-018-0412-8 PMID: 30022440

Raghupathi, W., & Raghupathi, V. (2014). Big Data Analytics in Healthcare: Promise and potential. *Health Information Science and Systems*, *2*(1), 3. Advance online publication. DOI: 10.1186/2047-2501-2-3 PMID: 25825667

Raj, A. (2022). Healthcare Innovation in India: Addressing challenges, understanding progress and offering opportunities. *The National Medical Journal of India*, *35*, 38–40. https://nmji.in/healthcare-innovation-in-india-addressing-challenges-understanding-progress-and-offering-opportunities/. DOI: 10.25259/NMJI_110_20 PMID: 36039626

Rajan Jeyaraj, P., & Nadar, E. R. S. (2019). Smart-monitor: Patient monitoring system for IoT-based healthcare system using deep learning. *Journal of the Institution of Electronics and Telecommunication Engineers*, •••, 1–8.

Rajeswari, A. M., Sridevi, M., & Deisy, C. (2014). Outliers detection on educational data using fuzzy association rule mining. In *Proceedings of International Conference on Advanced in Computer Communication and Information Science (ACCIS-14)* (pp. 1–9).

Rajkomar, A., Oren, E., Chen, K., Dai, A. M., Hajaj, N., Hardt, M., Liu, P. J., Liu, X., Marcus, J., Sun, M., Sundberg, P., Yee, H., Zhang, K., Zhang, Y., Flores, G., Duggan, G. E., Irvine, J., Le, Q., Litsch, K., & Dean, J. (2018). Scalable and accurate deep learning with electronic health records. *NPJ Digital Medicine*, *1*(1), 1–10. DOI: 10.1038/s41746-018-0029-1 PMID: 31304302

Ramachandran, N., Krishnan, P. H., Nair, S. S., & Padmanabhan, R. K. (2018). IoT-based patient monitoring and diagnostic system: An integrated approach. In *2018 International Conference on Circuits and Systems in Digital Enterprise Technology (ICCSDET)* (pp. 1-5). IEEE.

Ramos-Lopez, O., Milagro, F. I., Allayee, H., Chmurzynska, A., Choi, M. S., Curi, R., De Caterina, R., Ferguson, L. R., Goni, L., Kang, J. X., Kohlmeier, M., Marti, A., Moreno, L. A., Pérusse, L., Prasad, C., Qi, L., Reifen, R., Riezu-Boj, J. I., San-Cristobal, R., & Martínez, J. A. (2017). Guide for current nutrigenetic, nutrigenomic, and nutriepigenetic approaches for precision nutrition involving the prevention and management of chronic diseases associated with obesity. *Lifestyle Genomics*, *10*(1-2), 43–62. DOI: 10.1159/000477729 PMID: 28689206

Ramos-Lopez, O., Samblas, M., Milagro, F. I., Riezu-Boj, J. I., Crujeiras, A. B., Martinez, J. A., & Project, M. E. N. A. (2018). Circadian gene methylation profiles are associated with obesity, metabolic disturbances and carbohydrate intake. *Chronobiology International*, *35*(7), 969–981. DOI: 10.1080/07420528.2018.1446021 PMID: 29580070

Randeree, E. (2009). Exploring technology impacts of Healthcare 2.0 initiatives. *Telemedicine Journal and e-Health*, *15*(3), 255–260. DOI: 10.1089/tmj.2008.0093 PMID: 19382863

Rao, A. (2020). India's Aarogya Setu contact tracing app flawed and raises privacy concerns. *MIT Technology Review*.

Rathore, Y., Sinha, U., Haladkar, J. P., Mate, N. R., Bhosale, S. A., & Chobe, S. V. (2023). Optimizing Patient Flow and Resource Allocation in Hospitals using AI. *2023 International Conference on Artificial Intelligence for Innovations in Healthcare Industries (ICAIIHI)*, 1–6. DOI: 10.1109/ICAIIHI57871.2023.10489698

Rauch, E., Linder, C., & Dallasega, P. (2020). The anthropocentric perspective of production before and within Industry 4.0. *Computers & Industrial Engineering*, *139*, 105644. DOI: 10.1016/j.cie.2019.01.018

Rautaray, S. S., & Agrawal, A. (2015). Vision based hand gesture recognition for human computer interaction: A survey. *Artificial Intelligence Review*, *43*(1), 1–54. DOI: 10.1007/s10462-012-9356-9

Rawat, A. (2024, December 2). 7 Telemedicine Trends Shaping the Future of Healthcare. Appinventiv. https://appinventiv.com/blog/top-telehealth-trends/

Ray, P. P. (2018). A survey on Internet of Things architectures. *Journal of King Saud University. Computer and Information Sciences*, *30*(3), 291–319. DOI: 10.1016/j.jksuci.2016.10.003

Reboucas Filho, P. P., Sarmento, R. M., Holanda, G. B., & de Alencar Lima, D. (2017). New approach to detect and classify stroke in skull CT images via analysis of brain tissue densities. *Computer Methods and Programs in Biomedicine*, *148*, 27–43. DOI: 10.1016/j.cmpb.2017.06.011 PMID: 28774437

Reddy, C., Kishore, K., Doss, S., Bhatia, S., & Alqhatani, A. (2024). *Evolution and Advances in Computing Technologies for Industry 6.0*. Routledge. DOI: 10.1201/9781003503934

Redman, T. C. (2018). Seizing Opportunity in Data Quality. *Harvard Business Review*.

Reid, S. E., & de Brentani, U. (2004). The fuzzy front end ofnew product development for discontinuous innovations: A theoretical model. *Journal of Product Innovation Management*, *21*(3), 170–184. DOI: 10.1111/j.0737-6782.2004.00068.x

Reinertsen, D. (1994). Streamlining the fuzzy front-end. *World Class Design to Manufacture*, *1*(5), 4–8. DOI: 10.1108/09642369210069751

Reinertsen, D. G., & Smith, P. G. (1991). The strategist's role in shortening product development. *The Journal of Business Strategy*, *12*(4), 18–22. DOI: 10.1108/eb039425 PMID: 10113668

Renner, B., Buyken, A. E., Gedrich, K., Lorkowski, S., Watzl, B., Linseisen, J., Daniel, H., Conrad, J., Ferrario, P. G., Holzapfel, C., Leitzmann, M., Richter, M., Simon, M.-C., Sina, C., & Wirsam, J. (2023). Perspective: A conceptual framework for adaptive personalized nutrition advice systems (APNASs). *Advances in Nutrition*, *14*(5), 983–994. DOI: 10.1016/j.advnut.2023.06.009 PMID: 37419418

Reporter, S. (2023, September 20). BPJS Kesehatan wins big at the Asian Technology Excellence Awards. Asian Business Review. https://asianbusinessreview.com/event-news/bpjs-kesehatan-wins-big-asian-technology-excellence-awards

Riboli, E., Hunt, K. J., Slimani, N., Ferrari, P., Norat, T., Fahey, M., Charrondière, U. R., Hémon, B., Casagrande, C., Vignat, J., Overvad, K., Tjønneland, A., Clavel-Chapelon, F., Thiébaut, A., Wahrendorf, J., Boeing, H., Trichopoulos, D., Trichopoulou, A., Vineis, P., & Saracci, R. (2002). European Prospective Investigation into Cancer and Nutrition (EPIC): Study populations and data collection. *Public Health Nutrition*, *5*(6b), 1113–1124. DOI: 10.1079/PHN2002394 PMID: 12639222

Rice, M., Kelley, D., Peters, L., & Colarelli O'Connor, G. (2001). Radical innovation: Triggering initiation of opportunity recognition and evaluation. *R & D Management*, *31*(4), 409–420. DOI: 10.1111/1467-9310.00228

Riksdag, S. (2016). *Lag (2016:1145) om offentlig upphandling*. https://www.riksdagen.se/sv/dokument-lagar/dokument/svensk-forfattningssamling/lag-20161145-om-offentlig-upphandling_sfs-2016-1145

Ringel, Y., Maharshak, N., Ringel-Kulka, T., Wolber, E. A., Sartor, R. B., & Carroll, I. M. (2015). High throughput sequencing reveals distinct microbial populations within the mucosal and luminal niches in healthy individuals. *Gut Microbes*, *6*(3), 173–181. DOI: 10.1080/19490976.2015.1044711 PMID: 25915459

Ristevski, B., & Chen, M. (2018). Big Data Analytics in Medicine and Healthcare. *Journal of Integrative Bioinformatics*. https://www.ncbi.nlm.nih.gov/pmc/articles/PMC6340124/

Rizova, P. S., Gupta, S., Maltz, E. N., & Walker, R. W. (2018). Overcoming equivocality on projects in the fuzzy front end: Bringing social networks back in. *Technovation*, *78*, 40–55. DOI: 10.1016/j.technovation.2018.05.006

Robbins, P., O'Gorman, C., & Huff, A. S. (2021). The impact of team goal orientation in the fuzzy front end of the innovation process. *International Journal of Innovation Management*, *25*(6), 2150071. DOI: 10.1142/S1363919621500717

Robert, E. (2020). *Security flaw in Aarogya Setu app could expose user data*. Security Research Blog.

Roberts, J. P., Fisher, T. R., Trowbridge, M. J., & Bent, C. (2016). A design thinking framework for healthcare management and innovation. *Healthcare (Amsterdam, Netherlands)*, *4*(1), 11–14. DOI: 10.1016/j.hjdsi.2015.12.002 PMID: 27001093

Rojas, J. C., Teran, M., & Umscheid, C. A. (2023). Clinician Trust in Artificial Intelligence: What is Known and How Trust Can Be Facilitated. [PubMed]. *Critical Care Clinics*, *39*(4), 769–782. DOI: 10.1016/j.ccc.2023.02.004 PMID: 37704339

Rönnberg Sjödin, D., Frishammar, J., & Eriksson, P. E. (2016). Managing uncertainty and equivocality in joint process development projects. *Journal of Engineering and Technology Management*, *39*, 13–25. DOI: 10.1016/j.jengtecman.2015.12.001

Ross, C., &Swetlitz, I. (2018). IBM pitched its Watson supercomputer as a revolution in cancer care. It's nowhere close. STAT News.S69

Roy, S., Dan, P. K., & Modak, N. (2019). Leveraging new product innovation through R&D practices in engineering manufacturing sector: A study in Indian context. *International Journal of Innovation and Sustainable Development*, *13*(3–4), 275–295. DOI: 10.1504/IJISD.2019.100418

Rtc. (2023, December 25). Digital Transformation in Action: e-Invoicing in Estonia - RTC Suite. RTC Suite. https://rtcsuite.com/digital-transformation-in-action-e-invoicing-in-estonia/

Ruiz, M. D., Martin-Bautista, M. J., Sánchez, D., Vila, M. A., & Delgado, M. (2014). Anomaly detection using fuzzy association rules. *International Journal of Electronic Security and Digital Forensics*, *96*(1), 25–37. DOI: 10.1504/IJESDF.2014.060171

Rusnak, S., & Charney, P. (2019). Position of the Academy of Nutrition and Dietetics: Nutrition informatics. *Journal of the Academy of Nutrition and Dietetics*, *119*(8), 1375–1382. DOI: 10.1016/j.jand.2019.06.004 PMID: 31353011

Russell, R. K., & Tippett, D. D. (2008). Critical success factors for the fuzzy front end of innovation in the medical devices device industry. *Engineering Management Journal*, *20*(3), 36–43. DOI: 10.1080/10429247.2008.11431775

Sætre, A. S., & Brun, E. (2012). Strategic management of innovation: Managing exploitation by balancing creativity and constraint. *International Journal on Management of Innovation & Technology*, *09*(04), 1250025. DOI: 10.1142/S0219877012500253

Salsabila, N. N., Yusrani, N. K. G., Annajah, N. S., Azzahra, N. K. A., & Sabrina, N. R. S. N. (2023). The Comparative Analysis of inpatient service at public hospitals and private hospitals in order to Improve Patient Satisfication : A literature review. *Usada Nusantara Jurnal Kesehatan Tradisional*, *1*(2), 65–78. DOI: 10.47861/usd.v1i2.250

Salvetti, F., Gardner, R., Minehart, R., & Bertagni, B. (2023). Intelligent Avatars, Holographic Tools, Digitized Objects: An Extended Reality Simulation Demonstration. [iJAC]. *International Journal of Advanced Corporate Learning*, *16*(3), 73–81. DOI: 10.3991/ijac.v16i3.35739

Santra, S., Kukreja, P., Saxena, K., Gandhi, S., & Singh, O. V. (2024). Navigating regulatory and policy challenges for AI enabled combination devices. *Frontiers in Medical Technology*, *6*, 1473350. DOI: 10.3389/fmedt.2024.1473350 PMID: 39669903

Satriana, S. (2019). Easing Access to the National Health Insurance through a Mobile Application. In ILO Social Protection Department. ILO. Retrieved August 5, 2024, from https://www.social-protection.org/gimi/Media.action?id=16856

Saunders, M. N. K., Lewis, P., & Thornhill, A. (2019). *Research Methods for Business Students* (8th ed.). Pearson.

Savage, G. T., Buche, J., & Batchelor, J. (2018). Academic-practice partnerships: A win-win proposition. *Nursing Management*, *49*(11), 40–43.

Scala, B., & Lindsay, C. F. (2021). Supply chain resilience during pandemic disruption: Evidence from healthcare. *Supply Chain Management*, *26*(6), 672–688. DOI: 10.1108/SCM-09-2020-0434

Schesinger, L. A., & Hskett, J. L. (1991). Customer Satisfaction is Rooted in Employee Satisfaction. *Harvard Business Review*, (Nov/Dec), 148–149. https://hbr.org/1991/09/the-service-driven-service-company

Schoenfeld, A. J., & Mafi, J. N. (2018). Improving access to care in the US healthcare system: An Aesculapian perspective. *BMJ Quality & Safety*, *27*(11), 851–854.

Schoonmaker, M., Carayannis, E., & Rau, P. (2013). The role of marketing activities in the fuzzy front end of innovation: A study of the biotech industry. *The Journal of Technology Transfer*, *38*(6), 850–872. DOI: 10.1007/s10961-012-9296-1

Schweitzer, F., Palmié, M., & Gassmann, O. (2018). Beyond listening: The distinct effects of proactive versus responsive customer orientation on the reduction of uncertainties at the fuzzy front end of innovation. *R & D Management*, *48*(5), 534–551. DOI: 10.1111/radm.12252

Schweitzer, F., Roeth, T., & Gillier, T. (2020). The eye of the beholder: The influence of intuition, rationality, and leeway on the assessment of an Idea's market-creation potential. *Industrial Marketing Management*, *91*, 274–284. DOI: 10.1016/j.indmarman.2020.09.018

Scriver, C. R., Beaudet, A. L., Sly, W. S., Valle, D., Childs, B., Kinzler, K. W., & Vogelstein, B. (Eds.). (2001). The metabolic and molecular bases of inherited disease (8th ed.). McGraw-Hill. Biochemistry (Moscow), *67*(5), 611–612.https://doi.org/ DOI: 10.1023/A:1017418800320

Seal, V., Raha, A., Maity, S., Mitra, S. K., Mukherjee, A., & Naskar, M. K. (2012). A simple flood forecasting scheme using wireless sensor networks. *International Journal of Ad Hoc* [IJASUC]. *Sensor & Ubiquitous Computing*, *3*(1), 45–60. DOI: 10.5121/ijasuc.2012.3105

Sebek, M., & Menichetti, G. (2024). Network Science and Machine Learning for Precision Nutrition. In *Precision Nutrition* (pp. 367–402). Academic Press. DOI: 10.1016/B978-0-443-15315-0.00012-2

Seh, A. H., Zarour, M., Eisa, M., El-Qawasmeh, E., Saleem, K., & Khan, M. K. (2020). Healthcare data breaches: Insights and challenges. *Computers & Security*, *99*, 102011.

Serban, R. C., Campolo, D., Laschi, C., & Moser, E. (2020). Robots in healthcare: Past, present, and future. *SMC Benchmark*, *1*(1), 9–31.

Shah, S. H. H., Karlsen, A. S. T., Solberg, M., & Hameed, I. A. (2024). An efficient and lightweight multiperson activity recognition framework for robot-assisted healthcare applications. *Expert Systems with Applications*, *241*, 122482. DOI: 10.1016/j.eswa.2023.122482

Shaik, F., Yelchuri, R., Gudur, N. A., & Dash, J. K. (2024). ML Applications in Healthcare. *How Machine Learning is Innovating Today's World: A Concise Technical Guide*, 201-220.

Shalini, T. G., Ganeshabu, L., Chemudugunta, P., Yamsani, N., Kumar, Ch. A., & Athiraja, A. (2024). Exploring Innovations in Autonomous Robotics and Mechatronics: Application in Manufacturing and Healthcare. *2024 5th International Conference on Smart Electronics and Communication (ICOSEC)*, 336–342. DOI: 10.1109/ICOSEC61587.2024.10722417

Sharma, A. E., Willard-Grace, R., Hessler, D., Bodenheimer, T., & Thom, D. H. (2016). What happens after health coaching? Observational study 1 year following a randomized controlled trial. *Annals of Family Medicine*, *14*(3), 200–207. DOI: 10.1370/afm.1924 PMID: 27184989

Sharma, D., Bhagat, L., & Sharma, S. (2024). Regulating Children's Personal Data Protection in India: No Child's Play. *Development*, *67*(1-2), 28–33. Advance online publication. DOI: 10.1057/s41301-024-00402-w

Sharma, S., Chen, K., & Sheth, A. (2018). Toward practical privacy-preserving analytics for IoT and cloud-based healthcare systems. *IEEE Internet Computing*, *22*(2), 42–51. DOI: 10.1109/MIC.2018.112102519

Sharma, S., Malakar, S., Yadav, V., & Kak, S. M. (2023).. . *AI-Based Healthcare System.*, *IRSD2024*, 181.

Sheltami, T. R., Bala, A., & Shakshuki, E. M. (2016). Wireless sensor networks for leak detection in pipelines: A survey. *Journal of Ambient Intelligence and Humanized Computing*, *7*(3), 347–356. DOI: 10.1007/s12652-016-0362-7

Shilaskar, P. (2024). Multi Modal AI-Driven System for Enhanced Neurological Detection Using EEG, Retinal, and Brain Imaging Data. *International Journal for Research in Applied Science and Engineering Technology*, *12*(11), 876–882. DOI: 10.22214/ijraset.2024.65229

Shin, J. H., Lee, B., & Park, K. S. (2011). Detection of abnormal living patterns for Elderly living alone using support vector data description. *IEEE Transactions on Information Technology in Biomedicine*, *15*(3), 438–448. DOI: 10.1109/TITB.2011.2113352 PMID: 21317086

Siciliani, L., McKee, M., Garcia-Altes, A., De Maeseneer, J., Gruson, D., Kringos, D., Lehtonen, L., Lionis, C., Murauskiene, L., Nuti, S., Pita Barros, P., Rogers, H.-L., Wieczorowska-Tobis, K., Zacharov, S., Zaletel, J., & Stahl, D. (2021). Public Procurement in Healthcare Systems; Opinion of the Expert Panel on Effective Ways of Investing in Health (EXPH). *European Union.*

Siemens Healthineers. (2020). Predictive Maintenance for Medical Devices. Retrieved from https://www.siemens-healthineers.com/services/predictive-maintenance

Singh, B. (2024). Digital Twins as New Paradigm for Bridging the Gap from Personalized Medicine to Specific Rural Public Health. In P. K. Dutta, P. Raj, B. Sundaravadivazhagan, & C. P. Selvan, *Artificial Intelligence Solutions for Cyber-Physical Systems* (1st ed., pp. 286–309). Auerbach Publications. DOI: 10.1201/9781032694375-16

Singh, C. (2024). Healthcare delivery and beneficiary satisfaction: A focused study on AB-PMJAY beneficiaries at a tertiary care hospital of North India. Research Review. DOI: 10.52845/CMRO/2024/7-11-1

Singh, J., Shelke, N. A., Upreti, K., Divakaran, P., Lingareddy, N., & Deepika, S. (2024). Enhancing Patient Well-Being in Healthcare Through the Integration of IoT and Neural Network. *2024 International Conference on Emerging Innovations and Advanced Computing (INNOCOMP)*, 241–246. DOI: 10.1109/INNOCOMP63224.2024.00047

Sjoding, M. W., Dickson, R. P., Iwashyna, T. J., Gay, S. E., & Valley, T. S. (2020). Racial Bias in Pulse Oximetry Measurement. *The New England Journal of Medicine*, *383*(25), 2477–2478. DOI: 10.1056/NEJMc2029240 PMID: 33326721

Skinner, B. F. (1953). *Science and human behavior*. Macmillan.

Slight, S. P., Seger, D. L., Nanji, K. C., Cho, I., Maniam, N., Dykes, P. C., & Bates, D. W. (2013). Are we heeding the warning signs? Examining providers' overrides of computerized drug–drug interaction alerts in primary care. *PLoS One*, *8*(12), e85071. DOI: 10.1371/journal.pone.0085071 PMID: 24386447

Smith, A. B., Patel, N., & Thomas, K. (2020). Robotic-assisted laparoscopic prostatectomy: A review of the current state and future prospects. *The New England Journal of Medicine*, *382*(1), 88–95. PMID: 32343497

Smith, A. B., Patel, N., & Thomas, K. (2021). Robotic-assisted laparoscopic prostatectomy: A review of the current state and future prospects. *Journal of Robotic Surgery*, *15*(1), 5–12.

Sosa, R. A. (1983). Some observations on effect of a supportive companion during labor and delivery. *The Journal of the Florida Medical Association*, *70*(9), 761–763. PMID: 6631389

Srivastava, L. (2006, March). Pervasive, ambient, ubiquitous: the magic of radio. In *European Commission Conference "From RFID to the Internet of Things", Bruxelles, Belgium.*

Stahl, M., Srivastava, S., Majakari, D., Dutta, A., Liu, R., & Chin, B. (2021). *Digital technologies for government-supported health insurance systems in Asia and the Pacific*. Asian development bank., DOI: 10.22617/TCS210526

Stange, K. C. (2009). The problem of fragmentation and the need for integrative solutions. *Annals of Family Medicine*, *7*(2), 100–103. DOI: 10.1370/afm.971 PMID: 19273863

Stetler, K. L., & Magnusson, M. (2015). Exploring the tension between clarity and ambiguity in goal setting for innovation: Clarity and ambiguity in goal setting for i Dnnovation. *Creativity and Innovation Management*, *24*(2), 231–246. DOI: 10.1111/caim.12102

Stevens, E. (2014). Fuzzy front-end learning strategies: Exploration of a high-tech company. *Technovation*, *34*(8), 431–440. DOI: 10.1016/j.technovation.2013.12.006

Stick, K. (n.d.). Behavioral economics in action. Retrieved from https://www.stickk .com

Stilinović, M., Sabolić, I., Papeš, D., Pasini, N. M., Škrljak-šoša, D., & Luetić, T. (2021). PATIENT SATISFACTION. *Paediatria Croatica*, *65*(2), 90–94. DOI: 10.13112/pc.390

Strava. (n.d.). Social interaction in fitness. Retrieved from https://www.strava.com

Stuer, C., Husig, S., & Biala, S. (2010). How to create and sustain an open and radical innovation capability in the fuzzy front end: The case of Vodafone Group R&D Germany and selected ongoing radical innovation projects. *International Journal of Product Development*, *11*(3/4), 196. DOI: 10.1504/IJPD.2010.033958

Sulistyowati, W. T., Suryani, N. L., & Harokan, N. A. (2024). ANALYSIS OF PATIENT SATISFACTION WITH INPATIENT SERVICES IN REGIONAL GENERAL HOSPITALS. Cendekia Medika Jurnal Stikes Al-Ma`Arif Baturaja, 9(2), 255–264. DOI: 10.52235/cendekiamedika.v9i2.382

Summary of the HIPAA Security Rule. (n.d.). *US Department of Health and Human Services*. https://www.hhs.gov/hipaa/for-professionals/security/laws-regulations/index.html

Sundar, S. S., & Marathe, S. S. (2010). Personalization vs. customization: The importance of agency, privacy, and power usage. *Human Communication Research*, *36*(3), 298–322. DOI: 10.1111/j.1468-2958.2010.01377.x

Suryadevara, N. K., Gaddam, A., Mukhopadhyay, S. C., & Rayudu, R. K. (2011, November). Wellness determination of inhabitant based on daily activity behaviour in real-time monitoring using Sensor Networks. In Sensing Technology (ICST), 2011 Fifth International Conference on (pp. 474-481). IEEE. DOI: 10.1109/ICSensT.2011.6137025

Suryadevara, N. K., Mukhopadhyay, S. C., & Rayudu, R. K. (2012, December). Applying SARIMA time series to forecast sleeping activity for wellness model of Elderly monitoring in smart home. In Sensing Technology (ICST), 2012 Sixth International Conference on (pp. 157-162). IEEE.

Suryadevara, N. K., Mukhopadhyay, S. C., Rayudu, R. K., & Huang, Y. M. (2012, May). Sensor data fusion to determine wellness of an Elderly in intelligent home monitoring environment. In Instrumentation and Measurement Technology Conference (I2MTC), 2012 IEEE International (pp. 947-952). IEEE. DOI: 10.1109/I2MTC.2012.6229645

Suryadevara, N. K., Mukhopadhyay, S. C., Wang, R., Rayudu, R. K., & Huang, Y. M. (2013, May). Reliable measurement of Wireless Sensor Network data for forecasting wellness of Elderly at smart home. In Instrumentation and Measurement Technology Conference (I2MTC), 2013 IEEE International (pp. 16-21). IEEE. DOI: 10.1109/I2MTC.2013.6555372

Suryadevara, N. K., Quazi, M. T., & Mukhopadhyay, S. C. (2012, June). Intelligent Sensing Systems for Measuring Wellness Indices of the Daily Activities for the Elderly. In Intelligent Environments (IE), 2012 8th International Conference on (pp. 347-350). IEEE. DOI: 10.1109/IE.2012.49

Suryadevara, N. K., & Mukhopadhyay, S. C. (2011, September). Wireless sensors network based safe home to care Elderly people: A realistic approach. In *Recent Advances in Intelligent Computational Systems (RAICS), 2011 IEEE (pp. 001-005)*. IEEE. DOI: 10.1109/RAICS.2011.6069262

Suryadevara, N. K., & Mukhopadhyay, S. C. (2012). Wireless sensor network-based home monitoring system for wellness determination of Elderly. *IEEE Sensors Journal*, *12*(6), 1965–1972. DOI: 10.1109/JSEN.2011.2182341

Suryanto, S., Plummer, V., & Boyle, M. (2016). Financing Healthcare in Indonesia. *Asia Pacific Journal of Health Management*, *11*(2), 33–38. DOI: 10.24083/apjhm.v11i2.185

Susarla, A., Gopal, R., Thatcher, J. B., & Sarker, S. (2023). The Janus effect of generative AI: Charting the path for responsible conduct of scholarly activities in information systems. *Information Systems Research*, *34*(2), 399–408. DOI: 10.1287/isre.2023.ed.v34.n2

Tavana, M., Nazari-Shirkouhi, S., & Farzaneh Kholghabad, H. (2021). An integrated quality and resilience engineering framework in healthcare with Z-number data envelopment analysis. *Health Care Management Science*, *24*(4), 768–785. DOI: 10.1007/s10729-021-09550-8 PMID: 33834321

Taylor, R., Nguyen, T., & Wilson, K. (2024). Perceived threats to patient rights and safety with AI integration in healthcare: A scoping review. *Archives of Public Health = Archives Belges de Santé Publique*, *82*(4).

Technologies used on Mobile JKN - Fork.ai, https://fork.ai/lookup/ai-doc-7960137

Thaler, R. H., & Sunstein, C. R. (2008). *Nudge: Improving decisions about health, wealth, and happiness*. Yale University Press.

Thanasopon, B., Papadopoulos, T., & Vidgen, R. (2016). The role of openness in the fuzzy front-end of service innovation. *Technovation*, *47*, 32–46. DOI: 10.1016/j.technovation.2015.11.007

The Mobile Economy. (2020). GSMA. https://www.gsma.com/solutions-and-impact/connectivity-for-good/mobile-economy/wp-content/uploads/2020/03/GSMA_MobileEconomy2020_Global

The role of digital claims management for Estonia's health insurance: A leverage for making healthcare purchasing more strategic. (2023, February 14). World Health Organization (WHO). https://www.who.int/publications/i/item/9789240066687

Thombre, S., Islam, R. U., Andersson, K., & Hossain, M. S. (2016). Performance analysis of an IP based protocol stack for WSNs. In *Proceedings of the 2016 IEEE Conference on Computer Communications Workshops (INFOCOM WKSHPS)* (pp. 691–696). DOI: 10.1109/INFCOMW.2016.7562102

Thomke, S., & Manzi, J. (2014). The new science of building great teams. *Harvard Business Review*, *92*(4), 60–70.

Tibor, B., Mark, H., Michel, C. A. K., & Jan, T. (2011). An ambient agent model for monitoring and analysing dynamics of complex Elderly behavior. *Journal of Ambient Intelligence and Smart Environments*, *3*(4), 283–303. DOI: 10.3233/AIS-2011-0117

Tkachenko, N. (2023). Machine Learning in Healthcare: 12 Real-World Use Cases to Know. *NIX United*. https://nix-united.com/blog/machine-learning-in-healthcare-12-real-world-use-cases-to-know/

Tonga launches Pacific Islands first integrated national health information system. (2021, December 17). Matangi Tonga. https://matangitonga.to/2021/11/30/tonga-launches-pacific-islands-first-integrated-national-health-information-system

Tonga's experience in implementing national digital health. (2023). Pacific Health Information Network.

Topol, E. J. (2019). High-performance medicine: The convergence of human and artificial intelligence. *Nature Medicine*, *25*(1), 44–56. DOI: 10.1038/s41591-018-0300-7 PMID: 30617339

Tornhagen, L., & Ekstén, E. (2020). *Revisionsrapport: Granskning av anskaffning av medicinteknisk utrustning: Region Halland* [Audit Report]. PWC.

Tornhagen, L., & Fornstedt, C. (2019). *Revisionsrapport: Granskning av anskaffning av medicinteknisk utrustning: Region Gävleborg*. PWC. [Audit Report]

Tornhagen, L., Fornstedt, C., & Olausson, C. (2019). *Revisionsrapport: Anskaffning av medicinteknisk utrustning: Region Norrbotten* [Audit Report]. PWC.

Tornhagen, L., & Horstmann, H. (2020). *Granskning av anskaffning av medicinteknisk utrustning: Region Örebro* [Audit Report]. PWC.

Tornhagen, L., & Norén, S. (2018). *Revisionsrapport: Granskning av anskaffning av medicinteknisk utrustning: Region Västmanland* [Audit Report]. PWC.

Töyrä, A., Monfors, J., & Bern, A.-B. (2020). Upphandlingsmyndigheten och Konkurrensverket December 2020. *Swedish Competition Authority*, 216.

Tran, M. K., Goulding, C., & Shiu, E. (2018). The orchestra of ideas: Using music to enhance the 'fuzzy front end' phase of product innovation. *Journal of Business Research, 85*, 504–513. DOI: 10.1016/j.jbusres.2017.10.029

Tsai, J., & Bond, G. R. (2008). A comparison of electronic records to paper records in mental health centers. *International Journal for Quality in Health Care : Journal of the International Society for Quality in Health Care, 20*(2), 136–143. DOI: 10.1093/intqhc/mzm064 PMID: 18079127

Tsakiri, E. (2024). Measuring patient satisfaction in a general hospital. *Health Review, 35*(192), 21–28. DOI: 10.54042/hr3266hhsma

Tschumi, P., & Mayer, H. (2024). How does co-creation influence healthcare regulations? An analysis of co-creation in social innovation. *Innovation (Abingdon), 37*(1), 85–117. DOI: 10.1080/13511610.2023.2296380

Tsolakidis, D., Gymnopoulos, L. P., & Dimitropoulos, K. (2024, August). Artificial Intelligence and Machine Learning Technologies for Personalized Nutrition: A Review. []. MDPI.]. *Informatics (MDPI), 11*(3), 62. DOI: 10.3390/informatics11030062

Tuli, S., Basumatary, N., Gill, S. S., Kahani, M., Arya, R. C., Wander, G. S., & Buyya, R. (2020). HealthFog: An ensemble deep learning based Smart Healthcare System for Automatic Diagnosis of Heart Diseases in integrated IoT and fog computing environments. *Future Generation Computer Systems, 104*, 187–200. DOI: 10.1016/j.future.2019.10.043

Turchetti, G., Pierotti, F., Caldarelli, V., Cuschieri, A., & Micali, S. (2021). Robotic surgery: Ethical, legal, and regulatory issues. *Minimally Invasive Therapy & Allied Technologies, 30*(1), 9–17.

Turchin, A., Jaffe, C., & Hamid, M. (2018). Effect of a clinical decision support system on adherence to diabetes treatment guidelines. *JAMA Network Open, 1*(7), e185887.

Tyagi, A. K., Arumugam, S. K., Prasad, P. R., & Sharma, A. (2024). The Position of Digital Society, Healthcare 5.0, and Consumer 5.0 in the Era of Industry 5.0. In *Advancing Software Engineering Through AI, Federated Learning, and Large Language Models* (pp. 262-280). IGI Global. DOI: DOI: 10.4018/979-8-3693-3502-4.ch017

Umayal, K. M. (2024). *Strategic integration of digital health technologies for enhanced patient-centered care in modern healthcare management.* Shanlax International Journal of Management, 11(S1-Jan), 68-73. https://doi.org/DOI: 10.34293/management.v11iiS1-Jan.7142

United Nations Development Programme. (2024). Global Multidimensional Poverty Index 2024: Poverty amid conflict. Accessed from https://hdr.undp.org/system/files/documents/hdp-document/mpireport2024en.pdf

Unlu, O. (2024, October 25). 11 Big Data In Healthcare Statistics [Trends and Overall Market]. Edge Delta. https://edgedelta.com/company/blog/big-data-in-healthcare-industy-overview

Uns, H. (2022, March 11). UNS Hospital-BPJS Kesehatan Launched JKN Mobile-Connected Online Queue System. Universitas Sebelas Maret. https://uns.ac.id/en/uns-hospital-bpjs-kesehatan-launched-jkn-mobile-connected-online-queue-system/

Uscher-Pines, L., Kahn, J. M., Li, J., Luft, H. S., & Mehrotra, A. (2021). Behavioral Health Impacts of the COVID-19 Pandemic: Evidence for the Promise of Telehealth. *Psychiatric Services (Washington, D.C.)*, *72*(10), 1193–1202. PMID: 33622042

Using OCR to Search and Edit Scanned Documents. (2022, September 28). Foxit PDF Blog. https://www.foxit.com/blog/search-and-edit-scanned-documents-with-ocr/

Vaid, A., Jaladanki, S. K., Xu, J., Teng, S., Kumar, A., Lee, S., Somani, S., Paranjpe, I., De Freitas, J. K., Wanyan, T., Johnson, K. W., Bicak, M., Klang, E., Kwon, Y. J., Costa, A., Zhao, S., Miotto, R., Charney, A. W., Böttinger, E., & Glicksberg, B. S. (2021c). Federated Learning of Electronic Health Records to Improve Mortality Prediction in Hospitalized Patients With COVID-19: Machine Learning Approach. *JMIR Medical Informatics*, *9*(1), e24207. DOI: 10.2196/24207 PMID: 33400679

Vaigandla, K. K., Vanteru, M. K., & Siluveru, M. (2024). An Extensive Examination of the IoT and Blockchain Technologies in Relation to their Applications in the Healthcare Industry. *Mesopotamian Journal of Computer Science*, *2024*, 1–14. DOI: 10.58496/MJCSC/2024/001

Vallès-Peris, N., Barat-Auleda, O., & Domènech, M. (2021). Robots in Healthcare? What Patients Say. *International Journal of Environmental Research and Public Health*, *18*(18), 9933. DOI: 10.3390/ijerph18189933 PMID: 34574861

Vamathevan, J., Clark, D., Czodrowski, P., Dunham, I., Ferran, E., Lee, G., Li, B., Madabhushi, A., Shah, P., Spitzer, M., & Zhao, S. (2019). Applications of machine learning in drug discovery and development. *Nature Reviews. Drug Discovery, 18*(6), 463–477. DOI: 10.1038/s41573-019-0024-5 PMID: 30976107

Van Aken, J. E., & Weggeman, M. P. (2000). Managing learning in informal innovation networks: Overcoming the Daphne-dilemma. *R & D Management, 30*(2), 139–150. DOI: 10.1111/1467-9310.00164

Vaquero Martín, M., Reinhardt, R., & Gurtner, S. (2016). Stakeholder integration in new product development: A systematic analysis of drivers and firm capabilities: Stakeholder integration in NPD. *R & D Management, 46*(S3), 1095–1112. DOI: 10.1111/radm.12220

Vaquero Martín, M., Reinhardt, R., & Gurtner, S. (2021). The dilemma of downstream market stakeholder involvement in NPD: Untangling the effects of involvement and capabilities on performance. *Journal of Business Research, 124*, 136–151. DOI: 10.1016/j.jbusres.2020.11.040

Vayed, D. A., Nurmandi, A., Muallidin, I., & Loilatu, M. J. (2022). Utilization of the JAKI Application in Realizing Smart Living in the COVID-19 Pandemic Era (Case Study of DKI Jakarta Government, Indonesia). In Lecture notes in networks and systems (pp. 399–410). https://doi.org/DOI: 10.1007/978-981-19-2397-5_38

Vayena, E.. (2018). *Ethical challenges of big data in healthcare*. Health Ethics and Policy Lab.

Veeramakali, T., Siva, R., Sivakumar, B., Senthil Mahesh, P. C., & Krishnaraj, N. (2021). An intelligent internet of things-based secure healthcare framework using blockchain technology with an optimal deep learning model. *The Journal of Supercomputing, 77*(9), 9576–9596. DOI: 10.1007/s11227-021-03637-3

Venter, J. C., Adams, M. D., Myers, E. W., Li, P. W., Mural, R. J., Sutton, G. G., Smith, H. O., Yandell, M., Evans, C. A., Holt, R. A., Gocayne, J. D., Amanatides, P., Ballew, R. M., Huson, D. H., Wortman, J. R., Zhang, Q., Kodira, C. D., Zheng, X. H., Chen, L., & Zhu, X. (2001). The sequence of the human genome. *Science, 291*(5507), 1304–1351. DOI: 10.1126/science.1058040 PMID: 11181995

Verworn, B. (2009). A structural equation model of the impact of the "fuzzy front end" on the success of new product development. *Research Policy, 38*(10), 1571–1581. DOI: 10.1016/j.respol.2009.09.006

Vettorello, M., Eisenbart, B., & Ranscombe, C. (2022). The innovation system roadmap: A novel approach to instil futures-oriented reasoning in strategic decision making. *Creativity and Innovation Management*, *31*(1), 5–18. DOI: 10.1111/caim.12472

Vincent, A. C., Furman, H., Slepian, R. C., Ammann, K. R., Di Maria, C., Chien, J. H., Siu, K.-C., & Slepian, M. J. (2022). Smart phone-based motion capture and analysis: Importance of operating envelope definition and application to clinical use. *Applied Sciences (Basel, Switzerland)*, *12*(12), 6173. DOI: 10.3390/app12126173

Virtual Reality In Healthcare Market. (2023). Grand View Research. https://www.grandviewresearch.com/press-release/global-virtual-reality-vr-healthcare-market#
Waldie, P., Attef, M., Trudel, C., Chan, A. D. C., & Wallace, B. (2023). Implementation and Use of Real-Time Location Systems in Hospital Environments – Rapid Scoping Review of Human Factors Considerations. *Proceedings of the International Symposium on Human Factors and Ergonomics in Health Care*, *12*(1), 164–168. DOI: 10.1177/2327857923121038

Vladimirova, T., & Yuhaniz, S. (2011). An intelligent decision-making system for flood monitoring from space. *Soft Computing*, *15*(1), 13–24. DOI: 10.1007/s00500-009-0514-1

von Geibler, J., Piwowar, J., & Greven, A. (2019). The SDG-Check: Guiding open innovation towards sustainable development goals. *Technology Innovation Management Review*, *9*(3), 20–37. DOI: 10.22215/timreview/1222

Vroom, V. H. (1964). *Work and motivation*. Wiley.

Wagner, S. M. (2012). Tapping supplier innovation. *The Journal of Supply Chain Management*, *48*(2), 37–52. DOI: 10.1111/j.1745-493X.2011.03258.x

Wagrell, S., & Baraldi, E. (2019). The joys and sorrows of a start-up's interactions with the public sphere: A case from medical technology. *Journal of Business and Industrial Marketing*, *34*(1), 267–283. DOI: 10.1108/JBIM-11-2018-0326

Wahyuni, N., Triharini, M., & Has, E. M. M. (2022). STRATEGY TO PROMOTE PATIENT CENTERED CARE PCC FOR IMPROVING PATIENT SATISFACTION: A LITERATURE REVIEW. *Nurse and Health Jurnal Keperawatan*, *11*(1), 10–21. DOI: 10.36720/nhjk.v11i1.306

Wang, Z., Gerstein, M., & Snyder, M. (2009). RNA-Seq: A revolutionary tool for transcriptomics. *Nature Reviews. Genetics*, *10*(1), 57–63. DOI: 10.1038/nrg2484 PMID: 19015660

Wasir, R., Bahar, M. A., Irawati, S., & Wasir, R. (2020). Moving forward to achieve universal health coverage in Indonesia. https://doi.org/DOI: 10.33612/diss.124431881

Weaver, W. L., Mattke, T. L., & Cahill, T. F. (2021). Sustainability and the future of healthcare. *World Medical & Health Policy*, *13*(2), 266–280.

Weidener, L., & Fischer, M. (2024). Artificial intelligence in medicine: Cross-sectional study among medical students on application, education, and ethical aspects. *JMIR Medical Education*, *10*(1), e51247. DOI: 10.2196/51247 PMID: 38180787

Weissler, E. H., Naumann, T., Andersson, T., Ranganath, R., Elemento, O., Luo, Y., Freitag, D. F., Benoit, J., Hughes, M. C., Khan, F., Slater, P., Shameer, K., Roe, M., Hutchison, E., Kollins, S. H., Broedl, U., Meng, Z., Wong, J. L., Curtis, L., & Ghassemi, M. (2021). The role of machine learning in clinical research: Transforming the future of evidence generation. *Trials*, *22*(1), 1–15. DOI: 10.1186/s13063-021-05489-x PMID: 34399832

Weng, C. H. (2011). Mining fuzzy specific rare itemsets for education data. *Knowledge-Based Systems*, *24*(5), 697–708. DOI: 10.1016/j.knosys.2011.02.010

Werbach, K., & Hunter, D. (2012). *For the win: How game thinking can revolutionize your business*. Wharton Digital Press. Retrieved from https://books.google.com/books?hl=en&lr=&id=ywxq_c4XSHMC

What is GDPR, the EU's new data protection law? (n.d.). *GDPR.EU*. https://gdpr.eu/what-is-gdpr/

WHO, Barcelona Office for Health Systems Financing. (2023). How can digital technologies be used to enhance health financing? Claims management in Estonia. In Health Financing Policy Papers (Report WHO/EURO:2023-7340-47106-68912). World Health Organization. https://iris.who.int/bitstream/handle/10665/367965/WHO-EURO-2023-7340-47106-68912-eng.pdf?sequence=1 (Original work published 2023)

WHO, Patient safety. Available from Patient safety (who.int) Assessed on 25-06-2024

WHO, Universal Health Coverage. (2019, July 16). https://www.who.int/health-topics/universal-health-coverage#tab=tab_1

WHO. (n.d.). Health technology assessment. *WHO Health Topics*. https://www.who.int/health-topics/health-technology-assessment/

Wiens, J., Spector-Bagdady, K., & Mukherjee, B. (2024). Toward Realizing the Promise of AI in Precision Health Across the Spectrum of Care. *Annual Review of Genomics and Human Genetics*, *25*(1), 141–159. Advance online publication. DOI: 10.1146/annurev-genom-010323-010230 PMID: 38724019

Wijsen, J., & Meersman, R. (1998). On the complexity of mining quantitative association rules. *Data Mining and Knowledge Discovery*, *2*(3), 263–281. DOI: 10.1023/A:1009755120593

Wolbring, G., & Leopatra, V. (2013). Sensors: Views of Staff of a Disability Service Organization. *Journal of Personalized Medicine*, *3*(1), 23–39. DOI: 10.3390/jpm3010023 PMID: 25562409

World Bank and WHO. Half the world lacks access to essential health services, 100 million still pushed into extreme poverty because of health expenses. (2017, December 13). World Health Organization (WHO). https://www.who.int/news/item/13-12-2017-world-bank-and-who-half-the-world-lacks-access-to-essential-health-services-100-million-still-pushed-into-extreme-poverty-because-of-health-expenses

World Economic Forum. (2021). "Global AI Action Alliance: A Framework for Responsible AI."

World Health Organization. (2009). *WHO Patient Safety Curriculum Guide: Multi-professional Edition*. WHO.

World Health Organization. (2021). *Ethics and Governance of Artificial Intelligence for Health*. World Health Organization.

Wosik, J., Fudim, M., & Cameron, B.. (2020). Telehealth transformation: COVID-19 and the rise of virtual care. *Journal of the American Medical Association*, *323*(12), 1167–1168. PMID: 32311034

Wosik, J., Fudim, M., Cameron, B., Gellad, Z. F., Cho, A., Phinney, D., Curtis, S., Roman, M., Poon, E. G., Ferranti, J., Katz, J. N., & Tcheng, J. (2020). Telehealth transformation: COVID-19 and the rise of virtual care. *Journal of the American Medical Informatics Association : JAMIA*, *27*(6), 957–962. DOI: 10.1093/jamia/ocaa067 PMID: 32311034

Wright, S. P., Hall Brown, T. S., Collier, S. R., & Sandberg, K. (2019). How consumer physical activity monitors could transform human physiology research and healthcare. *JMIR mHealth and uHealth*, *5*(2), e4.

Wright, T.. (2022). Impact of wearable devices on patient engagement and chronic disease management: A systematic review. *JMIR mHealth and uHealth*.

Xu, X., Ren, C., Wu, R., & Yan, H. (2017) Sliced Inverse Regression With Adaptive Spectral Sparsity for Dimension Reduction. *IEEE transactions on cybernetics*. Volume 47 (3), Pp. 759-771. ISSN: 2168-2267. DOI: DOI: 10.1109/TCYB.2016.2526630

Xu, J., We, Z., Wang, C., & Jia, X. (2024). Machine Unlearning: Solutions and Challenges. *IEEE Transactions on Emerging Topics in Computational Intelligence*, *8*(3), 2150–2168. DOI: 10.1109/TETCI.2024.3379240

Yadav, N., Pandey, S., Gupta, A., Dudani, P., Gupta, S., & Rangarajan, K. (2023). Data Privacy in Healthcare: In the Era of Artificial Intelligence. *Indian Dermatology Online Journal*, *14*(6), 788–792. DOI: 10.4103/idoj.idoj_543_23 PMID: 38099022

Yadav, S. (2024). Transformative frontiers: A comprehensive review of emerging technologies in modern healthcare. *Cureus*, *16*(3). Advance online publication. DOI: 10.7759/cureus.56538 PMID: 38646390

Yang, A., & Yang, E. (2024). *A Multimodal Approach to The Detection and Classification of Skin Diseases* (Version 1). arXiv. DOI: 10.48550/ARXIV.2411.13855

Yap, C., Aiyegbusi, O. L., Alger, E., Basch, E., Bell, J., Bhatnagar, V., Cella, D., Collis, P., Dueck, A. C., Gilbert, A., Gnanasakthy, A., Greystoke, A., Hansen, A. R., Kamudoni, P., Kholmanskikh, O., King-Kallimanis, B. L., Krumholz, H., Minchom, A., O'Connor, D., & Peipert, J. D. (2024). Advancing patient-centric care: Integrating patient reported outcomes for tolerability assessment in early phase clinical trials – insights from an expert virtual roundtable. *EClinicalMedicine*, *76*, 102838. DOI: 10.1016/j.eclinm.2024.102838 PMID: 39386161

Yazici, A., Zhumabekova, D., Nurakhmetova, A., Yergaliyev, Z., Yatbaz, H. Y., Makisheva, Z., Lewis, M., & Ever, E. (2023). A smart e-health framework for monitoring the health of the elderly and disabled. *Internet of Things : Engineering Cyber Physical Human Systems*, *24*, 100971. DOI: 10.1016/j.iot.2023.100971

Yekeen, I. A., Adejumo, P., & Kolawole, I. O. (2024). Patient-Centered care as an optimal solution for enhancing the quality of healthcare delivery. International Journal of Innovative Science and Research Technology (IJISRT), 2606–2612. DOI: 10.38124/ijisrt/IJISRT24AUG1534

Yin, R. K. (2018). *Case Study Research and Applications: Design and Methods* (6th ed.). SAGE.

Young, F., Zhang, L., Jiang, R., Liu, H., & Wall, C. (2020, December). A deep learning based wearable healthcare IoT device for ai-enabled hearing assistance automation. In 2020 international conference on machine learning and cybernetics (ICMLC) (pp. 235-240). IEEE.

Yuan, Y., Chen, K., Zhu, Y., Yu, Y., Hu, M., Chu, Y., Hsu, Y., Hu, J., Yue, Q., & Liu, M. (2024). Exploring the feasibility of integrating ultra-high field magnetic resonance imaging neuroimaging with multimodal artificial intelligence for clinical diagnostics. *iRadiology*, *2*(5), 498–509. DOI: 10.1002/ird3.102

Yu, D., Yang, Y., Long, J., Xu, W., Cai, Q., Wu, J., Cai, H., Zheng, W., & Shu, X. O. (2021). Long-term diet quality and gut microbiome functionality: A prospective, shotgun metagenomic study among urban Chinese adults. *Current Developments in Nutrition*, *5*(4), nzab026. DOI: 10.1093/cdn/nzab026 PMID: 33937616

Zack, M. H. (2001). If managing knowledge is the solution, then what's the åroblem? *Knowledge Management and Business Model Innovaiton, IGI Global*, 16–36.

Zack, M. H. (2007). The role of decision support systems in an indeterminate world. *Decision Support Systems*, *43*(4), 1664–1674. DOI: 10.1016/j.dss.2006.09.003

Zahay, D., Griffin, A., & Fredericks, E. (2011). Information use in new product development: An initial exploratory empirical investigation in the chemical industry. *Journal of Product Innovation Management*, *28*(4), 485–502. DOI: 10.1111/j.1540-5885.2011.00821.x

Zakaria, H., Said, Y., Aleabova, S., Bangayan, J., Dandan, M., Debs, J., Dahlstrom, N., Divino, D., Hashemi, A., & Almarzooqi, I. (2024). Measuring the effectiveness of hybrid diabetes care over 90 days through continuous data monitoring in type 2 diabetic patients. *Frontiers in Endocrinology*, *15*, 1355792. Advance online publication. DOI: 10.3389/fendo.2024.1355792 PMID: 38774233

Zhang, H., Nakamura, T., Isohara, T., & Sakurai, K. (2023). A Review on Machine Unlearning. *SN Computer Science*, *4*(4), 337. Advance online publication. DOI: 10.1007/s42979-023-01767-4

Zhang, N., Feng, Y., Huo, R., & Zhao, Y. (2023). Design of Intelligent Hospital Information Service System Based on Intelligent Internet of Things. *2023 International Conference on Industrial IoT, Big Data and Supply Chain (IIoTBDSC)*, 16–22. DOI: 10.1109/IIoTBDSC60298.2023.00013

Zhang, Q., Cao, M., & Doll, W. (2019). Fuzzy front end of innovation: A dual theoretical rationale. *Journal of Business and Industrial Marketing*, *34*(1), 176–191. DOI: 10.1108/JBIM-06-2017-0144

Zhang, W., Jiang, Y., & Zhang, W. (2021). Capabilities for collaborative innovation of technological alliance: A knowledge-based view. *IEEE Transactions on Engineering Management*, *68*(6), 1734–1744. DOI: 10.1109/TEM.2019.2936678

Zhang, Y., Qiu, M., Tsai, C. W., Hassan, M. M., & Alamri, A. (2015). Health-CPS: Healthcare cyber-physical system assisted by cloud and big data. *IEEE Systems Journal, 11*(1), 88–95. DOI: 10.1109/JSYST.2015.2460747

Zhao, A. P., Li, S., Cao, Z., Hu, P. J. H., Wang, J., Xiang, Y., Xie, D., & Lu, X. (2024). AI for science: Predicting infectious diseases. *Journal of Safety Science and Resilience = An Quan Ke Xue Yu Ren Xing (Ying Wen).*

Zhao, P., Xu, J., & Han, M. (2024). Patient-Centric Care: Unveiling the potential of wearable electronics in clinical practice. *Wearable Electronics., 1*, 119–136. DOI: 10.1016/j.wees.2024.07.001

Zhao, Y., Yang, R., Chevalier, G., Xu, X., & Zhang, Z. (2018). Deep residual bidir-LSTM for human activity recognition using wearable sensors. *Mathematical Problems in Engineering, 2018*(1), 7316954. DOI: 10.1155/2018/7316954

Zhou, Z., Dai, W., Eggert, J., Giger, J. T., Keller, J., Rantz, M., & He, Z. (2009, September). A real-time system for in-home activity monitoring of elders. In Engineering in Medicine and Biology Society, 2009. EMBC 2009. Annual International Conference of the IEEE (pp. 6115-6118). IEEE.

Zhou, X., Liang, W., Kevin, I., Wang, K., Wang, H., Yang, L. T., & Jin, Q. (2020). Deep-learning-enhanced human activity recognition for Internet of healthcare things. *IEEE Internet of Things Journal, 7*(7), 6429–6438. DOI: 10.1109/JIOT.2020.2985082

Ziqitza, (2023), https://analyticsindiamag.com/how-surgical-robot-assistants-are-becoming-areality-in-indian-hospitals-and-healthcare-sector/

Zou, F. W., Tang, Y. F., Liu, C. Y., Ma, J. A., & Hu, C. H. (2020). Concordance Study Between IBM Watson for Oncology and Real Clinical Practice for Cervical Cancer Patients in China: A Retrospective Analysis. *Frontiers in Genetics, 11*, 200. Advance online publication. DOI: 10.3389/fgene.2020.00200 PMID: 32265980

About the Contributors

Piyush Kumar With over 17 years of extensive experience within the healthcare industry, Piyush has made significant contributions across the domains of healthcare and life sciences. Following a substantial tenure in the industry from 2007 to 2019, he decided to pursue his passion for academia. Presently, Piyush Kumar holds the position of Associate Professor at IILM University, Gurugram. Previously, he has been working as Associate Professor and Associate Dean, Trainings at Institute of Health Management Research, Bangalore, a role he has assumed since 2020. He has also managed the Institution Innovation Council (IIC) and was a core team member for the Center for Advancing Digital Health, Management, Innovation, Research, and Entrepreneurship (ADMIRE) at IIHMR, Bangalore During 2019 to 2020, Piyush served as an Assistant Professor in the Department of Management at Banasthali Vidyapith (NAAC A++ University). Between 2013 and 2019, he held a pivotal role in healthcare consulting as a Program Manager for the healthcare and life sciences practice, covering the South Asia, Middle East, and Africa region at Frost & Sullivan. During the period from 2007 to 2013, Piyush Kumar also made significant contributions to prominent healthcare chains in India, assuming various strategic leadership roles. Furthermore, he headed the medical services division of the 'Buddh International Circuit,' India's sole Formula One racing track. Piyush Kumar's academic journey commenced with the attainment of a master's degree in health and Hospital Administration from IIHMR University in 2007. Presently, he is pursuing his Ph.D. in Management from Banasthali Vidyapith, Rajasthan. His research interests encompass the realms of healthcare management and digital healthcare. Driven by a passion for writing, Piyush has authored numerous articles pertaining to the healthcare industry, which have been featured in esteemed healthcare publications. Additionally, he has presented his research findings at various national and international conferences. His expertise has been recognized by prestigious organizations, leading to invitations to speak at events hosted by the Ministry of Labor in Taiwan, CSR India, and the Consortium of Accredited

Healthcare Organizations (CAHO) in India. Much of his work has centred around enhancing healthcare management through the application of diverse tools and cutting-edge technologies. Mr. Piyush is credited as a co-author of two notable works: "Implementing Six Sigma to Enhance the Hospital Discharge Process" published in the International Journal of Pharmaceutical Sciences Research, and "Innovation in Healthcare Marketing Strategies in India" featured in the Innovative Journal of Business and Management.

Kirti Udayai boasts a remarkable career spanning over 17 years, seamlessly blending expertise in healthcare and academia. Presently, she holds the position of Head Academics at Max Healthcare Institute Limited, where she imparts knowledge in Hospital Management, a role she has embraced for over a decade. Dr. Udayai's professional journey pivots around her profound interest in hospital management where she has made significant research contributions. Her scholarly endeavours shine through her prolific publication record in both national and international journals. Beyond academia and research, Dr. Udayai's impact extends to the corporate realm, where she actively collaborates with organizations to mentor and enhance workforce skills. Her dedication to bridging the academia-industry gap resonates with her commitment to human resource development within the healthcare sector. On the global stage, Dr. Udayai has left her mark as a leader, having chaired International Conferences on Public Health in Sri Lanka and Malaysia. Her exceptional skills and experience converge in her role as a certified National Assessor for the National Quality Assurance Standard (NQAS), an initiative under the Ministry of Health and Family Welfare, India. In this capacity, she plays a pivotal role in assessing and ensuring the quality of public healthcare facilities across India, contributing significantly to the nation's healthcare landscape. Acknowledging her contributions, Dr. Udayai has received the prestigious Education Leadership award, a testament to her unwavering dedication to healthcare education excellence. Her multifaceted career epitomizes her unwavering commitment to advancing healthcare quality, research, education, and workforce development, making her a true luminary in the field.

Prashant Singh is a veteran of Air Force with over two decades of service in frontline combat squadrons and has flown over 2500 hours on various fighter and trainer aircraft. He has been actively engaged in operational and training roles and has held staff positions at different levels in the organization. During his tenure in the National Cadet Corps, he led the training of over 1000 cadets for a sound development of character and a sense of service to the nation. He has been awarded on multiple occasions for his service to the organization and holds a Masters degree in Human Resource Management and a Post Graduate Diploma in

Training and Development. Post his active years with the Indian Air Force, he has transitioned to the corporate world and has worked with startups and SMEs, sharing his experience and knowledge in the fields of Organizational Development and Strategy; Human Resource Development; Enterprise Resource Planning and Management; Data Analytics; Quality Management & Control; and Risk, Safety & Risk Management. He has a deep interest in applications of future technologies, especially, machine learning and artificial intelligence in the D&A sector. An ardent advocate for technological advancement, Prashant's writings reflect his deep interest in lifelong-learning, human resource development and future technologies. Currently, he collaborates with leading firms continuing to influence the intersection of technology, strategy, and leadership.

Shiv Dutt Gupta is a leading Public Health professional with a distinguished academic and research career. He obtained his M.D. (Preventive & Social Medicine) from India, and Ph.D. (Epidemiology) from Johns Hopkins University, Baltimore, USA. He was conferred Fellowship of Academy of Medical Science, India (FAMS) for his outstanding contribution in the field of public health. He has done pioneering work of creating and establishing new discipline of health management, and promoting research in health policy and health systems and programmes. Currently Dr. Gupta is Distinguished Professor, IIHMR University, Adjunct Professor, Epidemiology, Johns Hopkins University School of Public Health, Gates Leadership Fellow and Trustee Secretary, Indian Institute of Health Management Research (IIHMR), India. He was the Former Chairman, IIHMR University, and Director of IIHMR Jaipur for one and a half decade. He was the first President of the IIHMR University in 2014. He served as the Director of WHO Collaborating Centre for District Health Systems at IIHMR facilitating management research and interventions in the health systems to improve efficiency and effectiveness of health care. Dr Gupta is Adjunct Professor at the Johns Hopkins University, USA and Visiting Professor at University of Chester, UK. He was the President of WHO SEARO's South East Asia Public Health Education Network (SEAPHEIN). Dr. Gupta also served as Temporary Advisor to SEARO WHO on several consultation processes. He was member of the Technical Review Panel of the Global Fund. Dr Gupta is member of several research advisory committees of the Indian Council of Medical Research (ICMR) and Chairs Project Review Committee of Department of Health Research, Ministry of Health and Family Welfare, Government of India. He has championed the cause of quality improvement and capacity building in health care in India and South East Asia. Dr. Gupta is the recipient of QIMPRO Gold Standard Award 2009 for quality of Healthcare. Over the past three and a half decades of his distinguished career, he has completed more than 100 research studies and projects supported by various organizations/agencies and have more than 100 research publications to his credit. The areas of research include: public health, epidemiology, health systems and management.

Pankaj Rahi has completed his M.Phil in Computer Science from Vinayaka Mission University, Salem (NAAC A+, UGC & DSIR accredited) in 2009 and Ph.D in Computer Application from Chandigarh University(NAAC A+, NIRF 27th Rank), Mohali, Punjab India. He has also qualified with Post Graduate Diploma in Hospital Management from Madurai Kamaraj University, Madhurai with Specialisation in Community Health Demography and Biostatistics, Medical Record Management. His core research areas are Simulation Modeling of Smart eHealth Systems, eHealth Informatics, mHealth and Predictive Modeling and Data Mining, Telemedicine. Dr. Pankaj Rahi is a State Awardee of Chandigarh Administration, Chandigarh and conferred the State-level Commendation Certification from Hon'ble Governor of Punjab and Administrator of U.T-Chandigarh on 15th August 2020 for his best contributions as COVID-Warrior in the area of implementations of IT Systems, eGovernance initiatives in Health. He is also active team member of bringing out the eGovernance-Innovations of online Aadhar-enabled Birth Registration of Infants at hospitals in U.T Chandigarh, Implementations of online Direct Benefit Transfer Scheme through Public Financial Management System, Implementation of eSanjeevani- National Tele-Consultations Services at Health and Wellness Centres in UT Chandigarh. He has attains heights in academia by published 15 research Article in the Scopus-Indexed International Journals, Scopus index-Books/Conferences Published 10 Scientific Utility Patents and Granted 3-Scientific Designed Patens, issued by Office of Controller General of Patents, Design -Intellectual Property Rights, Trademark, Dept of Promotion of Industry & Trademark, Govt of India. He has also granted 2- International Scientific- Patents (South Africa, Australian) and 1- Copy Right for the ML based concept. He has participated and contributed as Member of Scientific and Reviewing Committee in many International Conferences.

***

Meshal AlHarbi Dean College of Computer Engineering & Sciences Prince Sattam Bin Abdulaziz University Office: Ground Floor – G6 P.O.BOX 151 Alkharj 11942 Kingdom of Saudi Arabia Email: mg.alharbi@psau.edu.sa

Henrik Barth is an associate professor in innovation sciences with a focus on innovation management, and he is currently leading several research projects addressing sustainable business model innovation (specifically the transformation phase from conventional to digital solutions), developed in close collaboration with client companies, students and researchers at FabLab Halmstad. Henrik's teaching experience includes over 4200 hours at international universities, focusing on courses in organisation, management, innovation, and entrepreneurship at bachelors and masters levels in the disciplines of innovation management, business administration, and engineering. Henrik has also been awarded "Excellent teaching practitioner" . Previously, Henrik Barth was Head of the Business Department and Dean for the School of Business, Engineering, and Science at Halmstad University for a total period of nine years. His research contributions include over 30 research projects and additionally 40 peer-reviewed publications. Henrik has published in journals such as Small Business Economics, Journal of Cleaner Production, Journal of Small Business Management, Journal of Rural Studies, Production Planning and Control, Journal of Agricultural Education and Extension, and British Food Journal.

Biswadip Basu Mallik is presently an Associate Professor of Mathematics in the Department of Basic Science & Humanities at the Institute of Engineering & Management, University of Engineering & Management, Kolkata, India. He has been involved in teaching and research for more than 22 years and has published several research papers and book chapters in various scientific journals from reputed international publishers like CRC Press, Apple, Wiley, IGI Global, and Springer. He has written five books at undergraduate levels in Engineering Mathematics, Quantitative Methods, and Computational Intelligence. He has also published five Indian patents along with fifteen edited books. His fields of research work are Computational Fluid Dynamics, Mathematical Modelling, Optimization and Machine Learning. Dr. Basu Mallik is a Series Editor of the Book series titled "Mathematics and Computer Science" from Wiley-Scrivener, USA and a Managing editor of the Journal of Mathematical Sciences & Computational Mathematics (JMSCM), USA. He is also an Editorial board member and reviewer of several scientific journals. He is a senior life member of Operational Research Society of India (ORSI) and a life member of Calcutta Mathematical Society (CMS), Indian Statistical Institute (ISI), Indian Science Congress Association (ISCA), and International Association of Engineers (IAENG).

Sukanti Bhattacharyya is an accomplished medical professional with a diverse background in medical education and research. He currently serves as an Associate Professor in the Department of Medical Physiology at ICARE Institute of Medical Sciences and Research & Dr. B.C. Roy Hospital in Haldia, West Bengal, India. Dr. Bhattacharyya began his educational journey by earning his MBBS degree from the University of Calcutta in 1991. He went on to obtain a Diploma in Public Health and an MD in Medical Physiology from the West Bengal University of Health Sciences. Currently, he is pursuing a PhD in the Faculty of Modern Medicine at the same university. Throughout his career, Dr. Bhattacharyya has made significant contributions to the field of medical education. He has served as a faculty member for both undergraduate and postgraduate students, teaching medical physiology and guiding research projects. Additionally, he has taken on various administrative roles, being an active member in the Death Review Committee, Medical Education Unit, and Institutional Ethics Committee at his institution. Dr. Bhattacharyya's research efforts have resulted in the publication of 6 original research articles, 5 review articles, and 1 book chapter. His dedication to the medical profession and passion for continuous learning make him a valuable asset to the healthcare community.

Susanta Das is a seasoned educator with a proven record of teaching and mentoring diverse students, working at multiple institutions, and providing service to the various initiatives of organizations. He received his Ph.D. and M.A. degrees from Western Michigan University (WMU), USA, and M.Sc. degree from Banaras Hindu University (BHU), India all in Physics. He continued his research as a Marie-Curie post-doctoral fellow at Stockholm University, Stockholm, Sweden on beam diagnostics for the DESIREE (Double ElectroStatic Ion Ring ExpEriment) in the project DITANET (Diagnostic Techniques for particle Accelerators – a Marie-Curie initial training NETwork), at the Indian Institute of Science Education and Research-Kolkata, India on high-pressure physics as a Project Scientist-B, and at the University of Electro-Communications, Tokyo, Japan on ion-surface interactions as a Post-doctoral fellow. Throughout his career, Dr. Das worked and collaborated with many researchers, Ph.D., master, and visiting students from different countries. He further visited many countries to discuss research and an international conference participant (UK, Italy, Germany, Greece, Belgium, Bulgaria, Romania, Brazil etc.). He co-authored several research articles in WoS/Scopus indexed international journals, conference proceedings, and scholarly book chapters published by renowned international publishing houses. Beyond his research endeavors, Dr. Das has a storied history of service to academic and administrative committees, exhibiting his commitment to the growth and development of educational institutions. His experience includes tenure at Central University South Bihar, Sri Sri University, and P.K. University before assuming his current role at Ajeenkya DY Patil University. He received the Marie-Curie post-doctoral fellowship in Sweden, Science Academies' Summer Research Fellowship in India, Gwen Frostic Doctoral Fellowship, Department Graduate Research and Creative Scholar Award by WMU, and Leo R. Parpart Doctoral Fellowship by Dept. of Physics, WMU, among many others, throughout his academic journey. At present, Dr. Das continues to delve into cutting-edge fields, with a keen interest in nanotechnology, UN SDGs, and data science. His multifaceted contributions, spanning teaching, research, and administrative leadership, showcase a dedicated professional who is instrumental in advancing the vision and mission of the institutions he serves.

Jayathra Datla is a public health specialist with over 5+ years of experience in implementing health systems strengthening projects and evaluating public health insurance schemes. She holds a Master's in public health and is a certified state level quality assessor. She has worked with prominent Central Government organizations, including NHSRC, NHA, health departments of Chhattisgarh, Andhra Pradesh, and Tamil Nadu and eminent client like WHO, ADB and WB. She facilitated national quality accreditation of public health facilities, developed treatment guidelines, and implemented fraud control measures under AB-PMJAY. She evaluated health insurance schemes in Mizoram, Meghalaya, Rajasthan, and Chhattisgarh. She implemented a project on using innovative digital technologies to enhance health financing in Asia and the Pacific.

Pooja Dehankar is working in the department of Artificial Intelligence and Data Science, Ajeenkya DY Patil School of Engineering, Affiliated by Savitribai Phule Pune University, Pune. She has completed BE in Computer Engineering from Priyadarshini College of Engineering, Nagpur, and ME in Information Technology from Sinhgad College of Engineering, Pune. She has done Post Graduate Diploma in Advance Computing. She has 16 years of experience in academics. Her areas of interest are Artificial Intelligence, Cyber Security, and Data Mining. She has published papers in Scopus Journals. She actively participates in workshops, faculty development programs, short-term training programs, conferences, and webinars. She is currently pursuing Ph.D. from Symbiosis Center for Research and Innovation, Symbiosis International (Deemed University).

Teesta Dey is currently pursuing Masters degree in Food Science and Nutrition from Mount Carmel College, Bangalore. She has completed Bachelor's great interest in recent advances in nutrition informatics, nutrigenomics, nano-nutrition for cancer treatment and public health. She is currently working on an original research on integration and adoption of telenutrition in dietary practice and has presented a paper on the same at WUACD's 2025 international conference held at Avinashilingam University, Tamil Nadu.

Kanishak Gautam is a Health Financing expert currently working at IQVIA. He has a Fellowship in Public Health (Health Financing) from IIHMR, New Delhi, where he also completed PG diploma in health and hospital management. His professional experience spans over several countries, including India, Armenia, Qatar, Bangladesh, Iraq, Sudan, Tunisia, Korea, Mongolia, Indonesia, and Libya. He has worked across health insurance, hospital planning and operations, market intelligence in the pharmaceutical sector, and health system reforms. He has worked on significant projects including Using Digital Technology to Improve

National Health Financing in Asia and the Pacific & UHC study for Bangladesh, Mandatory Health Insurance program in Qatar, Ayushman Bharat in India, Universal health coverage scheme evaluation. His roles have involved designing project frameworks, policy development, stakeholder engagement, and health benefit package implementation. He has worked with clients including national & state governments, WHO, ADB, World Bank, other multi-lateral and bi-lateral agencies.

Parul Goela is a public health specialist and has comprehensive knowledge in the implementation of several projects across domains such as maternal & child nutrition, health financing, pharmaceutical, sustainability & climate change. She has done MBA in hospital & health management from IIHMR Jaipur. She has 6 years of experience and has worked closely with donor agencies, central & state governments, NGOs across geographies India, Mongolia, Armenia & Bangladesh along with SEARO region. She has implemented & supported several projects including Using Digital Technology to Improve National Health Financing in Asia and the Pacific, UHC study for Bangladesh, health insurance scheme evaluation for Mizoram, POSHAN Abhiyaan (Delhi). She has worked with eminent clients including WHO, World Bank, IFC, ADB.

Avishek Gupta received his Bachelor of Technology degree in Computer Science and Engineering in the year 2006 from Asansol Engineering College, Asansol, West Bengal, under West Bengal University of Technology. He has received his Master of Technology degree in Computer Science and Engineering in the year of 2014 from JIS College of Engineering, Kalyani, West Bengal, under West Bengal University of Technology. At present, he is working as Assistant Professor of Computer Science and Engineering Department (B.Tech) in ABACUS Institute of Engineering and Management, Magra, West Bengal. Prior to this, he was engaged as Software Developer in various organizations since August,2006 without any break. His current areas of Interest are Data Analysis .

Monalisa Halder (PhD, B.Ed., M.Ed.) is currently working as an Assistant Professor of Physics and HOD of Dept. of BSHU in ABACUS Institute of Engineering and Management, Mogra, West Bengal, India. Till date, Dr. Halder has authored in 24 SCI indexed, peer reviewed international journal publications and 15 book chapter publications. She attended more than 24 international conferences, national seminars/workshops in India as well as in abroad so far. Her research interests lie in materials science, polymer nanotechnology, bio-waste management, early childhood education. educational technology and women empowerment. Dr. Halder is voluntarily serving as a peer reviewer for the journals of Elsevier and

Springer Nature. She is a lifetime member of Forum of Scientists, Engineers and Technologists (FOSET) and Indian Society for Technical Education (ISTE).

Aileen J A trained Hospital Administrator with decade plus of experience in Healthcare/Academics from reputed Institutions in the capacity of teaching, project/ dissertation guidance, guide for hospital internship, student mentoring, curriculum development and other academic coordination Hospital project Management, quality development projects |patient safety advocate with green belt in lean six sigma, PhD in the area of Patient Safety Culture, Fellowship in Developing Healthcare Leaders in Quality and Safety Worldwide, Quality in Healthcare and Safety, Institute of Healthcare Improvement

Lambodar Jena is currently working as Associate Professor in the Center for Data Science of the Department of Computer Science and Engineering, ITER, Siksha 'O' Anusandhan (Deemed to be) University, Bhubaneswar, Odisha. He has around 24 years of work experience in academics and research. He holds a Ph.D. from Utkal University, Odisha, India and an M.Tech in Computer Science and Application from IIT(ISM) Dhanbad,India. He received the MCA degree from Sambalpur University, Odisha, India. Dr. Jena's research interests include Data Mining, Machine Learning, Theoretical Computer Science, Wireless Sensor Networks, Artificial Intelligence and Data Science. He has published more than 50 research papers in peer-reviewed journals & conferences of national and international repute including 08 Patents. He has also served as reviewer to many reputed international/national journals and conferences. He is currently supervising 04 research scholars under him in the area of machine learning, recommender system and IOT.

Jesper Johansson holds a Bachelor's degree in Innovation Engineering from Halmstad University, where his thesis focused on leveraging technology to enhance healthcare systems. He continued his academic journey at the same institution, earning a Master of Science in Industrial Management and Innovation with a research focus on navigating the challenges of innovation in the Swedish medical device industry. Currently, Jesper works as a Strategic Sourcing Leader in the supply chain sector, specializing in category management and strategic sourcing processes. With over two and a half years of professional experience, he combines his academic background with practical expertise to drive innovation and efficiency. His research and professional interests include supply chain innovation, early-stage product development, and integrating sustainable and technological advancements into industrial processes. Jesper is passionate about fostering innovation at the intersection of technology and management, solving complex challenges, and driving sustainable progress in industrial operations. He is particularly motivated by opportunities to improve processes, collaborate across disciplines, and contribute to the development of solutions that create long-term value for organizations and society alike.

Varun Kumar is a seasoned public health professional and Erasmus Mundus scholar (2024-26) with diverse experience in the global health space, including health technology design, evaluations, reviews, strategy/policy development, technical advisory, and implementation research. He has worked extensively with the ministries of health and various international development partners in 20+ countries across Europe, Asia, and Africa, obtaining a strong knowledge of Global Health Policy, Information Systems, and Governance. He is an expert in the review and design of health management information systems (particularly, DHIS2) and as a specialist, he has led health technology assessments and implementations in multiple Asian and African countries. He was tasked as a core team member for the assessment of TB surveillance systems in 19 Global Fund Strategic Initiative countries and has also led country-level HIS enterprise architecture assessments in Bangladesh and Afghanistan. He is also the author of a Chapter "Lessons from India's Digital Public Infrastructure Transformation" in the book "Accelerating Global Health: Pathways to Health Equity for the G20" and as the founding member of YO.DH (Youth Ownership of Digital Health) - a youth-focused community for Digital Health professionals, he has been a lead author for a publication with Digital Square. In his education, he is trained in Biomedical Science from the University of Delhi and has also pursued an MBA in Health and Hospital Management from IIHMR Delhi. He has been a passionate researcher and through his academic & professional engagements, he has actively contributed to research work in the domains of Health Information Technology, Microbiology, Maternal and Child Health, Nutrition, Antimicrobial Resistance, and Disease Surveillance. Varun is currently associated with Dure Technologies as a Manager for Strategic Partnerships (part-time) and studying public health as an Erasmus Mundus Scholar with the University of Sheffield (UK).

Niladri Neel Majumder A seasoned Digital Health professional and entrepreneur, Neel Majumder brings over a decade of global experience in designing, implementing, and adopting advanced clinical informatics solutions for leading healthcare providers across Asia and North America. Recognized by the World Health Organization's Digital Health Technical Advisory Group, Majumder holds a Master of Health Informatics from the University of Toronto and an MBA in Healthcare Management from the Indian Institute of Health Management Research in Jaipur. His career features impactful roles with esteemed institutions, including Stanford University Medical Center, University Health Network Canada, Peter

Munk Cardiac Research Center, the Government of Canada Health Services, and Sidra Medical & Research Center. His expertise encompasses digital health strategy development, EHR design and implementation (Epic and Cerner), healthcare analytics, and product leadership in digital and virtual health. Additionally, Majumder serves as an Adjunct Faculty member of Health Informatics at the University of Toronto and a Digital Health Program Partner at BCIT Canada and Faculty of Health Informatics at the Higher Colleges of Technology, United Arab Emirates. Majumder is the founder of HealthTechX Academy, a unique training and mentorship platform for digital health professionals led by global health informatics experts. Committed to mentoring emerging professionals, he emphasizes empathy and user-centric design in technology development. He has also contributed to health system strengthening projects for India's National Rural Health Mission and has been recognized by the World Health Organization and the Canadian Government for his innovative contributions to healthcare technology.

Nilamadhab Mishra is an Associate Professor in the School of Computer Science and Engineering, AI-ML Division, at VIT Bhopal University, India. He received his Doctor of Philosophy (Ph.D.) in Computer Science and Information Engineering with a specialization in AI-data science and machine learning from Chang Gung University, Taiwan. He has over 23 years of national and international involvement in academic teaching and research at recognized Indian, Taiwanese, and African universities. He has over 100 publications in SCI/SCIE and SCOPUS-indexed journals, ISBN books and chapters, Indian and Australian patents, IEEE conference proceedings, etc. He has been a reviewer, associate editor, and editorial board member for SCI/SCIE-indexed journals and conferences. He has been involved with several professional bodies: "Fellow Member of "ISROSET"; Fellow Member of "ISRD"; Senior Member of "ASR" (Hong Kong); Senior Member of "IEDRC" (Hong Kong); and Member of "IEEE Collabratec". He is currently an Associate Editor for two SCOPUS-indexed journals, and his research interests span the areas of AI, Data Science, Machine Learning, and Cognitive Analytics & Applications.

Hitesh Mohapatra received the B.E. degree in Information Technology from Biju Patnaik University of Technology (BPUT), Odisha in 2006, and the MTech. Degree in CSE from Odisha University of Technology and Research (OUTR) University, Odisha in 2009. He received his Ph.D. in Computer Science & Engineering in 2021 from Veer Surendra Sai University of Technology (VSSUT), Burla, India. He has contributed 30 SCI and Scopus indexed research papers, 21 international/national conferences and books on Software Engineering and C Programming respectively. He has 15 years of teaching experience both in industry and academia. He has served the research community with various capacities like session chair, technical chair, keynote speaker etc. His research interests include wireless sensor network, smart city, smart grid and smart water. Currently he is working as Associate professor at School of Computer Engineering, KIIT DU, Bhubaneswar, and Odisha.

Santosh Moses in his role as the Director, Public Health for South and Central Asia, heads the Health Financing and Digital Health businesses for IQVIA Consulting. With an undergraduate degree in medicine and a post-graduate degree in public health and health care administration and currently pursuing a PhD in public health, he has over 20 years of experience in consulting and not for profit sectors in Asia and Africa. He has worked across several domains such as eyecare, health financing, community health, nutrition, and pharmaceuticals. He has led several PMUs such as in Qatar for Mandatory Health Insurance program, National Health Authority for Ayushman Bharat mission, National Centre for Disease Control, India, and several other. He has worked across several geographies such as India, Mongolia, Amenia, Bangladesh, South Korea, Indonesia, Qatar and Pakistan. He has worked with clients including national & state governments, WHO, ADB, World Bank, other multi-lateral and bi-lateral agencies.

Anshit Mukherjee is presently pursuing Bachelor of Technology (Hons.) in Computer Science and Engineering from the Abacus Institute of Engineering and Management, which is affiliated with Maulana Abul Kalam Azad University of Technology, and is presently in final year. He was the zonal topper of the AMBIKA KALNA zone in I.C.S.E. 2019 (10 TH STANDARD) and the second zonal topper in I.S.C. 2021 (12 TH STANDARD). He is also awarded with NPTEL Discipline Star in July–December 2023 and Motivated Learner in January-June 2024.

Rudra Kalyan Nayak serves as a Senior Assistant Professor in the School of Computing Science & Engineering at VIT Bhopal University. He has more than 14 years of expertise in teaching, mentoring and research. His Doctorate in Computer Science & Engineering was awarded by Siksha 'O' Anusandhan University in Bhubaneswar, Odisha, where he conducted research in the field of Financial Engineering. At the same university, he earned his M. Tech. in information technology. Dr. Nayak possesses nine patents total, two of which are granted Australian design patents and two of which are granted Indian design patents. In addition, he has written three book chapters and two books. He boasts over 45 international papers to his name, appearing in reputable journals and IEEE/ Springer conference proceedings. Additionally, he wrote an article for the IEEE India Council Newsletter. Speaking with expertise, Dr. Nayak has participated in faculty development programs. He has reviewed papers for a number of conferences and peer-reviewed journals. His areas of interest in research are Artificial Intelligence, Machine Learning, Financial Engineering, Bioinformatics and Computer Vision. A number of honors have been bestowed upon him, including the I2OR International Teaching Excellence Award 2023, I2OR National Elite Teacher Award 2022, 100 Eminent Academicians of 2021, Dynamic Teacher of the Year 2019, I2OR Preeminent Researcher Award 2019 and Green ThinkerZ Bright Educator Award 2019. A professional member of ACM, CSTA, IAENG, ICSES, theIRED, SDIWC, and a life member of ISTE, Dr. Nayak holds these memberships. He was also a London Journals Press Honorary Rosalind Member.

Konrad Obermann is a physician and economist with more than 30 years of experience in clinical work, research, strategic planning, and consulting. His work focuses on international health economics, development of health systems and financing of the health care system / social health insurance as well as empirical quantitative and qualitative health system research. He has 20+ years of experience in international cooperation in more than 25 countries in Europe, North Africa, Sub-Saharan Africa and Central, South and Southeast Asia. Clients include WHO, European Commission, GIZ, KfW, ADB, UNICEF, World Bank, KPMG, IQVIA as well as a number of non-profit organizations. Since 2008, he has been a Senior Lecturer at the Mannheim Center for Preventive Medicine and Digital Health at Heidelberg University.

Preethi Prabhakaran is currently working as head and assistant professor in the Department of BBA (Hospital Administration) in Auxilium College (Autonomous) affiliated to Thiruvalluvar University. Her research focuses on multidimensions aspects which focuses on managerial aspects and how these aspects are linked with healthcare sector. Dr. Preethi has over eight articles in peer-reviewed journals of WOS and UGC Care. She extends her expertise to various organizations as a trainer, outsider her academic commitments.

Ashwini Kumar Pradhan is currently working as Assistant Professor in the School of Computing Science and Engineering. He has a total experience of more than 9 years of teaching. He has been associated with Galgotias University since 2023. He completed his B. Tech (CSE) from (SOA University) in 2012 and M. Tech (CSE) from CET, Bhubaneswar, in 2016, and Ph.D. (CSE) from SOA University, Bhubaneswar, INDIA in 2023. His area of research is Machine Learning, Deep learning, AI.He is a firm believer in productivity and efficiency at work. . He has convened/organized more than 40 co-curricular/extracurricular events for the benefit of students in the past 5 years. He has 4 SCI Q1 journals and 6 conference paper.

Soumi Ray is an accomplished academic and healthcare professional with over 13 years of experience. She currently serves as an Assistant Professor in the Department of Hospital Management at Dr. B.C. Roy Academy of Professional Courses, Durgapur, India. Prior to her academic role, Dr. Ray held various leadership positions in the healthcare industry. She worked as a Quality Assurance Manager and In-Charge at the NABH accredited Mayo Medical Centre in Lucknow. She also served as an Administrator and Quality Assurance Expert at other NABH accredited hospitals in New Delhi and Lucknow. In addition to her professional experience, Dr. Ray is an active researcher and publisher. She has published several manuscripts in reputable journals, including the Acta Journal, Academy of Marketing Studies Journal, and Journal of Current Science and Technology. Her research interests span diverse topics such as social communication, lifestyle disease management, and virtual assistance-based healthcare interventions. Dr. Ray is also an accomplished presenter, having participated in numerous national and international conferences. She has presented papers on sustainable learning spaces, student well-being, and tech-enabled healthcare practices. Her dedication to the field of healthcare management and her extensive experience make her a valuable asset to the academic and healthcare communities.

David Rosendal holds a Bachelor's degree in Mechatronic Engineering and a Master of Science in Industrial Management and Innovation. With a strong foundation in both technical and managerial disciplines, David's academic work focuses on bridging the gap between innovation theory and practical application. His master's research delved into the "fuzzy front end" of product development, examining the unique challenges faced by companies in the Swedish medical devices industry, particularly in navigating public procurement processes and regulatory complexities. David currently serves as an Application Manager in the finance sector, where he leverages his technical expertise and strategic leadership to enhance business intelligence frameworks and support data-driven decision-making. His work involves creating structured reporting processes, improving data validation, and aligning financial systems with organizational strategies to foster innovation and growth. Passionate about connecting academic insights with real-world challenges, David continues to explore how technology and innovation can be harnessed to drive sustainable development and operational efficiency.

Saroja Kumar Rout (Senior Member, IEEE) received M.Tech (CS) from Utkal University in the year 2007 and a Ph.D. in Computer Science in the year 2018 from Siksha 'O' Anusandhan University for work in the field of Wireless Sensor Networks. Currently working as Associate Professor in the Department of Information Technology, Vardhaman College of Engineering (Autonomous), Hyderabad, India.

Contributed more than 60 research-level papers to many National and International journals and conferences. Also having 8 Indian patents. Research interests include Sensor Networks, Machine Learning, Cloud computing, and Health Informatics.

Dipanjan Roy is a senior public health professional, academician, and implementation expert with three decades of experience. He is a medical doctor with advanced degrees in internal medicine, public health and HIV medicine. He has more than 25 years of international experience spanning over three continents, Asia, Africa and Europe. He has worked in WHO, US CDC, UNAIDS, UNICEF, IIHMR, Delhi and international NGOs as well as government of India. He served as the focal point for resilient and sustainable systems in health, technical review panel, the Global Fund for AIDS, tuberculosis and malaria and currently serves as senior advisor for UNAIDS RST, Bangkok and a visiting professor of Global Health, Jodhpur School of Public Health. He is the former director of IIHMR, Delhi and CEO LEHS/ WISH Foundation India. He currently also serves as one of the directors for SRCMF and Regional Director Public Health, Dure Technologies. He has several publications to his credit and has authored couple of books. He was awarded the "Global Health Achievement - India" award by US CDC for his contributions towards leadership in developing and adopting Global public health policies in developing countries in 2009 and Excellence in Global Public Health Practice by Jodhpur School of Public Health in 2019.

Sudamini Saproo is an MBA in Hospital and Health Management and has over 5 years of experience in the field of market research and public health. She has worked with eminent clients like WHO, GIZ, ADB, Boston Consulting Group, Central & State governments etc. Her market research experience includes roles where she conducted qualitative and quantitative research, analyzed pharmaceutical and biotechnological markets, and provided detailed reports on market trends and drug developments. In public health, she has contributed to projects such as the Ayushman Bharat Digital Mission, Pandemic Preparedness in Armenia, and the evaluation of health schemes in Chhattisgarh. Her expertise spans healthcare consulting, secondary & primary research, project management, public health surveillance, and program implementation.

Sanghamitra Sharma, B.Pharm, MBA, is Assistant Professor for PGDM Healthcare Management program at S.P. Mandali's Prin. L.N.Welingkar Institute of Management Development and Research, Mumbai. She has work experience of 15 years which includes 9 years in academia and 7 years with the pharmaceutical industry, working in various departments such as quality assurance, regulatory, brand management and international marketing and has worked with both Indian and multi-national companies. Her domain expertise lies in the field of marketing, brand building, understanding of consumer research and the role of digital in marketing. She has published one national level paper. She has mentored student teams for hackathons including Maharashtra Health hackathon, Hackathons conducted by MIT RedX. She is an avid reader and enjoys watching movies.

Angela Shresta holds a BSc in Applied Nutrition, Botany, and Chemistry and is currently pursuing a Master's in Food Science and Nutrition. She conducted a study at Christel House, Bangalore, as part of a community development program, gaining valuable insights into public health. Additionally, completed a 45-day internship at IIHMR Bangalore, further enhancing her practical knowledge in the field with a strong academic foundation and hands-on experience.

Amit Thakur is a passionate scholar currently pursuing a Ph.D. in Machine Learning at VIT BHOPAL University. With a background in computer science and a fascination for artificial intelligence, Amit's research focuses on developing innovative algorithms for natural language processing and computer vision applications. Throughout his academic journey, Amit has demonstrated a strong aptitude for theoretical and applied research in machine learning. His work combines advanced mathematical techniques with practical implementations to address real-world challenges in data analysis and pattern recognition. In addition to his research endeavors, Amit is actively involved in teaching and mentoring undergraduate students, sharing his knowledge and enthusiasm for machine learning. He volunteers his time to organize workshops and seminars, fostering a collaborative learning environment within the academic community. Driven by a desire to harness the power of machine learning for societal benefit, Amit is dedicated to pushing the boundaries of AI research and developing intelligent systems that can positively impact people's lives. Through his interdisciplinary approach and commitment to excellence, Amit strives to be a leading figure in the field of machine learning and contribute to its continued advancement.

Akhilesh Kumar Tripathi Assistant Professor in CSE Department, Galgotias University, Greater Noida, has received M. Tech degree in CSE from MMM University of Technology, Gorakhpur. He is currently pursuing Ph.D. from KNIT Sultanpur, UP, India. He has 10 years of teaching experience. He has Published 5+ international and conference papers. His research interest includes deep learning, neurological disorder, image processing.

Tatjana Prenđa Trupec is International Expert coming from Croatia with 26+ years of experience. She is computing engineer with MBA diploma, currently pursuing her PHD in health financing in Netherlands. She is working as an expert for the World Bank, European Commission and World Health Organization. She gained expertise in health financing being director of national health insurance fund, leading health reforms and managing health budget of the Republic of Croatia.

Gaurav Upadhyay is an undergraduate student currently pursuing engineering at Delhi Technological University, specializing in Electronics and Machine Learning. He has developed various machine learning models to assess health variables across 193 UN member states, establishing relationships between healthy life expectancy and various dependent variables. He has also contributed to a research paper on the role of the circular economy in finance and accounting. Additionally, he worked with the Centre for Science and Environment to develop a comprehensive course on the design, installation, and maintenance of solar mini-grid systems, helping village dwellers gain reliable access to electricity. He is passionate about leveraging technology for social impact and sustainability.

Jyoti Vijay Area of Expertise – Nutritional Assessment, Micronutrient deficiency Assessment, Micronutrient supplementation, Social behavior change communication, Program Impact Evaluation, Lifestyle Interventions, Dietary Pattern, Dietary Diversity and other areas of nutrition. Experience with Previous Organizations – AIIMS, New Delhi and IIHMR Jaipur Dr. Jyoti Vijay contributed significantly to various projects, demonstrating expertise in research and program management. As a team member, she played a crucial role in the "Impact Evaluation of ICDS program in the state of Karnataka," funded by Government of Karnataka, from March to December 2022. Additionally, she served as a Monitoring and Evaluation Officer in a UNICEF funded project titled "Technical Support to Accelerate the Promotion of COVID-19 Appropriate Behaviors (CAB) for the State of Karnataka" from Aug 2021 to April 2022. In this capacity, her responsibilities included overseeing the implementation of Social and Behavior Change Communication (SBCC) activities focusing on COVID specific behaviors, including nutrition and WASH, across 31 districts of Karnataka. She worked on assessments of malnutrition, IYCF practices, lifestyle behaviors, dietary patterns, and nutrient intake among infants, toddlers, and children aged 6 months to 18 years in six states of North and East India. Additionally, she assessed the iodine nutritional status among neonates, school age children, adolescent girls, and pregnant mothers in Himachal Pradesh and Rajasthan, funded by ICMR and DBT, Government of India. Her work also involved evaluating iodine content in food and water samples across various cooking methods. She worked on the management system of Iron and Folic Acid (IFA) tablets and liquid, Vitamin A supplements, and zinc dispersible tablets in five states of India, funded by ICMR. Her role included identifying bottlenecks in the procurement and distribution of IFA, vitamin A, and zinc dispersible tablets, contributing to improved program implementation strategies

Arvind Yadav received the B. Tech. degree from the Biju Patnaik University of Technology, Odisha, in 2011 and Ph.D. degree from the National Institute of Technology, Rourkela, Odisha, in 2019. He is currently working as an Associate Professor with the Department of Computer Science and Engineering, Galgotias University, Greater Noida, Uttar Pradesh, India. He worked as an Associate Professor with the Department of Computer Science and Engineering, Koneru Lakshmaiah Education Foundation, Vaddeswaram, Andhra Pradesh, India and SRM University, Sonepat, India. He is involved in teaching of machine learning, artificial intelligence, mathematics, database management system, Python, C Programming, Object Oriented Programming, Java etc. subjects. He has around twelve years of teaching and research experiences, and contributed a number of research articles in several standard journals and conference proceedings of National and International. His main research interests include artificial intelligence, machine learning and soft computing. He has applied these techniques in hydrology and other interdisciplinary domains.

Index

A

AI 1, 2, 3, 5, 7, 13, 14, 21, 24, 25, 26, 27, 28, 32, 34, 39, 40, 41, 42, 43, 44, 45, 48, 49, 50, 55, 57, 58, 60, 62, 65, 67, 68, 78, 98, 120, 122, 125, 131, 141, 151, 158, 160, 164, 168, 169, 170, 175, 176, 177, 178, 179, 180, 181, 182, 183, 184, 185, 186, 187, 188, 189, 190, 191, 192, 193, 194, 195, 196, 198, 208, 209, 212, 213, 220, 224, 225, 231, 243, 244, 246, 248, 268, 275, 276, 277, 278, 280, 281, 282, 283, 295, 296, 297, 298, 299, 300, 301, 304, 314, 315, 317, 319, 322, 325, 326, 328, 341, 349, 350, 356, 361, 362, 364, 366, 368, 375, 382, 383, 385, 391, 392, 393, 394, 395, 396, 397, 398, 399, 400, 402, 403, 404, 405, 406, 407, 408, 409, 410, 411, 412, 413, 414, 415, 416, 417, 418, 424, 426, 432, 433, 434, 436, 440
Analytical dashboards 141, 160
Analytics 5, 6, 7, 8, 9, 13, 14, 15, 21, 23, 25, 26, 27, 28, 36, 40, 41, 42, 44, 45, 48, 49, 50, 54, 55, 56, 58, 59, 61, 65, 67, 121, 122, 125, 127, 135, 137, 139, 150, 157, 159, 160, 169, 175, 176, 181, 190, 192, 193, 200, 207, 212, 219, 221, 222, 223, 227, 243, 244, 246, 274, 301, 304, 318, 319, 322, 324, 327, 329, 341, 345, 349, 350, 373, 383, 395, 402, 403, 410, 415, 424, 426, 436, 437
Anomaly Detection 221, 222, 223, 224, 225, 226, 227, 228, 229, 230, 231, 232, 233, 236, 238, 239, 240, 241, 242, 244, 245, 247, 248, 267, 310
Application Program Interface 149
Apps 26, 28, 57, 105, 106, 107, 108, 109, 110, 112, 116, 117, 118, 119, 120, 121, 122, 123, 124, 125, 126, 128, 129, 130, 131, 133, 163, 174, 175, 181, 184, 187, 201, 215, 274, 282, 339, 373, 398, 433
Artificial Intelligence 1, 2, 5, 7, 26, 31, 32, 34, 38, 40, 43, 48, 50, 55, 57, 62, 68, 69, 120, 135, 137, 151, 168, 169, 177, 179, 180, 182, 183, 184, 185, 186, 190, 191, 192, 194, 195, 196, 198, 212, 217, 219, 221, 225, 246, 248, 254, 268, 270, 273, 277, 278, 283, 285, 286, 299, 300, 301, 302, 319, 327, 328, 330, 341, 345, 350, 356, 359, 362, 366, 373, 382, 383, 391, 394, 395, 400, 402, 404, 407, 409, 414, 415, 416, 417, 418, 422, 424, 425, 432, 436, 438, 440

B

Backpropagation algorithm 254, 256, 257, 262, 268
Behavior 107, 108, 109, 110, 112, 113, 114, 115, 116, 117, 118, 119, 120, 121, 123, 125, 127, 129, 130, 131, 132, 133, 185, 191, 214, 229, 232, 241, 255, 256, 257, 260, 266, 271, 276, 283, 346, 347
Biases in AI 182, 391, 395, 400, 408
Big Data 36, 42, 65, 69, 135, 137, 160, 167, 171, 181, 182, 188, 190, 192, 193, 196, 208, 212, 220, 238, 274, 301, 321, 327, 328, 345, 349, 357, 368, 373, 403, 410, 418, 426
big data analysis 167, 208

C

Change 6, 17, 21, 33, 50, 59, 62, 63, 105, 106, 107, 108, 109, 110, 111, 113, 114, 115, 116, 117, 118, 119, 126, 128, 129, 130, 131, 148, 156, 185, 188, 196, 198, 223, 229, 278, 346, 347, 365, 415, 437
clinical decision support 7, 43, 46, 48, 49, 50, 55, 62, 99, 167, 178, 191, 397, 398, 401, 417, 418
Clinical Decision Support Systems 43, 46, 48, 49, 50, 62, 178, 191, 397, 398, 401

Clinicians 8, 14, 15, 24, 26, 29, 41, 49, 57, 176, 181, 187, 188, 227, 245, 274, 366, 393, 397, 398, 400, 401, 406, 410, 414, 433, 434
complexity 21, 23, 53, 71, 72, 78, 79, 80, 81, 82, 84, 87, 88, 89, 91, 92, 169, 180, 183, 184, 185, 203, 211, 234, 235, 236, 239, 240, 241, 243, 249, 281, 292, 295, 308, 312, 331, 393
Cybersecurity 8, 15, 20, 23, 35, 42, 59, 362, 369, 370, 371, 373, 375, 376, 377, 379, 381, 382, 384, 385, 387, 388, 398, 400, 409, 417

D

Data Fusion 212, 215, 221, 222, 223, 224, 226, 227, 229, 230, 231, 232, 236, 238, 239, 240, 241, 244, 245, 246, 248, 271
Data Integrity 8, 60, 142, 177, 223, 294, 362, 377, 383, 396
Data Protection 54, 122, 158, 182, 188, 190, 273, 276, 287, 288, 289, 297, 298, 300, 301, 302, 303, 307, 313, 315, 316, 317, 318, 321, 323, 324, 363, 368, 369, 370, 371, 372, 373, 374, 378, 379, 380, 381, 382, 384, 385, 387, 404, 407, 410, 411, 412, 413, 415, 417, 436
Data Quality 49, 222, 227, 236, 240, 336, 393, 394, 402, 403, 404, 417
Data Security 15, 29, 46, 59, 60, 63, 135, 142, 156, 181, 203, 273, 275, 277, 278, 305, 314, 316, 362, 363, 367, 369, 371, 372, 373, 374, 375, 378, 379, 380, 381, 382, 384, 385, 395, 396, 397, 398, 402, 406, 410, 413
Deep Learning 37, 48, 49, 168, 169, 172, 182, 185, 191, 192, 193, 195, 198, 216, 217, 218, 219, 220, 225, 267, 299, 307, 338, 354, 414
Design 11, 13, 19, 29, 31, 39, 40, 41, 69, 80, 81, 83, 92, 94, 95, 96, 97, 99, 100, 103, 105, 106, 107, 108, 109, 111, 114, 115, 116, 122, 123, 124, 125, 128, 130, 131, 132, 133, 151, 179, 190, 195, 208, 222, 231, 244, 254, 255, 260, 261, 262, 268, 313, 325, 331, 343, 344, 352, 391, 392, 393, 394, 396, 397, 398, 404, 406, 424, 431, 432, 438
Diet 129, 330, 331, 334, 335, 340, 341, 342, 344, 345, 351, 357, 359
Digital 1, 3, 5, 6, 8, 12, 13, 15, 17, 21, 22, 24, 26, 27, 28, 29, 32, 34, 36, 37, 38, 39, 40, 44, 54, 62, 63, 66, 67, 68, 97, 105, 106, 107, 108, 109, 111, 113, 116, 117, 118, 130, 131, 132, 134, 135, 136, 137, 138, 139, 140, 141, 142, 143, 144, 145, 146, 147, 151, 153, 154, 155, 156, 157, 158, 159, 160, 161, 162, 163, 164, 165, 168, 173, 175, 181, 183, 189, 191, 193, 195, 201, 203, 212, 248, 269, 274, 275, 276, 277, 289, 290, 297, 300, 301, 304, 329, 330, 332, 335, 336, 340, 346, 348, 356, 362, 363, 364, 365, 366, 367, 368, 370, 373, 374, 379, 382, 384, 385, 394, 395, 397, 407, 408, 409, 413, 415, 416, 417, 426, 428, 432, 433
Digital Technology 26, 136, 137, 289, 301, 362, 363, 367, 368, 370
Digital Tools 329, 346, 348, 408, 413
Digital transformation 5, 27, 63, 156, 158, 162, 164, 195, 275, 290, 385
DPDPA 273, 276, 289

E

Elderly Health activity supervision 251, 252, 254, 256, 257, 263, 268
Engagement 9, 11, 12, 14, 15, 18, 21, 31, 42, 44, 46, 53, 55, 56, 58, 63, 105, 106, 107, 108, 109, 110, 111, 112, 116, 117, 118, 119, 120, 121, 122, 123, 124, 125, 128, 129, 130, 131, 142, 161, 186, 274, 346, 365, 366, 394, 395, 404, 408, 409, 419, 422, 424, 426, 428, 430, 431, 433, 434, 435, 438
equivocality 71, 78, 79, 80, 81, 82, 84, 88, 89, 91, 92, 95, 96, 100
Explainable AI 180, 181, 191, 193, 275, 295, 299, 317, 325, 408

F

Fitness 106, 109, 112, 115, 117, 120, 123, 129, 130, 133, 201, 203, 261, 383, 395, 401, 407, 409
Fuzzy front end 71, 72, 73, 75, 76, 82, 90, 94, 95, 96, 97, 98, 99, 100, 101, 102, 103, 104

G

Gamification 105, 106, 107, 108, 109, 110, 111, 112, 113, 114, 115, 116, 117, 120, 121, 122, 123, 124, 125, 126, 127, 128, 129, 130, 131, 132, 133, 434
Gamified 47, 105, 107, 109, 110, 112, 115, 116, 118, 120, 121, 122, 123, 125, 126, 127, 128, 129, 130, 131
GDPR 173, 182, 189, 273, 276, 278, 288, 289, 290, 293, 294, 298, 302, 307, 313, 315, 317, 318, 321, 324, 363, 368, 371, 372, 374, 381, 384, 387, 402, 404, 411, 412, 413, 415, 416

H

Health 1, 2, 5, 6, 7, 8, 9, 11, 12, 13, 14, 15, 16, 17, 19, 21, 24, 26, 27, 28, 31, 32, 33, 34, 35, 36, 37, 38, 40, 41, 43, 44, 46, 47, 48, 49, 50, 51, 52, 54, 55, 56, 57, 58, 59, 60, 61, 62, 63, 65, 66, 67, 68, 72, 73, 89, 94, 99, 101, 102, 105, 106, 107, 108, 109, 110, 111, 112, 113, 114, 116, 117, 118, 120, 121, 122, 123, 124, 125, 126, 127, 128, 129, 130, 131, 132, 133, 134, 135, 136, 137, 138, 139, 140, 141, 142, 143, 144, 145, 146, 147, 148, 149, 150, 151, 152, 153, 154, 156, 157, 158, 159, 160, 161, 162, 163, 164, 165, 167, 169, 170, 173, 174, 175, 176, 177, 178, 179, 180, 181, 182, 183, 185, 186, 189, 190, 191, 192, 193, 194, 195, 196, 198, 201, 202, 203, 205, 206, 207, 208, 209, 210, 211, 212, 214, 215, 217, 218, 219, 220, 221, 222, 223, 224, 225, 226, 227, 232, 243, 244, 245, 246, 247, 248, 251, 252, 253, 254, 255, 256, 257, 258, 259, 260, 261, 262, 263, 264, 265, 266, 267, 268, 269, 271, 273, 274, 275, 276, 277, 282, 284, 286, 287, 288, 289, 291, 298, 299, 300, 301, 302, 304, 311, 317, 318, 319, 320, 321, 322, 324, 327, 328, 329, 330, 331, 332, 333, 334, 335, 337, 338, 339, 340, 341, 342, 343, 344, 345, 346, 347, 349, 350, 351, 352, 354, 355, 356, 357, 358, 359, 362, 363, 364, 365, 366, 367, 368, 369, 370, 371, 372, 374, 378, 379, 381, 383, 384, 387, 388, 391, 392, 393, 395, 397, 398, 399, 400, 401, 402, 404, 405, 407, 408, 409, 410, 412, 413, 414, 415, 416, 417, 418, 421, 427, 428, 431, 432, 433, 434, 439, 441
healthcare 1, 2, 3, 5, 6, 7, 8, 9, 10, 11, 12, 13, 14, 15, 16, 17, 18, 19, 20, 21, 22, 23, 24, 25, 26, 27, 28, 29, 30, 31, 32, 33, 34, 35, 36, 37, 38, 39, 40, 41, 42, 43, 44, 45, 46, 47, 48, 49, 50, 51, 52, 53, 54, 55, 56, 57, 58, 59, 60, 61, 62, 63, 64, 65, 66, 67, 68, 72, 73, 75, 83, 86, 89, 90, 92, 97, 99, 100, 101, 102, 105, 106, 107, 109, 110, 111, 122, 127, 130, 131, 132, 133, 136, 139, 140, 141, 144, 145, 146, 147, 148, 149, 150, 151, 152, 153, 154, 156, 158, 159, 160, 161, 163, 164, 167, 168, 169, 170, 172, 173, 174, 175, 176, 177, 178, 179, 180, 181, 182, 183, 184, 185, 186, 187, 188, 189, 190, 191, 192, 193, 194, 195, 196, 197, 198, 199, 201, 202, 203, 204, 205, 206, 207, 208, 209, 210, 211, 212, 213, 214, 215, 216, 217, 218, 219, 220, 221, 222, 223, 224, 226, 227, 231, 233, 241, 242, 243, 244, 245, 246, 248, 254, 255, 256, 259, 267, 268, 269, 270, 273, 274, 275, 276, 277, 278, 279, 280, 283, 284, 285, 286, 287, 288, 289, 290, 291, 292, 293, 294, 295, 296, 297, 298,

299, 300, 301, 302, 303, 304, 305, 307, 308, 309, 310, 311, 312, 313, 314, 317, 318, 319, 320, 321, 322, 323, 324, 325, 326, 327, 328, 329, 330, 331, 332, 335, 348, 349, 350, 354, 357, 361, 362, 363, 364, 365, 366, 367, 368, 369, 370, 371, 372, 373, 374, 375, 376, 377, 378, 379, 380, 381, 382, 383, 384, 385, 386, 387, 388, 389, 391, 392, 393, 394, 395, 396, 397, 398, 399, 400, 401, 402, 404, 405, 406, 407, 408, 409, 410, 411, 412, 413, 414, 416, 417, 418, 419, 421, 422, 423, 424, 425, 426, 427, 428, 429, 430, 431, 432, 433, 434, 435, 436, 437, 438, 439, 440, 441
Healthcare 6.0 1, 2, 3, 5, 6, 14, 17, 18, 19, 20, 29, 34, 39, 72, 75, 90, 105, 131, 136, 175, 196, 273, 274, 275, 277, 278, 290, 292, 296, 297, 298, 303, 304, 329, 330, 331, 350, 363, 422, 424, 426, 438
Healthcare Analytics 244
Healthcare Technology 34, 289, 317, 382, 383, 384, 391, 393, 394, 396, 397, 398, 401, 409, 416
hidden correlations 167
HIPAA 174, 182, 189, 223, 273, 276, 287, 289, 290, 293, 294, 298, 301, 317, 324, 363, 368, 371, 372, 374, 378, 381, 384, 387, 402

I

Incentives 20, 115, 121, 129, 130, 137, 139, 148
innovation 6, 9, 10, 12, 13, 14, 15, 18, 21, 23, 28, 33, 34, 36, 40, 43, 44, 63, 64, 65, 71, 72, 73, 74, 75, 76, 77, 78, 79, 80, 81, 83, 86, 87, 88, 90, 91, 92, 93, 94, 95, 96, 97, 98, 99, 100, 101, 102, 103, 104, 106, 131, 144, 145, 146, 154, 161, 163, 175, 180, 186, 222, 245, 246, 292, 296, 298, 317, 321, 362, 374, 384, 391, 396, 402, 405, 406, 409, 410, 413, 426, 437, 440
Integration of the Internet of Things 46
Intelligent Hospital 43, 69
intelligent sensing framework 251, 252, 254, 256, 257, 259, 263, 265, 266, 268
Interoperability 3, 8, 20, 23, 35, 50, 54, 59, 60, 62, 63, 107, 136, 137, 139, 141, 142, 143, 149, 151, 158, 159, 176, 177, 184, 192, 217, 274, 275, 289, 295, 297, 363, 365, 371, 383
IoMT 175, 184, 196, 269
IT Ecosystem 149

L

least square method 254, 256, 257, 260, 261, 263, 268

M

Machine learning 7, 8, 32, 43, 48, 50, 59, 61, 131, 137, 147, 148, 155, 158, 167, 168, 169, 170, 171, 172, 173, 174, 176, 177, 178, 180, 182, 186, 187, 188, 190, 191, 192, 193, 194, 195, 196, 197, 198, 205, 216, 218, 220, 221, 224, 225, 226, 246, 248, 256, 266, 267, 275, 276, 277, 278, 279, 280, 281, 283, 285, 286, 290, 291, 292, 293, 296, 297, 299, 300, 301, 302, 303, 304, 305, 307, 308, 312, 313, 314, 315, 316, 318, 321, 323, 324, 326, 327, 328, 337, 338, 341, 342, 345, 350, 352, 354, 356, 359, 362, 375, 382, 395, 400, 402, 405, 406, 414, 424, 426, 436, 438
Machine Unlearning 273, 275, 276, 277, 278, 280, 282, 283, 284, 285, 286, 290, 291, 292, 294, 295, 296, 297, 298, 299, 300, 301, 302, 303, 304, 305, 307, 308, 313, 314, 315, 316, 317, 318, 321, 324, 325, 326, 327, 328
medical devices industry 71, 72, 75, 83, 85, 88, 89, 90, 91, 92, 93
Medical Errors 392, 400
Medical Image 48, 187, 218, 224
ML models 147, 216, 273, 276, 280, 281, 282, 283, 284, 285, 286, 290, 294, 296
Mobile applications 44, 47, 56, 135, 137,

139, 144, 210, 337, 347, 350
model interpretability 167, 185
Motivation 106, 109, 110, 111, 112, 113, 115, 116, 119, 121, 125, 129, 131, 134, 346

N

Nutrition Informatics 329, 330, 331, 332, 334, 335, 349, 350, 351, 355, 357, 358

O

Optical Character Recognition 154

P

Patient Care 2, 5, 6, 14, 15, 24, 25, 27, 28, 30, 35, 40, 41, 43, 44, 49, 50, 51, 52, 53, 55, 56, 57, 58, 59, 60, 61, 64, 66, 148, 160, 162, 176, 177, 178, 180, 195, 221, 244, 246, 275, 277, 284, 285, 286, 297, 298, 307, 318, 319, 320, 321, 322, 324, 325, 330, 335, 362, 363, 364, 366, 369, 370, 382, 383, 387, 393, 394, 396, 399, 400, 402, 405, 406, 407, 410, 413, 422, 427, 431, 434, 439
Patient-centric care 16, 29, 55, 421, 441
Patient Privacy 8, 15, 29, 142, 282, 287, 320, 323, 324, 367, 374, 384, 410
Patient Safety 49, 57, 223, 244, 285, 286, 289, 297, 363, 364, 370, 384, 391, 392, 393, 394, 396, 397, 398, 399, 400, 401, 406, 410, 411, 412, 413, 415, 418
Patient Satisfaction 11, 42, 54, 56, 223, 245, 364, 385, 395, 401, 421, 422, 423, 424, 425, 426, 427, 428, 429, 430, 431, 432, 433, 434, 435, 436, 437, 438, 440, 441
Physician 34, 178, 198, 319, 421, 423, 433, 435
Precision Medicine 7, 170, 177, 192, 195, 196, 275, 357, 395
Precision Nutrition 329, 330, 331, 340, 341, 343, 344, 345, 346, 347, 348, 349, 350, 352, 354, 358, 359
Predictive Analytics 5, 14, 25, 27, 40, 45, 48, 49, 50, 58, 59, 127, 169, 175, 176, 318, 319, 322, 324, 383, 395, 402
Privacy 8, 15, 16, 20, 23, 29, 40, 41, 42, 45, 46, 50, 54, 59, 60, 62, 63, 121, 134, 142, 143, 156, 157, 167, 175, 177, 181, 182, 189, 190, 193, 207, 208, 211, 219, 222, 223, 224, 227, 253, 255, 267, 268, 273, 275, 276, 277, 278, 281, 282, 283, 286, 287, 288, 289, 290, 293, 295, 296, 297, 298, 299, 300, 302, 304, 305, 307, 308, 310, 312, 313, 314, 315, 317, 318, 320, 321, 323, 324, 326, 327, 349, 357, 362, 363, 366, 367, 368, 371, 373, 374, 378, 380, 384, 385, 387, 394, 395, 397, 398, 399, 401, 402, 403, 404, 406, 410, 411, 412, 413, 416, 417, 433, 436
Psychology 109, 129, 131, 133, 177, 190, 406
public sector 34, 71, 72, 73, 74, 83, 84, 85, 88, 89, 90, 91, 154, 163

R

Real-Time Location Systems 45, 66, 68
Regulations 16, 23, 42, 54, 60, 71, 73, 74, 86, 102, 122, 138, 151, 188, 189, 203, 267, 273, 276, 278, 282, 287, 288, 289, 290, 293, 294, 297, 301, 307, 313, 315, 316, 317, 318, 321, 323, 324, 326, 362, 363, 365, 366, 368, 371, 372, 373, 384, 387, 402, 404, 409, 410, 411
Regulatory Compliance 55, 122, 156, 167, 292, 293, 297, 298, 315, 316, 324, 363, 369, 375
Rewards 107, 109, 110, 112, 113, 115, 116, 117, 120, 121, 123, 125, 129, 130, 133

S

Sensor Data 25, 203, 212, 221, 222, 223, 226, 227, 228, 229, 230, 231, 232, 233, 236, 238, 239, 240, 241, 243, 244, 245, 246, 271, 310

sickness diagnosis 167
Smart healthcare 65, 67, 210, 217, 220, 224, 248, 426
Smart Hospital 24, 27, 35, 39, 40, 41, 44, 55, 63, 64
Strategy 18, 19, 28, 33, 63, 100, 111, 125, 131, 132, 157, 158, 181, 185, 187, 207, 208, 212, 238, 274, 280, 295, 323, 370, 378, 417, 421, 441

T

Technique 172, 204, 207, 212, 226, 230, 256, 261, 280, 281, 290, 293, 294, 308, 309, 312, 321, 323
Technology 7, 9, 10, 14, 15, 17, 21, 23, 26, 27, 31, 32, 34, 35, 37, 39, 40, 41, 47, 48, 50, 51, 54, 55, 56, 58, 59, 60, 63, 66, 67, 68, 72, 86, 95, 96, 97, 98, 99, 100, 101, 103, 106, 109, 120, 121, 122, 131, 133, 136, 137, 141, 143, 145, 151, 154, 155, 156, 164, 167, 168, 175, 177, 178, 179, 181, 186, 187, 193, 195, 196, 198, 201, 207, 208, 220, 223, 224, 227, 244, 246, 247, 248, 252, 254, 257, 266, 268, 269, 270, 271, 274, 275, 277, 280, 285, 289, 292, 294, 296, 297, 298, 301, 302, 303, 317, 320, 323, 324, 325, 326, 327, 329, 330, 331, 332, 339, 340, 342, 343, 350, 351, 353, 361, 362, 363, 366, 367, 368, 369, 370, 371, 374, 375, 377, 378, 382, 383, 384, 385, 391, 392, 393, 394, 396, 397, 398, 401, 402, 404, 405, 407, 408, 409, 410, 411, 413, 414, 415, 416, 417, 421, 428, 429, 430, 432, 433, 434, 439, 441
Technology Design 109, 392
Telemedicine 2, 5, 6, 14, 16, 17, 29, 47, 72, 145, 160, 175, 177, 201, 274, 282, 301, 330, 339, 361, 362, 364, 365, 366, 373, 382, 383, 387, 388, 389, 394, 395, 401, 402, 404, 406, 407, 408, 410, 416, 422, 425, 438
Tools 6, 9, 11, 13, 14, 29, 42, 44, 47, 52, 57, 58, 59, 61, 68, 94, 95, 106, 126, 127, 131, 136, 137, 145, 151, 160, 168, 172, 173, 178, 182, 187, 189, 198, 201, 224, 225, 227, 244, 251, 252, 254, 257, 263, 268, 275, 282, 289, 290, 291, 301, 304, 308, 313, 326, 329, 331, 334, 335, 337, 338, 340, 341, 342, 346, 347, 348, 349, 352, 353, 354, 355, 357, 364, 365, 366, 376, 379, 383, 392, 393, 396, 397, 401, 404, 405, 407, 408, 410, 413, 429, 433, 434, 436, 437

U

uncertainty 71, 72, 78, 79, 80, 81, 82, 84, 85, 86, 88, 89, 91, 92, 95, 96, 97, 99, 100
Unlearning 273, 275, 276, 277, 278, 280, 281, 282, 283, 284, 285, 286, 288, 290, 291, 292, 294, 295, 296, 297, 298, 299, 300, 301, 302, 303, 304, 305, 306, 307, 308, 309, 312, 313, 314, 315, 316, 317, 318, 321, 324, 325, 326, 327, 328

V

Value-based care 16, 29, 136, 424

W

Wearable Technology 50, 120, 175, 181, 207, 339, 383, 407, 416
Wellness 12, 30, 112, 129, 133, 253, 255, 263, 270, 271

www.ingramcontent.com/pod-product-compliance
Lightning Source LLC
Chambersburg PA
CBHW080851220726
48556CB00005B/59